5. Microsurgery

坎贝尔骨科手术学
关节镜与显微外科

Campbell's Operative Orthopaedics

第 14 版
（影印版）

Frederick M. Azar, MD

James H. Beaty, MD

人民卫生出版社
·北 京·

图书在版编目（CIP）数据

坎贝尔骨科手术学．关节镜与显微外科：英文 /
（美）弗雷德里克·M. 阿扎尔（Frederick M. Azar），
（美）詹姆斯·H. 比蒂（James H. Beaty）主编 . —影印
本 . —北京：人民卫生出版社，2021.12
　　ISBN 978-7-117-32519-6

　　Ⅰ. ①坎… 　Ⅱ. ①弗… ②詹… 　Ⅲ. ①骨科学 – 外科
手术 – 英文②关节镜 – 外科手术 – 英文③骨疾病 – 显微外
科手术 – 英文 　Ⅳ. ①R68

中国版本图书馆 CIP 数据核字（2021）第 241274 号

人卫智网　**www.ipmph.com**	医学教育、学术、考试、健康，	
	购书智慧智能综合服务平台	
人卫官网　**www.pmph.com**	人卫官方资讯发布平台	

图字：01–2021–6747 号

坎贝尔骨科手术学
关节镜与显微外科
Kanbeier Guke Shoushuxue
Guanjiejing yu Xianwei Waike

主　　编：Frederick M. Azar　James H. Beaty
出版发行：人民卫生出版社（中继线 010-59780011）
地　　址：北京市朝阳区潘家园南里 19 号
邮　　编：100021
E - mail：pmph @ pmph.com
购书热线：010-59787592　010-59787584　010-65264830
印　　刷：三河市宏达印刷有限公司（胜利）
经　　销：新华书店
开　　本：889 × 1194　1/16　印张：18.5
字　　数：881 千字
版　　次：2021 年 12 月第 1 版
印　　次：2022 年 2 月第 1 次印刷
标准书号：ISBN 978-7-117-32519-6
定　　价：306.00 元

坎贝尔骨科手术学
关节镜与显微外科

Campbell's Operative Orthopaedics

第 14 版
（影印版）

Frederick M. Azar, MD

Professor

Department of Orthopaedic Surgery and Biomedical Engineering University of Tennessee–Campbell Clinic

Chief of Staff, Campbell Clinic

Memphis, Tennessee

James H. Beaty, MD

Harold B. Boyd Professor and Chair

Department of Orthopaedic Surgery and Biomedical Engineering University of Tennessee–Campbell Clinic

Memphis, Tennessee

Editorial Assistance

Kay Daugherty *and* **Linda Jones**

人民卫生出版社
·北 京·

Elsevier (Singapore) Pte Ltd.
3 Killiney Road,
#08-01 Winsland House I,
Singapore 239519
Tel: (65) 6349-0200; Fax:(65) 6733-1817

This English Reprint of Parts ⅩⅣ and ⅩⅦ from Campbell's Operative Orthopaedics, 14E by Frederick M. Azar and James H. Beaty was undertaken by People's Medical Publishing House and is published by arrangement with Elsevier (Singapore) Pte Ltd.

Parts ⅩⅣ and ⅩⅦ from Campbell's Operative Orthopaedics, 14E by Frederick M. Azar and James H. Beaty由人民卫生出版社进行影印,并根据人民卫生出版社与爱思唯尔(新加坡)私人有限公司的协议约定出版。

Notice

Practitioners and researchers must always rely on their own experience and knowledge in evaluating and using any information, methods, compounds or experiments described herein. Because of rapid advances in the medical sciences, in particular, independent verification of diagnoses and drug dosages should be made. To the fullest extent of the law, no responsibility is assumed by Elsevier, authors, editors or contributors in relation to the adaptation or for any injury and/or damage to persons or property as a matter of products liability, negligence or otherwise, or from any use or operation of any methods, products, instructions, or ideas contained in the material herein.

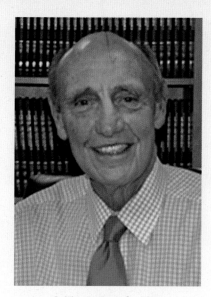

S. Terry Canale, MD

It is with humble appreciation and admiration that we dedicate this edition of *Campbell's Operative Orthopaedics* to Dr. S. Terry Canale, who served as editor or co-editor of five editions. He took great pride in this position and worked tirelessly to continue to improve "The Book." As noted by one of his co-editors, "Terry is probably the only person in the world who has read every word of multiple editions of *Campbell's Operative Orthopaedics*." He considered *Campbell's Operative Orthopaedics* an opportunity for worldwide orthopaedic education and made it a priority to ensure that each edition provided valuable and up-to-date information. His commitment to and enthusiasm for this work will continue to influence and inspire every future edition.

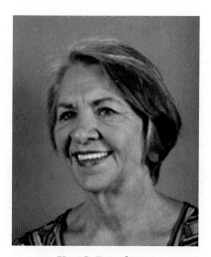

Kay C. Daugherty

It is with equal appreciation and regard that we dedicate this edition to Kay C. Daugherty, the managing editor of the last nine editions *Campbell's Operative Orthopaedics*. Over the last 40 years, she has faithfully and tirelessly edited, reshaped, and overseen all aspects of publication from manuscript preparation to proofing. She has a profound talent to put ideas and disjointed words into comprehensible text, ensuring that each revision maintains the gold standard in readability. Each edition is a testament to her dedication to excellence in writing and education. A favorite quote of Mrs. Daugherty to one of our late authors was, "I'll make a deal. I won't operate if you won't punctuate." We are grateful for her many years of continual service to the Campbell Foundation and for the publications yet to come.

CONTRIBUTORS

FREDERICK M. AZAR, MD
Professor
Director, Sports Medicine Fellowship
University of Tennessee–Campbell Clinic
Department of Orthopaedic Surgery and
    Biomedical Engineering
Chief-of-Staff, Campbell Clinic
Memphis, Tennessee

JAMES H. BEATY, MD
Harold B. Boyd Professor and Chair
University of Tennessee–Campbell Clinic
Department of Orthopaedic Surgery and
    Biomedical Engineering
Memphis, Tennessee

MICHAEL J. BEEBE, MD
Instructor
University of Tennessee–Campbell Clinic
Department of Orthopaedic Surgery and
    Biomedical Engineering
Memphis, Tennessee

CLAYTON C. BETTIN, MD
Assistant Professor
Director, Foot and Ankle Fellowship
Associate Residency Program Director
University of Tennessee–Campbell Clinic
Department of Orthopaedic Surgery and
    Biomedical Engineering
Memphis, Tennessee

TYLER J. BROLIN, MD
Assistant Professor
University of Tennessee–Campbell Clinic
Department of Orthopaedic Surgery and
    Biomedical Engineering
Memphis, Tennessee

JAMES H. CALANDRUCCIO, MD
Associate Professor
Director, Hand Fellowship
University of Tennessee–Campbell Clinic
Department of Orthopaedic Surgery and
    Biomedical Engineering
Memphis, Tennessee

DAVID L. CANNON, MD
Associate Professor
University of Tennessee–Campbell Clinic
Department of Orthopaedic Surgery and
    Biomedical Engineering
Memphis, Tennessee

KEVIN B. CLEVELAND, MD
Instructor
University of Tennessee–Campbell Clinic
Department of Orthopaedic Surgery and
    Biomedical Engineering
Memphis, Tennessee

ANDREW H. CRENSHAW JR., MD
Professor Emeritus
University of Tennessee–Campbell Clinic
Department of Orthopaedic Surgery and
    Biomedical Engineering
Memphis, Tennessee

JOHN R. CROCKARELL, MD
Professor
University of Tennessee–Campbell Clinic
Department of Orthopaedic Surgery and
    Biomedical Engineering
Memphis, Tennessee

GREGORY D. DABOV, MD
Assistant Professor
University of Tennessee–Campbell Clinic
Department of Orthopaedic Surgery and
    Biomedical Engineering
Memphis, Tennessee

MARCUS C. FORD, MD
Instructor
University of Tennessee–Campbell Clinic
Department of Orthopaedic Surgery and
    Biomedical Engineering
Memphis, Tennessee

RAYMOND J. GARDOCKI, MD
Assistant Professor
University of Tennessee–Campbell Clinic
Department of Orthopaedic Surgery and
    Biomedical Engineering
Memphis, Tennessee

BENJAMIN J. GREAR, MD
Instructor
University of Tennessee–Campbell Clinic
Department of Orthopaedic Surgery and
    Biomedical Engineering
Memphis, Tennessee

JAMES L. GUYTON, MD
Associate Professor
University of Tennessee–Campbell Clinic
Department of Orthopaedic Surgery and
    Biomedical Engineering
Memphis, Tennessee

JAMES W. HARKESS, MD
Associate Professor
University of Tennessee–Campbell Clinic
Department of Orthopaedic Surgery and
    Biomedical Engineering
Memphis, Tennessee

ROBERT K. HECK JR., MD
Associate Professor
University of Tennessee–Campbell Clinic
Department of Orthopaedic Surgery and
    Biomedical Engineering
Memphis, Tennessee

MARK T. JOBE, MD
Associate Professor
University of Tennessee–Campbell Clinic
Department of Orthopaedic Surgery and
    Biomedical Engineering
Memphis, Tennessee

DEREK M. KELLY, MD
Professor
Director, Pediatric Orthopaedic Fellowship
Director, Resident Education
University of Tennessee–Campbell Clinic
Department of Orthopaedic Surgery and
    Biomedical Engineering
Memphis, Tennessee

SANTOS F. MARTINEZ, MD
Assistant Professor
University of Tennessee–Campbell Clinic
Department of Orthopaedic Surgery and
    Biomedical Engineering
Memphis, Tennessee

ANTHONY A. MASCIOLI, MD
Assistant Professor
University of Tennessee–Campbell Clinic
Department of Orthopaedic Surgery and
    Biomedical Engineering
Memphis, Tennessee

BENJAMIN M. MAUCK, MD
Assistant Professor
Director, Hand Fellowship
University of Tennessee–Campbell Clinic
Department of Orthopaedic Surgery and
    Biomedical Engineering
Memphis, Tennessee

MARC J. MIHALKO, MD
Assistant Professor
University of Tennessee–Campbell Clinic
Department of Orthopaedic Surgery and
    Biomedical Engineering
Memphis, Tennessee

WILLIAM M. MIHALKO, MD PhD
Professor, H.R. Hyde Chair of Excellence in
    Rehabilitation Engineering
Director, Biomedical Engineering
University of Tennessee–Campbell Clinic
Department of Orthopaedic Surgery and
    Biomedical Engineering
Memphis, Tennessee

ROBERT H. MILLER III, MD
Associate Professor
University of Tennessee–Campbell Clinic
Department of Orthopaedic Surgery and
Biomedical Engineering
Memphis, Tennessee

G. ANDREW MURPHY, MD
Associate Professor
University of Tennessee–Campbell Clinic
Department of Orthopaedic Surgery and
Biomedical Engineering
Memphis, Tennessee

ASHLEY L. PARK, MD
Clinical Assistant Professor
University of Tennessee–Campbell Clinic
Department of Orthopaedic Surgery and
Biomedical Engineering
Memphis, Tennessee

EDWARD A. PEREZ, MD
Associate Professor
University of Tennessee–Campbell Clinic
Department of Orthopaedic Surgery and
Biomedical Engineering
Memphis, Tennessee

BARRY B. PHILLIPS, MD
Professor
University of Tennessee–Campbell Clinic
Department of Orthopaedic Surgery and
Biomedical Engineering
Memphis, Tennessee

DAVID R. RICHARDSON, MD
Associate Professor
University of Tennessee–Campbell Clinic
Department of Orthopaedic Surgery and
Biomedical Engineering
Memphis, Tennessee

MATTHEW I. RUDLOFF, MD
Assistant Professor
Co-Director, Trauma Fellowship
University of Tennessee–Campbell Clinic
Department of Orthopaedic Surgery and
Biomedical Engineering
Memphis, Tennessee

JEFFREY R. SAWYER, MD
Professor
Co-Director, Pediatric Orthopaedic
Fellowship
University of Tennessee–Campbell Clinic
Department of Orthopaedic Surgery and
Biomedical Engineering
Memphis, Tennessee

BENJAMIN W. SHEFFER, MD
Assistant Professor
University of Tennessee–Campbell Clinic
Department of Orthopaedic Surgery and
Biomedical Engineering
Memphis, Tennessee

DAVID D. SPENCE, MD
Assistant Professor
University of Tennessee–Campbell Clinic
Department of Orthopaedic Surgery and
Biomedical Engineering
Memphis, Tennessee

NORFLEET B. THOMPSON, MD
Instructor
University of Tennessee–Campbell Clinic
Department of Orthopaedic Surgery and
Biomedical Engineering
Memphis, Tennessee

THOMAS W. THROCKMORTON, MD
Professor
Co-Director, Sports Medicine Fellowship
University of Tennessee–Campbell Clinic
Department of Orthopaedic Surgery and
Biomedical Engineering
Memphis, Tennessee

PATRICK C. TOY, MD
Associate Professor
University of Tennessee–Campbell Clinic
Department of Orthopaedic Surgery and
Biomedical Engineering
Memphis, Tennessee

WILLIAM C. WARNER JR., MD
Professor
University of Tennessee–Campbell Clinic
Department of Orthopaedic Surgery and
Biomedical Engineering
Memphis, Tennessee

JOHN C. WEINLEIN, MD
Assistant Professor
Director, Trauma Fellowship
University of Tennessee–Campbell Clinic
Department of Orthopaedic Surgery and
Biomedical Engineering
Memphis, Tennessee

WILLIAM J. WELLER, MD
Instructor
University of Tennessee–Campbell Clinic
Department of Orthopaedic Surgery and
Biomedical Engineering
Memphis, Tennessee

A. PAIGE WHITTLE, MD
Associate Professor
University of Tennessee–Campbell Clinic
Department of Orthopaedic Surgery and
Biomedical Engineering
Memphis, Tennessee

KEITH D. WILLIAMS, MD
Associate Professor
University of Tennessee–Campbell Clinic
Department of Orthopaedic Surgery and
Biomedical Engineering
Memphis, Tennessee

DEXTER H. WITTE III, MD
Clinical Assistant Professor in
Radiology
University of Tennessee–Campbell Clinic
Department of Orthopaedic Surgery and
Biomedical Engineering
Memphis, Tennessee

When Dr. Willis Campbell published the first edition of *Campbell's Operative Orthopaedics* in 1939, he could not have envisioned that over 80 years later it would have evolved into a four-volume text and earned the accolade of the "bible of orthopaedics" as a mainstay in orthopaedic practices and educational institutions all over the world. This expansion from some 400 pages in the first edition to over 4,500 pages in this 14th edition has not changed Dr. Campbell's original intent: "to present to the student, the general practitioner, and the surgeon the subject of orthopaedic surgery in a simple and comprehensive manner." In each edition since the first, authors and editors have worked diligently to fulfill these objectives. This would have not been possible without the hard work of our contributors who always strive to present the most up-to-date information while retaining "tried and true" techniques and tips. The scope of this text continues to expand in the hope that the information will be relevant to physicians no matter their location or resources.

As always, this edition also is the result of the collaboration of a group of "behind the scenes" individuals who are involved in the actual production process. The Campbell Foundation staff—Kay Daugherty, Linda Jones, and Tonya Priggel—contributed their considerable talents to editing often confusing and complex author contributions, searching the literature for obscure references, and, in general, "herding the cats." Special thanks to Kay and Linda who have worked on multiple editions of *Campbell's Operative Orthopaedics* (nine editions for Kay and six for Linda). They probably know more about orthopaedics than most of us, and they certainly know how to make it more understandable. Thanks, too, to the Elsevier personnel who provided guidance and assistance throughout the publication process: John Casey, Senior Project Manager; Jennifer Ehlers, Senior Content Development Specialist; and Belinda Kuhn, Senior Content Strategist.

We are especially appreciative of our spouses, Julie Azar and Terry Beaty, and our families for their patience and support as we worked through this project.

The preparation and publication of this 14th edition was fraught with difficulties because of the worldwide pandemic and social unrest, but our contributors and other personnel worked tirelessly, often in creative and innovative ways, to bring it to fruition. It is our hope that these efforts have provided a text that is informative and valuable to all orthopaedists as they continue to refine and improve methods that will ensure the best outcomes for their patients.

Frederick M. Azar, MD
James H. Beaty, MD

CONTENTS

PART I

ARTHROSCOPY

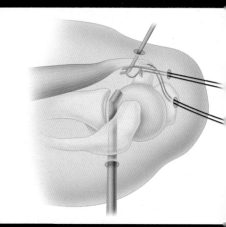

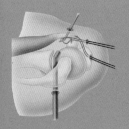

CHAPTER 1

GENERAL PRINCIPLES OF ARTHROSCOPY

Barry B. Phillips

During the past five decades, arthroscopy has dramatically changed the orthopaedic surgeon's approach to the diagnosis and treatment of a variety of joint ailments. A high degree of clinical accuracy, combined with low morbidity, has encouraged the use of arthroscopy to assist in diagnosis, to determine prognosis, and often to provide treatment. Arthroscopic procedures should serve as adjuncts to and not as replacements for thorough clinical evaluation; arthroscopy is not a substitute for clinical skills.

Progressive improvements in the lens systems of arthroscopes and fiberoptic systems, in miniaturization, and in the accessory operative instruments have made advanced arthroscopic operative techniques possible for virtually every joint in the body, including the knee, shoulder, hip, ankle, elbow, wrist, hand, and foot. Even spinal procedures are increasingly performed using endoscopic techniques. Although many arthroscopic procedures have proved superior to previous open techniques, surgical results should not be sacrificed to expand the indications for arthroscopic procedures.

INSTRUMENTS AND EQUIPMENT
ARTHROSCOPE

An arthroscope is an optical instrument. Three basic optical systems have been used in rigid arthroscopes: (1) the classic thin lens system, (2) the rod-lens system designed by Professor Hopkins of Reading, England, and (3) the graded index (GRIN) lens system. Fiberoptic technology, the use of magnifying lenses, and digital monitors have allowed advancements in arthroscope design. Newer arthroscopes offer an increased field of view with smaller scope diameters, better depth of field with improved optics, and better flow through the sheath.

Certain features determine the optical characteristics of an arthroscope. Most important are the diameter, angle of inclination, and field of view. The angle of inclination, which is the angle between the axis of the arthroscope and a line perpendicular to the surface of the lens, varies from 0 to 120 degrees. The 25- and 30-degree arthroscopes are most commonly used. The 70- and 90-degree arthroscopes are useful for seeing around corners, such as the posterior compartments of the knee through the intercondylar notch, but have the disadvantage of making orientation by the observer more difficult.

Field of view refers to the viewing angle encompassed by the lens and varies according to the type of arthroscope. The 1.9-mm scope has a 65-degree field of view; the 2.7-mm scope, a 90-degree field of view; and the 4.0-mm scope, a 115-degree field of view. Wider viewing angles make orientation by the observer much easier. Rotation of the forward oblique viewing (25- and 30-degree) arthroscopes allows a much larger area of the joint to be observed (Fig. 1.1). Rotation of 70-degree arthroscopes produces an extremely large field of view but may create a central blind area directly in front of the scope (Fig. 1.2).

TELEVISION CAMERAS

McGinty and Johnson were among the first to introduce a television camera to the arthroscopy system. The advantages of this addition included a more comfortable operating position for the surgeon, avoidance of contamination of the operative field by the surgeon's face, and involvement of the rest of the surgical team in the procedure. Early cameras were bulky and inconvenient, but small, solid-state cameras have been developed that can be connected directly to the arthroscope. In these camera systems, improvements in the chip and electronic circuitry have allowed reductions in size and better high-definition digital resolution. Cableless arthroscopic systems also are available in which the video signal is transmitted to the monitor from an arthroscope that contains its own miniature light source. Cameras using three-chip technology allow even greater color resolution, and digitalization of the video signal has resulted in advancements in high-quality imaging.

ACCESSORY INSTRUMENTS

The basic instrument kit consists of the following: arthroscopes (30- and 70-degree); probe; scissors; basket forceps; grasping forceps; arthroscopic knives; motorized meniscus cutter and shaver; electrosurgical, laser, and radiofrequency instruments; and miscellaneous equipment. These instruments are used to perform most routine arthroscopic surgical procedures. Additional instruments are available and are occasionally used in special circumstances. Procedure-specific instrumentation has also been developed for cruciate ligament reconstruction, meniscal repair, osteochondral transplantation, hip arthroscopy, and small joint arthroscopy, among others. Each surgeon has personal preferences regarding the type, design, and manufacturer of each instrument.

Many new instruments have been redesigned for use in advanced shoulder procedures. Instruments to pass, retrieve, and tie sutures have greatly advanced soft-tissue repair procedures of the capsule, labrum, and rotator cuff (Fig. 1.3).

■ PROBE

The probe is perhaps the most used and important diagnostic instrument after the arthroscope. The probe has become known over the years as "the extension of the arthroscopist's finger." It is used in both diagnostic and operative arthroscopy, and is the safest instrument that one can use when learning triangulation techniques (Fig. 1.4). The probe is essential for palpating intraarticular structures and planning the approach to a surgical procedure. A tactile sensation regarding what is normal and what is abnormal soon develops. It is better to

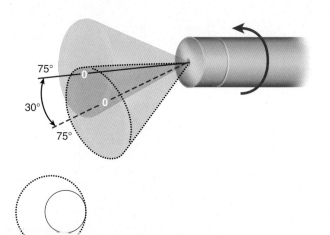

FIGURE 1.1   Rotation of arthroscope with 30-degree angle of inclination, which causes a scanning effect that increases the field of view by about threefold. *Dotted circle* shows field of view and is compared at lower left with *small circle* that shows field of view of the 0-degree arthroscope.

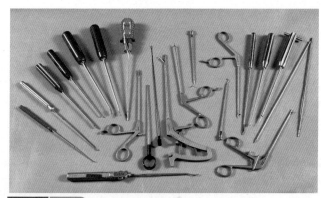

FIGURE 1.3   Arthroscopic instruments for shoulder procedures.

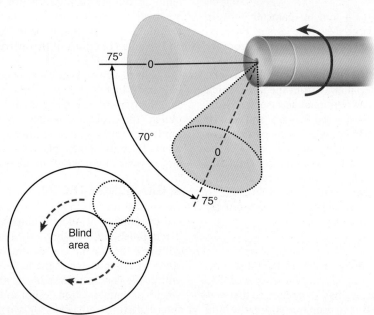

FIGURE 1.2   Rotation of arthroscope with 70-degree angle of inclination. This scans a large circle but creates a blind area directly ahead of it in which nothing can be seen.

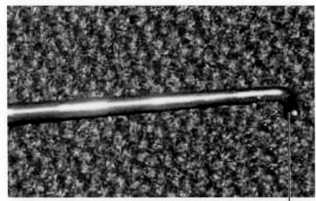

Rounded, blunt tip

FIGURE 1.4   Arthroscopic probe used in exploring intraarticular structures during arthroscopic triangulation techniques.

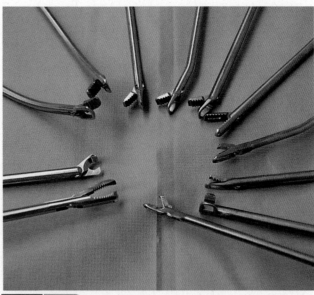

FIGURE 1.5   Commonly used arthroscopic instruments (see text).

"see and feel" rather than to "see" alone. The probe can be used to feel the consistency of a structure, such as the articular cartilage; to determine the depth of chondromalacic areas; to identify and palpate loose structures within the joint, such as tears of the menisci; to maneuver loose bodies into more accessible grasping positions; to palpate the anterior cruciate ligament (ACL) and determine the tension in the ligamentous and synovial structures within the joint; to retract structures within the joint for exposure; to elevate a meniscus so that its undersurface can be viewed; and to probe the fossae and recesses, such as the popliteal hiatus within the joint. Most probes are right angled with a tip size of 3 to 4 mm, and this known size of the hook can be used to measure the size of intraarticular lesions. The arthroscope magnifies, and the closer the arthroscope, the greater the magnification. Care should be taken in using the tip of the probe; much of the palpation with the probe within the joint is actually done with the elbow of the probe rather than the tip or toe of the instrument.

■ SCISSORS

Arthroscopic scissors are 3 to 4 mm in diameter and are available in both small and large sizes. The jaws of the scissors may be straight or hooked (Fig. 1.5). Hooked scissors are preferred because the configuration of the jaws tends to hook the tissue and pull it between the cutting edges of the scissors, rather than pushing the material away from the jaws, which can occur with straight scissors. Optional accessory scissors designs include right- and left-curved scissors and angled cutting scissors. The difference between these two designs is based on the location of the angulation. The shank of the curved scissors is gently curved to accommodate right and left positioning, whereas the angled scissors, usually with a rotating type of jaw mechanism, actually cut at an angle to the shaft of the scissors. These accessory designs are useful for detaching difficult-to-reach meniscal fragments.

■ BASKET FORCEPS

The basket or punch biopsy forceps is one of the most commonly used operative arthroscopic instruments (see Fig. 1.5). The standard basket forceps has an open base that permits each punch or bite of tissue to drop free within the joint and does not require the instrument to be removed from the joint and cleaned with each bite. Small fragments of

tissue that drop free within the joint through the open-floor punch or basket forceps can be irrigated out or subsequently removed from the joint by suction. This instrument is available in 3- to 5-mm sizes with a straight or curved shaft. It is useful for trimming the peripheral rim of the meniscus or can be used instead of scissors to cut across meniscal or other tissue. Wide, low-profile baskets are excellent for meniscal work. The configuration of the jaws of the basket forceps may be straight or hooked; again, the hooked configuration is preferred. Baskets are available in an assortment of angles, including 30, 45, and 90 degrees, which are especially useful for trimming the anterior portions of the meniscus. They also are available in 15-degree down-biting and up-biting curves to make it easier to get around the femoral condyle during resection of the posterior meniscal horn. As with other arthroscopic instruments, the proper technique is to make small bites to avoid excessive pressure on the joints and pins of the instrument and to prevent frequent breakage.

Hinged, jawed suction punches are available to cleanly bite small bits of meniscus or other small tissues and suction them from the joint through a channel in the shaft of the punch. This prevents fragments of tissue from floating in the joint, blocking vision, and ensures removal of all free fragments from the joint. This instrument, however, often is too large to reach tight posterior areas.

■ GRASPING FORCEPS

Grasping forceps (see Fig. 1.5) are useful for retrieving material from the joint, such as loose bodies or synovium, or for placing meniscal flaps and other tissues under tension while cutting with a second instrument. Most grasping forceps have some type of ratchet closure on the handle to secure the tissue within the jaws. The jaws of the grasping forceps may be of single- or double-action design and may have regular serrated interdigitating teeth or one or two sharp teeth to better secure the grasped tissue. The double-action grasping forceps, of which both jaws open, are especially preferred for securing an

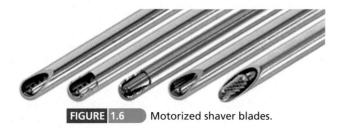

FIGURE 1.6 Motorized shaver blades.

osteocartilaginous loose body because the single-action types frequently allow it to slip from between the jaws.

KNIFE BLADES

Most arthroscopic knives currently used are disposable, single-use instruments. A variety of disposable blade designs are available: hooked or retrograde blades; regular down-cutting blades, both straight and curved; and Smillie-type end-cutting blades. Magnetic properties are also helpful in retrieving the blade if it is inadvertently broken inside the joint. These blades should be inserted through cannula sheaths or encased within a retractable sheath mechanism so that the cutting portion of the blade is only exposed when it enters the field of arthroscopic vision and not as it enters through the entry portal.

MOTORIZED SHAVING SYSTEMS

The motorized shaving systems are all basically of similar design, consisting of an outer, hollow sheath and an inner, hollow rotating cannula with corresponding windows (Fig. 1.6). The window of the inner sheath functions as a two-edged, cylindrical blade that spins within the outer hollow tube. Suction through the cylinder brings the fragments of soft tissue into the window, and as the blade rotates, the fragments are amputated, sucked to the outside, and collected in a suction trap. Numerous cutting tips have been developed for specific situations and functions. The diameter of the cutting tip is usually 3 to 5.5 mm, and many of the tips have variable sizes to allow access to smaller or tighter joints. Special blades have been designed for meniscal cutting or trimming, synovial resection, and shaving of articular cartilage. Special burrs and abraders have been designed for arthroscopic acromioplasty and ACL reconstructions. Most systems use a foot pedal to control the motor and allow for variable speed and direction. Reversing the rotation of the cutting blade intermittently often improves cutting efficiency and minimizes clogging with debris. Motorized shavers have been developed for small joints with a 2-mm shaver and burr.

Finally, the cutting tip should always be positioned within the visual field, and the position of the window should be located before activating the rotary motion of the blade.

ELECTROSURGICAL, LASER, AND RADIOFREQUENCY INSTRUMENTS

Electrocautery has been used as an arthroscopic tool for cutting and hemostasis most often after arthroscopic synovectomy and subacromial decompression. It also has been used for both cutting and hemostasis in lateral retinacular release for malalignment of the patella.

At a much lower cost, radiofrequency systems have been reported to produce heat energy similar to that of lasers which have fallen out of favor. The two types available are monopolar and bipolar. Monopolar devices use a grounding pad and draw energy through the body; with bipolar devices, energy is transferred between electrodes at the site of treatment. Current controversies include the depth of tissue penetration, the amount of cell death, and the ability of the devices to monitor and to control temperature. Reported complications of radiofrequency meniscal ablation include articular cartilage damage, osteonecrosis, and tissue damage caused by the irrigant.

IMPLANTS

A variety of implants, both metal and biodegradable, have been developed for use in arthroscopic procedures, including suture anchors, meniscal repair devices, and devices for tendon and ligament fixation and articular cartilage repair.

Suture anchors are used to attach ligaments and tendons to bone without the need for creating a bony tunnel for the passage of sutures. Instead, sutures are passed through an eyelet on the suture anchor, which is inserted into the bone. According to Barber and Richards, desirable characteristics of a suture anchor are that it must fix the suture to the bone, not pull out of the bone, permit an easy surgical technique (the ability to tie an arthroscopic slip knot), and not cause long-term problems; other desirable features include biocompatibility, adequate strength, easy insertion, and the ability to allow early rehabilitation. Suture anchors are used most often for arthroscopic procedures around the shoulder. Small-diameter all-suture anchors, polyetheretherketone (PEEK) biocomposite or metal anchors can be used; these have less potential for producing osteolytic reactions that have been associated with bioabsorbable implants.

Meniscal repair devices, of varying designs and materials, allow an all-inside meniscal repair without the need for arthroscopic knot-tying, accessory portals, or incisions. The first-generation meniscal repair devices were solid flexible devices placed across the tear to hold the meniscal fragments in place. Today's fourth-generation devices are low profile, have a suture tension construct, and provide much greater fixation strength. The techniques for use of specific meniscal repair devices are discussed in other chapters.

Depending on the graft chosen, cruciate ligament fixation devices can be used for bone-to-bone fixation or for soft tissue-to-bone fixation. They may be made from either biodegradable or nonbiodegradable materials.

MISCELLANEOUS EQUIPMENT

A variety of sheaths and trocars are required for arthroscopic surgery, and they must accommodate the arthroscope and accessory equipment being used. When possible, sharp instruments should be placed through sheaths to protect the soft tissues of the skin portals. Motorized instruments can be used with or without a sheath. The initial perforation through the capsular and synovial tissue may be made with a No. 11 blade and blunt trocar or with a sharp trocar carefully passed through the appropriate instrument sheath. Some systems allow cannulas to be interchanged for inflow, arthroscope, and motorized shaver systems. Disposable plastic cannulas with sealed ends reduce fluid extravasation.

As arthroscopic surgery procedures have advanced to cater for more joints, additional instruments have been developed. "Switching sticks" are simple rods placed through the cannula to maintain the portal while the cannula is exchanged. For a larger operating cannula, a dilator is used before exchange. The Wissinger rod was designed to assist in establishing a portal on the opposite side of a joint from a previously established portal. Traction devices have been developed for use in the shoulder, elbow, and ankle for better exposure. There has also been an explosion of procedure-specific instruments, many of which are described in the pertinent operative sections in other chapters.

CARE AND STERILIZATION OF INSTRUMENTS

Arthroscopy equipment that is heat stable may be autoclaved for sterility. Heat- or moisture-sensitive equipment may be sterilized with a low-temperature hydrogen peroxide gas plasma. Low-temperature sterilization processes, gas sterilization, and activated glutaraldehyde have been shown to be less effective and have more potential side effects.

IRRIGATION SYSTEMS

Irrigation and distention of the joint are essential to all arthroscopic procedures. Joint distention is maintained by using lactated Ringer solution during arthroscopy. The inflow may pass directly through the arthroscopic sheath or through a separate portal by means of a cannula. For adequate flow, a 6.0- or 6.2-mm sheath should be used with the scope. We routinely use lactated Ringer solution because it is physiologic and results in minimal synovial and articular surface changes. Shinjo et al. determined that lactated Ringer solution was better at maintaining meniscal cell integrity than isotonic sodium chloride solution.

Usually, two 5-L plastic bags of lactated Ringer solution, interconnected with a Y-connector, are suspended for use with the arthroscopic pump (Fig. 1.7). Once the inflow and outflow cannulas are established, the joint is lavaged until the

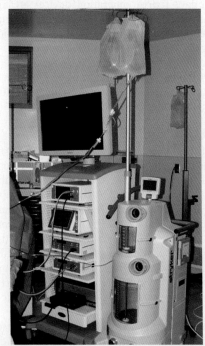

fluid is clear. When a pump is not used, joint distention can be increased by elevating the fluid bag, using large-diameter tubing, or decreasing the size and number of outflow portals. For each foot of elevation of the solution bag above the level of the joint, 22 mm Hg of pressure is produced. The bag usually is placed 3 feet (~1 m) above the level of the joint, thus producing approximately 66 mm Hg of pressure. Arthroscopic pumps should be used carefully, and the tightness of muscle compartments and soft-tissue spaces, such as the popliteal fossa, should be monitored closely. Pump pressures should be varied according to the joint being treated and the type of pump used. When a pressure inflow system is used, joint distention pressures in the knee generally should be 45 to 60 mm Hg. Vision and hemostasis in the shoulder usually are best when the distention pressure is maintained approximately 40 mm Hg below the systolic blood pressure. In healthy patients, hypotensive anesthesia may be used to reduce the systolic pressure to approximately 100 mm Hg, at which level a pump pressure of 55 to 60 mm Hg usually provides safe distention and clear vision. In a prospective, double-blinded, randomized study, Olszewski et al. found that the addition of epinephrine (1 mg/L of saline) significantly increased visibility and reduced the need for tourniquet inflation by 50% compared with a placebo group of patients who had not received epinephrine. In patients with hypertension or cardiac problems, we forgo the use of epinephrine. Karaoglu et al. also found that adding a small amount of epinephrine (50 µg/10 mL) to the local anesthetic mixture just before portal site injection improved arthroscopic visibility.

Because of the increased likelihood of extravasation, distention pressures in the elbow and ankle should be maintained at approximately 40 to 45 mm Hg using gravity inflow. The surgeon should be aware of individual variations relating to different pump flow and sensor mechanisms. We do not use pumps for distention in small joints.

TOURNIQUET

During arthroscopic procedures of the knee, ankle, elbow, and other distal joints, a tourniquet is almost always applied and is inflated as needed. Contraindications to the use of a tourniquet include a history of thrombophlebitis and significant peripheral vascular disease. Advantages of tourniquet use are increased visibility and no significant increase in postoperative morbidity with tourniquet times of less than 90 minutes. The disadvantages of routine tourniquet use include blanching of the synovium (which makes differentiation and diagnosis of various synovial disorders difficult) and the possibility of ischemic damage to muscle and nervous tissue with prolonged tourniquet times of greater than 90 to 120 minutes. Many of the commercial leg holders used in knee arthroscopy require the tourniquet to be placed within them. These holders may function satisfactorily whether or not the tourniquet is inflated.

In a prospective, randomized clinical trial, Kirkley et al. found no significant differences between patients in whom a tourniquet was used and those without tourniquet use. There was a trend for less early postoperative pain and slightly better isokinetic strength testing at 2 weeks in patients without tourniquet use, but visibility was rated by the surgeons as being three times better with tourniquet use. The authors concluded that the use of a tourniquet at 300 mm Hg did not significantly affect overall functional outcome. In a prospective, randomized trial including 109 patients who had undergone arthroscopic knee surgery with or without a tourniquet, Johnson et al. found no significant differences between the two groups with respect to operative view, duration of operation, pain scores, analgesic requirement, or complications. Because the use of a tourniquet did not appear to improve the operative view, these authors recommended against routine use of a tourniquet for arthroscopic knee surgery.

LEG HOLDERS

The greatest advantage of a leg holder is that it permits application of stress, primarily to open the posteromedial compartment for better viewing, manipulation of the meniscus, and posterior horn meniscal surgery, especially in tight knees. Because the thigh is firmly held by the leg holder, the number of different positions in which the leg can be placed is somewhat limited. An alternative to an encompassing leg holder is a lateral post attached to the side rail of the operating table (Fig. 1.8). The lateral aspect of the distal thigh can be levered against this post for opening of the posteromedial compartment. The post does not confine or prevent the knee from being positioned in an almost unlimited number of positions, including flexion and the figure-four position, and therefore has advantages over many of the expensive commercial leg-holding devices. We use this for major knee reconstructive procedures.

Routine use of a leg holder, especially one that incorporates a tourniquet within the confines of the holder, may present other difficulties. In such an arrangement, wide fluctuations in the tourniquet pressures may occur when stress is applied to the leg; however, we have had no specific complications related to this. Also, the leg-holding device may fix the distal femur so securely that the applied stress can result in fractures around the knee or tearing of the ligamentous structures; such occurrences have been reported.

Thus if the clinical evaluation suggests medial compartment meniscal disease, a leg holder can be of significant

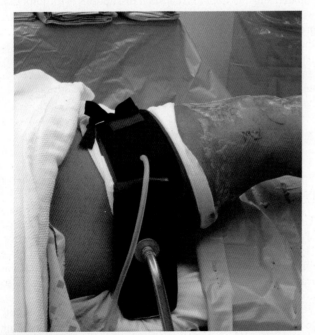

FIGURE 1.8 Lateral post attached to the side rail of the operating table.

assistance. However, if a patellofemoral joint or a lateral compartment problem is anticipated, a valgus stress post may be chosen to make viewing of these compartments easier. For endoscopic repair of the ACL, a lateral post should be used or the end of the table should be flexed to allow full, unobstructed knee flexion.

ANESTHESIA

Diagnostic arthroscopy can be performed with the patient under local, regional, or general anesthesia. Some intraarticular operative procedures can be performed with regional and local anesthetics.

Local anesthesia can be used for many arthroscopic procedures around the knee and ankle in a cooperative patient. Intravenous sedation is used to complement the local injection. Articles by Hansen et al., Chu et al., Petty et al., and many others have brought to light the chondrotoxicity of lidocaine and bupivacaine, particularly when combined with epinephrine, which alters the local pH. When used, lower-volume and lower-concentration injections (i.e., 1% lidocaine and 0.25% bupivacaine) are safer alternatives. Prolonged presence of local agents provided through intraarticular pain pumps should be avoided.

Ultrasound-guided regional blocks for postoperative pain management are safe and effective in most patients and are used routinely. Interscalene blocks affect the phrenic nerve, which is in close proximity, and thus should be avoided or used with caution in respiratory-compromised patients. When used in overhead athletes, the potential for postinjection neuritis should be considered and discussed with the patient. Saphenous nerve blocks provide excellent pain relief after ACL surgery and have the added benefit of being a purely sensory block. We do not use femoral blocks because of the loss of motor function and occasional prolonged quadriceps weakness.

General anesthesia is used or indicated more often in an acutely injured knee, when pain is an important factor, when significant intraarticular surgery is anticipated, or when the patient is not cooperative or is especially apprehensive. Allergy to local anesthetics, of course, requires that a general anesthetic be administered. Arthroscopic surgeons who are less experienced and unfamiliar with all of the techniques are best advised to select a general anesthetic. If the need for a tourniquet to control bleeding is anticipated, such as for partial or complete synovectomies or excision of adhesions, general anesthesia is recommended. Most arthroscopic procedures performed at our clinic are performed with general anesthesia.

If a local anesthetic is chosen, the tourniquet is not inflated. Yoshiya et al. reported the use of a 1:1 mixture of 1% lidocaine and 0.25% bupivacaine. Usually, 50 mL of the mixture was injected intraarticularly before the procedure. When a long procedure was expected, a small amount of epinephrine was added to the mixture to help maintain hemostasis and to increase the duration of action of the anesthetic agents. The authors recommended taking care not to exceed the maximal dosage when using bupivacaine (2 mg/kg of body weight). At each anticipated portal, an additional 5 mL of the lidocaine-bupivacaine mixture was injected. There was only one report of nausea and no other reports of toxic reactions or central nervous system or cardiovascular complications.

Postoperative pain may be diminished by treatment with oral nonsteroidal antiinflammatory medication preoperatively and postoperatively, or intraoperatively through intramuscular or intravenous administration. The use of nonsteroidal antiinflammatory medication has also been shown to reduce swelling and to increase range of motion in the early postoperative period. The use of oral corticosteroids has not proved effective. Beneficial analgesic effects have been documented for administration of 30 mL of 0.25% bupivacaine with or without the addition of 3 mg of morphine. We do not recommend the use of intraarticular pain pump catheters because of the potential for chondrocyte toxicity.

DOCUMENTATION

A systematic examination of the operative joint should be recorded using digital photographs, video clips, or both. Preoperative and postoperative photographs are valuable elements of a patient's record and can be used to critically analyze and teach operative procedures.

ADVANTAGES

The advantages of arthroscopic procedures far outweigh the disadvantages. Some advantages of arthroscopic procedures compared with arthrotomy are as follows:

- *Reduced postoperative morbidity.* The patient can return to sedentary work almost immediately and to more vigorous work activities within 2 to 3 weeks after most simple procedures.
- *Smaller incisions.* Arthroscopic diagnostic and operative procedures can be carried out through multiple small incisions around the joint, which are less likely to produce disfiguring scars.
- *Less intense inflammatory response.* The small incisions through the capsule and synovium result in a much less intense inflammatory response than with standard arthrotomy. This results in less postoperative pain, faster rehabilitation, and faster return to work.
- *Improved visualization.* Better visualization is particularly important in shoulder procedures where pathology is common and can be repaired concomitantly through the use of common arthroscopic portals.
- *Absence of secondary effects.* The secondary effects of arthrotomy around the joints, such as neuroma formation, painful disfiguring scars, and potential functional imbalance (e.g., of the extensor mechanism of the knee), are eliminated by arthroscopic techniques.
- *Reduced hospital stay.* Most arthroscopic procedures are performed on an outpatient basis.
- *Reduced complication rate.* Only infrequent complications of arthroscopic procedures have been reported.
- *Improved follow-up evaluation.* The minimal morbidity associated with arthroscopy allows the effects of a previous operative procedure, such as meniscal repair, to be reevaluated if persistent symptoms warrant further evaluation. These are often referred to as *relook* or *second-look* procedures.
- *Possibility of performing surgical procedures that would be difficult or impossible to perform through open arthrotomy.* A number of surgical procedures are more easily performed with arthroscopic techniques than through open arthrotomy incisions. Many menisci that can be repaired are accessible only with arthroscopic techniques and cannot be satisfactorily viewed through arthrotomy.

DISADVANTAGES

The disadvantages of arthroscopy are few but may be significant to the individual arthroscopic surgeon. Not every surgeon has the temperament to perform arthroscopic surgery because it requires working through small portals with delicate and fragile instruments. The need to maneuver the instruments within the tight confines of intraarticular spaces may produce significant scuffing and scoring of the articular surfaces, especially by an inexperienced surgeon. The procedures can be extremely time-consuming early in one's experience with arthroscopy. Also, the specialized equipment that is required is extensive and expensive.

Although these disadvantages can be significant, the advantages to patients generally far outweigh them.

INDICATIONS AND CONTRAINDICATIONS

Intraarticular or periarticular pathologic conditions can be examined and treated arthroscopically. However, previous experience and the skillset of the operating surgeon should determine whether an arthroscopic or open technique would ensure the best possible treatment for the patient. The contraindications are few. Arthroscopy should not be used in a minimally damaged joint that will respond to the usual conservative methods of treatment. Furthermore, the surgeon should not consider arthroscopy before careful evaluation of the patient's history, thorough physical examination, and standard noninvasive diagnostic procedures have been performed. Arthroscopy is contraindicated when the risk of joint sepsis from a local skin condition is present or when a remote infection may be seeded in the operative site. Partial or complete ankylosis around the joint is a relative contraindication, although the use of arthroscopy for lysis of adhesions around the knee, shoulder, elbow, and ankle can be beneficial. Major collateral ligamentous and capsular disruptions of the joint that will permit excessive extravasation of fluids into the soft tissues are relative contraindications to arthroscopy. In this situation, the capsule should be allowed to "stick down" or should be repaired primarily before any arthroscopic procedure. Gravity inflow should be used, and outflow should be maintained to help prevent increased compartmental fluid pressures.

BASIC ARTHROSCOPIC TECHNIQUES

Proficiency in arthroscopic techniques requires a great deal of patience and persistence.

Techniques are best learned by assisting with and performing surgical procedures alongside an experienced arthroscopist during residency or fellowship or in practice. Hands-on learning sources by the American Academy of Orthopaedic Surgeons and by specialty societies are excellent ways to learn new procedures. Internet surgical videos also are available at many vendor websites.

Patients' expectations regarding the use of arthroscopic techniques have placed tremendous demands on practicing orthopaedic surgeons. A surgeon should not be persuaded by these pressures to perform a difficult arthroscopic procedure for which sufficient skills have yet to be developed. If an arthroscopic procedure is not progressing as expected, it may be wise to abort the procedure and return to an open method that has given good results in the past. As arthroscopic procedures become better defined and results continue to improve, the number of arthroscopic procedures is increasing steadily. There is a steep learning curve to successful completion of complicated procedures, such as shoulder stabilization and rotator cuff repair. The practicing surgeon should keep up with the literature, attend workshops, and observe these procedures being performed by highly skilled arthroscopists. Orthopaedic surgeons should perform procedures concurrent with their skill levels, keeping in mind that a skillfully performed procedure through an open arthrotomy is preferable to a poorly performed arthroscopic procedure.

TRIANGULATION TECHNIQUE

Triangulation involves the use of one or more instruments inserted through separate portals and brought into the optical field of the arthroscope, with the tip of the instrument and the arthroscope forming the apex of a triangle. The principle of triangulation is the basis for operative arthroscopy. Triangulation separates the arthroscope from the operating instrument, allowing the viewing arthroscope to be enlarged and increasing the field of view. The angle of inclination can be varied to allow improved visual access to more areas of the joint. Separation of the instruments from the arthroscope improves depth perception and, perhaps the most significant advantage, permits independent movement of the arthroscope and the surgical instrument, which is essential for operative arthroscopy.

To begin triangulation, the arthroscope should be placed at a sufficient distance from the area to be probed to give a wide field of vision. When the instrument is positioned, the scope and instrument are advanced together toward the intended area, reducing the field of vision while increasing the magnification. A mistake commonly made by arthroscopists early on is placement of the scope too close to objects, thus losing the larger field of vision necessary to maintain constant visual orientation.

If the surgeon becomes disoriented and has difficulty in triangulation, the accessory instrument may be brought into the joint to contact the sheath of the arthroscope. By sliding the instrument down the sheath to the arthroscope tip, the surgeon may bring the instrument into the field of vision. With practice, a surgeon will develop a stereoscopic sense that allows placement of the instrument into the field of view immediately.

COMPLICATIONS

Complications during or after arthroscopy are infrequent and fortunately are usually minor. Most are preventable with good preoperative and intraoperative planning and attention to the details of basic techniques. Familiarity with local anatomy and gaining familiarity with new techniques through learning centers, operating with colleagues, videos, and staying current with specialty journals allow the surgeon to gain valuable information from the experiences of other colleagues. Before operative procedures, having all office notes and radiographs available is similarly beneficial. Also, before entering the operating room, reviewing the surgical procedure with the patient and having the patient write the word "wrong" on the

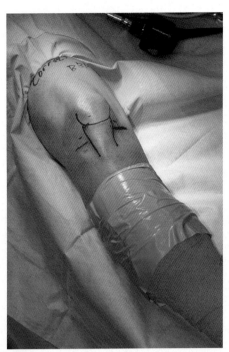

FIGURE 1.9 Operative extremity has been marked by the patient and by the surgeon.

nonoperative extremity can alleviate possible confusion on a long operative day. The *Sign Your Site* program of the American Academy of Orthopaedic Surgeons and the Universal Protocol recommendations of the Joint Commission on Accreditation of Healthcare Organizations include preoperative verification of the operative site, marking of the operative site by the surgeon (Fig. 1.9), and a "time out" before the procedure is begun for final verification and a final checklist.

Overall complication rates for arthroscopy are reported to be between 1% and 4.7%. The complication rate is proportional to experience, operating time, tourniquet time, procedure complexity, multi-ligament and posterior cruciate ligament (PCL) injuries, number of procedures, and meniscal repairs. The most commonly reported complications include return to the operating room and superficial infections. Careful preparation before the procedure can prevent many of the potential complications. In their review of complications reported by surgeons sitting for part II of the American Board of Orthopaedic Surgeons examinations, Salzler et al. found 4305 complications reported in approximately 92,565 arthroscopic knee procedures, a 4.7% complication rate. Procedure complexity was correlated with an increase in adverse outcomes. PCL reconstruction had the highest complication rate, which was 20%. Basques et al. showed that comorbidities and smoking increased the risk of complications after arthroscopic meniscectomy.

DAMAGE TO INTRAARTICULAR STRUCTURES

Damage to intraarticular structures probably is the most common complication of knee arthroscopy. Scuffing of the articular cartilage surfaces by the tip of the arthroscope or the operating instrument occurs most often when the arthroscopist is inexperienced, when the joint is tight, or when the procedure is long and particularly difficult. Forcing the arthroscope or other instruments between articular surfaces,

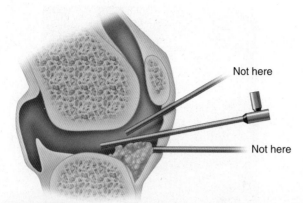

FIGURE 1.10   Ideal placement of cannula. If it is positioned too high, the angle of obliquity is such that the posterior horn cannot be seen; if it is too low, the cannula can go through the meniscus and limit view or mobility. Ideal placement is directly in the slot between the femur and tibia.

such as the femoral and tibial condyles or the humeral head and glenoid cavity, may severely score their surfaces and lead to progressive chondromalacic changes and degenerative arthritis. The joint should be opened with leverage or traction first and the arthroscope allowed to slide into the space created. Use of a leg holder or a leverage post during knee surgery, as well as traction or distraction devices during shoulder, hip, and ankle procedures, is helpful. Once the arthroscope has been inserted between the articular surfaces, distraction should be maintained. If distraction is released and the scope is then retracted, the articular cartilage will be severely scored. Finally, a poorly placed portal frequently makes instrument passage and maneuvering more difficult. It is better to change the portal site or to make an accessory portal than to scuff the articular surface by forcing the instrument.

DAMAGE TO MENISCI AND FAT PAD

The anterior horn of either meniscus of the knee can be damaged by incision or penetration if the anterior portals are located too inferiorly (Fig. 1.10). If the portals are too close to the patellar tendon, they may traverse the fat pad. Repeated penetration of the fat pad causes swelling of the pad and obstruction of view, and may also result in hemorrhage, hypertrophy, or fibrosis of that structure.

DAMAGE TO CRUCIATE LIGAMENTS

Either cruciate ligament may be damaged during meniscal excision when an intercondylar attachment is cut. With knee ligament reconstructions, the intact cruciate is susceptible to injury when motorized instruments are debriding the intercondylar notch. Thus, the shaver blade should always be directed away from the intact ligament.

DAMAGE TO EXTRAARTICULAR STRUCTURES
■ BLOOD VESSELS

Damage to the blood vessels around the joint may be the most serious and devastating arthroscopic complication. Vascular injury most often occurs as a result of direct penetration or laceration but may occur from pressure caused by excessive fluid extravasation. Small's 1986 report included 12 vascular

injuries, all in knee surgery; no vascular complications were reported in his 1988 study. The popliteal artery is at risk during meniscectomy when intercondylar attachments are cut, especially when arthroscopic knives are used. Both the popliteal artery and vein have been damaged during meniscal repairs as the sutures are placed posteriorly. Most surgeons now recommend a posteromedial or posterolateral incision, with exposure of the capsule and placement of a suitable retractor to protect the popliteal vessels during meniscal repairs and for PCL reconstructions. When large, complicated procedures are performed, constant awareness of the posterior vascular structures is necessary and having the availability of a vascular surgeon is desirable. The vessels are also vulnerable if there is uncontrolled penetration during establishment of the posteromedial or posterolateral knee portals. Extensive arthroscopic synovectomies have been associated with injury to the genicular arteries, with subsequent arteriovenous fistula or pseudoaneurysm formation.

The anterior tibial artery is at risk during anterior approaches for ankle arthroscopy, especially with the anterocentral approach. Likewise, posteromedial portals are not recommended because of the proximity of the posterior artery. During elbow arthroscopy, the brachial artery may be damaged when establishing either the anteromedial or anterolateral portal. Fluid extravasation may also compress this vessel in the antecubital fossa. In shoulder arthroscopy, the axillary artery may be injured by an arthroscopic instrument plunging through the axillary pouch. More often, axillary vessel occlusion is caused by fluid extravasation or excessive arm traction.

During shoulder arthroscopy, the acromial branch of the coracoacromial artery can be transected just lateral to the acromioclavicular joint during resection of the coracoacromial ligament.

Major superficial veins may be lacerated by improper portal selection. In the knee, the saphenous vein may be penetrated by poor posteromedial portal location. In the shoulder, the cephalic vein may be penetrated by poor anterior portal site selection.

■ COMPARTMENT SYNDROMES

Increased compartment pressure may occur during surgery from fluid extravasations and should be monitored during all extensive procedures. By using gravity inflow or lower pump pressures and ensuring adequate outflow, most of these complications can be avoided. When excessive extravasations occur, stopping fluid inflow, releasing any constricting dressing or tourniquets, and placing the extremity at the level of the heart are recommended. Wrapping with an Esmarch tourniquet from a distal to proximal direction and then removing it may help remove the extravasated fluid. Persistence of elevated pressure should be evaluated and treated following the guidelines set for compartment syndrome.

■ NERVES

Nerve injuries may be caused by direct trauma from a scalpel or sharp trocar, traction from overdistraction, mechanical compression or compression from fluid extravasation, prolonged ischemia from excessive tourniquet use, or a poorly defined mechanism of injury to the anatomic nervous system that results in reflex sympathetic dystrophy. Many of these complications can be avoided by marking the portals appropriately, making sure the scalpel penetrates the skin only, using a hemostat to spread down to the joint capsule in the proximity of a nerve, and routinely using blunt trocars. Maintaining proper joint distention and distraction, padding nerve and bony prominences, and proper patient positioning also greatly reduce the chances of nerve complications. Familiarity with techniques and anatomy allows proper portal placement and improves surgical technique, thus minimizing tourniquet time.

Sensory and motor nerves near the joint may also be damaged. The inferior branches of the saphenous nerve or sartorial branches of the femoral nerve are the most commonly injured cutaneous nerves. The location of each of these numerous cutaneous branches varies, and therefore occasional injury to one may be unavoidable, especially if multiple portals are used. In most instances, the hypesthesia produced is of minor consequence and causes no problem. On occasion, a painful neuroma may require subsequent resection. In Small's report (1986), 229 nerve injuries were reported during knee arthroscopies.

During shoulder arthroscopy, the branches of the axillary nerve that course along the deep surface of the deltoid may be injured if either anterior or posterior portal sites are too far inferior. Traction neurapraxia of the brachial plexus may occur when strong traction and distraction of the shoulder have been used. The position that appears to result in the greatest traction on the brachial plexus is 30 degrees of forward elevation and 70 degrees of abduction. In 1986, Small reported one axillary nerve injury and three brachial plexus injuries in 14,329 shoulder arthroscopies. In 1988, there were no nerve injuries in 1184 shoulder procedures. Arthroscopy of the smaller joints, elbow and ankle, requires even greater attention to detail and general principles than in the more familiar knee arthroscopy. Neurovascular injury is the major risk of elbow arthroscopy: anterior portals place the radial and posterior interosseous nerves at risk on the lateral side and the median nerve at risk on the medial side; posteromedial portals place the ulnar nerve at risk. However, nerve palsies after elbow arthroscopy usually are transient and result from local anesthetic, tourniquet use, or blunt injury. Kelly et al. reported 12 transient nerve palsies in 473 elbow arthroscopies and identified rheumatoid arthritis and contractures as significant risk factors for the development of temporary nerve palsy.

Regardless of the site of the arthroscopic procedure, a thorough understanding of local anatomy and precise marking of tendons and neurovascular structures are essential. Exact portal placement and proper distention before blunt entry into the joint decrease nerve vulnerability. Careful use of less aggressive motorized shavers is important in working close to neurovascular structures.

■ LIGAMENTS AND TENDONS

The medial collateral ligament (MCL) may be injured by accessory medial portals around the knee, or it may be torn by severe valgus stress in an attempt to open up the medial compartment. This is a real possibility if a rigid leg holder is used and a strong valgus stress is applied.

HEMARTHROSIS

Hemarthrosis is the most common postoperative complication, occurring most frequently after lateral retinacular releases and synovectomies. The superior lateral geniculate vessels usually are cut in lateral retinacular releases, and the inferior lateral geniculate vessels may be lacerated just anterior to the popliteal hiatus during lateral meniscectomy and synovectomy. Persistent unexplained hemarthrosis is an indication for appropriate vascular studies and hematologic clotting studies to help determine appropriate treatment.

THROMBOPHLEBITIS

Thrombophlebitis is potentially the most dangerous postoperative complication. In a meta-analysis of patients who had not received prophylactic antithrombotic medication, Ilahi et al. found the overall rate to be 9.9% for deep vein thrombosis (DVT) and 2.1% for proximal DVT after knee arthroscopy. Although rates of pulmonary emboli after arthroscopic surgery have been reported to be less than 1%, a meta-analysis by Sun et al. found an average rate of 6.8% for DVT in patients without low molecular weight heparin (LMWH) prophylaxis; 29 of 136 DVTs were proximal. In patients who received LMWH prophylaxis, the DVT rate was 1.8%; 4 of 36 DVTs were proximal. Two studies evaluating DVT after ACL reconstruction reported DVT rates of 14% (Ye et al.) and 9% (Struijk-Mulder et al.). Ye et al. found age of greater than 35 years and female sex to be associated with an increased risk of DVT. In a later study of 537 patients who were examined with venography after knee arthroscopy, Sun et al. found venous thromboemboli in 80 patients (15%), only 20 of whom had clinical signs of DVT. Advanced age and complex procedures were significantly associated with DVT.

DVT of the upper extremity is rare. Randelli et al. reported only six occurrences of DVT in 9385 shoulder arthroscopies (0.06%). In a series of 1908 patients with shoulder arthroscopy reported by Kuremsky et al., six patients (0.3%) had thromboembolic complications involving both the ipsilateral upper and lower extremities; four of the six patients had pulmonary emboli.

Based on the currently available data, we recommend use of lower extremity serial compression devices during extensive arthroscopic shoulder surgery, especially in at-risk patients. The risks of DVT prophylaxis should be weighed against the benefits when ligament or meniscal repair is performed, particularly in patients with known risk factors for thromboembolic complications, such as female sex, age over 35 years, comorbidities, use of birth control, and factor V Leiden thrombophilia. An age greater than 70 years increases thromboembolic risk 10 times; body mass index greater than 29, smoking, and oral contraception increase the risk three times; and diabetes and hypertension increase the risk two times. Medical consultation is indicated for these patients. In general, early active range of motion of the extremity is encouraged, and then use of aspirin postoperatively for prophylaxis should be considered when weight bearing status is altered. Finally, prolonged travel, especially by air, is best avoided in the immediate postoperative period.

INFECTION

Despite early fears of infection, the actual number of reported infections after arthroscopy has remained extremely low. Numerous investigators have reported large series, all with infection rates of less than 0.2%. This low incidence is undoubtedly the result of several factors, including limited incisions, young and healthy patients, short operating times, and irrigation and dilutional effects of the irrigating solutions. Babcock et al. noted, however, that when such infections occur, they can cause significant morbidity. As risk factors, they cited the use of intraarticular corticosteroids, prolonged tourniquet time, patient age of greater than 50 years, failure to prepare the surgical site again before conversion to arthrotomy, procedure complexity, and history of previous procedures. They also noted that several reported outbreaks of infection after arthroscopy were related to breaks in infection control or contaminated instruments.

The use of prophylactic antibiotics is still controversial. Citing the development of septic arthritis in nine patients after knee arthroscopy, D'Angelo and Ogilvie-Harris suggested that the use of prophylactic antibiotics may be cost beneficial, considering the unpredictability of this complication and its serious consequences. However, Bert et al. reviewed 3231 arthroscopic knee surgeries and found infection rates of 0.15% in patients who received antibiotics and 0.16% in those who did not. These authors concluded that there was no value in administering antibiotics before routine arthroscopic knee surgery. Kurzweil noted that prophylactic antibiotics may be appropriate to reduce the risk of infection in "high-risk" patients, such as those with diabetes, immune problems, and skin disorders. Judd et al. reported an infection rate of 0.68% in 1615 patients who had undergone arthroscopic ACL reconstructions, and associated previous knee surgery, especially previous ACL reconstruction and tibial graft fixation with a post and washer, with an increased risk of infection. Routine use of postoperative intraarticular steroids has been associated with an increased incidence of postoperative infection.

In a literature review of infections after arthroscopic ACL reconstruction, Saper et al. found an 86% success rate in 90 infections treated with early arthroscopic irrigation and debridement and intravenous antibiotics. Infections involving *Staphylococcus aureus* and allografts were less likely to be successfully treated with this regimen.

Infection rates after arthroscopy of other joints are equally low. Clarke et al. reported only one case of septic arthritis in 1054 consecutive patients who underwent hip arthroscopy, and infections have been reported to occur in less than 1% of patients after shoulder arthroscopy and after arthroscopy of the ankle. Kelly et al. reported an infection rate of 0.8% in 473 consecutive elbow arthroscopy patients.

We recommend that surgical sites be cleansed and clippers be used in a preoperative area for hair removal. The entire extremity is cleansed with Hibiclens (Mölnlycke Health Care, Norcross, GA) and then painted with DuraPrep (3M, St Paul, MN). A sterile technique is used while draping and isolating the surgical site with a waterproof seal. Sterile handling of the surgical site is also mandatory after surgery.

Antibiotics are given as recommended by the American Academy of Orthopaedic Surgeons' Advisory Statement for Total Joints, which recommends intravenous administration of 1 g cefazolin or 2 g for patients over 80 kg be given to the patient within 1 hour of the skin incision. Patients who are allergic to cephalosporins are treated with alternative antibiotic prophylaxis.

TOURNIQUET PARESIS

Temporary paresis in the extremity has been observed after tourniquet use to control bleeding in diagnostic or operative arthroscopy, usually after prolonged procedures. If a tourniquet is required, it should be deflated after 90 to 120 minutes. Careful monitoring of the tourniquet pressure and testing the accuracy of the tourniquet gauges minimize these problems.

Fortunately, tourniquet paresis is usually mild and resolves within a few days.

SYNOVIAL HERNIATION AND FISTULAS

Small globules of fat and synovial tissue may herniate through any of the arthroscopic portals. Usually, the larger the portal, the greater the chance of this complication occurring. Rarely, a large fluid-filled cystic herniation may occur. These fat and synovial herniations are usually small and become asymptomatic over several weeks and do not require any specific treatment. If a herniation persists and remains symptomatic, excision of the herniated portion with careful closure of the capsule may be required.

Synovial fistulas are rare but have occurred after suture reactions or stitch abscesses. Fistulas are more commonly associated with posteromedial knee and ankle portals. To improve closure, these portals should be routinely sutured rather than closed with adhesive strips. Fistulas do not usually produce significant intraarticular infections, but the patient should probably receive antibiotics, and the knee should be immobilized for 7 to 10 days to allow the fistula to close spontaneously. Surgical closure is rarely required.

INSTRUMENT BREAKAGE

If an instrument breaks, the surgeon should immediately close the outflow cannula, but the inflow should be left open to keep the joint distended. Stopping the outflow reduces turbulence, and holding the joint still helps to prevent the fragment from falling out of sight into another part of the joint. If the broken instrument is located in the visual field, it is essential to focus total attention on keeping it within view and removing it. Broken instruments tend to gravitate into the medial or lateral gutters of the knee, to hide beneath the menisci, or to drop by gravity into the posterior or most dependent part of the joint. If the fragment cannot be located by thorough examination and probing of the joint, a radiograph of the joint should be made. If the broken piece is located, a suction apparatus or magnet may be introduced through an accessory portal to stabilize and remove the small broken fragment, or an additional grasping instrument can be inserted through a third portal to secure and extract the piece.

IMPLANT COMPLICATIONS

Suture anchors, sutures, and knots can cause chondral damage, synovitis, osteolysis, and chondrolysis. Persistence of mechanical symptoms, reproducible knot impingement, and persistence of synovitis should be evaluated by MRI and by aspiration if indicated. Arthroscopic examination is indicated for painful mechanical catching or impingement for which another cause cannot be found.

REFERENCES

American Academy of Orthopaedic Surgeons: Advisory statement: recommendations for the use of intravenous antibiotic prophylaxis in primary total joint arthroplasty. Available online at http://www.aaos.org/about/papers/advistmt/1027.asp.

American Academy of Orthopaedic Surgeons: Advisory statement: wrong-site surgery. Available online at www.aaos.org/wordhtml/papers/advistmt/1015.htm.

Ashraf A, Luo TD, Christophersen C, et al.: Acute and subacute complications of pediatric and adolescent knee arthroscopy, *Arthroscopy* 30:710, 2014.

Bhattacharyya R, Davidson DJ, Sugand K, et al.: Knee arthroscopy simulation: a randomized controlled trial evaluating the effectiveness of the Imperial Knee Arthroscopy Cognitive Task Analysis (IKACTA) tool, *J Bone Joint Surg Am* 99(19):e103, 2017.

Basques BA, Gardner EC, Varthi AG, et al.: Risk factors for short-term adverse events and readmission after arthroscopic meniscectomy. Does age matter? *Am J Sports Med* 43:169, 2015.

Cancienne JM, Brockmeier SF, Carson EW, Werner BC: Risk factors for infection after shoulder arthroscopy in a large Medicare population, *Am J Sports Med* 46(4):809, 2018.

Cancienne JM, Mahon HS, Dempsey IJ, Miller MD, Werner BC: Patient-related risk factors for infection following knee arthroscopy: an analysis of over 700,000 patients from two large databases, *Knee* 24(3):594, 2017.

Cancienne JM, Miller MD, Browne JA, Werner BC: Not all patients with diabetes have the same risks: perioperative glycemic control is associated with postoperative infection following knee arthroscopy, *Arthroscopy* 34(5):1561, 2018.

Carter CW, Moros C, Ahmad CS, Levine WN: Arthroscopic anterior shoulder instability repair: techniques, pearls, pitfalls, and complications, *Instr Course Lect* 57:125, 2008.

Chapelle C, Rosencher N, Zuffery PJ, et al.: Prevention of venous thromboembolic events with low-molecular-weight heparin in the non-major orthopaedic setting: meta-analysis of randomized controlled trials, *Arthroscopy* 30:987, 2014.

Chong AC, Pate RC, Prohaska DJ, Bron TR, Wooley PH: Validation of improvement of basic competency in arthroscopic knot tying using a bench top simulator in orthopaedic residency education, *Arthroscopy* 32(7):1389, 2016.

Dhwan A, Ghodadra N, Karas V, et al.: Complications of bioabsorbable suture anchors in the shoulder, *Am J Sports Med* 40:1424, 2012.

Dragoo JL, Korotkova TA, Kanwar R, Wood B: The effect of local anesthetics administered via pain pump on chondrocyte viability, *Am J Sports Med* 36:1484, 2008.

Grutter PW, McFarland EG, Zikria BA, et al.: Techniques for suture anchor removal in shoulder surgery, *Am J Sports Med* 38:1706, 2010.

Kuo LT, Yu PA, Chen CL, Hsu WH, Chi CC: Tourniquet use in arthroscopic anterior cruciate ligament reconstruction: a systematic review and meta-analysis of randomized controlled trials, *BMC Musculoskelet Disord* 18(1):358, 2017.

Kuremsky MA, Cain EL, Fleischli JE: Thromboembolic phenomena after arthroscopic shoulder surgery, *Arthroscopy* 27:1614, 2011.

Ladner B, Nester K, Cascio B: Abdominal fluid extravasation during hip arthroscopy, *Arthroscopy* 26:131, 2010.

Martin KD, Patterson DP, Cameron KL: Arthroscopic training courses improve trainee arthroscopy skills: a simulation-based prospective trial, *Arthroscopy* 32(11):2228, 2016.

Matthews B, Wilkinson M, McEwen P, et al.: In vivo arthroscopic temperatures: a comparison between 2 types of radiofrequency ablation systems in arthroscopic anterior cruciate ligament reconstruction – a randomized controlled trial, *Arthroscopy* 33(1):165, 2017.

Memon M, Kay J, Gholami A, Simunovic N, Ayeni OR: Fluid extravasation in shoulder arthroscopic surgery: a systematic review, *Orthop J Sports Med* 6(5):2325967118771616, 2018.

Noticewala MS, Trofa DP, Vance DD, Jobin CM, Levine WN, Ahmad CS: Elbow arthroscopy: 30-day postoperative complication profile and associated risk factors, *Arthroscopy* 34(2):414, 2018.

Pauzenberger L, Brieb A, Hexel M, et al.: Infections following arthroscopic rotator cuff repair: incidence, risk factors, and prophylaxis, *Knee Surg Sports Traumatol Arthrosc* 25(2):595, 2017.

Randelli P, Castagna A, Cabitza F, et al.: Infectious and thromboembolic complications of arthroscopic shoulder surgery, *J Shoulder Elbow Surg* 19:97, 2010.

Romeo AA, Ghodadra NS, Salata MJ, Provencher MT: Arthroscopic suprascapular nerve decompression: indications and surgical technique, *J Shoulder Elbow Surg* 19:118, 2010.

Salzler MJ, Lin A, Miller CD, et al.: Complications after arthroscopic knee surgery, *Am J Sports Med* 42:292, 2014.

Saper M, Stephenson K, Helsey M: Arthroscopic irrigation and debridement in the treatment of septic arthritis after anterior cruciate ligament reconstruction, *Arthroscopy* 30:747, 2014.

Steiner SRH, Cancienne JM, Werner BC: Narcotics and knee arthroscopy: trends in use and factors associated with prolonged use and postoperative complications, *Arthroscopy* 34(6):1931, 2018.

Struijk-Mulder MC, Ettema HB, Verheyen CCPM, Büller MR: Deep vein thrombosis after arthroscopic anterior cruciate ligament reconstruction: a prospective cohort study of 100 patients, *Arthroscopy* 29:1211, 2013.

Sun Y, Chen D, Xu Z, et al.: Deep venous thrombosis after knee arthroscopy: a systematic review and meta-analysis, *Arthroscopy* 30:406, 2014.

Syed HM, Gillham SB, Jobe CM, et al.: Fenestrated cannulae with outflow reduces fluid gain in shoulder arthroscopy, *Clin Orthop Relat Res* 468:158, 2010.

Thorsness R, Thirukumaran C, Zhang L, et al.: Defining risk factors for perioperative complications following shoulder arthroscopy: an analysis of the National Surgical Quality Improvement Program database, *Arthroscopy* 30(Suppl):e36, 2014.

Ye S, Dongyang C, Zhihong X, et al.: The incidence of deep venous thrombosis after arthroscopically assisted anterior cruciate ligament reconstruction, *Arthroscopy* 29:742, 2013.

The complete list of references is available online at Expert Consult.com.

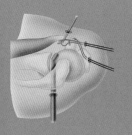

CHAPTER 2

ARTHROSCOPY OF THE FOOT AND ANKLE

G. Andrew Murphy

ANKLE ARTHROSCOPY

The most common current indications for ankle arthroscopy include soft-tissue or bony impingement and treatment of osteochondral lesions of the talus. These patients often have continuing ankle pain after injuries such as sprains that have not responded to the usual conservative therapy, and tenderness is noted specifically at the ankle joint line on physical examination. A definite diagnosis should be made before arthroscopy is performed; purely diagnostic arthroscopy has a low success rate. If magnetic resonance imaging (MRI) is not helpful with the diagnosis, a diagnostic intraarticular injection can be used. Significant relief from an intraarticular anesthetic suggests the presence of an intraarticular pathologic process, for which ankle arthroscopy and debridement may be beneficial. Arthroscopy also has been used to treat ankle instability, septic arthritis, arthrofibrosis, and loose bodies. Werner et al. examined trends in ankle arthroscopy from 2007 to 2011 and found that this modality had significantly increased, especially for repair of the lateral ligament or for peroneal tendon subluxation.

Several anatomic structures are at risk during anterior ankle arthroscopy, with most of the risk of injury occurring during portal placement. In addition, the anterior tibial artery is at risk of injury when working in the anterior aspect of the ankle. In an MRI study, a branch of the anterior tibial artery was near the anterolateral portal in 6.2% of patients, and the artery was an average of 2.3 mm from the anterior capsule. In a cadaver study, the mean distance from the distal tibia to the anterior tibial artery was 0.9 cm when the ankle was in dorsiflexion, and the distance decreased to 0.7 cm when noninvasive distraction was applied to the ankle; thus the safe anterior working area is decreased with distraction. The superficial peroneal nerve often is marked preoperatively with the foot in plantarflexion and inversion. A cadaver study found that the nerve moves laterally when the foot is moved from plantarflexion and inversion to neutral or dorsiflexion (which is the usual position of the foot when creating the anterolateral portal); the authors therefore advise to stay medial to the preoperative marking when making the portal to lessen the risk of injury to the nerve.

There is a wide variation in this nerve's location near the ankle, and transillumination has been found to be of no benefit in showing its position, so extreme caution must be exercised. Another cadaver study found that two or more branches of the superficial peroneal nerve crossed the ankle in 83% of specimens, 68% of ankles had a branch near the anterolateral portal, and 12% had a branch near the anteromedial portal.

The use of a tourniquet for ankle arthroscopy is still common practice. Although Dimnjakovic et al. found that anterior ankle arthroscopy can be adequately performed without a tourniquet, we recommend its use, especially early in a surgeon's experience, because it allows a clearer view of the joint.

In addition to adequate visualization, accessibility of lesions of the ankle joint during arthroscopy is an important consideration. Tonogai et al. recommended a 70-degree arthroscope for best visualization of the posterior medial talar gutter. We recommend this for posterior lesions, lateral and medial gutter lesions, and deltoid lesions.

A posterior approach arthroscopy has been shown to improve working space in talar dome lesions. As these are difficult to access, noninvasive distraction or maximal plantarflexion can be used. Barg et al. compared noninvasive distraction with wire-based distraction for both anterior and posterior arthroscopy (Fig. 2.1A,B). Access to the talar dome could be achieved in both anterior and posterior arthroscopy with these techniques, but in anterior arthroscopy accessibility was not better with wire-based distraction. In a posterior approach, however, wire-based distraction significantly improved accessibility (Fig. 2.2) over noninvasive distraction.

Inadequate pain management before, during, and after arthroscopic techniques can lead to greater morbidity, lower satisfaction scores, and even chronic pain syndromes. Use of preemptive local anesthesia before surgery can substantially reduce postoperative pain and avoid neuropathic pain. Liszka et al. found that operative site infiltration of local anesthetics decreased the level of postoperative pain during the first day after arthroscopic surgery, lowering the amount of analgesics required.

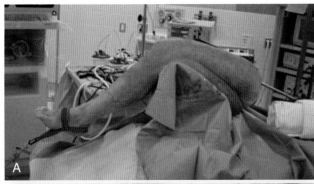

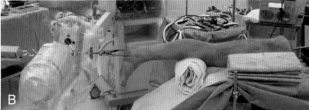

FIGURE 2.1   **A,** Specimen positioned for anterior ankle arthroscopy with noninvasive distraction. **B,** Specimen positioned for posterior ankle arthroscopy with wire-based distraction. (From Barg A, Saltzman CL, Beals TC, et al: Arthroscopic talar dome access using a standard versus wire-based traction method for ankle joint distraction, *Arthroscopy J Arthrosc Relat Surg* 32:1367, 2016.)

ARTHROSCOPIC EXAMINATION AND DEBRIDEMENT OF THE ANKLE JOINT

TECHNIQUE 2.1

- For routine ankle arthroscopy, place the patient supine, with the operative extremity in a leg holder such that the hip and knee are flexed, with the foot hanging free, resulting in gravity-assisted distraction. This also allows free ankle range of motion, which can assist in access to different parts of the ankle (Fig. 2.3).
- Mark portal placement after establishing the path of the superficial peroneal nerve, which can be seen subcutaneously after plantarflexion and inversion of the foot (Fig. 2.4).
- Mark anterolateral and anteromedial portals at the joint line, which can be palpated, staying away from the peroneal nerve (Fig. 2.5).
- After Esmarch exsanguination of the extremity and inflation of the thigh tourniquet, establish the anteromedial portal by inserting an 18-gauge spinal needle at the marked site and insufflating the joint with saline to ensure intraarticular placement and to provide more space for introduction of the blunt trocar (Fig. 2.6). Successful insufflation occurs when there is minimal resistance to the introduction of saline, when the foot dorsiflexes as the joint capsule becomes tight, and when there is backflow of the saline into the syringe after the joint is maximally distended. The anteromedial portal is established first because there are fewer structures at risk than with the anterolateral portal.

- After localization of the anteromedial portal with the spinal needle, make a skin incision just large enough to insert the cannula. A large incision allows more extravasation of fluid into the surrounding soft tissues and can make the procedure more difficult.
- Further penetrate the joint with a blunt straight hemostat to avoid damage to the saphenous nerve, which is at risk in this area.
- Place a 2.7-mm 30-degree arthroscope into the anteromedial portal, and establish the anterolateral portal by direct visualization of a spinal needle introduced at the site of the anticipated portal placement.
- When appropriate needle placement is seen, make the skin incision for the anterolateral portal and penetrate the joint with a blunt instrument (Fig. 2.7); then introduce the arthroscopic shaver in this portal.
- Inspect the lateral aspect of the joint with use of instruments in the anterolateral portal as needed for debridement (Fig. 2.8), and then switch portals (arthroscope in the anterolateral portal and instruments in the anteromedial portal) for treatment of the medial side of the joint (Fig. 2.9).
- Noninvasive distraction can be used if needed to access the deeper aspects of the joint (Fig. 2.10). Occasionally, a posterolateral portal is needed to treat pathologic processes in the posterior aspect of the ankle that cannot be reached even after distraction is applied.
- After the procedure is completed, close the portals with suture to avoid the development of a fistula, which is a reported complication of ankle arthroscopy.

POSTOPERATIVE CARE Patients are placed in a walking boot and can bear weight as tolerated but should be cautioned against excessive activity, because this could cause the ankle to become inflamed. Physical therapy should be started once the wounds have healed and postoperative pain is minimal.

COMPLICATIONS

Complication rates vary from 9% to 17%, with the most common complication being neurologic injury. More recent studies have reported lower complication rates of 3.5% to 6.8%, presumably related to the use of noninvasive distraction or dorsiflexion with minimal distraction. Other complications include vascular injury with pseudoaneurysms, joint fistula, infection, chronic regional pain syndrome, instrument breakage, deep venous thrombosis, and compartment syndrome. Iatrogenic cartilage damage has been reported in 31% of cases, with severe damage in 6.7%; however, there were no symptoms in these patients at follow-up. Blázquez Martín et al. reported a total of 31 complications in 257 ankle or hindfoot arthroscopies. Neurologic injury occurred in 14 patients (eight from superficial peroneal nerve injury), persistent drainage in 10, infection in four, and complex regional pain syndrome in three. Yammine et al., in a systematic review, found 23 case reports of patients who developed pseudoaneurysms after ankle arthroscopy. Although this is a rare complication, it is associated with synovectomy, removal of large anterior osteophytes, hypocoagulability, and arterial injury. Venous thromboembolism also is a rare complication

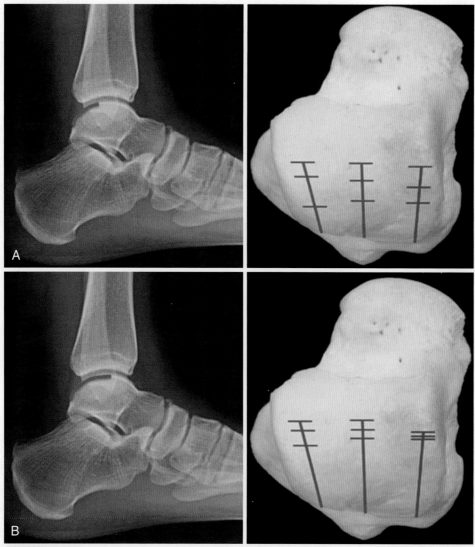

FIGURE 2.2 Accessibility of talar dome by posterior ankle arthroscopy. **A,** Noninvasive strap distraction. **B,** Calcaneal wire-based distraction. Middle hash mark represents mean value; upper and lower hash marks represent maximal and minimal values. (From Barg A, Saltzman CL, Beals TC, et al: Arthroscopic talar dome access using a standard versus wire-based traction method for ankle joint distraction, *Arthroscopy J Arthrosc Relat Surg* 32:1367, 2016.)

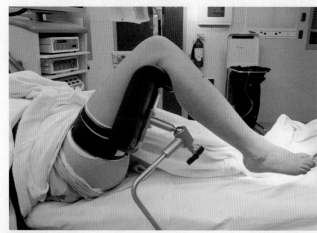

FIGURE 2.3 Leg holder for ankle arthroscopy. **SEE TECHNIQUE 2.1.**

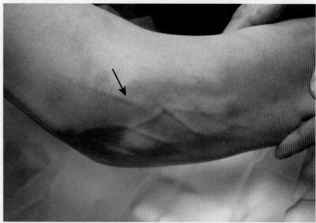

FIGURE 2.4 Path of superficial peroneal nerve is marked on ankle. **SEE TECHNIQUE 2.1.**

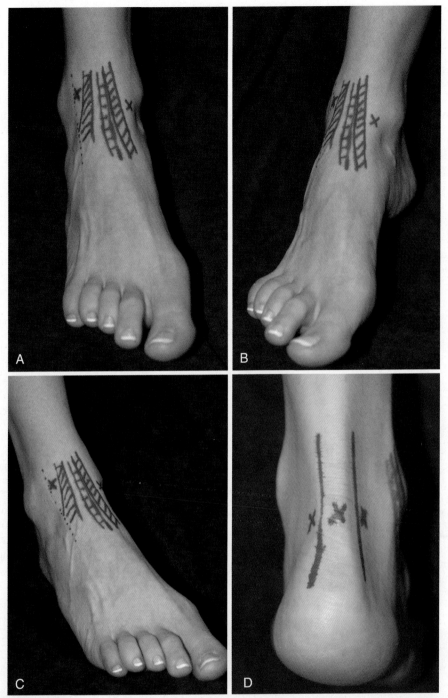

FIGURE 2.5   **A,** Two anterior portals for ankle arthroscopy are marked in relation to anterior tibial and other extensor tendons where they cross anterior aspect of ankle. **B,** Anteromedial portal site. **C,** Anterolateral portal site. **D,** Posterior portals. **SEE TECHNIQUE 2.1.**

that has been reported to occur in 0.6% of patients after foot surgery and arthroscopy. Huntley et al. reported significant associations with nonelective surgery, obesity, older age, and female sex. Although infection rates are relatively low in arthroscopic surgery, a significant correlation was found between intraoperative corticosteroid injections and infection rates after arthroscopy (Werner et al.).

After arthroscopic surgery, many patients ask when they may return safely to driving. Sittapairoj et al. studied this in 36 patients (17 with right-sided ankle or subtalar

arthroscopy and 19 in the control group). They tested preoperative and postoperative brake reaction times and found that emergency braking improves by 2 weeks postoperatively.

ANKLE IMPINGEMENT SYNDROMES
■ ANTERIOR ANKLE IMPINGEMENT

Anterior ankle impingement can be caused by anterior tibial and talar osteophytes and by anterior soft tissue that becomes compressed with dorsiflexion of the ankle. Patients

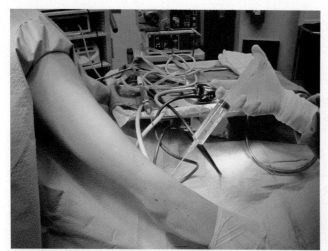

FIGURE 2.6 Establishment of anteromedial portal using 18-gauge spinal needle. **SEE TECHNIQUE 2.1.**

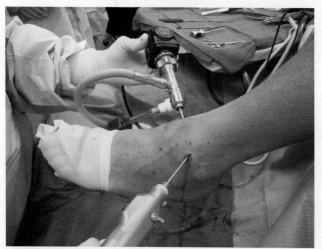

FIGURE 2.7 Anterolateral portal is made with blunt instrument, followed by insertion of arthroscopic shaver. **SEE TECHNIQUE 2.1.**

present with pain localized to the anterior aspect of the ankle and have tenderness at the joint line anteriorly. Lateral radiographs may not show the osteophytes; an anteromedial view of the ankle is often helpful. MRI can show osteophytes but is not very sensitive for soft-tissue impingement; MR arthrography or contrast-enhanced, fat-suppressed, three-dimensional (3D), fast-gradient recalled acquisition in the steady state with radiofrequency spoiling (CE 3D-FSPGR) . MRI is more sensitive and specific but is less practical. MRI may be helpful; however, in one study, 58% of patients had an associated diagnosis, which changed the surgical plan in 33%. Careful physical examination and diagnostic injection can help to pinpoint the diagnosis. The use of intraarticular injections has been questioned because of the potential cytotoxicity to chondrocytes; however, these are all in-vitro studies, and there are no studies substantiating the effects in the clinical setting.

If symptoms persist despite activity modification, immobilization, and rehabilitation, arthroscopic debridement can be helpful in alleviating symptoms. Reported success rates for this procedure range from 73% to 96% in level II to IV studies. In a 2015 systematic review, patient satisfaction was good or excellent in 74% to 100%, with a complication rate of 5.1%, although most studies did not differentiate between types of impingement. When separating out the different types of impingement, level IV studies show that ankle arthroscopy is successful for anteromedial impingement, anterolateral impingement, and anterior bony impingement. Patients with a poorer prognosis include those without a clear diagnosis and those with higher grades of arthritic changes of the ankle. Osteophytes may recur but usually are not symptomatic. There is currently a grade B recommendation (fair evidence) to support use of ankle arthroscopy for ankle impingement according to a systematic review from 2009. According to a national database study, the frequency of ankle arthroscopy has increased from 2814 cases in 2007 to 3314 cases in 2011, the rate of increase being greater than that for shoulder, knee, and elbow arthroscopy. Some level IV studies have described arthroscopic debridement for persistent pain after supramalleolar osteotomy and ankle fracture and for rheumatoid arthritis.

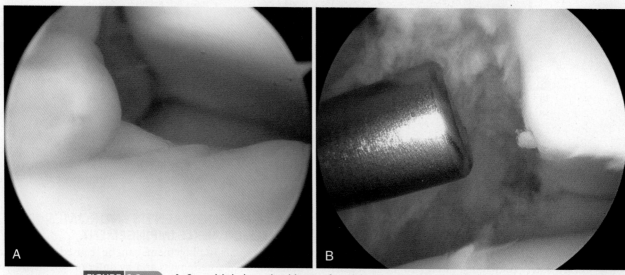

FIGURE 2.8 A, Synovitis in lateral ankle. B, After debridement. **SEE TECHNIQUE 2.1.**

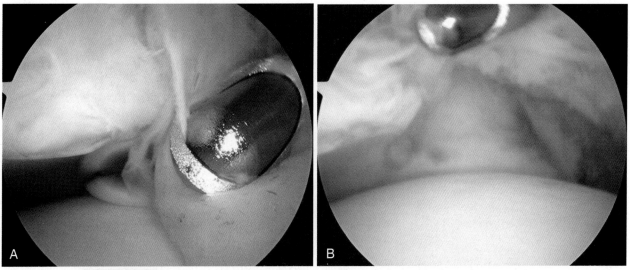

FIGURE 2.9   **A,** Synovitis in medial ankle. **B,** After debridement. **SEE TECHNIQUE 2.1.**

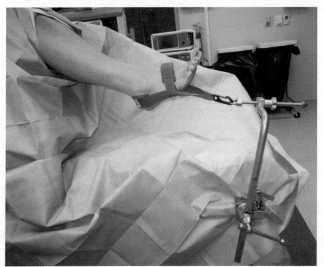

FIGURE 2.10   Noninvasive ankle distraction. **SEE TECHNIQUE 2.1.**

OUTCOMES

Good clinical and radiographic outcomes after arthroscopic treatment of anterior ankle impingement are being reported. McCrum et al. noted significant improvements on visual analog pain scores, AOFAS hindfoot scores, and range of motion in 29 National Football League players after anterior arthroscopic ankle debridement. In 42 patients with a mean age of 32.6 years, the AOFAS score improved from 40.6 preoperatively to 82.6, 78.4, and 74.8 at 2, 4, and 6 years postoperatively, respectively. A body mass index of greater than 26 and male sex were associated with worse outcomes. In a systematic review of 20 articles, Zwier et al. reported 74% to 100% good-to-excellent satisfaction scores, with a low complication rate of 4.6%; major complications were 1.1%. Walsh et al. reported 5-year outcomes in 46 patients with anterior impingement without ankle osteoarthritis. Limited improvement was noted in ankle dorsiflexion; however, functional outcome scores considerably improved, even though there was recurrence of radiographic osteophytes.

POSTERIOR ANKLE IMPINGEMENT

Patients with posterior ankle impingement point to the back of the ankle as the area of pain and have tenderness in the deep posterior aspect of the ankle and pain with a forced plantarflexion test (Fig. 2.11). Studies may show an os trigonum or hypertrophic posterior process of the talus, and patients obtain relief with a fluoroscopic-guided injection in the area.

OUTCOMES

Good and excellent outcomes have been reported in 91% to 100% of patients with this procedure. Multiple level IV studies demonstrate the efficacy of this procedure for symptomatic os trigonum and bony impingement, flexor hallucis longus tenosynovitis, and for patients with both diagnoses. Posterior debridement enabled all 27 elite professional soccer players to return to training at an average of 5 weeks; it can result in significant reduction in pain. Outcomes after arthroscopic and open posterior debridement are similar, but earlier return to sports is possible with arthroscopic treatment, with lower complication rates. Complication rates range from 4% to 20%; complications include neurologic symptoms of the tibial and sural nerves, infection, chronic regional pain syndrome, Achilles tightness, and wound problems.

A systematic review suggested a grade C recommendation (poor quality evidence) for arthroscopic treatment of posterior ankle impingement, given the level of studies available in the literature. Georgiannos and Bisbinas compared open and arthroscopic excision of a symptomatic os trigonum for the treatment of posterior ankle impingement syndrome in 52 athletes (26 in each group). The arthroscopic group had significantly greater improvement in the AOFAS hindfoot score and in the mean time to return training and to sport engagement. The overall complication rate was also lower in the arthroscopic group. Carreira et al. prospectively followed 20 patients who had posterior arthroscopy for posterior impingement. The Tegner score remained the same, but the AOFAS hindfoot scores significantly improved. Complications were minimal, although 15% of patients reported postoperative neuritis. Miyamoto et al. noted that this complication may be reduced by making the posterolateral portal just lateral to the Achilles tendon and performing the procedure lateral to the flexor hallucis longus tendon.

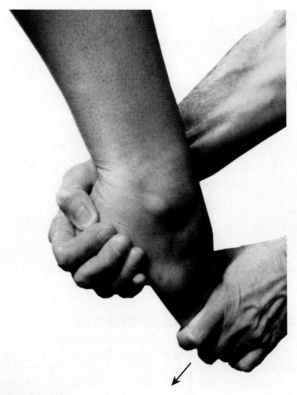

FIGURE 2.11 Forced plantarflexion test for diagnosis of posterior ankle impingement.

POSTERIOR DEBRIDEMENT FOR ANKLE IMPINGEMENT

TECHNIQUE 2.2

- Place the patient prone with the foot at the end of the bed and a support under the lower leg so that the foot hangs freely (Fig. 2.12A). Keeping the foot in neutral with respect to dorsiflexion/plantarflexion and varus/valgus is the safest position in which to avoid neurovascular damage.
- Make the posterolateral portal just superior to a line from the tip of the lateral malleolus to the Achilles tendon, just lateral to the tendon (Fig. 2.12B). Insert a hemostat through a small skin incision, aiming along a line directed to the first web space of the forefoot, until it hits bone (Fig. 2.12C).
- Make the posteromedial portal at the same level, just medial to the Achilles tendon, and insert a hemostat through the skin incision, directing it to contact the arthroscope at a 90-degree angle (Fig. 2.12D). Once the hemostat contacts the arthroscope, move it down the shaft until it hits bone and can be seen through the scope. If desired, use fluoroscopy to confirm appropriate placement.
- Place a shaver in this portal and remove the posterior subtalar capsule (Fig. 2.12E). Take care to stay lateral to the flexor hallucis longus tendon to avoid damage to the neurovascular bundle (see Fig. 2.12F).

- To remove the os trigonum, partially detach the posterior talofibular ligament and posterior talocalcaneal ligament and release the flexor retinaculum to expose the bone to be removed (Fig. 2.12G).
- If distraction is needed, a transcalcaneal traction pin can be hooked to a traction device.

◼ ANTERIOR AND POSTERIOR IMPINGEMENT

If access to both anterior and posterior aspects of the joint is necessary, changing the setup to switch the patient from supine to prone can be cumbersome but can have good results. An alternative to this is to perform anterior ankle arthroscopy as described earlier, and then rotate the leg to place two posteromedial portals, or to place the patient in the lateral position for the posterior surgery and externally rotate the leg for the anterior surgery. Alternatively, posterior arthroscopy can be done with the patient prone, and the knee can be flexed to 90 degrees to access the anterior ankle arthroscopically. Song et al. combined standard anteromedial and anterolateral approaches with dual posterolateral approaches for anterior and posterior ankle impingement. The technique proved to be safe and effective and avoided having to reposition the patient and redrape the limb. This significantly reduced their operating time as well.

OSTEOCHONDRAL LESIONS OF THE TALUS

Osteochondral lesions of the talus can be treated arthroscopically, and the current grade of recommendation is grade B (fair evidence), according to the literature that is currently available. Ankle arthroscopy is performed as described earlier; noninvasive distraction often is necessary to allow room for the instruments for subchondral penetration. Noninvasive distraction has been shown to increase arthroscopic visualization in both anterior and posterior arthroscopy. Akoh et al. found that posterior arthroscopy improved the working space compared with anterior arthroscopy. However, a cadaver study by Phisitkul et al. showed areas that are difficult to access in both approaches. The posterior third of the talus was not as accessible during anterior arthroscopy and the anterior third was not as accessible during posterior arthroscopy. Ankle plantarflexion up to 30 degrees significantly improved access to the dome of the talus in anterior arthroscopy but dorsiflexion did not significantly improve accessibility in posterior arthroscopy. The frequencies of inaccessible areas were 55% for the posterior third during anterior arthroscopy and 83% for the anterior third in posterior arthroscopy, data suggesting that posterior lesions are best approached posteriorly and that lesions in the central third are best approached anteriorly.

Aside from the arthroscopic and positioning techniques used, the main determining factor in the treatment of osteochondral lesions of the talus is lesion size. Smaller lesions (<1 cm^3) for which conservative measures have failed can be treated with arthroscopic excision, curettage, and bone stimulating techniques, as opposed to large lesions that may require autologous osteochondral transplantation. MRI is frequently used in preoperative evaluation of lesions, but Yasui et al. cautioned that it can overestimate the size, and this should be a consideration when making treatment decisions.

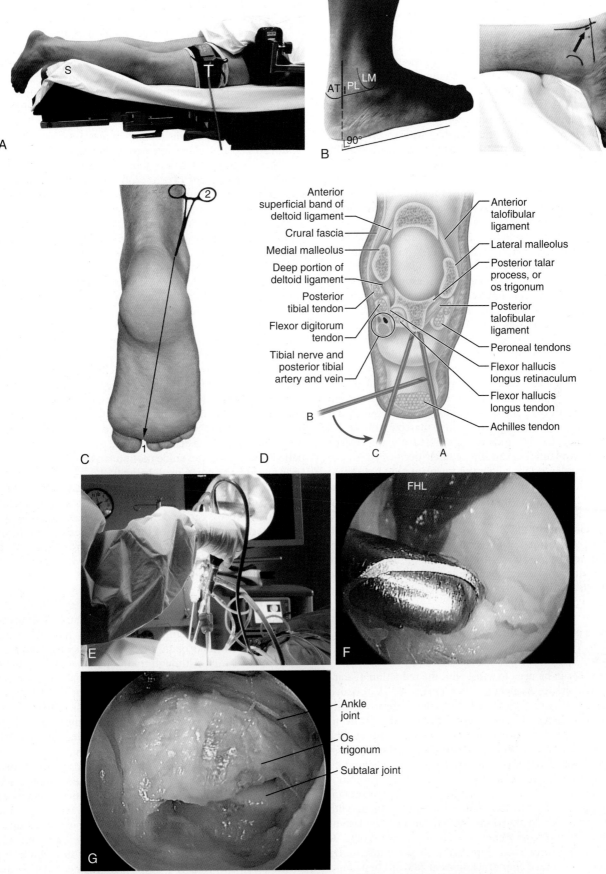

FIGURE 2.12 Posterior debridement for ankle impingement. **A,** Patient positioning. **B,** Postero-lateral portal. **C,** Insertion of hemostat aimed along line directed to first web space. **D,** Insertion of arthroscope through posteromedial portal. **E,** Insertion of arthroscopic shaver. **F,** Identification of flexor hallucis longus. **G,** Exposure of os trigonum. **SEE TECHNIQUE 2.2.**

As Ahmad et al. pointed out, treatment for small osteochondral lesions is not without problems. Reported success rates are only around 46% to 86%. Van Eekeren et al. performed a 5- to 24-year follow-up study on 93 patients who had arthroscopic debridement and bone marrow stimulation for osteochondral defects of the talus to determine how many had returned to their sport after treatment. They found that 76% had continued participating in sports; however, the activity level never returned to preinjury levels.

Curettage of osteochondral talar lesions leaves a void in cartilage that will fill with fibrocartilage if microfracture or drilling of the subchondral plate is done. However, fibrocartilage is different from normal talar hyaline articular cartilage in that it is less yielding and its wear properties are worse. To solve this problem, tissue that is more similar to hyaline articular cartilage is being used. Ahmad et al. evaluated the use of allograft cartilage extracellular matrix after arthroscopic excision and microfracture in 30 patients, finding good results and decrease in pain. DeSandis et al. used juvenile articular cartilage allograft and autologous bone marrow aspirate, reporting improved functional outcome scores; however, they noticed that reparative tissue was still composed mostly of fibrocartilage on radiographs and stated that long-term studies are necessary. D'Ambrosi et al. reported that autologous bone graft and autologous matrix-induced chondrogenesis was safe and effective to use in young patients (<20 years). They noted a significant decrease in lesion size on imaging and an increase in outcome scores. Usuelli et al. had similar results in 20 patients, and Lee et al. reported good clinical results even in the presence of a cyst. If primary bone marrow stimulation techniques fail, Georgiannos et al. pointed out that osteochondral transplantation can still be safely performed.

In larger talar lesions, allograft transplantation has shown utility in improving functional status and delaying or even avoiding the need for arthrodesis or total ankle arthroplasty. However, VanTiendcren et al. reported clinical failure in 13%, the need for reoperation in 25%, and the need for revision surgery in 9%. Guney et al. compared medium-term outcomes between mosaicplasty and arthroscopic microfracture with and without platelet-rich plasma in 54 patients. All had good results, but mosaicplasty may be preferred in patients in whom pain control is important.

A more thorough discussion of osteochondral lesions of the talus is provided in other chapter.

ANKLE FRACTURES

Arthroscopy can be used to assist with the reduction of fractures of the ankle. A meta-analysis by Lee et al. revealed that functional outcomes were better after arthroscopically assisted open reduction and internal fixation than conventional open reduction in patients with ankle fractures. The most likely reason for this is that arthroscopy allows assessment of fracture severity and treatment of concomitant intraarticular injuries, such as disruption of the syndesmosis, ligament injury, and osteochondral lesions. Concomitant injuries have been reported in up to 80% of patients with ankle fractures. Chan et al. found that osteochondral lesions were present in 26% of Weber B fractures, 24% of Weber C fractures, and 20% of isolated medial malleolar fractures. Da Cunha et al. identified chondral lesions in 78% of 116 patients with acute ankle fracture and talar dome chondral lesions in 43%. All patients with dislocations had a chondral lesion, and

patients with complete syndesmosis disruption and instability were more likely to have chondral injury. Patients younger than 30 were less likely to have a chondral injury.

Arthroscopic evaluation of the joint before fixation of an ankle fracture can detect chondral injuries and latent syndesmosis injuries. It has been found to be more sensitive than MRI and stress radiographs of the syndesmosis in detecting instability. A cadaver study showed that stress radiographs were inadequate in distinguishing between an intact ligament and a single disrupted ligament, whereas arthroscopy better demonstrated an isolated ligament disruption.

There is some controversy in the literature, however, as to whether treatment of these otherwise unknown pathologic processes can improve outcomes. In a systematic review of the English literature, Gonzalez et al. found fair-quality evidence for use of ankle arthroscopy in detecting intraarticular injuries; however, there was insufficient evidence for improvement of functional outcome, reduction in complication rates, or operative time. Fuchs et al. also found no statistically significant improvement in patients with unstable ankle fractures who had concomitant ankle arthroscopy but also found no increased complications. Average operative time was increased by only 15 minutes. There is a grade I (incomplete) recommendation for supplementing ankle fracture fixation with arthroscopy.

Primary arthroscopic reduction of talar neck fractures has been reported. Wagener et al. were able to achieve primary reduction in six of seven patients; one patient required removal of a fracture fragment through a small arthrotomy. Six of seven patients were pain free, and excellent functional outcomes were achieved in five patients. However, two patients had restricted ankle motion, and a reduction in subtalar motion was noted in all patients.

In patients with chronic syndesmosis injuries, arthroscopic debridement of the associated intraarticular pathologic process can be done without screw fixation if there is no lateral displacement of the talus. Patients with chronic widening of the syndesmosis can benefit from arthroscopic debridement and percutaneous placement of screws across the syndesmosis after reduction.

◼ TILLAUX FRACTURES

The goal of treatment in intraarticular Tillaux-Chaput fractures is to reestablish alignment and stability. Internal fixation usually is performed open when fragment displacement is greater than 2 mm. Although traditional open reduction and internal fixation obtains excellent results in most patients, it requires a large incision, places blood supply at risk, and does not define any cartilage injury. Because of the anatomy of the ankle, the alignment of fracture fragments and articular surface cannot be seen during open reduction even with C-arm radiography, which can lead to malalignment and missed injuries to cartilage. Feng et al. examined an all-inside ankle arthroscopy for treatment of this injury in 19 patients and reported excellent results in 14 and good results in five. None of the patients had decreased ankle range of motion or pain at 12 to 25 months' follow-up. To obtain comparable results, they recommended that attention be directed at (1) preserving the integrity of the anterior tibiofibular ligament, (2) preserving the periosteal fragment periosteum, (3) avoiding the epiphysis in children when inserting screws, and (4) removing all fragments or tissue. The authors recognized their nonrandomized study design and small sample size as limitations and recommended future study of this technique.

■ CALCANEAL FRACTURES

Recently, the sinus tarsi approach has been advocated in the treatment of intraarticular calcaneal fractures. Confirming adequate reduction of the posterior facet is challenging, however, because of the limited exposure due to the shape of the calcaneus. Subtalar arthroscopy has been used in extensile lateral approaches for intraarticular calcaneal fractures but not so much in the sinus tarsi approach. Park et al. evaluated whether arthroscopy combined with fluoroscopy would be more effective in restoring joint congruity than intraoperative fluoroscopy alone during a sinus tarsi approach for Sanders type 2 calcaneal fractures. They reported that this combined approach allowed better reduction of the posterior facet than fluoroscopy alone. Posterior facet reduction was graded as excellent or good in 95% of patients in the combined approach, compared with 74% in the fluoroscopy-only approach ($p < 0.04$).

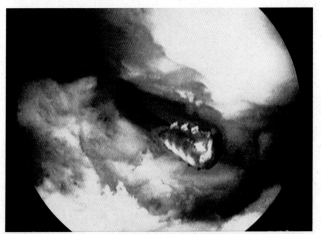

FIGURE 2.13 Ankle arthrodesis. Motorized burr used to remove thin layer of subchondral bone (≈2 mm).

ANKLE ARTHRODESIS

Arthrodesis of the ankle can be done arthroscopically, avoiding large incisions in patients with a poor soft-tissue envelope and minimal deformity. Once standard anterolateral and anteromedial portals have been established and noninvasive distraction applied, curets and shavers are used to remove articular cartilage. An arthroscopic burr is then used to abrade the subchondral bone (Fig. 2.13). Complete joint preparation can be time consuming and tedious, but care should be taken to be thorough and complete. Percutaneous 6.5-mm or 7.0-mm screws can be placed across the joint with the help of fluoroscopy (Fig. 2.14). Goetzmann et al. compared fusion rates in patients who had two or three screws for fixation. Adding a third screw seemed to lower the risk of nonunion, and time to union was shorter.

Fusion rates are similar to those with open ankle arthrodesis, and some studies have reported shorter times to fusion and less morbidity. Quayle et al. compared 29 open with 50 arthroscopic ankle arthrodeses to determine their ability to correct the deformity. Higher complication rates were noted in the open arthrodesis group (31%) compared with the arthroscopic group (8%). Also, a longer time to fusion and lower fusion rates occurred in the open ankle arthrodesis group. In another level III study, outcomes also were better in the arthroscopic arthrodesis group at 1 and 2 years, with shorter hospital stays. Results may be less optimal in patients with greater deformity, but ankle arthrodesis has been done in patients with more than 15 degrees of deformity with good results. In Quayle et al.'s study, most patients with severe deformity (>10 degrees) had correction to within 5 degrees of neutral, which was comparable to the open technique.

Although results are good from this procedure, the complication rate has been reported to be as high as 55%, although most of these complications are minor. A systematic review of the literature showed complication rates of 0% to 23.8% after arthroscopic arthrodesis, which was lower than complications after open arthrodesis (6.7% to 47.1%). Quayle et al. also reported an 8% complication rate, and Jones et al. reported no cases of

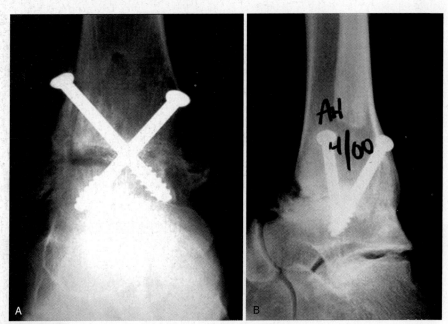

FIGURE 2.14 Fixation with two 6.5-mm cannulated screws.

deep infection or other serious problems in 120 ankles after arthroscopic arthrodesis. They too noted a good or excellent result in these patients at 86 months' follow-up. Park et al. noted higher clinical scores, less blood loss, shorter hospital stays, and fewer complications with arthroscopic arthrodesis compared with open arthrodesis, but union and reoperation rates were similar.

Vilá-Rico et al. examined arthroscopic subtalar joint arthrodesis for posttraumatic arthritis after calcaneal fractures in 37 patients. They reported a 16.2% complication rate (2.7% superficial wound infection, 5.4% symptomatic hardware, and 8.1% nonunion), but AOFAS scores improved significantly at final follow-up. They recommended arthroscopic subtalar arthrodesis because it preserves the soft-tissue envelope. Arthroscopic ankle arthrodesis has also been determined to be safe and reliable with minimal complications for patients who have advanced symptomatic talar osteonecrosis.

A grade B recommendation (fair evidence) exists for arthroscopic arthrodesis of ankles without deformity of more than 15 degrees. There is incomplete evidence for its use in ankles with greater deformity. Regardless, care should be taken in patients who smoke or who have neuromuscular problems. Jain et al. emphasized smoking cessation in patients before arthroscopic arthrodesis because union can be significantly delayed in these patients. They also suggested keeping patients with neuromuscular problems immobilized longer and using more rigid fixation to achieve better union rates.

POSTERIOR ARTHROSCOPIC SUBTALAR ARTHRODESIS

Devos Bevernage et al. performed the following arthrodesis technique in 41 subtalar joints with isolated subtalar arthritis or talocalcaneal coalition without any major hindfoot arthritis. All but two joints fused at an average of 6.7 weeks. The mean AOFAS hindfoot score improved from 49 to 81 points at latest follow-up (mean, 22 months). Two joints had nonunion and required a second procedure with bone grafting. Indications for this procedure included primary or posttraumatic arthritis, osteochondral lesions of the posterior subtalar facet, symptomatic talocalcaneal synostosis or synchondrosis, inflammatory systemic diseases, and subtalar joint arthritis. Contraindications included posterior subtalar joint bone loss, lateral wall impingement, malrotation of the talus on the calcaneus, dislocation of the Chopart joint, active septic arthritis, and problems with prone positioning. Vilá-Rico reported early results (average of 12 weeks) after arthroscopic posterior arthrodesis in 65 patients. They noted a 95.4% union rate with improvement in AOFAS scores and a 12.3% complication rate, which included superficial wound infections, nonunion, and symptomatic hardware.

TECHNIQUE 2.3

(DEVOS-BEVERNAGE ET AL.)
- Place the patient prone on a radiolucent table, making sure the ankle is straight and perpendicular to the floor. Apply a tourniquet and place a support under the foot to allow free motion of the ankle.

- Identify the lateral malleolus and lateral border of the Achilles tendon, drawing a line between the two. Make a vertical stab incision proximal to this line (Fig. 2.15A). Direct a closed mosquito clamp anteriorly toward the first and second toes to the posterior aspect of the talus. Exchange the mosquito clamp for a 4.5-mm arthroscope with a blunt trocar (open the mosquito clamp during extraction).

- Extend the line that was drawn earlier in a medial direction to cross the Achilles tendon. Create the posteromedial portal medial to the Achilles tendon at the same level as the posterolateral portal (Fig. 2.15B). Make a skin incision and insert a mosquito clamp directed toward the arthroscopic shaft. Using the shaft as a guide, travel anteriorly toward the ankle joint until it reaches bone. This avoids the neurovascular bundle. Exchange the trocar for a 4.0-mm 30-degree arthroscope. Exchange the mosquito clamp for a 5-mm full-radius shaver.

- With the shaver, remove tissue and part of the posterior joint capsule, looking for landmarks while moving from the posterolateral part of the subtalar joint toward the medially located flexor hallucis longus tendon. Remove the subtalar joint capsule to view the posterior compartment of the subtalar joint and identify the posterior tibiofibular and talofibular ligaments. The posterior talofibular ligament can be removed for better visualization. Remove the os trigonum and osseous avulsions and reduce the posterolateral process as indicated. Release the flexor hallucis longus tendon through its retinaculum (Fig. 2.15C).

- If a total synovectomy or capsulectomy of the posterior subtalar joint is performed, retain the intermalleolar ligament and the fibers of the posterior tibiofibular ligament to avoid debris entering the tibiotalar joint during debridement.

- Debride the subtalar articular surface with curets and full-radius 5-mm shaver to subchondral bleeding bone and perform microfracturing of the subchondral bone, using the interosseous talocalcaneal ligament in the sinus tarsi as the end point (Fig. 2.15D). To debride the anteromedial aspect of the posterior subtalar facet articular surface, an additional anterolateral portal in front of the lateral malleolus may be necessary. The middle and anterior subtalar articular surfaces are not approached. Devos-Bevernage et al. removed as much as possible of the middle facet. No invasive traction is necessary.

- If bone graft is to be used, apply it at this point and slightly impact the graft. Obtain subtalar joint fixation with two cannulated screws with the aid of fluoroscopy as follows: make an incision in the center of the heel (Fig. 2.15E). Position Kirschner wires from the posterior calcaneal tuberosity to the talar body and check mobility of the tibiotalar joint. Once positioned, close the skin to maintain reaming materials before drilling the screws. Check the screw positions fluoroscopically (Fig. 2.15F).

POSTOPERATIVE CARE Apply a short leg posterior splint to be worn for 10 days. At 2 weeks a non–weight-bearing cast is applied and worn for 4 weeks, after which time a removable boot is used for night and while walking. Flexion and extension exercises should be performed regularly, but rotatory movement is discouraged. Patients are allowed to bear weight after 8 weeks as tolerated.

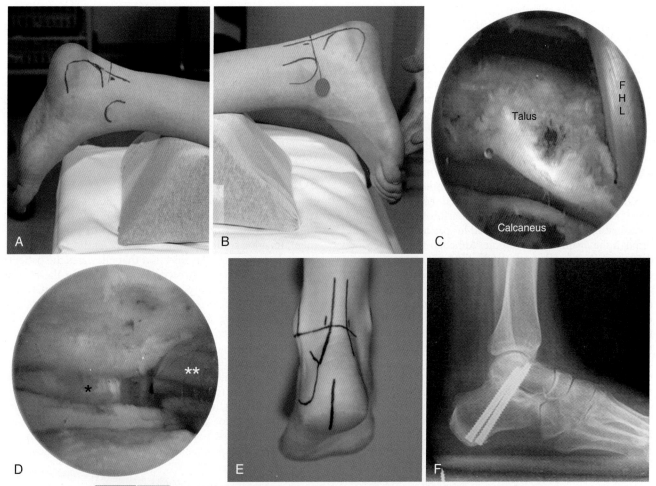

FIGURE 2.15   **A,** Mark tip of lateral malleolus and lateral border of Achilles tendon. While holding ankle in neutral, draw a line between these two landmarks. Make incision on lateral border of Achilles tendon, proximal to line. Orange oval indicates location of anterolateral portal. **B,** Postero-medial portal made medial to Achilles tendon at same level as posterolateral portal. **C,** Tibiotalar and subtalar joints after removal of fatty tissue, part of posterior joint capsule, intermalleolar ligament, and posterolateral tubercle of talus (*FHL*, flexor hallucis longus). **D,** Debridement of posterior subtalar facet performed from posterior to anterior until interosseous talocalcaneal ligament is reached (*black asterisk,* interosseous talocalcaneal ligament; *two white asterisks,* full-radius shaver). **E,** Incision made in center of heel to allow placement of cannulated screws from posterior tuberosity of calcaneus to talar body. **F,** Subtalar joint arthrodesis with cannulated stabilization screws placed from posterior tuberosity of calcaneus to talar body.   (From Devos Bevernage B, Goubau L, Deleu PA, et al. Posterior arthroscopic subtalar arthrodesis, *JBJS Essential Surg Tech* 5[4]:e27, 2015.) **SEE TECHNIQUE 2.3.**

ANKLE INSTABILITY

Since concomitant intraarticular pathologic processes are often associated with chronic ankle instability, arthroscopy is recommended before open lateral ankle ligament surgery. Arthroscopic-assisted procedures for lateral ligament repair have been described. There is ongoing debate about whether arthroscopy should be routinely performed with lateral ligament reconstruction. Yasui et al. investigated reoperation rates and complications after ankle ligament reconstruction, with and without arthroscopic procedures, in 16,069 patients. Ankle arthroscopy did not decrease the rate of reoperations required; however, there was a lower rate of ankle arthrodesis as a second procedure and lower complications in the patients who had arthroscopy. Based on their findings they recommended ankle arthroscopy for lateral ligament reconstruction.

Lopes et al. reported 286 patients undergoing arthroscopic ligament repair or reconstruction for chronic ankle instability. They noted significant improvements in AOFAS and Karlsson scores at a mean 10-month follow-up (range, 6 to 43 months) in both. Neurologic complications occurred in 10% of patients (transient dysesthesia and neuroma), and cutaneous complications and infection in 4.2% that required surgical revision. The rate of cutaneous complications, however, was at least half that of open surgery. Although arthroscopic techniques appear reliable, the authors recommended further study to determine long-term outcomes.

Li et al. compared arthroscopic repair with open repair of the talofibular ligament in 60 patients. No significant differences were found between the two in AOFAS score, Karlsson Ankle Functional Score, and the Tegner activity score. They noted that arthroscopic anterior talofibular ligament repair provided favorable outcomes at rates similar to open repair. Two systematic reviews (Brown et al. and Guelfi et al.) and one study of 119 patients (Araoye et al.) showed complication rates to be between 11.5% and 18%. Although short-term outcomes were favorable, long-term data showing an advantage of arthroscopic technique over an open procedure were lacking. Two-stage arthroscopy was associated with significantly higher complication rates compared with single-stage arthroscopy, and higher complications were noted with suture anchor fixation (29%) compared with suture fixation (9%; Araoye et al.). The complication rate of arthroscopic ligament repair or reconstruction is a concern; however, it did not seem to affect patient satisfaction in some studies.

Techniques for ligament repair are discussed in other chapter. Suture anchors are placed into the fibula arthroscopically, and an accessory anterolateral portal is used for passage of the sutures through the ligament and capsule. Although these procedures only correct laxity of the anterior tibiofibular ligament, good outcomes have been reported with their use. All-inside arthroscopic techniques have been described as well for the Broström procedure and lateral ligament reconstruction with gracilis autograft. A cadaver study showed no difference in the strength of the repair with open or arthroscopic Broström techniques. In a systematic review of level IV studies, all patients had subjective improvement of instability with arthroscopic Broström techniques, but there was a 17% complication rate. Entrapment of the peroneus tertius, extensor tendons, and the superficial peroneal nerve can occur when tying sutures for the anterior talofibular ligament. Yeo et al. compared an open modified Broström procedure with an all-inside arthroscopic modified Broström in 48 patients to determine best clinical and radiographic outcomes. The AOFAS ankle-hindfoot score, visual analog scale, and Karlsson score were used to determine clinical outcomes at 6 weeks, 6 months, and 12 months postoperatively. Anterior talar translation and talar tilt were used to determine radiographic outcomes at 1 year postoperatively. No significant differences were noted between outcome scores, anterior talar translation, or talar tilt between the two groups. These authors emphasized that an all-inside arthroscopic modified Broström technique can be safely done in patients with lateral ankle instability. Yeo et al. later evaluated if generalized ligamentous laxity affected the results of an arthroscopic modified Broström procedure; they found it to be successful regardless of whether generalized ligamentous laxity was present. A study by Rigby and Cottom of 62 patients showed similar findings. The authors noted the added advantage of earlier weight bearing in arthroscopically treated patients.

Anterolateral impingement is a less frequent finding in chronic lateral ankle instability. It can present with synovitis and fibrosis; 12% of patients with chronic ankle instability have anterior bony impingement.

Thermal capsular shrinkage has been suggested to be helpful for ankle instability; however, there is sparse evidence in the orthopaedic literature that supports this intervention, leading to a grade C recommendation (poor evidence) for this procedure.

OTHER INDICATIONS
■ SEPTIC ARTHRITIS

There is sparse literature regarding the use of arthroscopy for treatment of septic arthritis of the ankle. In one series of 78 infected joints that included five ankles, there was a 91% cure rate. In another series of 89 infected joints, three

of which were ankles, there were 61% good/excellent, 20% satisfactory, and 19% poor functional outcomes. There is a grade C (poor evidence) for the use of arthroscopy for this indication.

■ ARTHROFIBROSIS

There are only small series (level IV studies) on the use of arthroscopy to treat arthrofibrosis of the ankle, most of which report promising results. There is, however, only a grade C recommendation (poor evidence) for the use of ankle arthroscopy in the treatment of arthrofibrosis.

SUBTALAR ARTHROSCOPY

Patients with sinus tarsi syndrome or subtalar synovitis localize their pain to the lateral hindfoot and have tenderness at the subtalar joint on examination. As with ankle impingement, imaging studies may be negative and the diagnosis can be made with a subtalar injection that alleviates the patient's symptoms. Subtalar arthroscopy, when done for therapeutic and not diagnostic purposes, has good or excellent results in 86% to 94% of patients, and 97% of patients are satisfied with the procedure. Arthroscopic debridement can be helpful for symptoms after calcaneal fractures, with 80% of patients experiencing considerable relief of pain and 82% satisfied with their outcomes. Subtalar arthroscopy can be used in conjunction with fluoroscopy for percutaneous reduction and fixation of calcaneal fractures. Arthrodesis of the subtalar joint can be performed through a lateral or posterior approach or a combined posterior and lateral approach. Complications are rare, and most commonly are neurologic complications that resolve over time, similar to those after ankle arthroscopy.

SUBTALAR ARTHROSCOPY

TECHNIQUE 2.4

- The setup for subtalar arthroscopy is similar to that for ankle arthroscopy, with the operative extremity placed in a leg holder, the hip and knee flexed, and the foot hanging free. Alternatively, the patient can be placed in the lateral decubitus position with the foot hanging off a bump.
- After insufflation of the joint, establish the central portal and then the anterolateral portal by direct visualization using a spinal needle (Fig. 2.16).
- Often, visualization of the joint is difficult when the arthroscope first enters the joint because of the synovitis that fills the sinus tarsi (Fig. 2.17A). After triangulation to place portals, continue debridement until the joint can be visualized.
- Debride the anterior aspect of the posterior facet, including the often attenuated interosseous talocalcaneal ligament (Fig. 2.17B).
- Rotate the instruments to the lateral aspect of the posterior facet, where debridement of synovitis often is necessary (Fig. 2.18). Switch portals as needed for better access. Occasionally, a posterolateral portal is necessary for posterior access.

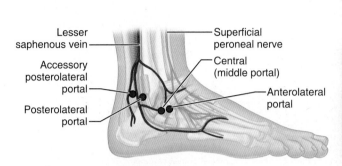

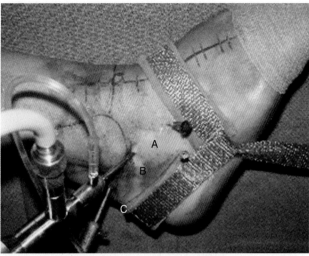

FIGURE 2.16 Subtalar portals must be made carefully to avoid neurovascular injury. *A,* Antero-lateral portal. *B,* Central portal. *C,* Posterolateral portal. **SEE TECHNIQUE 2.4.**

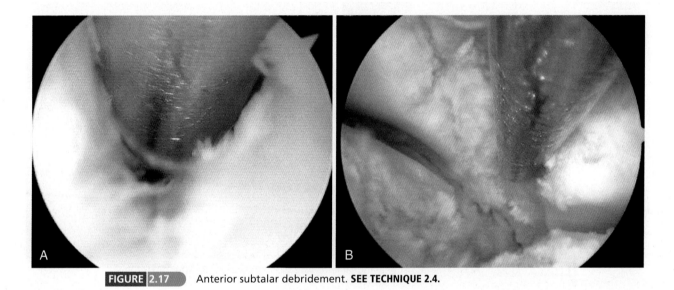

FIGURE 2.17 Anterior subtalar debridement. **SEE TECHNIQUE 2.4.**

- The subtalar joint can also be approached through posterior portals, similar to that described for posterior ankle arthroscopy.

POSTOPERATIVE CARE Postoperative care is similar to that after ankle arthroscopy.

FIRST METATARSOPHALANGEAL JOINT ARTHROSCOPY

First metatarsophalangeal joint arthroscopy can be used to treat osteochondral lesions of the first metatarsal head (Fig. 2.19), early osteophytosis, chondromalacia, loose bodies, arthrofibrosis, synovitis, and gouty arthritis. Arthroscopic or arthroscopic-assisted techniques have been described for first metatarsophalangeal joint arthrodesis, with a soft-tissue release for hallux valgus before a distal first metatarsal osteotomy. Significant improvement in pain and AOFAS hindfoot scores have also been reported in a

small group of patients with hallux rigidus and early focal osteochondral lesions of the first metatarsophalangeal joint after arthroscopic microdrilling procedures (Kuyucu et al.).

A recent cadaver study evaluated the ability of arthroscopy to visualize the articular surface of the metatarsophalangeal joint and found that a complete view of the proximal phalangeal base was achievable. Only 49% to 65% of the metatarsal head could be seen, but the authors stressed that this may have been due to their technique.

FIRST METATARSOPHALANGEAL JOINT ARTHROSCOPY

TECHNIQUE 2.5

- Place the patient supine and place a finger trap on the hallux for distraction; suspend the foot from a tower such as those used for wrist arthroscopy (Fig. 2.20A).

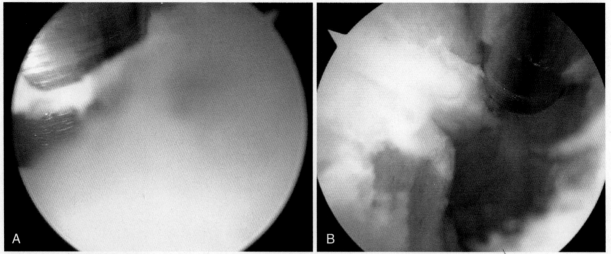

FIGURE 2.18   **A,** Synovitis in lateral aspect of posterior facet. **B,** After debridement. **SEE TECH-NIQUE 2.4.**

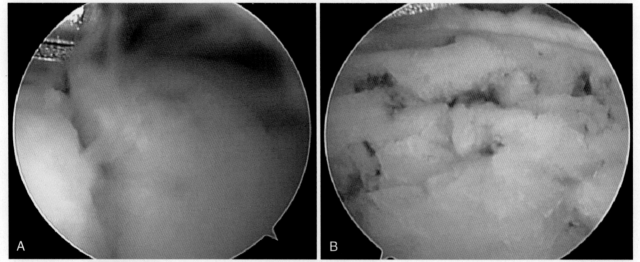

FIGURE 2.19   **A,** First metatarsophalangeal joint osteochondral lesion. **B,** After debridement and microfracture.

- Make portals on either side of the extensor hallucis longus tendon at the level of the joint (Fig. 2.20B).
- Use a 1.9-mm arthroscope and 2.0-mm shavers as needed.

Lesser metatarsophalangeal joint arthroscopy also has been described for synovectomy, arthroscopic-assisted plantar plate tenodesis, and interpositional arthroplasty for Freiberg infraction. A cadaver study confirmed the accuracy of arthroscopic evaluation of lesser metatarsophalangeal joints.

TENDOSCOPY/ENDOSCOPY OF TENDONS

Tendoscopy of the peroneal tendons (Fig. 2.21) and posterior tibial tendons (Fig. 2.22) has been described and can be used for tenosynovectomy for tendinitis and groove deepening for peroneal dislocation. Posterior tibial tendoscopy also can be performed through a posterior approach. According to a systematic review, there was weak evidence (grade C) for use of tendoscopy of the Achilles tendon, flexor hallucis longus, and peroneal tendons, and insufficient evidence to support tendoscopy of the posterior tibial tendon, anterior tibial tendon, flexor digitorum longus, extensor hallucis longus, and extensor digitorum longus. However, more recent studies are demonstrating good outcomes. In an evidence-based update, Bernasconi et al. noted efficacy of tendoscopy in the treatment of chronic and acute tendon disorders in the ankle. Recently, Urguden et al. found tendoscopy useful in the diagnosis and treatment of peroneal tendon pathologies, with improvement in AOFAS scores seen at 2 years postoperatively in 20 ankles. Another study of 16 patients (level of evidence IV) showed improved pain and SF-36 scores at 26 months after tendoscopy treatment of stage II posterior tibial tendon dysfunction.

Tendoscopic calcaneoplasty with debridement of the retrocalcaneal space has good to excellent results in 80% to 100% of patients. There have also been reports of tendoscopy to treat unicameral bone cysts of the calcaneus, talar cysts, calcaneofibular impingement after calcaneal fractures, and tarsal coalitions. These procedures can be helpful for conditions around the Achilles tendon as well (Fig. 2.23). Opdam et al. reported good functional outcomes of endoscopic release of the paratendon and transection of the plantaris tendon in 45 patients with mid-portion Achilles tendinopathy. One recurrence was noted in their study.

In the diagnosis of tendon disorders, tendoscopy may be a more sensitive diagnostic tool than MRI. Kennedy et al. found good correlation between tendoscopic findings and preoperative MRI findings in patients with peroneal tendon pathology, which supports the use of MRI when a peroneal tendon disorder is suspected. However, Gianakos et al. found MRI to be in agreement with tendoscopy findings in only eight of 12 patients.

In patients with gastrocnemius equinus deformity, endoscopic gastrocnemius recession is an effective procedure. It can be done open or endoscopically, although both procedures

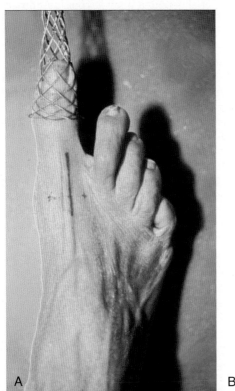
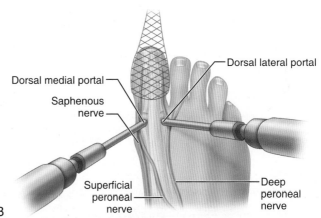

FIGURE 2.20 **A,** Distraction of first metatarsophalangeal joint with sterile finger trap. **B,** Placement of dorsal medial and dorsal lateral portals. **SEE TECHNIQUE 2.5.**

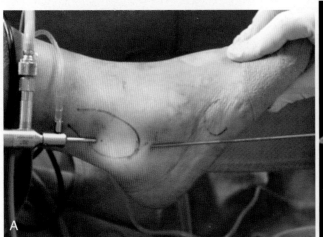
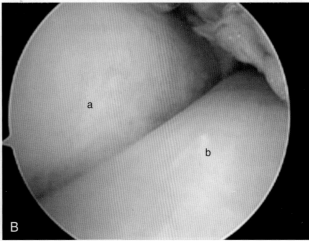

FIGURE 2.21 Peroneal tendoscopy. **A,** Portal placement approximately 4 cm apart. **B,** Peroneal brevis tendon (*a*) medial and deep to peroneus longus tendon (*b*) as seen from portal proximal to fibula. (From Ferkel RD, Hommen JP: Arthroscopy of the ankle and foot. In Coughlin MJ, Mann RA, Saltzman CL, editors: *Surgery of the foot and ankle*, ed 8, Philadelphia, 2007, Elsevier.)

have associated complications. Harris et al. assessed complications and compared endoscopic with open gastrocnemius recession in 74 patients (80 procedures: 41 open and 39 endoscopic). Overall postoperative complications occurred in 12 of the 80 procedures (10 in the open group and one in the tendoscopic group). The 10 complications in the open group included scar pain, dehiscence, infection, calf abscess, and nerve injury. In the tendoscopic technique one dehiscence was noted.

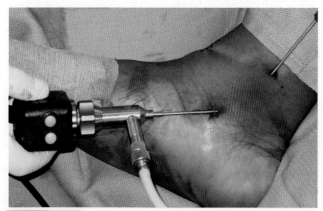

FIGURE 2.22 Tendoscopy of posterior tibial tendon. Arthroscope is in distal portal, and shaver is in proximal portal in right ankle. (From Ferkel RD, Hommen JP: Arthroscopy of the ankle and foot. In Coughlin MJ, Mann RA, Saltzman CL, editors: *Surgery of the foot and ankle*, ed 8, Philadelphia, 2007, Elsevier.)

TENDOSCOPIC RECESSION OF THE GASTROCNEMIUS TENDON

Phisitkul et al. reported a tendoscopic gastrocnemius tendon recession technique, and in a separate prospective study of 320 patients found improvement in ankle dorsiflexion, pain, and validated outcome scores at 1-year follow-up. Active infection over the area or an earlier open gastrocnemius recession at the same level are contraindications to this technique. Both open and tendoscopic techniques are contraindicated in competitive athletes who require maximal push-off strength because ankle plantarflexion weakness can be expected after this technique. Potential complications with the tendoscopic technique include intraoperative bleeding, incomplete release of the tendon, and sural nerve neuralgia. In patients with a severe contracture, the ankle may not achieve 15 degrees of dorsiflexion even with complete release, and percutaneous lengthening may be required after the gastrocnemius release.

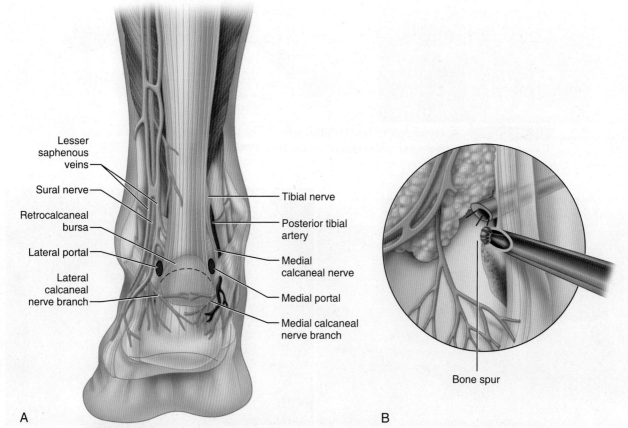

A

B

FIGURE 2.23 **A,** Achilles tendoscopy portals. **B,** Excision of Haglund deformity with scope through medial portal and burr laterally. (From Ferkel RD, Hommen JP: Arthroscopy of the ankle and foot. In Coughlin MJ, Mann RA, Saltzman CL, editors: *Surgery of the foot and ankle*, ed 8, Philadelphia, 2007, Elsevier.)

TECHNIQUE 2.6

- Position the patient supine or prone, depending on additional procedures required, and apply a thigh tourniquet. A standard 4-mm arthroscope is used without fluid irrigation. Keep the ankle slightly dorsiflexed by leaning against the sole of the foot.
- Create a portal on the medial aspect of the calf, 2 cm distal to the distal aspect of the gastrocnemius muscle belly. This should be anterior to the medial edge of the gastrocnemius tendon. Puncture the crural fascia and dilate it with a hemostat (Fig. 2.24A).

- Introduce a clear cannula and trocar from the medial portal and pass it deep to the crural fascia but superficial to the gastrocnemius tendon (Fig. 2.24B). Palpate the medial border of the gastrocnemius tendon with the trocar tip. The correct plane lies beneath the skin and subcutaneous tissue. The cannula should be palpable.
- Advance the trocar laterally, relaxing the ankle in plantarflexion for less resistance. When the plane is correct, the trocar can easily be swiveled sideways. The sural nerve, dorsal to the cannula, may be palpable in some patients.

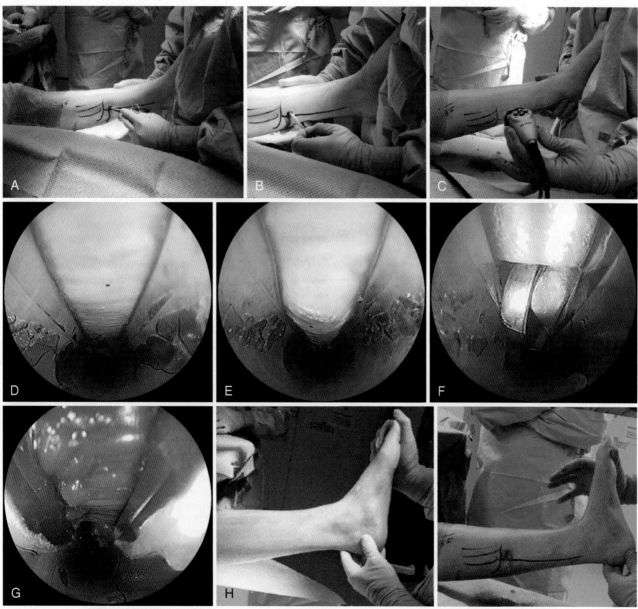

FIGURE 2.24 **A,** Hemostat used to dilate crural fascia from medial portal. **B,** Clear cannula and trocar introduced while ankle held in dorsiflexion. **C,** A 30-degree 4-mm arthroscopic introduced from medial portal. **D,** Cannula inserted dorsal to crural fascia. **E,** Plane finder used to dissect between gastrocnemius tendon and crural fascia. **F,** Release of gastrocnemius tendon from midline laterally. **G,** Soleus muscle shown from lateral portal after completion of gastrocnemius recession. **H,** Ankle dorsiflexion improved to 15 degrees from 5 degrees of equinus preoperatively. (From Phisitkul P, Barg A, Amendola A: Endoscopic recession of gastrocnemius tendon, *Foot Ankle Int* 38:4567, 2017.) **SEE TECHNIQUE 2.6.**

- Create a lateral portal with an inside-out technique. Pass the cannula into the lateral portal. Keeping the open slot directed anteriorly, remove the trocar and clean the cannula.
- Insert a 4-mm 30-degree arthroscope (Fig. 2.24C) for direct visualization of the gastrocnemius tendon and its fibers. If the cannula is positioned too anteriorly into the soleus muscle, withdraw it until its tip is correctly placed. Advance the cannula through the lateral portal. Take care that it is not dorsal to the crural fascia (Fig. 2.24D) because this will risk injury to the lesser saphenous vein and sural nerve. If the cannula is dorsal to the crural fascia, introduce a plane finder into the lateral portal and use the beveled tip to puncture the crural fascia laterally. Then under direct visualization, advance the plane finder between the gastrocnemius tendon and the crural fascia (Fig. 2.24E). The plane finder is then used as a switching-stick for reinserting the cannula from the medial portal into the correct plane.
- Hold the ankle in dorsiflexion. With a retrograde knife inserted through the lateral portal, release the gastrocnemius tendon from its midline to its lateral border (Fig. 2.24F). For a partial release, leave 1 to 2 cm of the tendon intact.
- Switch the arthroscope to the lateral portal and insert the retrograde knife through the medial portal. Release the gastrocnemius tendon from the midline toward the medial edge (Fig. 2.24G). Move the ankle into 15 degrees of dorsiflexion (Fig. 2.24H). For additional anterior reach, a curved knife may be used. Close the portals with sutures or Steri-Strips.

POSTOPERATIVE CARE After gastrocnemius tendon release without additional procedures, the ankle is immobilized in a boot day and night, but patients may start bearing weight immediately after surgery. Gentle ankle motion out of the boot should be performed several times a day. Sutures are removed at 2 weeks, and the patient is encouraged to ambulate in the boot and to wear a splint at night. At 4 to 6 weeks, patients may wean from the boot, and a compressive stocking can be used to control swelling. Ankle strengthening exercises are begun at 6 weeks for 12 weeks. If additional procedures were performed, postoperative care must take these into account.

REFERENCES

ANKLE ARTHROSCOPY
General
Abdelatif NMN: Combined arthroscopic management of concurrent posterior and anterior ankle pathologies, *Knee Surg Sports Traumatol Arthrosc* 22:2837, 2014.

Akoh CC, Dibbern K, Amendola A, et al.: Effect of ankle position and noninvasive distraction on arthroscopic accessibility of the distal tibial plafond, *Foot Ankle Int* 38(10):1152, 2017.

Allegra F, Maffulli N: Double posteromedial portals for posterior ankle arthroscopy, *Clin Orthop Relat Res* 468:996, 2010.

Amendola N: Not using a tourniquet during anterior ankle arthroscopy did not affect postoperative intraarticular bleeding or function at six months, *J Bone Joint Surg Am* 100(4):344, 2018.

Aurich M, Bedi HS, Smith PJ, et al.: Arthroscopic treatment of osteochondral lesions of the ankle with matrix-associated chondrocyte implantation: early clinical and magnetic resonance imaging results, *Am J Sports Med* 39:311, 2011.

Barg A, Saltzman CL, Beals TC, et al.: Arthroscopic talar dome access using a standard versus wire-based traction method for ankle joint distraction, *Arthroscopy* 32(7):1367, 2016.

Darland AM, Kadakia AR, Zeller JL: Branching patterns of the superficial peroneal nerve: implications for ankle arthroscopy and for anterolateral surgical approaches to the ankle, *J Foot Ankle Surg* 54(3):332, 2015.

Dimnjaković D, Hrabač P, Bojanić I: Value of tourniquet use in anterior ankle arthroscopy: a randomized controlled trial, *Foot Ankle Int* 38(7):716, 2017.

Epstein DM, Black BS, Sherman SL: Anterior ankle arthroscopy: indications, pitfalls, and complications, *Foot Ankle Clin* 20:41, 2015.

Glazebrook MA, Ganapathy V, Bridge MA, et al.: Evidence-based indications for ankle arthroscopy, *Arthroscopy* 25:1478, 2009.

Grishko V, Xu M, Wilson G, Pearsall AW 4th: Apoptosis and mitochondrial dysfunction in human chondrocytes following exposure to lidocaine, bupivacaine, and ropivacaine, *J Bone Joint Surg* 92A:609, 2010.

Hampton CB, Shawen SB, Keeling JJ: Technique for combined anterior, lateral, and posterior ankle procedures: technique tip, *Foot Ankle Int* 31:348, 2010.

Harnroongroj T, Chuckpaiwong B: Is the arthroscopic transillumination test effective in localizing the superficial peroneal nerve? *Arthroscopy* 33(3):647, 2017.

Hirtler L, Schuh R: Accessibility of the talar dome-anatomic comparison of plantarflexion versus noninvasive distraction in arthroscopy, *Arthroscopy* 34(2):573, 2018.

Jacobs TF, Vansintjan PS, Roels N, et al.: The effect of lidocaine on the viability of cultivated mature human cartilage cells: an in vitro study, *Knee Surg Sports Traumatol Arthrosc* 19:1206, 2011.

Kim HN, Park YJ, Lee SY, Park YW: Ankle arthroscopy in prone position with ankle suspended: technique tip, *Foot Ankle Int* 33:1027, 2012.

Kim YS, Young HK, Kim BS, et al.: Arthroscopic evaluation of persistent pain following osteotomy for varus ankle osteoarthritis, *Knee Surg Sports Traumatol Arthrosc* 24:1860, 2016.

Liszka H, Gądek A: Preemptive local anesthesia in ankle arthroscopy, *Foot Ankle Int* 37(12):1326, 2016.

Lui TH: Ankle arthroscopy with patient in prone position, *Arch Orthop Trauma Surg* 128:1283, 2008.

Lui TH, Chan WK, Chan KB: The arthroscopic management of frozen ankle, *Arthroscopy* 22:283, 2006.

Lui TH, Tse LF: Peroneal tendoscopy, *Foot Ankle Clin* 20(1):15, 2015.

Lui TH, Yuen CP: Small joint arthroscopy in foot and ankle, *Foot Ankle Clin* 20(1):123, 2014.

Muñoz G, Eckholt S: Subtalar arthroscopy: indications, technique, and results, *Foot Ankle Clin* 20(1):93, 2015.

Osti L, Del Buono A, Maffulli N: Arthroscopic debridement of the ankle for mild to moderate osteoarthritis: a midterm follow-up study in former professional soccer players, *J Orthop Surg Res* 11:37, 2016.

Piper SL, Kramer JD, Kim HT, Feeley BT: Effects of local anesthetics on articular cartilage, *Am J Sports Med* 39:2245, 2011.

Sittapairoj T, Anthony CA, Rungprai C, et al.: *Brake reaction time after ankle and subtalar arthroscopy* 33(12):2231, 2017.

Tonogai I, Hayashi F, Tsuruo Y, Sairyo K: Comparison of ankle joint visualization between the 70° and 30° arthroscopes: a cadaveric study, *Foot Ankle Spec* 11(1):72, 2018.

Vega J, Dalmau-Pastor M, Malagelada F, et al.: Ankle arthroscopy an update, *J Bone Joint Surg Am* 99(16):1395, 2017.

Werner BC, Burrus T, Park JS, et al.: Trends in ankle arthroscopy and its use in the management of pathologic conditions of the ankle in the United States: a national database study, *Arthroscopy* 31:1330, 2015.

Zhang K, Jiang Y, Du J, et al.: Comparison of distraction arthroplasty alone versus combined with arthroscopic microfracture in treatment of post-traumatic ankle arthritis, *J Orthop Surg Res* 12(1):45, 2017.

ANATOMY

Darland AM, Kadakia AR, Zeller ML: Branching patterns of the superficial peroneal nerve: implications for ankle arthroscopy and for anterolateral surgical approaches to the ankle, *J Foot Ankle Surg* 54:332, 2015.

de Leeuw PA, Golanó P, Blankevoort L, et al.: Identification of the superficial peroneal nerve: anatomical study with surgical implications, *Knee Surg Sports Traumatol Arthrosc* 24:1381, 2016.

de Leeuw PA, Golanó P, Clavero JA, van Dijk CN: Anterior ankle arthroscopy, distraction or dorsiflexion? *Knee Surg Sports Traumatol Arthrosc* 18:594, 2010.

de Leeuw PAJ, Golanó P, Sierevelt IN, van Dijk CN: The course of the superficial peroneal nerve in relation to the ankle position: anatomical study with ankle arthroscopic implications, *Knee Surg Sports Traumatol Arthrosc* 18:612, 2010.

Drakos M, Behrens SB, Mulcahey MK, et al.: Proximity of arthroscopic ankle stabilization procedures to surrounding structures: an anatomic study, *Arthroscopy* 29:1089, 2013.

Son KH, Cho JH, Lee JW, et al.: Is the anterior tibial artery safe during ankle arthroscopy? Anatomic analysis of the anterior tibial artery at the ankle joint by magnetic resonance imaging, *Am J Sports Med* 39:2452, 2011.

Urguden M, Cevikol C, Dabak K, et al.: Effect of joint motion on safety of portals in posterior ankle arthroscopy, *Arthroscopy* 25:1442, 2009.

COMPLICATIONS

Aim F, Delambre J, Bauer T, Hardy P: Efficacy of arthroscopic treatment for resolving infection in septic arthritis of native joints, *Orthop Traumatol Surg Res* 101(1):61, 2015.

Blázquez Martín T, Iglesias Durán E, San Miguel Campos M: Complications after ankle and hindfoot arthroscopy, *Rev Esp Cir Orthop Traumatol* 60(6):387, 2016.

Deng DE, Hamilton GA, Lee M, et al.: Complications associated with foot and ankle arthroscopy, *J Foot Ankle Surg* 51:281, 2012.

Huntley SR, Abyar E, Lehtonen EJ, et al.: Incidence of and risk factors for venous thromboembolism after foot and ankle surgery, *Foot Ankle Spec*, 2018, [Epub ahead of print].

Imade S, Takao M, Miyamoto W, et al.: Leg anterior compartment syndrome following ankle arthroscopy after Maisonneuve fracture, *Arthroscopy* 25:215, 2009.

Jang EC, Kwak BK, Song KS, et al.: Pseudoaneurysm of the anterior tibial artery after ankle arthroscopy treated with ultrasound-guided compression therapy, *J Bone Joint Surg* 90A: 2235, 2008.

Kashir A, Kiely P, Dar W, D'Souza L: Pseudoaneurysm of the dorsalis pedis artery after ankle arthroscopy, *Foot Ankle Surg* 16:151, 2010.

Nickisch F, Barg A, Saltzman CL, et al.: Postoperative complications of posterior ankle and hindfoot arthroscopy, *J Bone Joint Surg* 94A:439, 2012.

Vega J, Golanó P, Peña F: Iatrogenic articular cartilage injuries during ankle arthroscopy, *Knee Surg Sports Traumatol Arthrosc* 24:1304, 2016.

Werner BC, Cancienne JM, Burrus MT, et al.: Risk of infection after intra-articular steroid injection at the time of ankle arthroscopy in a Medicare population, *Arthroscopy* 32(2):350, 2016.

Yammine K, Kheir N, Daher J, et al.: Pseudoaneurysm following ankle arthroscopy: a systematic review of case series, *Eur J Orthop Surg Traumatol*, 2018, [Epub ahead of print].

Young BH, Flanigan RM, DiGiovanni BF: Complications of ankle arthroscopy utilizing a contemporary noninvasive distraction technique, *J Bone Joint Surg* 93:963, 2011.

Zengerink M, van Dijk CN: Complications in ankle arthroscopy, *Knee Surg Sports Traumatol Arthrosc* 20:1420, 2012.

IMPINGEMENT

Baums MH, Kahl E, Schultz W, Klinger HM: Clinical outcome of the arthroscopic management of sports-related "anterior ankle pain": a prospective study, *Knee Surg Sports Traumatol Arthrosc* 14:482, 2006.

Buda R, Baldassarri M, Parma A, et al.: Arthroscopic treatment and prognostic classification of anterior soft tissue impingement of the ankle, *Foot Ankle Int* 37(1):33, 2016.

Calder JD, Sexton SA, Pearce CJ: Return to training and playing after posterior ankle arthroscopy for posterior impingement in elite professional soccer, *Am J Sports Med* 38:120, 2010.

Carreira DS, Vora AM, Hearne KL, Kozy J: Outcome of arthroscopic treatment of posterior impingement of the ankle, *Foot Ankle Int* 37:394, 2016.

Choi WJ, Lee JW, Han SH, et al.: Chronic lateral ankle instability: the effect of intra-articular lesions on clinical outcome, *Am J Sports Med* 36:2167, 2008.

Dinato MC, Luques IU, Freitas Mde F, et al.: Endoscopic treatment of the posterior ankle impingement syndrome on amateur and professional athletes, *Knee Surg Sports Traumatol Arthrosc* 24(4):1396, 2016.

Ferkel RD, Tyorkin M, Applegate GR, Heinen GT: MRI evaluation of anterolateral soft tissue impingement of the ankle, *Foot Ankle Int* 31:654, 2010.

Galla M, Lobenhoffer P: Technique and results of arthroscopic treatment of posterior ankle impingement, *Foot Ankle Surg* 17:79, 2011.

Georgiannos D, Bisbinas I: Endoscopic versus open excision of os trigonum for the treatment of posterior ankle impingement syndrome in an athletic population: a randomized controlled study with 5-year follow-up, *Am J Sports Med* 45(6):1388, 2017.

López Valerio V, Seijas R, Alvarez P, et al.: Endoscopic repair of posterior ankle impingement syndrome due to os trigonum in soccer players, *Foot Ankle Int* 36(1):70, 2015.

Mardani-Kivi M, Mirbolook A, Khajeh-Jahromi S, et al.: Arthroscopic treatment of patients with anterolateral impingement of the ankle with and without chondral lesions, *J Foot Ankle Surg* 52:188, 2013.

McCrum CL, Arner JW, Lesniak B, Bradley JP: Arthroscopic anterior ankle decompression is successful in National Football League Players, *Am J Orthop (Belle Mead NJ)* 47(1), 2018, https://doi.org/10.12788/ajo.2018.0001.

Miyamoto W, Takao M, Matsui K, Matsushita T: Simultaneous ankle arthroscopy and hindfoot endoscopy for combined anterior and posterior ankle impingement syndrome in professional athletes, *J Orthop Sci* 20:642, 2015.

Miyamoto W, Takao M, Matsushita T: Hindfoot endoscopy for posterior ankle impingement syndrome and flexor hallucis longus tendon transfers, *Foot Ankle Clin* 20(1):139, 2015.

Morelli F, Mazza D, Serlorenzi P, et al.: Endoscopic excision of symptomatic os trigonum in professional dancers, *J Foot Ankle Surg* 56(1):22, 2017.

Murawski CD, Kennedy JG: Anteromedial impingement in the ankle joint: outcomes following arthroscopy, *Am J Sports Med* 38:2010, 2017.

Noguchi H, Ishii Y, Takeda M, et al.: Arthroscopic excision of posterior ankle bony impingement for early return to the field: short-term results, *Foot Ankle Int* 31:398, 2010.

Parma A, Buda R, Vannini F, et al.: Arthroscopic treatment of ankle anterior bony impingement: the long-term clinical outcome, *Foot Ankle Int* 35:148, 2014.

Smyth NA, Murawski CD, Levine DS, Kennedy JG: Hindfoot arthroscopic surgery for posterior ankle impingement: a systematic surgical approach and case series, *Am J Sports Med* 41:1869, 2013.

Song B, Li C, Shen Z, et al.: Combined anterior and dual posterolateral approaches for ankle arthroscopy for posterior and anterior ankle impingement syndrome, *Foot Ankle Int* 37(6):605–610, 2016.

Tey M, Monllau JC, Centenera JM, Pelfort X: Benefits of arthroscopic tuberculoplasty in posterior ankle impingement syndrome, *Knee Surg Sports Traumatol Arthrosc* 15:1235, 2007.

Walsh SJ, Twaddle BC, Rosenfeldt MP, Boyle MJ: Arthroscopic treatment of anterior ankle impingement: a prospective study of 46 patients with 5-year follow-up, *Am J Sports Med* 42(11):2722, 2014.

Wang X, Zhao Z, Liu X, et al.: Combined posterior and anterior ankle arthroscopy for posterior and anterior ankle impingement syndrome in a switching position, *Foot Ankle Int* 35:829, 2014.

Willits K, Sonneveld H, Amendola A, et al.: Outcome of posterior ankle arthroscopy for hindfoot impingement, *Arthroscopy* 24:196, 2008.

Zwiers R, Wiegerinck JI, Murawski CD, et al.: Arthroscopic treatment for anterior ankle impingement: a systematic review of the current literature, *Arthroscopy* 31:1585, 2015.

Zwiers R, Wiegerinck JI, Murawski CD, et al.: Surgical treatment for posterior ankle impingement, *Arthroscopy* 29:1263, 2013.

OSTEOCHONDRAL LESIONS OF THE TALUS

Ahmad J, Maltenfort M: Arthroscopic treatment of osteochondral lesions of the talus with allograft cartilage matrix, *Foot Ankle Int* 38(8):855, 2017.

Becher C, Malahias MA, Ali MM, et al.: Arthroscopic microfracture vs. arthroscopic autologous matrix-induced chondrogenesis for the treatment of articular cartilage defects of the talus, *Knee Surg Sports Traumatol Arthrosc*, 2018, https://doi.org/10.1007/s00167-018-5278-7.

Choi JI, Lee KB: Comparison of clinical outcomes between arthroscopic subchondral drilling and microfracture for osteochondral lesions of the talus, *Knee Surg Sports Traumatol Arthrosc* 24(7):2140, 2016.

D'Ambrosi R, Maccario C, Ursino C, et al.: Combining microfractures, autologous bone graft, and autologous matrix-induced chondrogenesis for the treatment of juvenile osteochondral talar lesions, *Foot Ankle Int* 38(5):485, 2017.

De Sandis BA, Haleem AM, Sofka CM, et al.: Arthroscopic treatment of osteochondral lesions of the talus using juvenile articular cartilage allograft and autologous bone marrow aspirate concentration, *J Foot Ankle Surg* 57(2):273, 2018.

Georgiannos D, Bisbinas I, Badekas A: Osteochondral transplantation of autologous graft for the treatment of osteochondral lesions of talus: 5- to 7-year follow-up, *Knee Surg Sports Traumatol Arthrosc* 24(12):3722, 2016.

Guney A, Yurakakul E, Karaman I, et al.: Medium-term outcomes of mosaicplasty versus arthroscopic microfracture with or without platelet-rich plasma in the treatment of osteochondral lesions of the talus, *Knee Surg Sports Traumatol Arthrosc* 249(4):1293, 2016.

Hannon CP, Ross KA, Murawski CD, et al.: Arthroscopic bone marrow stimulation and concentrated bone marrow aspirate for osteochondral lesions of the talus: a case-control study of functional and magnetic resonance observation of cartilage repair tissue outcomes, *Arthroscopy* 32(2):339, 2016.

Lee KB, Park HW, Cho HJ, Seon JK: Comparison of arthroscopic microfracture for osteochondral lesions of the talus with and without subchondral cyst, *Am J Sports Med* 43(8):1951, 2015.

Phisitkul P, Akoh CC, Rungprai C, et al.: Optimizing arthroscopy for osteochondral lesions of the talus: the effect of ankle positions and distraction during anterior and posterior arthroscopy in a cadaveric model, *Arthroscopy* 33(12):2238, 2017.

Ross AW, Murawski CD, Fraser EJ, et al.: Autologous osteochondral transplantation for osteochondral lesions of the talus: does previous bone marrow stimulation negatively affect clinical outcome? *Arthroscopy* 32(7):1377, 2016.

Usuelli FG, D'Ambrosi R, Maccario C, et al.: All-arthroscopic AMIC® (AT-AMIC®) technique with autologous bone graft for talar osteochondral defects: clinical and radiological results, *Knee Surg Sports Traumatol Arthrosc* 26(3):875, 2018.

Van Bergen CJA, Baur OL, Murawski CD, et al.: Diagnosis: history, physical examination, and arthroscopy: proceedings of the International Consensus Meeting on cartilage repair of the ankle, *Foot Ankle Int* 39(Suppl 1):3S.

Van Eekeren IC, van Bergen CJ, Sierevelt IN, et al.: Return to sports after arthroscopic debridement and bone marrow stimulation of osteochondral talar defects: a 5- to 24-year follow-up study, *Knee Sur Sports Traumatol Arthrosc* 24(4):1311, 2016.

VanTienderen RJ, Dunn JC, Kusnezov N, Orr JD: Osteochondral allograft transfer for treatment of osteochondral lesions of the talus: a systematic review, *Arthroscopy* 33(1):217, 2017.

Yasui Y, Hannon CP, Fraser EJ, et al.: Lesion size measured on MRI does not accurately reflect arthroscopic measurement in talar osteochondral lesions, *Orthop J Sports Med* 7(2):232–261, 2019.

INSTABILITY

Acevedo JI, Mangone P: Arthroscopic Broström technique, *Foot Ankle Int* 36(4):465, 2015.

Araoye I, De Cesar Netto C, Cone B, et al.: Results of lateral ankle ligament repair surgery in one hundred and nineteen patients: do surgical method and arthroscopy timing matter? *Int Orthop* 41(11):2289, 2017.

Brown AJ, Shimozono Y, Hurley ET, Kennedy JG: Arthroscopic repair of lateral ankle ligament for chronic lateral ankle instability: a systematic review, *Arthroscopy* 34(8):2497, 2018.

Corte-Real NM, Moriera RM: Arthoscopic repair of chronic lateral ankle instability, *Foot Ankle Int* 30:213, 2009.

Feller R, Borenstein T, Fantry AJ, et al.: Arthroscopic quantification of syndesmotic instability in a cadaveric model, *Arthroscopy* 33(2):436, 2017.

Ferkel RD, Chams RN: Chronic lateral instability: arthroscopic findings and long-term results, *Foot Ankle Int* 28(24), 2007.

Giza E, Shin EC, Wong SE, et al.: Arthroscopic suture anchor repair of the lateral ligament ankle complex: a cadaveric study, *Am J Sports Med* 41:2567, 2013.

Guelfi M, Zamperetti M, Pantalone A, et al.: Open and arthroscopic lateral ligament repair for treatment of chronic ankle instability: a systematic review, *Foot Ankle Surg* 24(1):11, 2018.

Guillo S, Archbold P, Perera A, et al.: Arthroscopic anatomic reconstruction of the lateral ligaments of the ankle with gracilis autograft, *Arthrosc Tech* 3:e593, 2014.

Han SH, Lee JW, Kim S, et al.: Chronic tibiofibular syndesmosis injury: the diagnostic efficiency of magnetic resonance imaging and comparative analysis of operative treatment, *Foot Ankle Int* 28:336, 2007.

Hua Y, Chen S, Li Y, et al.: Combination of modified Brostrom procedure with ankle arthroscopy for ankle instability accompanied by intra-articular symptoms, *Arthroscopy* 26:524, 2010.

Li H, Hua Y, Li H, et al.: Activity level and function 2 years after anterior talofibular ligament repair: a comparison between arthroscopic repair and open repair procedures, *Am J Sports Med* 45(9):2044, 2017.

Lopes R, Andrieu M, Cordier G, et al.: Arthroscopic treatment of chronic ankle instability: prospective study of outcomes in 286 patients, *Orthop Traumatol Surg Res* 104(8S):S199, 2018.

Lubberts B, Guss D, Vopat BG, et al.: The arthroscopic syndesmotic assessment tool can differentiate between stable and unstable ankle syndesmoses, *Knee Surg Sports Traumatol Arthrosc*, 2018, https://doi.org/10.1007/s00167-018-5229-3.

Lui TH: Arthroscopic-assisted lateral ligamentous reconstruction in combined ankle and subtalar instability, *Arthroscopy* 23, 554.e1, 2007.

Matsui K, Takao M, Miyamoto W, et al.: Arthroscopic Broström repair with Gould augmentation via an accessory anterolateral port for lateral instability of the ankle, *Arch Orthop Trauma Surg* 134:1461, 2014.

Nery C, Fonseca L, Raduan F, et al.: Prospective study of the "inside-out" arthroscopic ankle ligament technique: preliminary result, *Foot Ankle Surg* 24(4):320, 2018.

Nery C, Raduan F, Del Buono A, et al.: Arthroscopic-assisted Broström-Gould for chronic ankle instability: a long-term follow-up, *Am J Sports Med* 39:2381, 2011.

Odak S, Ahluwalia R, Shivarathre DG, et al.: Arthroscopic evaluation of impingement and osteochondral lesions in chronic lateral ankle instability, *Foot Ankle Int* 36(9):1045, 2015.

Rigby RB, Cottom JM: A comparison of the "all-inside" arthroscopic Broström procedure with traditional open modified Broström-Gould technique: a review of 62 patients, *Foot Ankle* 25(1):31, 2019.

Schuberth JM, Jenning MM, Lau AC: Arthroscopy-assisted repair of latent syndesmotic instability of the ankle, *Arthroscopy* 24:868, 2008.

Vega J, Galanó P, Pellegrino A, et al.: All-inside arthroscopic lateral collateral ligament repair for ankle instability with a knotless suture anchor technique, *Foot Ankle Int* 34:1701, 2013.

Ventura A, Terzaghi C, Legnani C, Borgo E: Arthroscopic four-step treatment for chronic ankle instability, *Foot Ankle Int* 33:29, 2012.

Vuurberg G, de Vries JS, Krips R, et al.: Arthroscopic capsular shrinkage for treatment of chronic lateral ankle instability, *Foot Ankle Int* 38(10):1078, 2017.

Wang J, Hua Y, Chen S, et al.: Systematic review. Arthroscopic repair of lateral ankle ligament complex by suture anchor, *Arthroscopy* 30:766, 2014.

Watson BC, Lucas DE, Simpson GA, et al.: Arthroscopic evaluation of syndesmotic instability in a cadaveric model, *Foot Ankle Int* 36(11):1362, 2015.

Yasui Y, Murawski CD, Wollstein A, Kennedy JG: Reoperation rates following ankle ligament procedures performed with and without concomitant arthroscopic procedures, *Knee Surg Sports Traumatol Arthrosc* 25(6):1908, 2017.

Yeo ED, Lee KT, Sung IH, et al.: Comparison of all-inside arthroscopic and open techniques for the modified Broström procedure for ankle instability, *Foot Ankle Int* 37(10):1037, 2016.

Yeo ED, Par JY, Kim JH, Lee YK: Comparison of outcomes in patients with generalized ligamentous laxity and without generalized laxity in the arthroscopic modified Broström operation for chronic lateral ankle instability, *Foot Ankle Int* 38(12):1318, 2017.

FRACTURE

Chan KB, Lui TH: Role of ankle arthroscopy in management of acute ankle fractures, *Arthroscopy* 32(11):2373, 2016.

Chen XZ, Chen Y, Liu CG, et al.: Arthroscopy-assisted surgery for acute ankle fractures: a systematic review, *Arthroscopy* 31(11):2224, 2015.

Dawe EJC, Jukes CP, Ganesan K, et al.: Ankle arthroscopy to manage sequelae after ankle fractures, *Knee Surg Sports Traumatol Arthrosc* 23:3393, 2015.

Da Cunha R, Karnovsky SC, Schairer W, Drakos MC: Ankle arthroscopy for diagnosis of full-thickness talar cartilage lesions in the setting of acute ankle fractures, *Arthroscopy* 34(6):1950, 2018.

Dodd A, Simon D, Wilkinson R: Arthroscopically assisted transfibular talar dome fixation with a headless screw, *Arthroscopy* 25:806, 2009.

Duramaz A, Bacca E: Microfracture provides better clinical results than debridement in the treatment of acute talar osteochondral lesions using arthroscopic assisted fixation of acute ankle fractures, *Knee Surg Sports Traumatol Arthrosc* 26(10):3089, 2018.

Feng SM, Sun QQ, Wang AG, Li CK: All-inside arthroscopic treatment of Tillaux-Chaput fractures: clinical experience and outcomes analysis, *J Foot ankle Surg* 57:56, 2018.

Fuchs DJ, Ho BS, LaBelle MW, Kelikian AS: Effect of arthroscopic evaluation of acute ankle fractures on PROMIS intermediate-term functional outcomes, *Foot Ankle Int* 37(1):51, 21016.

Gonzalez TA, Macaulay AA, Ehrlichman LK, et al.: Arthroscopically assisted versus standard open reduction and internal fixation techniques for the acute ankle fracture, *Foot Ankle Int* 2015, [Epub ahead of print].

Kim HN, Park YJ, Kim GL, Park YW: Arthroscopy combined with hardware removal for chronic pain after ankle fracture, *Knee Surg Sports Traumatol Arthrosc* 21:1427, 2013.

Lee KM, Ahmed S, Park MS, et al.: Effectiveness of arthroscopically assisted surgery for ankle fractures: a meta-analysis, *Injury* 48(10):2318, 2017.

Leontaritis N, Hinojosa L, Panchbhavi VK: Arthroscopically detected intra-articular lesions associated with acute ankle fractures, *J Bone Joint Surg* 91A:333, 2009.

McGillion S, Jackson M, Lahoti O: Arthroscopically assisted percutaneous fixation of triplane fractures of the distal tibia, *J Pediatr Orthop B* 16:313, 2007.

Panagopoulos A, van Niekerk L: Arthroscopic assisted reduction and fixation of a juvenile Tillaux fracture, *Knee Surg Sports Traumatol Arthrosc* 15:415, 2007.

Park CH, Yoon DH: Role of subtalar arthroscopy in operative treatment of Sanders type 2 calcaneal fractures using a sinus tarsi approach, *Foot Ankle Int* 39(4):443, 2018.

Sherman TI, Casscells N, Rabe J, McGuigan FX: Ankle arthroscopy for ankle fractures, *Arthrosc Tech* 16:e75, 2015.

Thaunat M, Billot N, Bauer T, Hardy P: Arthroscopic treatment of a juvenile Tillaux fracture, *Knee Surg Sports Traumatol Arthrosc* 15:286, 2007.

Utsugi K, Sakai H, Hiraoka H, et al.: Intra-articular fibrous tissue formation following ankle fracture: the significance of arthroscopic debridement of fibrous tissue, *Arthroscopy* 23:89, 2007.

Wagener J, Schweizer C, Zwicky L, et al.: Arthroscopically assisted fixation of Hawkins type II talar neck fractures, *Bone Joint Lett J* 100-B(4):461, 2018.

Wood DA, Christensen JC, Schuberth JM: The use of arthroscopy in acute foot and ankle trauma: a review, *Foot Ankle Spec* 7:495, 2014.

Yasui Y, Vig KS, Murawski CD, et al.: Open versus arthroscopic ankle arthrodesis: a comparison of subsequent procedures in a large database, *J Foot Ankle Surg* 2016, [Epub ahead of print].

ARTHRODESIS

Beals TC, Junko JT, Amendola A, et al.: Minimally invasive distraction technique for prone posterior ankle and subtalar arthroscopy, *Foot Ankle Int* 31:316, 2010.

Collman DR, Kaas MH, Schuberth JM: Arthroscopic ankle arthrodesis: factors influencing union in 39 consecutive patients, *Foot Ankle Int* 27:1079, 2006.

Dannawi Z, Nawabi DH, Patel A, et al.: Arthroscopic ankle arthrodesis: are results reproducible irrespective of pre-operative deformity? *Foot Ankle Surg* 17:294, 2011.

De Leuw PA, Hendrick RP, van Dijk CN, et al.: Midterm results of posterior arthroscopic ankle fusion, *Knee Surg Sports Traumatol Arthrosc* 24(4):1326, 2016.

Devos Bevernage B, Goubau L, Deleu PA, et al.: Posterior arthroscopic subtalar arthrodesis, *JBJS Essent Surg Techn* 5(4):327, 2015.

Elmlund AO, Winson IG: Arthroscopic arthrodesis, *Foot Ankle Clin* 20(1):71, 2015.

Goetzmann T, Molé D, Jullion S, et al.: Influence of fixation with two vs. three screws on union of arthroscopic tibio-talar arthrodesis: comparative radiographic study of 111 cases, *Orthop Traumatol Surg Res* 102(5):651, 2016.

Jain SK, Tiernan D, Kearns SR: Analysis of risk factors for failure of arthroscopic ankle fusion in a series of 52 ankles, *Foot Ankle Surg* 22(2):91, 2016.

Jones CR, Wong E, Applegate GR, Ferkel RD: Arthroscopic ankle arthrodesis: a 2-15 year follow-up study, *Arthroscopy* 34(5):1641, 2018.

Kendal AR, Cooke P, Sharp R: Arthroscopic ankle fusion for avascular necrosis of the talus, *Foot Ankle Int* 36(5):591, 2015.

Malekpour L, Rahali S, Duparc F, et al.: Anatomic feasibility study of posterior arthroscopic tibiotalar arthrodesis, *Foot Ankle Int* 36(10):1229, 2015.

Martin Oliva X, Falcao P, Fernandes Cerqueira R, Rodrigues-Pinto R: Posterior arthroscopic subtalar arthrodesis: clinical and radiologic review of 19 cases, *J Foot Ankle Surg* 5693:543, 2017.

Gougoulias NE, Agathangelidis FG, Parsons SW: Arthroscopic ankle arthrodesis, *Foot Ankle Int* 28:695, 2007.

Nielsen KK, Linde F, Jensen NC: The outcome of arthroscopic and open surgery ankle arthrodesis: a comparative retrospective study on 107 patients, *Foot Ankle Surg* 14:153, 2008.

Park JH, Kim HJ, Suh DH, et al.: Arthroscopic versus open ankle arthrodesis: a systematic review, *Arthroscopy* 34(3):988, 2018.

Quayle J, Shafafy R, Khan MA, et al.: Arthroscopic versus open ankle arthrodesis, *Foot Ankle Surg* 24(2):137, 2018.

Roster B, Kreulen C, Giza E: Subtalar joint arthrodesis: open and arthroscopic indications and surgical techniques, *Foot Ankle Clin* 20(2):319, 2015.

Townshend D, Di Silvestro M, Krause F, et al.: Arthroscopic versus open ankle arthrodesis: a multicenter comparative case series, *J Bone Joint Surg* 95:98, 2013.

Vilá-Rico J, Mellado-Romero MA, Bravo-Giménez B, et al.: Subtalar arthroscopic arthrodesis: technique and outcomes, *Foot Ankle Surg* 23(1):9, 2017.

Vilá-Rico J, Ojeda-Thies C, Mellado-Romero MA, et al.: Arthroscopic posterior subtalar arthrodesis for salvage of posttraumatic arthritis following calcaneal fractures, *Injury* 49(2):S64, 2018.

Vilá y R, Jiménez Díaz V, Bravo Giménez B, et al.: Results of arthroscopic subtalar arthrodesis for adult-acquired flatfoot deformity vs. posttraumatic arthritis, *Foot Ankle Int* 37(2):198, 2016.

SUBTALAR ARTHROSCOPY

Ahn JH, Lee SK, Kim KJ, et al.: Subtalar arthroscopic procedures for the treatment of subtalar pathologic conditions: 115 consecutive cases, *Orthopedics* 32:891, 2009.

Amendola A, Lee KB, Saltzman CL, Suh JS: Technique and early experience with posterior arthroscopic subtalar arthrodesis, *Foot Ankle Int* 28:298, 2007.

Guo QW, Hu YL, Jiao C, et al.: Open versus endoscopic excision of a symptomatic os trigonum: a comparative study of 41 cases, *Arthroscopy* 26:384, 2010.

Hammond AW, Crist BD: Arthroscopic management of C3 tibial plafond fractures: a technical guide, *J Foot Ankle Surg* 51:382, 2012.

Kim HN, Ryu SR, Park JM, Park YW: Subtalar arthroscopy with calcaneal skeletal traction in a hanging position, *J Foot Ankle Surg* 51:816, 2012.

Lee KB, Bai LB, Song EK, et al.: Subtalar arthroscopy for sinus tarsi syndrome: arthroscopic findings and clinical outcomes of 33 consecutive cases, *Arthroscopy* 24:1130, 2008.

Lee KB, Chung JY, Song EK, et al.: Arthroscopic release for painful subtalar stiffness after intra-articular fractures of the calcaneum, *J Bone Joint Surg* 90B:1457, 2008.

Lee KB, Park CH, Seon JK, Kim MS: Arthroscopic subtalar arthrodesis using a posterior 2-portal approach in the prone position, *Arthroscopy* 26:230, 2010.

Narita N, Takao M, Innami K, et al.: Minimally invasive subtalar arthrodesis with iliac crest autograft through posterior arthroscopic portals: a technical note, *Foot Ankle Int* 33:803, 2012.

Noh KC, Hong DY, Kim YT, et al.: Arthroscopic transfibular approach for removal of bone fragments in posterior malleolar fracture: technical tip, *Foot Ankle Int* 36:108, 2015.

Shazly OE, Nassar W, Badrawy AE: Arthroscopic subtalar fusion for posttraumatic subtalar arthritis, *Arthroscopy* 25:783, 2009.

Sitte W, Lampert C, Baumann P: Osteosynthesis of talar body shear fractures assisted by hindfoot and subtalar arthroscopy: technique tip, *Foot Ankle Int* 33:74, 2012.

Sivakumar BS, Wong P, Dick CG, et al.: Arthroscopic reduction and percutaneous fixation of selected calcaneus fractures: surgical technique and early results, *J Orthop Trauma* 28:569, 2014.

Swart EF, Vosseller JT: Arthroscopic assessment of medial malleolar reduction, *Arch Orthop Trauma Surg* 134:1287, 2014.

Woon CY, Chong KW, Yeo W, et al.: Subtalar arthroscopy and fluoroscopy in percutaneous fixation of intra-articular calcaneal fractures: the best of both worlds, *J Trauma* 71:917, 2011.

FIRST METATARSOPHALANGEAL JOINT ARTHROSCOPY

Ahn JH, Choy WS, Lee KW: Arthroscopy of the first metatarsophalangeal joint in 59 consecutive cases, *J Foot Ankle Surg* 51:161, 2012.

Debnath UK, Hemmady MV, Hariharan K: Indications for and technique of first metatarsophalangeal joint arthroscopy, *Foot Ankle Int* 27:1049, 2006.

Hull M, Campbell JT, Jeng CL, et al.: Measuring visualized joint surface in hallux metatarsophalangeal arthroscopy, *Foot Ankle Int* 39(8):978, 2018.

Hsu AR, Gross CE, Lee S, Carreira DS: Extended indications for foot and ankle arthroscopy, *J Am Acad Orthop Surg* 22(1):10, 2014.

Hunt KJ: Hallux metatarsophalangeal (MTP) joint arthroscopy for hallux rigidus, *Foot Ankle Int* 36(1):113, 2015.

Kuyucu E, Mutlu H, Mutlu S, et al.: Arthroscopic treatment of focal osteochondral lesions of the first metatarsophalangeal joint, *J Orthop Surg Res* 12(1):68, 2017.

Lui TH: First metatarsophalangeal joint arthroscopy in patients with hallux valgus, *Arthroscopy* 24:1122, 2008.

Lui TH, Yuen CP: Small joint arthroscopy in foot and ankle, *Foot Ankle Clin* 20:123, 2015.

Michels F, Guillo S, de Lavigne C, Van Der Bauwhede J: The arthroscopic Lapidus procedure, *Foot Ankle Surg* 17:25, 2011.

Nakajima K: Arthroscopy of the first metatarsophalangeal joint, *J Foot Ankle Surg* 57(2):357, 2018.

Nery C, Coughlin MJ, Baumfeld D, et al.: Lesser metatarsal phalangeal joint arthroscopy: anatomic description and comparative dissection, *Arthroscopy* 30:971, 2014.

Schmid T: Younger A: first metatarsophalangeal joint degeneration: arthroscopic treatment, *Foot Ankle Clin* 20(3):413, 2015.

Siclari A, Decantis V: Arthroscopic lateral release and percutaneous distal osteotomy for hallux valgus: a preliminary report, *Foot Ankle Int* 30:675, 2009.

Siclari A, Piras M: Hallux metatarsophalangeal arthroscopy: indications and techniques, *Foot Ankle Clin* 20:109, 2015.

Vaseeon T, Phisitkul P: Arthroscopic debridement for first metatarsophalangeal joint arthrodesis with a 2- versus 3-portal technique: a cadaveric study, *Arthroscopy* 26:1363, 2010.

ENDOSCOPY/TENDOSCOPY

Ballal MS, Roche A, Brodrick A, et al.: Posterior endoscopic excision of os trigonum in professional national ballet dancers, *J Foot Ankle Surg* 55(5):927, 2016.

Bauer T, Deranlot J, Hardy P: Endoscopic treatment of calcaneo-fibular impingement, *Knee Surg Sports Traumatol Arthrosc* 19:131, 2011.

Bernasconi A, Sadile F, Smeraglia F, et al.: Tendoscopy of Achilles, peroneal and tibialis posterior tendons: an evidence-based update, *Foot Ankle Surg* 24(5):374, 2018.

Bernasconi A, Sadile F, Welck M, et al.: Role of tendoscopy in treating stage II posterior tibial tendon dysfunction, *Foot Ankle Int* 39(4):433, 2018.

Bonasia DE, Phisitkul P, Amendola A: Endoscopic coalition resection, *Foot Ankle Clin* 20(1):81, 2015.

Bonasia DE, Phisitkul P, Saltzman CL, et al.: Arthroscopic resection of talocalcaneal coalitions, *Arthroscopy* 27:430, 2011.

Bulstra GH, Olsthoorn PGM, van Dijk N: Tendoscopy of the posterior tibial tendon, *Foot Ankle Clin* 11:421, 2006.

Carreira D, Ballard A: Achilles tendoscopy, *Foot Ankle Clin* 20(1):27, 2015.

Choi WJ, Choi GW, Lee JW: Arthroscopic synovectomy of the ankle in rheumatoid arthritis, *Arthroscopy* 29:133, 2013.

Chraim M, Alrabai HM, Krenn S, et al.: Short-term results of endoscopic percutaneous longitudinal tenotomy for noninsertional Achilles tendinopathy and the presentation of a simplified operative method, *Foot Ankle Spec* 12(1):73, 2019.

Corte-Real NM, Moreira RM, Guerra-Pinto F: Arthroscopic treatment of tenosynovitis of the flexor hallucis longus tendon, *Foot Ankle Int* 33:1108, 2012.

Cychosz CC, Phisitkul P, Barg A, et al.: Foot and ankle tendoscopy: evidence-based recommendations, *Arthroscopy* 30:755, 2014.

Gedam PN, Rushnaiwala FM: Endoscopy-assisted Achilles tendon reconstruction with a central turndown flap and semitendinosus augmentation, *Foot Ankle Int* 37(12):1333, 2016.

Georgiannos D, Bisbinas I: Endoscopic versus open excision of os trigonum for the treatment of posterior ankle impingement syndrome in an athletic population: a randomized controlled study with 5-year follow-up, *Am J Sports Med* 45(6):1388, 2017.

Gianakos AL, Ross KA, Hannon CP, et al.: Functional outcomes of tibialis posterior tendoscopy with comparison to magnetic resonance imaging, *Foot Ankle Int* 36(7):812, 2015.

Guo QW, Hu YL, Jiao C, et al.: Open versus endoscopic excision of a symptomatic os trigonum: a comparative study of 41 cases, *Arthroscopy* 26:384, 2010.

Harris 3rd RC, Strannigan KL, Piraino J: Comparison of the complication incidence in open versus endoscopic gastrocnemius recession: a retrospective medical record review, *J Foot Ankle Surg* 57(4):747, 2018.

Hua Y, Chen S, Li Y, Wu Z: Arthroscopic treatment for posterior tibial tendon lesions with a posterior approach, *Knee Surg Sports Traumatol Arthrosc* 23:879, 2015.

Hull M, Campbell JT, Jeng CL, et al.: Measuring visualized tendon length in peroneal tendoscopy, *Foot Ankle Int* 39(8):990, 2018.

Husebye EE, Molund M, Hvaal KH, Stodle AH: Endoscopic transfer of flexor hallucis longus tendon for Chronic Achilles tendon rupture: technical aspects and short-time experiences, *Foot Ankle Spec* 11(5):461, 2018.

Innami K, Takao M, Miyamoto W, et al.: Endoscopic surgery for young athletes with symptomatic unicameral bone cyst of the calcaneus, *Am J Sports Med* 39:575, 2011.

Jagodzinski NA, Hughes A, Davis NP, et al.: Arthroscopic resection of talocalcaneal coalitions—a bicentre case series of a new technique, *Foot Ankle Surg* 19:125, 2013.

Jerosch J: Endoscopic calcaneoplasty, *Foot Ankle Clin* 20(1):149, 2015.

Kennedy JG, van Dijk PA, Murawski CD, et al.: Functional outcomes after peroneal tendoscopy in the treatment of peroneal tendon disorders, *Knee Surg Sports Traumatol Arthrsc* 24(4):1148, 2016.

Khazen G, Khazen C: Tendoscopy in stage I posterior tibial tendon dysfunction, *Foot Ankle Clin* 17:399, 2012.

Komatsu F, Takao M, Innami K, et al.: Endoscopic surgery for plantar fasciitis: application of a deep-fascial approach, *Arthroscopy* 27:1105, 2011.

Lui TH: Endoscopic curettage and bone grafting of huge talar bone cyst with preservation of cartilaginous surfaces: surgical planning, *Foot Ankle Surg* 20:248, 2014.

Lui TH: Tendoscopy of the peroneus longus in the sole, *Foot Ankle Int* 34(2):299, 2013.

Lui TH, Chan KB, Chan LK: Endoscopic distal soft-tissue release in the treatment of hallux valgus: a cadaveric study, *Arthroscopy* 26:1111, 2010.

Lui TH, Tse LF: Peroneal tendoscopy, *Foot Ankle Clin* 20(1):15, 2015.

Miyamoto W, Takao M, Matsushita T: Hindfoot endoscopy for posterior ankle impingement syndrome and flexor hallucis longus tendon disorders, *Foot Ankle Clin* 20(1):139, 2015.

Monteagudo M, Maceira E: Posterior tibial tendoscopy, *Foot Ankle Clin* 20(1):1, 2015.

Opdam KTM, Baltes TPA, Zwiers R, et al.: Endoscopic treatment of midportion Achilles tendinopathy: a retrospective case series of patient satisfaction and functional outcome at 2- to 8-year follow-up, *Arthroscopy* 34(1):264, 2018.

Ogut T, Ayhan E: Hindfoot endoscopy for accessory flexor digitorum longus and flexor hallucis longus tenosynovitis, *Foot Ankle Surg* 17:e7, 2011.

Ortmann FW, McBryde AM: Endoscopic bony and soft-tissue decompression of the retrocalcaneal space for the treatment of Haglund deformity and retrocalcaneal bursitis, *Foot Ankle Int* 28:149, 2007.

Phisitkul P, Barg A, Amendola A: Endoscopic recession of the gastrocnemius tendon, *Foot Ankle Int* 38(4):457, 2017.

Scholten PE, van Dijk N: Endoscopic calcaneoplasty, *Foot Ankle Clin* 11:439–446, 2006.

Scholten PE, van Dijk N: Tendoscopy of the peroneal tendons, *Foot Ankle Clin* 11:415, 2006.

Singh AK, Parsons SW: Arthroscopic resection of calcaneonavicular coalition/malunion via a modified sinus tarsi approach: an early case series, *Foot Ankle Surg* 18:266, 2012.

Spennacchio P, Cucchi D, Randelli PS, van Dijk NC: Evidence-based indications for hindfoot endoscopy, *Knee Surg Sports Traumatol Arthrosc* 24(4):1386, 2016.

Syed TA, Perera A: A proposed staging classification for minimally invasive management of Haglund's syndrome with percutaneous and endoscopic surgery, *Foot Ankle Clin* 21(3):641, 2016.

Urguden M, Gulten IA, Civan O, et al.: Results of peroneal tendoscopy with a technical modification, *Foot Ankle Int* 40(3):356, 2019.

Valerio VL, Seijas R, Alvarez P, et al.: Endoscopic repair of posterior ankle impingement syndrome due to os trigonum in soccer players, *Foot Ankle Int* 36:70, 2015.

Vega J, Batista JP, Goalnó P, et al.: Tendoscopic groove deepening for chronic subluxation of the peroneal tendons, *Foot Ankle Int* 34(6):832, 2013.

Vega J, Vilá J, Batista J, et al.: Endoscopic flexor hallucis longus transfer for chronic noninsertional Achilles tendon rupture, *Foot Ankle Int* 39(12):1464, 2018.

Vilá J, Vega J, Mellado M, et al.: Hindfoot endoscopy for the treatment of posterior ankle impingement syndrome: a safe and reproducible technique, *Foot Ankle Surg* 20:174, 2014.

Wake J, Martin K: Posterior tibial tendon endoscopic debridement for stage I and II posterior tibial tendon dysfunction, *Arthrosc Tech* 6(5):e2019, 2017.

Wiegerinck JI, Kok AC, van Dijk N: Surgical treatment of chronic retrocalcaneal bursitis, *Arthroscopy* 28:283, 2012.

The complete list of references is available online at ExpertConsult.com.

CHAPTER 3

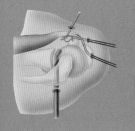

ARTHROSCOPY OF THE LOWER EXTREMITY

Barry B. Phillips, Marc J. Mihalko

KNEE

The knee is the joint in which arthroscopy has its greatest diagnostic and intraarticular surgical application. The usefulness of arthroscopic techniques in diagnosis and treatment of intraarticular pathology has been well documented.

Arthroscopy should be considered a diagnostic aid used in conjunction with a good history, complete physical examination, and appropriate radiographs. It should serve as an adjunct to, not as a replacement for, a thorough clinical evaluation. With increased proficiency in examination of extremities and more accurate adjuvant tests, including MRI, we rarely, if ever, perform simple "diagnostic arthroscopy." Surgical alternatives are discussed thoroughly with the patient before the procedure, and the definitive surgical procedure is performed at the time of a thorough arthroscopic examination. The general principles, instrumentation, indications, contraindications, and complications of arthroscopy are discussed in chapter 1.

BASIC DIAGNOSTIC TECHNIQUES
■ GENERAL PRINCIPLES

Arthroscopy of the knee can be done as the essential initial step before proceeding to operative arthroscopy or before an open arthrotomy. Anesthesia can be local, regional block, or general. If the procedure is uncomplicated and of short duration, it can be done using a regional block local anesthesia in cooperative patients, especially if the surgeon is experienced in arthroscopy. If local anesthesia is to be used, we prefer intravenous sedation for portal injection with 1% lidocaine and an intraarticular bolus of 30 mL of bupivacaine and 15 mL of lidocaine 20 minutes before starting the procedure. Diagnostic arthroscopy before arthrotomy or major intraarticular surgery generally is best done with the patient under general anesthesia, unless this type of anesthesia is contraindicated.

The procedure is performed in the operating room under strict sterile conditions. The seriousness of this surgical procedure must not be minimized. Although complications such as infection are infrequent (<1%), carelessness in surgical scrubbing, preparation, or draping or careless handling of the irrigating solutions, arthroscopes, and instruments can result in intraarticular infections just as devastating as those after arthrotomy. Sterilization of arthroscopy equipment and use of waterproof arthroscopy gowns and drapes are essential. Sealing the extremity proximal and distal to the arthroscopy site and use of a durable skin preparation (DuraPrep, 3M Healthcare, St. Paul, MN) and iodine-impregnated drape at the surgical site can help to minimize infections.

The scrub nurse uses a large table for instruments. This is positioned for the nurse's convenience, usually on the same side as the knee having surgery. A Mayo stand is placed over the operating table at the upper part of the patient's thighs, and the more commonly used instruments are placed on it. Power cords and light cables are attached to the appropriate sources and are placed on a side table. Irrigation bags are suspended from an intravenous stand at the head of the table and are raised 3 to 4 feet above the level of the patient. The use of an arthroscopic pump for inflow through the arthroscope sheath or a separate sheath helps keep flow and pressure constant. The pump may eliminate the need for a tourniquet, making arthroscopy using local anesthesia feasible.

A tourniquet is placed around the thigh but is not inflated in diagnostic arthroscopy unless troublesome bleeding occurs. Inflation of the tourniquet blanches the synovium and other vascularized tissue and makes diagnostic evaluation of these

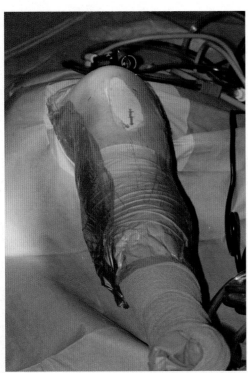

FIGURE 3.1 Waterproof outer drape with central rubberized opening seals unsterile proximal thigh from operative field.

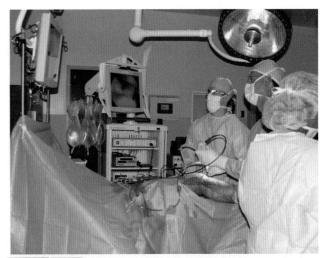

FIGURE 3.2 Technique of table-flat position. Surgeon and assistant stand at side of table.

structures more difficult. Meniscal vascularity and healing potential should be evaluated with the tourniquet deflated and the intraarticular hydrostatic pressure low. The tourniquet usually is inflated after exsanguination of the limb in acute traumatic disorders, or if the surgeon anticipates anything other than the simplest intraarticular surgical procedure. Tourniquet time should be minimized and not exceed 90 minutes for routine procedures to prevent possible deep vein thrombosis. For major complicated procedures, tourniquet times of up to 2 hours can be used, but times longer than this should be avoided to prevent ischemic neurovascular changes.

Stressing the knee to open up the various compartments is necessary for diagnostic or operative procedures. This can be accomplished by using a padded lateral post or a commercial leg-holding device. The use of a padded lateral post attached to the edge of the operating table can be effective for valgus stressing in or near full extension, but it does not control rotation. The commercial thigh holders are most effective, but some of their potential dangers must be kept in mind.

■ PATIENT POSITIONING

When the patient is anesthetized, and a tourniquet and leg holder are applied if desired, the limb from the ankle to the tourniquet is thoroughly scrubbed and surgically prepared, just as for an open arthrotomy. Excellent commercial arthroscopy draping systems are available that isolate the foot and lower leg and the distal thigh just below the tourniquet and leg holder (Fig. 3.1). Waterproof gowns also are imperative for the surgeon and assistant to prevent contamination.

The patient can be placed supine with the prepared and draped limb angled off the lateral aspect of the table. The use of a leg holder or a lateral post allows the surgeon to stand on the inside of the abducted leg, placing the patient's foot and ankle on the surgeon's hip and iliac crest area. Placing the surgeon's

outside foot on a small platform often helps maintain the patient's foot in the correct position. This position frees both of the surgeon's hands, and the surgeon can stress the leg into valgus by simply leaning against the leg in the leg holder. This maneuver opens up the medial compartment for examination and probing. When the patient is supine, examination of the lateral compartment requires the assistant to hold the leg in a figure-four position. The table-flat position can be used with the surgeon and assistant standing at the side of the table (Fig. 3.2).

The patient also can be placed supine on a standard operating table with the knee joint positioned slightly past the distal break point of the table. The end of the table is dropped so that both limbs dangle at 90 degrees. The opposite limb should be well padded to prevent potential pressure problems. Flexing the middle of the table and placing a padded bolster also flexes the hips to take the stretch off the femoral nerve and simultaneously flattens the lumbar spine. The use of a well-leg support for the uninvolved limb is another excellent technique. With either technique, it is recommended to wrap the uninvolved extremity with an elastic wrap or to use an elastic stocking to minimize venostasis (Fig. 3.3).

■ PORTAL PLACEMENT

Among the keys to success in arthroscopy are adequate light and distention of the joint and precise localization of the portals of entry for the arthroscope and accessory instruments. Without adequate illumination, clear vision is impossible; without adequate distention of the joint, the fat pad, synovium, and other soft tissues obliterate the view; and without precise location of the portals of entry, one would be unable to see adequately or to maneuver within all parts of the joint. Attempts to force a poorly placed arthroscope or instrument can result in articular scuffing, instrument damage, and other problems. Adequate illumination is ensured by proper care of the arthroscope and fiberoptic light cables, changing the light source bulbs when required, cleansing the arthroscope lens of film from frequent disinfectant soakings, and maintaining a clear irrigation medium. Any damage to the arthroscope tip, whether from motorized instrumentation or careless handling, can result in uneven light regulation and inability to focus the arthroscope properly. Precise entry portal location can be ensured best by

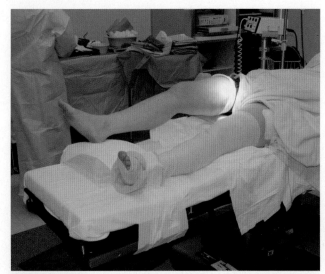

FIGURE 3.3   Placement of lateral post and taping of saline bag to table allow ease of leg positioning and full range of motion during ligament reconstruction.

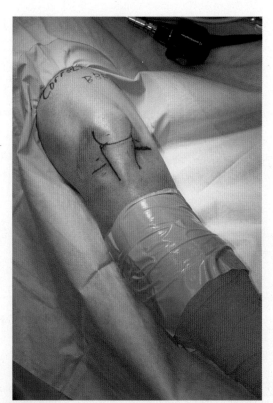

FIGURE 3.4   Landmarks drawn on knee before distention.

carefully drawing the joint lines and soft-tissue and bony landmarks with a skin-marking pen before joint distention. All standard and optional portals are marked. Typically, the outlines of the patella and patellar tendon are drawn, medial and lateral joint lines are palpated with the fingertip and drawn, and the posterior contours of the medial and lateral femoral condyles are marked. The surgeon should recheck these outlines after distention to ensure proper placement.

When the portals are carefully marked, a small outflow, needle-type cannula can be placed superomedially or superolaterally with inflow through the arthroscope. This generally is necessary for large procedures, such as anterior cruciate ligament reconstruction when hemarthrosis is present. For smaller procedures, such as a meniscectomy, an outflow cannula might not always be necessary. Avoiding going through the vastus medialis obliquus may help to accelerate rehabilitation.

▌STANDARD PORTALS
The standard portals for diagnostic arthroscopy are the anterolateral, anteromedial, posteromedial, and superolateral (Fig. 3.4).

Anterolateral Portal. If allowed only one approach for diagnostic arthroscopy of the knee joint, most arthroscopic surgeons would choose the anterolateral portal. With the use of a 4-mm-diameter, 30-degree oblique forelens arthroscope through the anterolateral portal, almost all of the structures within the knee joint can be seen. Through this portal, the posterior cruciate ligament (PCL), the anterior portion of the lateral meniscus, and, in tight knees, the periphery of the posterior horn of the medial meniscus cannot be viewed adequately, however. This portal is located approximately 1 cm above the lateral joint line and approximately 1 cm lateral to the margin of the patellar tendon. Palpation of the inferior pole of the patella helps to ensure that the anterior portals are not placed too high; the portal should be approximately 1 cm inferior to the patella. If the portal is placed too near the joint line, the anterior horn of the lateral meniscus can be lacerated or otherwise damaged. Also, an arthroscope inserted through such a portal can pass either through or beneath the anterior horn of the lateral

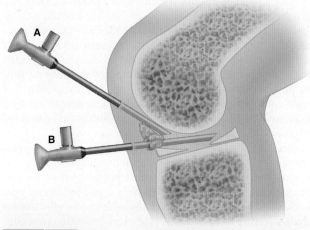

FIGURE 3.5   Placement of anterolateral portal. Arthroscope introduced through portal placed high above joint line *(A)* has advantages of avoiding fat pad and being easy to manipulate. It is difficult to reach posterior aspect of joint, however, where most meniscal pathology is located. With low portal placement *(B)*, posterior access is easier because femoral condyle does not get in the way, but instrumentation through fat pad is more difficult. Compromise should be made depending on location of intraarticular pathology and tightness of joint.

meniscus, resulting in damage to the anterior horn or difficulty in maneuvering the arthroscope within the joint because it is bound down by the overlying meniscus. A portal placement too superior to the joint line allows the arthroscope to enter the space between the femoral and tibial condyles and prevents viewing of the posterior horns of the menisci and other posterior structures (Fig. 3.5). An arthroscope placed immediately adjacent to the edge of the patellar tendon can penetrate the fat pad, causing difficulty in viewing and in maneuvering the arthroscope within the joint.

Anteromedial Portal. The anteromedial portal is most commonly used for additional viewing of the lateral compartment and for insertion of a probe for palpation of the medial and lateral compartment structures. This portal is located similarly to the anterolateral portal: 1 cm above the medial joint line, 1 cm inferior to the tip of the patella, and 1 cm medial to the edge of the patellar tendon. Precise placement can be confirmed by using a percutaneous spinal needle visualized from the anterolateral portal. A no. 11 blade with the cutting edge pointed away from the meniscus is visualized while making the portal.

Posteromedial Portal. The posteromedial portal is located in a small triangular soft spot formed by the posteromedial edge of the femoral condyle and the posteromedial edge of the tibia. Before distention of the joint, this small triangle can be palpated easily with the knee flexed to 90 degrees. The landmarks should be drawn on the skin before beginning the diagnostic arthroscopy. The posteromedial compartment is small, but any arthroscope can be inserted into it with proper care and technique. In this portal, a 30-degree angled arthroscope offers optimal viewing of all the structures in the posteromedial compartment. Three guidelines aid in the establishment of this portal: (1) the knee must be maximally distended with irrigating solution so that the posteromedial compartment balloons out like a bubble when the knee is flexed to 90 degrees; (2) the knee must be flexed as close to 90 degrees as possible; and (3) the bony landmarks must be drawn before the joint is distended. The location of the portals should be approximately 1 cm above the posteromedial joint line and approximately 1 cm posterior to the posteromedial margin of the femoral condyle. This portal is useful for repair or removal of displaced posterior horn meniscal tears and for removal of posterior loose bodies that cannot be displaced into the medial compartment and removed through an anterior portal. It is always used in PCL reconstruction.

Superolateral Portal. The superolateral portal is most useful diagnostically for viewing the dynamics of the patellofemoral articulation. It also is the best approach for visualization of the patellar tendon using a 70-degree scope. This portal is located just lateral to the quadriceps tendon and about 2.5 cm superior to the superolateral corner of the patella. With the arthroscope in this portal, the patellofemoral joint can be viewed with a 30- or 70-degree arthroscope, allowing evaluation of patellar tracking, patellar congruity, and lateral overhang of the patella as the knee is carried from extension into varying degrees of flexion.

OPTIONAL PORTALS

Posterolateral Portal. The knee should be flexed to 90 degrees, and the joint should be maximally distended. The landmark for the posterolateral portal is at the point where a line drawn along the posterior margin of the femoral shaft intersects a line drawn along the posterior aspect of the fibula. This is about 2 cm above the posterolateral joint line at the posterior edge of the iliotibial band and the anterior edge of the biceps femoris tendon. A 6-mm skin incision is made, and the distended posterior capsule is penetrated using the arthroscope sheath and a sharp trocar. The posterior edge of the femoral condyle is palpated with a trocar, slipping off the posterior condyle parallel to it. Directed slightly inferiorly, the sheath enters the posterolateral compartment. Care must be taken not to damage the articular surface of the posterior femoral condyle with this maneuver. Also, plunging in with a sharp trocar through the capsule and into the popliteal space must be avoided for fear of damaging neurovascular structures. The outflow of irrigation solution on removal of the sharp trocar confirms entry into the joint. This portal is useful for assisting with repair of lateral meniscal tears.

Proximal Midpatellar Medial and Lateral Portals. The optional midpatellar portal designations should not be confused with a central transpatellar tendon portal. These optional portals were described to improve the viewing of the anterior compartment structures, the lateral meniscocapsular structures, and the popliteus tunnel and to minimize accessory instrument crowding with the arthroscope during procedures requiring triangulation of several instruments into these compartments. Viewing of the posterior horns of the menisci and the tibial attachment of the PCL may be difficult through these portals.

These portals are located just off the medial and lateral edges of the midpatella at the broadest portion of the patella. The selection of the site is crucial. A site that is too far superior or inferior can jeopardize proper viewing. A 30-degree oblique arthroscope is ideal here. These are our preferred accessory portals for anterior compartment procedures.

Accessory Far Medial and Lateral Portals. These inferior optional portals often are used for triangulation of accessory instruments into the knee during operative arthroscopic procedures. They are located approximately 2.5 cm medial or lateral to the standard anteromedial and anterolateral portals. Medially, these portals are near the anterior edge of the medial collateral ligament; laterally, they should be well anterior to the lateral collateral ligament and popliteus tendon. An excellent technique is to insert a spinal needle through the skin and capsule and into the compartment under direct vision with the arthroscope. The needle should enter the joint above the superior surface of the meniscus, which would allow passage to its desired location. After the needle is directed to the desired location within the joint, the accessory instrument can be passed to this location with ease. If the needle cannot pass to the desired location, its point of entry is adjusted carefully before the portal incision is made. The margin for error is less through these accessory medial and lateral portals; the meniscus or the collateral ligament can be lacerated, or the articular margin of the femoral condyle can be damaged.

Central Transpatellar Tendon (Gillquist) Portal. The central transpatellar tendon portal is located approximately 1 cm inferior to the lower pole of the patella in the midline of the joint through the patellar tendon. With the patella in higher or lower locations than normal, or if the patellar tendon is located entirely lateral to the midline of the joint, adjustments in portal location must be made. We find this portal most helpful in anterior cruciate ligament reconstruction procedures after graft harvest has been completed, avoiding tendon damage.

If a transpatellar tendon portal is necessary for posterior compartment evaluation or anterior compartment triangulation, it is made with the knee in 90 degrees of flexion to keep the tendon under tension. A 6- to 7-mm vertical incision is made sharply with a no. 11 blade through the skin and subcutaneous tissues and the patellar tendon, approximately 1 cm from the inferior pole of the patella. In the case of fixation of osteochondritis dissecans fragments, in which a more distal portal might be necessary, a spinal needle should be used to localize the portal before making an incision. We do not advocate routine use of this portal because of patellar tendon damage from the incision and instrumentation through the tendon. In certain cases, this portal would allow better instrumentation of an anterior articular joint surface and can complement the standard arthroscopic portals.

■ INSERTION OF SCOPE

If the tourniquet is not to be inflated unless troublesome bleeding occurs, the portal sites should be infiltrated with 4 to 5 mL of a local anesthetic agent mixed with epinephrine, which reduces bleeding and postoperative pain. The use of more than 4 to 5 mL is not advised because a larger bolus, especially in the anterolateral and anteromedial portals, can distend the fat pads sufficiently to make viewing difficult. If inflation of the tourniquet is planned, the portals usually are not infiltrated.

ARTHROSCOPIC EXAMINATION OF THE KNEE

The key to successful, accurate, and complete diagnosis of lesions within the knee joint is a systematic approach to viewing. A methodical sequence of examination should be developed, progressing from one compartment to another and systematically carrying out this sequence in every knee. The exact sequence is not crucial, but it is important to develop the habit of following it every time. Failure to do so could compromise diagnostic accuracy and completeness.

The knee should be divided routinely into the following compartments for arthroscopic examination (Fig. 3.6):
1. Suprapatellar pouch and patellofemoral joint
2. Medial gutter
3. Medial compartment
4. Intercondylar notch
5. Posteromedial compartment
6. Lateral compartment
7. Lateral gutter and posterolateral compartment

The posteromedial compartment can be examined by passing the scope posteriorly through the intercondylar notch or through a separate posteromedial portal. The posterolateral compartment usually can be examined adequately from an anterior portal, but if this compartment is incompletely viewed, a direct posterolateral portal should be chosen.

ARTHROSCOPIC SURGERY OF THE MENISCUS
■ CLASSIFICATION OF MENISCAL TEARS

Classification of the types of meniscal tears encountered during diagnostic arthroscopy of the knee is essential in planning the subsequent arthroscopic resection or repair. Although numerous classifications of meniscal tears have been described, that of O'Connor has proved useful: (1) longitudinal tears; (2) horizontal tears; (3) oblique tears; (4) radial tears (Fig. 3.7); and (5) variations, which include flap tears, complex tears, and degenerative meniscal tears.
Longitudinal tears most commonly occur as a result of trauma to a reasonably normal meniscus. The tear usually is vertically oriented and may extend completely through the

thickness of the meniscus or may extend only partially or incompletely through it. The tear is oriented parallel to the edge of the meniscus; if the tear is complete, a displaceable inner fragment frequently is produced. When the inner fragment displaces over into the intercondylar notch, it commonly is referred to as a *bucket-handle tear* (Fig. 3.8). If the tear is near the meniscocapsular attachment of the meniscus, it commonly is referred to as a *peripheral tear.* A peripheral vertical tear in zone I, referred to as a red-red tear, and a tear between zone I and II, referred to as a red-white tear, are in the vascularized portion of the meniscus (Fig. 3.9). These peripheral tears should be repaired when feasible.
Horizontal tears tend to be more common in older patients, with the horizontal cleavage plane occurring from shear, which divides the superior and inferior surfaces of the meniscus. These are more commonly seen in the posterior half of the medial meniscus or the midsegment of the lateral meniscus. Many flap tears and complex tears begin with a horizontal cleavage component.
Oblique tears are full-thickness tears running obliquely from the inner edge of the meniscus out into the body of the meniscus. If the base of the tear is posterior, it is referred to as a *posterior oblique tear;* the base of an anterior oblique tear is in the anterior horn of the meniscus (Fig. 3.10).
Radial tears, similar to oblique tears, are vertically oriented, extending from the inner edge of the meniscus toward its periphery, and can be complete or incomplete, depending on the extent of involvement. These probably are similar in pathogenesis to oblique tears (Fig. 3.11). Tears posterior to the popliteal tendon may heal on their own or with local stimulation techniques (Fig. 3.12).
The possible variations include flap tears, complex tears, and degenerative meniscal tears. *Flap tears* are similar to oblique tears but usually have a horizontal cleavage element rather than being purely vertical in orientation. Tears containing a horizontal element often are referred to as superior or inferior flap tears, depending on where the flap is based on the surface of the meniscus.
Complex tears may contain elements of all of the just-mentioned types of tears and are more common in chronic meniscal lesions or in older degenerative menisci. These generally are caused by chronic, long-standing, altered mechanics of the meniscus, and the initial tear occurring in the meniscus may not be identifiable after several different planes of tearing have resulted.
Degenerative tears often refer to complex tears. These present with marked irregularity and complex tearing within the meniscus. These are most often seen in older patients.

■ TYPES OF MENISCAL EXCISIONS

O'Connor separated meniscal excisions into three categories depending on the amount of meniscal tissue to be removed (Fig. 3.13).

▌ PARTIAL MENISCECTOMY

In this type of meniscal excision, only the loose, unstable meniscal fragments are excised, such as the displaceable inner edge in bucket-handle tears, the flaps in flap tears, or the flaps in oblique tears. In partial meniscectomies, a stable and balanced peripheral rim of healthy meniscal tissue is preserved.

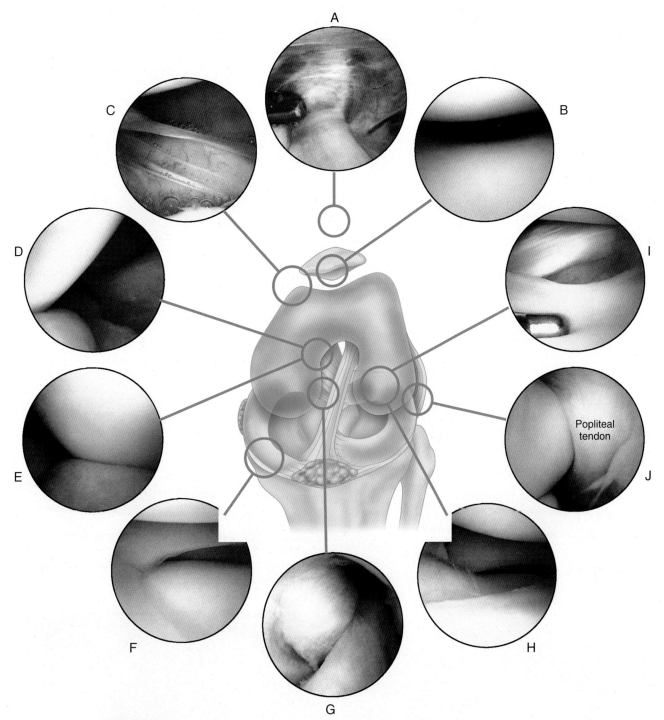

FIGURE 3.6 **A,** Suprapatellar pouch with view of undersurface of articularis genu. **B,** Tangential view of patellofemoral articulation. **C,** Normal medial parapatellar plica. **D,** Posteromedial compartment is seen by passing arthroscope through intercondylar notch after viewing medial compartment. **E,** Posteromedial compartment is seen through posteromedial portal, which is made after completion of routine examination if complete posteromedial view is unsatisfactory. **F,** Medial meniscus and medial compartment. **G,** Cruciate ligaments with fatty synovium covering posterior cruciate ligament. **H,** View of lateral meniscus and lateral compartment. **I,** View of posterior horn of lateral meniscus and popliteal tendon through hiatus. **J,** Posterolateral view of knee with arthroscope in anterolateral portal showing popliteal tendon insertion into femur in popliteal hiatus.

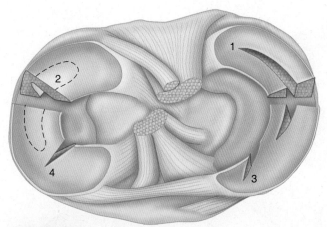

FIGURE 3.7 Four basic patterns of meniscal tears: *1,* longitudinal; *2,* horizontal; *3,* oblique; and *4,* radial.

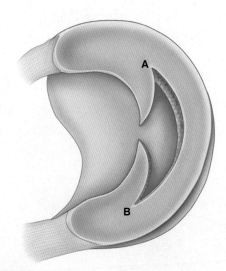

FIGURE 3.10 Diagram of posterior oblique *(A)* and anterior oblique *(B)* tears.

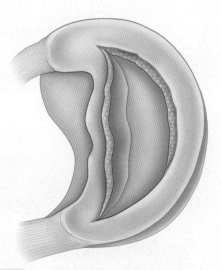

FIGURE 3.8 Bucket-handle tear, displaced centrally.

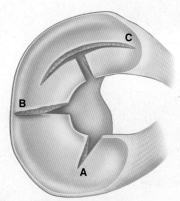

FIGURE 3.11 Radial tears: incomplete radial tear involves part of width of meniscus *(A)*; complete radial tear extends to periphery *(B)*; and incomplete tear, called "parrot beak tear," extends posteriorly or anteriorly *(C)*.

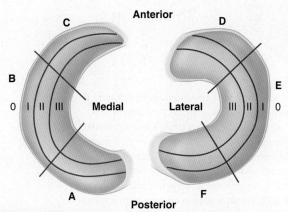

FIGURE 3.9 Zone classification of meniscus (modified from Cooper et al.). Most anterior zone of medial meniscus is labeled *C,* whereas most anterior zone of lateral meniscus is labeled *D. 0* is meniscosynovial junction; *I* is outer third, *II* is middle third, and *III* is inner third of each meniscus.

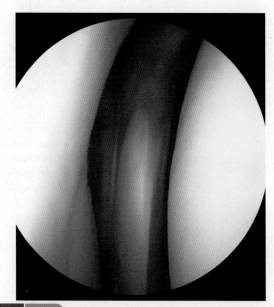

FIGURE 3.12 Healed posterior horn lateral meniscus.

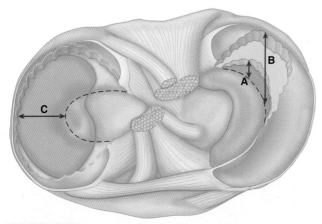

FIGURE 3.13 Types of meniscal excision: partial meniscectomy *(A)*; subtotal meniscectomy *(B)*; and total meniscectomy *(C)*.

SUBTOTAL MENISCECTOMY

In this type of meniscectomy, the type and extent of the tear require excision of a portion of the peripheral rim of the meniscus. This is most commonly required in complex or degenerative tears of the posterior horn of either meniscus. Resection of the involved portion by necessity extends out to and includes the peripheral rim of the meniscus. It is termed *subtotal* because in most cases most of the anterior horn and a portion of the middle third of the meniscus are not resected.

GENERAL PRINCIPLES

- Preserve functional meniscus; resect and contour the damaged tissue.
- When possible, repair horizontal tears in the vascular zone and longitudinal and radial tears in young patients.
- Repair the meniscus to protect the cartilage; protect the cartilage to repair the meniscus.
- Release the superficial medial collateral ligament with a spinal needle to allow joint opening and prevent articular damage when necessary to repair.
- Finally, check for a hypermobile lateral meniscus and any of the "3 Rs": rips, ramps, and roots. Wrisberg rips are tears of the attachment over the popliteus tendon that allows displacement of the lateral meniscus. A ramp lesion is a peripheral, posterior horn, medial meniscal tear associated with the pivot shift from an acute ACL tear. A posterior root tear must be identified and repaired in non-arthritic knees to prevent cartilage overload and degeneration.
- For partial meniscectomy use instrumentation in the ipsilateral portal with a straight or 15-degree up-curve instrument. For anterior tears, use curved or side-cutting instruments from the contralateral portal. Repairs are best performed outside-in for anterior tears and all-inside or inside-out for posterior tears, preferably from a contralateral portal to direct needles away from neurovascular structures.

SURGERY FOR SPECIFIC MENISCAL TEARS

As discussed earlier, tears of the menisci can be (1) longitudinal, either intrameniscal or peripheral, complete or incomplete, displaced (bucket-handle) or nondisplaced; (2) horizontal; (3) oblique; (4) radial; (5) flap; (6) complex; or (7) degenerative. No standard technique can be used in every case. The following techniques are useful in dealing with each of these types of tears through the anteroinferior portals. Even partial meniscectomy has been shown to increase joint wear; reasonable judgment must be used in planning meniscal surgery to preserve functional meniscal tissue. Planning begins in the preoperative period, ensuring the patient is fully informed as to the possibility of a partial meniscectomy versus meniscal repair and the postoperative course involved with each. Also, having the appropriate equipment and a thorough understanding of the incision and repair techniques are imperative.

As a whole, tears of the lateral meniscus are less common than tears of the medial meniscus. The radial tear configuration is almost unique to the lateral meniscus, occurring rarely in the medial meniscus. Also, the occasional discoid meniscus rarely is encountered in the medial compartment.

Most lateral meniscal excisions or repairs are done with the knee in the figure-four position: the hip slightly flexed, abducted, and externally rotated; the knee flexed at 30 to 90 degrees; and the tibia internally rotated. This position can be achieved with the foot of the table extended or flexed. With the end of the table extended, the ankle is placed on the table surface or on the opposite lower leg. In this position, the hip falls into external rotation, and a varus stress can be applied by pushing downward on the flexed knee. The figure-four position also can reduce overall joint distention by collapsing the suprapatellar pouch, making viewing and the use of suction and motorized cutters and trimmers in the lateral compartment more difficult. Inflow through the arthroscopic sheath allows for best visualization.

VERTICAL LONGITUDINAL (BUCKET-HANDLE) TEARS

This common tear usually occurs in young patients as a result of significant trauma. It frequently is associated with an anterior cruciate ligament injury, and the medial side is more commonly involved than the lateral side (approximately 3 : 1). Long tears that extend at least two thirds of the circumference of the meniscus produce an unstable fragment that locks into the joint by displacing in toward the notch (Fig. 3.14). The patient typically has episodes of locking in which the knee can be neither fully extended nor flexed. The fragment may displace and reduce with an audible and palpable clunk. There is associated pain and effusion. Occasionally, the bucket-handle fragment permanently displaces into the intercondylar notch. In these situations, the patient is gradually able to resume most activities but knows that something is wrong with the knee. The fragment may become distorted and fixed in place. Other bucket-handle tears divide in their central portion, creating two separate flaps, one based anteriorly and the other posteriorly.

A patient with a suspected bucket-handle tear who may be a candidate for meniscal repair should have this possibility discussed before arthroscopy. The most common criteria for meniscal repair include (1) a vertical longitudinal tear more than 1 cm in length located within the vascular zone, (2) a tear that is unstable and displaceable into the joint (Fig. 3.15A), (3) an informed and cooperative patient who is active and younger than 40 years old, (4) a knee that

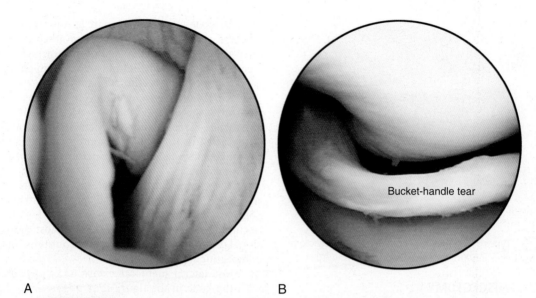

A   B

FIGURE 3.14 **A,** Bucket-handle tear of medial meniscus that has flipped into intercondylar notch; in this position, meniscus may cause intermittent symptoms. **B,** Locked bucket-handle tear of medial meniscus.

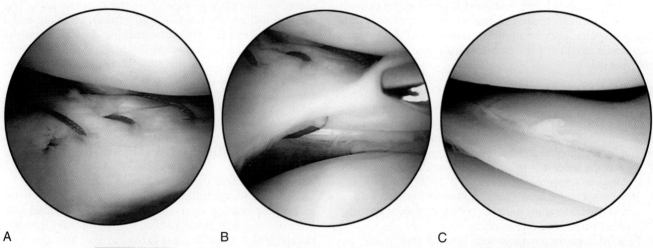

A   B   C

FIGURE 3.15 **A,** Unstable 2-cm peripheral tear of meniscus. Meniscus is being repaired with stacked vertical mattress suture. **B,** Incomplete undersurface tear of medial meniscus; this can be treated with abrasion to stimulate local healing followed by placement of one or two sutures. **C,** Complete 2-cm tear in avascular zone of meniscus; this type of tear generally is treated with excision, but if repair is attempted, use of fibrin clot and other local stimuli should be considered.

either is stable or would be stabilized with a ligamentous reconstruction simultaneously, and (5) a bucket-handle portion and remaining meniscal rim that are in good condition. Chronically deformed or degenerative menisci are not good candidates for repair. Most investigators report that only 10% to 15% of meniscal tears can be repaired and that most such repairs are done in association with an anterior cruciate ligament reconstruction.

Bucket-handle tears that cannot be repaired can be treated with partial meniscectomy. Early reports suggested that preserving a meniscal rim eventually would lead to better long-term results, particularly in stable joints with a normal weight-bearing axis.

Partially displaceable tears usually are shorter and confined to the posterior half of the meniscus. Often, these shorter tears are located peripherally and can be repaired. Tears that are less than 5 to 7 mm in length and stable to probing during which the tear does not displace more than 1 mm can have the edges and perimeniscal synovium freshened with a meniscal rasp. Talley and Grana noted a 21% failure rate at short-term follow-up of 19 patients with stable partial-thickness medial meniscal tears that were treated with perimeniscal rasping. For lateral tears, 4% failed. These authors recommended repair of partial-thickness medial tears. We also believe that an aggressive treatment approach should be used for medial meniscal tears.

When the decision has been made to perform a partial meniscectomy, the choice must be made as to whether to use a two-portal or three-portal technique. If the meniscal fragment has displaced into the notch, it should be reduced using either a probe or a blunt trocar. If the meniscal fragment is large or chronic, the medial compartment may have to be opened with flexion and a valgus stress to permit reduction of the fragment. The technique for resecting a displaced bucket-handle tear and the technique for resecting a nondisplaced, short, vertical, longitudinal tear are essentially the same. In each situation, a probe should be introduced and the tear should be examined with the probe to determine the anterior and posterior extents. The probe also can be used to plan the subsequent cuts. This examination usually is most easily conducted with the arthroscope in the anterior portal contralateral to the tear and the probe in the ipsilateral portal.

RESECTION OF BUCKET-HANDLE TEAR

TECHNIQUE 3.1

- For reduction of the meniscal fragment, use a probe or a blunt trocar to reduce the fragment to its normal position (Fig. 3.16A).
- Begin the technique with partial division of the posterior attachment of the meniscal fragment. This can be done with basket forceps, scissors, or an arthroscopic knife. Attempt to cut almost completely through the posterior attachment of the mobile fragment at its junction with the remaining normal meniscal rim (Fig. 3.16B). This cut should not be done blindly to prevent harm to the normal meniscus or articular cartilage or both. Exposure can be aided by passing the arthroscope through the intercondylar notch to look down onto the posterior horn of the meniscus while cutting, or a posteromedial portal can be made if necessary to look directly down onto the meniscus for visualization or to pass through the posterior compartment for cutting of the meniscus.
- Leave a small tag of meniscal tissue intact posteriorly to prevent the meniscus from floating freely in the posterior compartment after anterior release.
- Divide the anterior horn attachment with angled scissors, basket forceps, or an arthroscopic knife. Make the release of the anterior attachment flush with the intact anterior rim so that no stump or "dog ear" remains (Fig. 3.16C). If the approach is difficult from the ipsilateral portal, changing portal sites and approaching from the contralateral portal with the operating instrument often facilitates making this cut. Rarely, a midpatellar portal is necessary so that both anterior portals can be used for instrumentation.
- Use a hemostat to dilate the capsular incision before attempting meniscal removal.
- Insert a grasping clamp through the ipsilateral portal and grasp the meniscal fragment as close to its remaining posterior attachment as possible. Keep the meniscal fragment in view and twist and rotate the grasping forceps at least two revolutions while applying traction to avulse the small bridge previously created.
- If the meniscal fragment does not come loose as planned, use a grasper through the lateral portal for traction on the meniscus and pass arthroscopic scissors through the same

portal to complete the resection posteriorly. If it is still difficult with this technique, make an accessory portal, 1 cm from the anterior portal using the spinal needle. The other option is to make an accessory midpatellar portal for the arthroscope and use the two anterior portals for instrumentation.
- Observe the fragment as it exits the joint to ensure complete removal (Fig. 3.16D).
- Occasionally, the fragment is so large that it lodges within the subcutaneous tissues. In these circumstances, the skin incision may have to be enlarged to deliver the fragment. Additional longitudinal tears can be treated as previously described.
- If there are no further tears, use a motorized meniscal shaver to smooth the remaining rim.
- Before the procedure is completed, examine the posterior compartment with either a 30- or 70-degree arthroscope inserted through the intercondylar notch or a 30-degree oblique arthroscope inserted through the corresponding posterior portal.

POSTOPERATIVE CARE Partial weight bearing with the use of crutches is allowed for 48 hours until the patient is comfortable. Straight-leg raising exercises, ankle pumps, and range-of-motion exercises are started in the recovery room and repeated hourly during the early postoperative period. Wall sets are started 3 to 4 days after surgery. Stationary bike and progressive low-impact strengthening exercises are started when postoperative swelling has resolved. Return to sports is allowed around 3 to 4 weeks.

LONGITUDINAL INCOMPLETE INTRAMENISCAL TEARS

Longitudinal incomplete intrameniscal tears may extend from the superior surface into the body of the meniscus or may enter from the inferior surface. These often are extremely difficult to view and treat. This type of tear is commonly located in the posterior horn of the meniscus and may be only a few millimeters long. By the time such a tear extends more than 1 cm or 2 cm, it usually becomes complete and often displaceable. Usually a significant amount of stress must be applied to the knee to open up the appropriate compartment to view small tears. The first sign of such a tear may be a wrinkled or buckled inner meniscal border. If the incomplete tear begins from the superior surface, the probe tip passes into it but not through to the inferior surface. Inferior incomplete tears are even more difficult to view and explore, especially in a tight knee. The tip of the probe passes into the inferior tear but not through to the superior surface of the meniscus. Vigorous attempts to hook the probe into an unseen inferior tear should be avoided for danger of extending the tear. If such a tear exists, gentle probing can make the inner border of the meniscus buckle and evert (see Fig. 3.15B).

Stable peripheral one third tears in relatively healthy menisci should be treated by abrasion of the tear site and meniscal synovial tissue to stimulate healing, preserving meniscal function. If stability is in question, suturing may be indicated for most medial meniscal tears (see "Arthroscopic Surgery of the Meniscus," earlier).

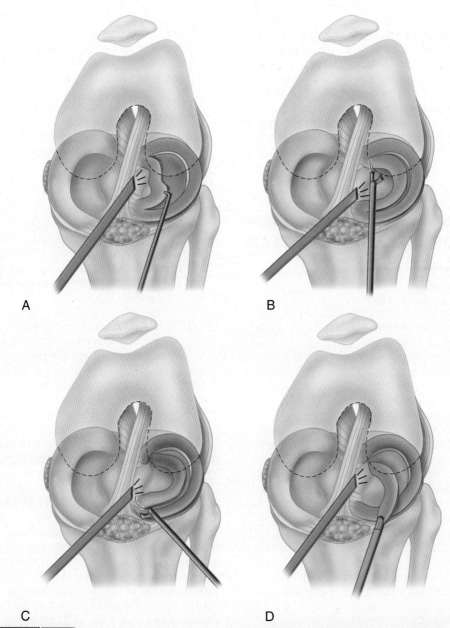

FIGURE 3.16 Two-portal technique for bucket-handle tears of lateral meniscus. **A,** Displaced bucket-handle tear of lateral meniscus probed. **B,** After reduction of displaced bucket-handle tear, posterior attachment is partially released with scissors. **C,** Anterior attachment is released with scissors. **D,** Tenuous remaining posterior attachment is avulsed with grasper and extracted. **SEE TECHNIQUE 3.1.**

REMOVAL OF POSTERIOR HORN TEAR

TECHNIQUE 3.2 *Figure 3.17*

- Use a 15-degree up-biting low-profile basket to make removal of a posterior horn tear easier.
- Carry the resection out through the ipsilateral portal, trimming back to a stable contoured peripheral rim.

POSTOPERATIVE CARE Postoperative care is the same as that described for Technique 3.1.

▌HORIZONTAL, OBLIQUE, RADIAL, AND COMPLEX TEARS

In evaluating horizontal, oblique, radial, and complex tears, it is imperative to evaluate and remove only damaged tissue while maintaining functional, healthy meniscal tissue. Ahn et al. reported successful repair of horizontal tears using a marrow stimulation technique and an all-inside suture device. With horizontal tears of long-term duration, a meniscal cyst may be present. This generally is evident on preoperative MRI and should be looked for during the arthroscopic examination. In most instances, the superior and the inferior leaves are resected back to relatively normal stable tissue. The cleft should be probed, and if there is a meniscal cyst present, a small curved curet can be placed through the cleft

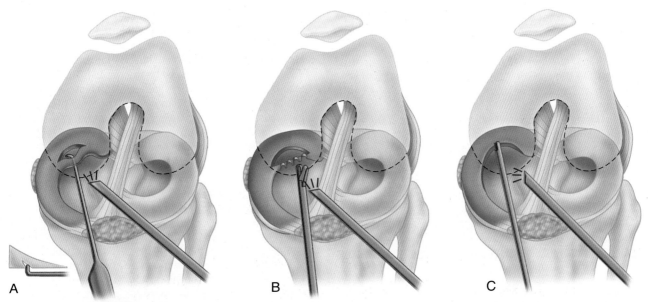

FIGURE 3.17 Technique for longitudinal incomplete intrameniscal tears. **A,** Probing longitudinal intrameniscal incomplete inferior surface tear. **B,** Fragment is removed bit by bit with basket forceps. **C,** Rim is smoothed and contoured with motorized trimmer. **SEE TECHNIQUE 3.2.**

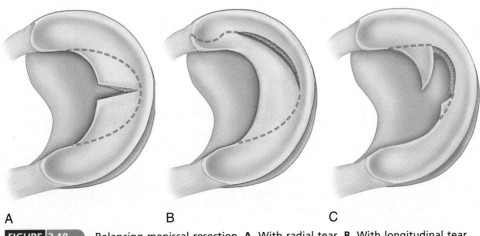

FIGURE 3.18 Balancing meniscal resection. **A,** With radial tear. **B,** With longitudinal tear. **C,** With flap tear.

aimed toward the surgeon's finger on the exterior extent of the meniscal cyst. This can be opened with a small curet, and the cyst can be drained into the knee. A shaver or suction without running the shaver also can be used to open and decompress the cyst. Localization also can be aided with the use of a spinal needle placed exteriorly to enter the cyst.

When evaluating flap tears, one must probe the meniscus in the tear site carefully. Often a flap can be rolled up under the normal portion of the meniscus and its size and contour are not apparent. Likewise, the flap can be posterior to the femoral condyle, and careful examination of the posterior compartments is necessary to evaluate these meniscal tears fully. Resection in the case of a flap tear or a complex tear generally is accomplished with a basket forceps to morcellize the tear, and careful probing is done to ensure that the meniscal tissue remaining is of relatively normal contour with a smooth transition at its edges.

Radial tears can be divided into partial and complete. A partial-depth tear of the meniscus is treated with saucerization,

balancing, and contouring of the edges (Fig. 3.18). Complete radial tears that go to the meniscosynovial junction are difficult problems. Many authors believe that horizontal mattress repair of the peripheral portion of the meniscus is indicated because resection would result in loss of the functional protective mechanism of the meniscus. This is discussed further in the section on meniscal repairs.

TREATMENT OF PARTIAL DEPTH MENISCAL TEARS

TECHNIQUE 3.3

- Examine the tear through the contralateral portal and probe it through the ipsilateral portal.
- Evaluate the extent of the tear.

- Use basket forceps or scissors to resect the torn and degenerative portion of the meniscus.
- Probe the stable meniscal rim to ensure there is no additional flap that is inverted under the meniscus or inverted behind the condyle. Horizontal-type tears should be resected back to a stable rim.
- If a meniscal cyst has been noted on MRI before surgery, open this area with a small curved curet passed from the contralateral portal, dilate the opening, and decompress the cyst. Localization can be accomplished with a spinal needle.
- Contour the meniscal fragment with a shaver after resection and remove small morcellized meniscal fragments.

POSTOPERATIVE CARE Postoperative care is the same as that described for Technique 3.1.

DISCOID LATERAL MENISCUS

Most discoid menisci are lateral; compared with other meniscal pathologic entities, discoid lateral meniscus is rare (0.4% to 5%). Bilateral discoid menisci generally are reported in less than 10% of patients. Discoid medial meniscus is reported to be present in less than 0.3% of knee arthroscopies. A discoid lateral meniscus may be discovered during a systematic examination of the knee in which another abnormality may be producing symptoms. The abnormality accounting for the symptoms should be appropriately corrected, and the discoid lateral meniscus should be left intact unless torn or degenerative. Careful evaluation of the superior and inferior surfaces of the meniscus is necessary to rule out a meniscal tear.

The most common method of classification of discoid lateral meniscus is that of Wantanabe et al., who described three types: complete or incomplete, based on the degree of coverage of the lateral tibial plateau, and the Wrisberg variant with absent or abnormal posterior meniscal tibial attachment. The current recommended treatment of a discoid lateral meniscus is based on this system of classification. Complete and incomplete lesions with tears of the discoid component are partially resected to a stable peripheral rim of lateral meniscus 6 to 8 mm wide. When healthy meniscal tissue is present, repair of the Wrisberg-type lateral meniscus is performed.

Good and excellent results have been reported in 55% to 94% of knees that have had a partial central meniscectomy or "saucerization." Preexisting degenerative changes, female gender, and age older than 20 years are associated with unsatisfactory results. We found at long-term follow-up that a significant percentage of patients had lateral joint symptoms after partial central meniscectomy, and others have reported similar findings. We try to preserve, contour, balance, and repair healthy meniscal tissue.

PARTIAL EXCISION OF THE DISCOID MENISCUS

The objective of partial excision of the discoid meniscus generally is to remove the central portion, leaving a balanced rim of meniscus about the width of the normal lateral meniscus. The width is dictated, however, by the location and extent of the tear within the meniscus. If the free inner edge of the meniscus is not noted in the systematic diagnostic arthroscopy of the lateral compartment, a discoid lateral meniscus may be responsible. The tibial plateau may be completely covered by the meniscus, and the lateral compartment may appear to be devoid of a lateral meniscus; alternatively, varying portions may be covered. If a discoid meniscus is suspected, careful exploration should be focused more centrally on the lateral compartment or over near the intercondylar eminence for a meniscal edge.

TECHNIQUE 3.4

- In young patients with small knees, use a 2.7-mm arthroscope and small joint instruments. In older individuals, use a medial midpatellar portal for the arthroscope and standard anteromedial and lateral portals for instrumentation.
- With direct vision of the meniscus, plan the resection so that a healthy peripheral meniscus of approximately 8 mm in width remains.
- With the knee in a figure-four position, use basket forceps to start the central resection of the discoid tissue (Fig. 3.19A and B).
- When the bulk has been resected, place arthroscopic scissors through the anterolateral portal to make a posterior, radially directed cut extending to the outer 8 mm of the meniscal tissue (Fig. 3.19C).
- From a lateral peripatellar portal, place a curved arthroscopic knife into the outer extent of the radial cut. Direct the incision anteriorly in a semicircular manner, preserving a peripheral rim of 6 to 8 mm of tissue. Complete the cut by changing the knife or scissors to the medial portal.
- When the desired amount of meniscal tissue has been removed and the rim is balanced, the thickness of the inner edge is much greater than that after routine partial meniscus excision.
- Thoroughly lavage and suction the joint.

POSTOPERATIVE CARE Postoperative care is the same as that described for Technique 3.1.

MENISCAL CYST

Meniscal cysts may develop from chronic medial or lateral degenerative meniscal tears; they most commonly involve the lateral meniscus. The site of the cyst usually can be differentiated intraarticularly by probing the meniscal tear fragments and opening the horizontal split in the meniscus with a small curved curet and passing it through the meniscal body into the central portion of the cyst. The cyst is curetted, and external digital palpation of the cyst is used to free up the cyst and decompress it into the joint. Suction may be used to remove the contents further. The meniscal fragments are removed and are cleaned up to relatively stable healthy meniscus.

Good to excellent results have been reported with arthroscopic partial meniscectomy and cyst decompression. If the cyst decompresses during the meniscectomy, no further

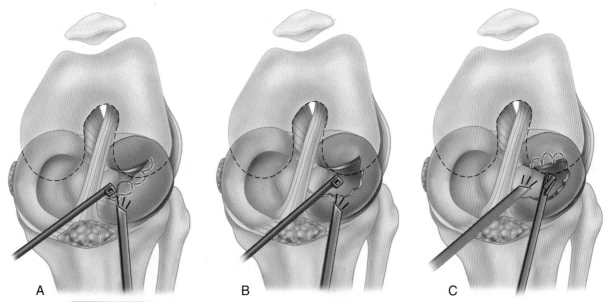

FIGURE 3.19   Technique for discoid lateral meniscus. **A,** Anterior portion of discoid lateral meniscus is removed with rotary basket forceps. **B,** Further contouring of anterior rim with 90-degree rotary basket forceps. **C,** Posterior discoid fragment is removed with arthroscopic scissors. **SEE TECHNIQUE 3.4.**

treatment is needed for the cyst. If the cyst does not spontaneously decompress, it can be percutaneously aspirated and does not require open excision.

■ ARTHROSCOPIC REPAIR OF TORN MENISCI

Although partial meniscectomy has yielded functionally better results than total meniscectomy, the ultimate outcome for partial meniscectomy remains suboptimal, with Fairbanks changes and functional deterioration much more frequent after partial and total meniscectomy than after meniscal repair. Multiple authors have found that joint deterioration after meniscectomy is accelerated with concomitant conditions of femoral and tibial chondromalacia, grade II or III anterior cruciate ligament instability, or tibiofemoral malalignment at the time of the initial meniscectomy. Partial lateral meniscectomies tend to do worse than partial medial meniscectomies. The lateral meniscus bears approximately 70% of the weight in that compartment, whereas the medial meniscus bears 50% of the weight in the medial compartment.

As noted earlier, only 10% to 15% of meniscal tears can be repaired, and these usually are associated with anterior cruciate ligament injuries. The only other positive correlations with healing have been found in patients who have a narrow peripheral meniscal rim (<4 mm) and when the repair is done within 8 weeks of injury. The length of the tear also has been associated with variations in healing, with failure to heal in over half of tears longer than 4 cm. The addition of a fibrin clot or marrow stimulation has been reported to increase the healing rate.

Arthroscopic repair techniques can be divided into four categories: (1) inside-out repairs; (2) outside-in repairs; (3) all-inside repairs; and (4) hybrid repairs, which combine the previous techniques. The inside-out technique can be done with double-lumen or single-lumen zone-specific repair cannulas, with absorbable or nonabsorbable sutures. The technique is rendered safe with the use of an incision for

BOX 3.1	
Repair Techniques and Indications	
Outside-in sutures	Anterior horn tears, midthird tears, radial tears, complex tears, reduction of bucket-handle tears
Inside-out sutures	Posterior horn tears, midthird tears, displaced bucket-handle tears, peripheral capsular tears, meniscal allografts
Fixator implants	Posterior horn tears, tears with > 2- to 3-mm rim width, vertical/longitudinal tears, midthird tears, radial tears

Modified from Sgaglione NA: Instructional course 206. The biological treatment of focal articular cartilage lesions in the knee: future trends? *Arthroscopy* 19:154, 2003.

exposure of the capsule and placement of retractors for safe retrieval of suture needles. The outside-in technique is most suitable for repairs of the middle and the anterior thirds of the meniscus.

All-inside repair techniques have been simplified by the development of suture fixators, which have pre-tied knots. These devices provide secure fixation and decrease the potential for chondral injury present in earlier devices. They are best used for securing tears that are 2 to 4 mm from the peripheral attachment. Because of the ease and speed of repair, greatly reduced patient morbidity, and midterm results that are equal to or better than those with outside-in sutures, most of our repairs are done with all-inside devices. Indications for the different repair techniques are listed in Boxes 3.1 and 3.2.

Regardless of the arthroscopic technique preferred by the surgeon, arthroscopic meniscal repairs consist of four

BOX 3.2
Authors' Preferred Techniques for Meniscal Repair
Meniscal body tears
—   All-inside devices
Meniscal capsular tears
—   Inside-out devices
Anterior root tears (8% of tears)
—   All suture anchors
Posterior root tears (10%-20% of tears)
—   Simple sutures, transtibial tunnel, and button fixation

TABLE 3.1

Meniscal Repair Versus Resection*

L—LOCATION FROM CAPSULE	<2 mm	0
	2-3 mm	1
	4-5 mm	2
A—AGE	<20	0
	20-40 years	1
	>40 years	2
S—SIZE	1-2 cm	0
	2-3 cm	1
	>4 cm	2
T—TISSUE QUALITY	Excellent	0
	Good	1
	Fair	2
QUALIFIERS	Unstable	2
	Malalignment	1
	Chondromalacia grade III	1
	Radial tear	2
	ACL reconstruction or fibrin clot	−1

*Higher scores associated with higher failure rates.
ACL, Anterior cruciate ligament.

important steps: (1) appropriate patient selection; the patient should have a documented meniscal tear that is able to heal, most often a single vertical longitudinal tear in the outer one third; (2) tear debridement and local synovial, meniscal, and capsular abrasion to stimulate a proliferative fibroblastic healing response; (3) use of marrow stimulation or orthobiologics to enhance healing; and (4) suture placement to reduce and stabilize the meniscus.

Tears can be categorized into (1) tears that can be rasped and left alone, (2) tears that definitely can be repaired, (3) tears that can be repaired under certain circumstances, and (4) tears that should be resected. Weiss et al. showed that peripheral tears of 7 mm or less heal without suture stabilization. Such tears should be probed to ensure less than 3 mm of displacement, and the tear and the meniscal synovium should be rasped to promote healing.

Tears that definitely can be repaired are single vertical tears in the peripheral vascular portion of the meniscus, the red-red zone at the meniscosynovial junction, or the red-white zone within 3 mm of the junction. These tears are displaceable, are more than 1 cm long, and involve minimal damage to the body of the meniscus. Generally, repair should be limited to patients aged 40 years or younger. A healing response is stimulated by rasping the tear and the perisynovial tissue. Tears that can be repaired under certain circumstances include tears 3 to 5 mm from the meniscosynovial junction. These tears, similar to all tears that can be repaired, should be evaluated with the tourniquet deflated to determine vascularity. In young, active patients with minimal damage to the meniscal body, suture repair in association with healing enhancement is most likely to be successful when anterior cruciate ligament reconstruction is performed concomitantly. If rasping produces bleeding, potential healing can be considered. Vascular access channels, achieved through meniscal trephination using an 18-gauge spinal needle to penetrate the peripheral meniscus to the synovium, can stimulate bleeding. When isolated tears are to be repaired, microfracture marrow stimulation of the intercondylar notch or addition of fibrin clot or platelet-rich plasma (PRP) should be considered. Resection is necessary for a meniscus with several tears, for tears involving damage or deformation of the body, and for tears that are definitely in an avascular (white-white) area (see Fig. 3.15C). Although complete radial tears are uncommon, they present particularly perplexing problems. When within the meniscal body, these tears disrupt all circumferential fibers. Although radial tears near the origin of the posterior horn of the lateral meniscus have been shown to heal, the biomechanical functionality of these repairs is in doubt. However, long-term results of repair may be better than those of a subtotal meniscectomy, especially in young patients (Table 3.1).

We often combine two or three basic arthroscopic techniques (suture-based meniscal fixator, inside-to-outside cannula technique, and outside-to-inside needle technique). If a large bucket-handle tear of the medial meniscus is suitable for repair, an initial stabilizing horizontal mattress suture can be inserted with a single-cannula or double-cannula technique in the midpoint of the tear near the posteromedial corner. Additional sutures can be placed posteriorly using the cannula technique from inside to outside or with a suture-based fixation device. The anterior portion of the tear, especially if this extends into the anterior half of the meniscus, is often best approached with an outside-to-inside technique.

If a patient has an unstable knee caused by an anterior cruciate ligament deficiency and a meniscal lesion that can be repaired, generally a ligament reconstruction and a meniscal repair should be done at the same time.

INSIDE-TO-OUTSIDE TECHNIQUE

TECHNIQUE 3.5

- Perform a systematic and complete diagnostic arthroscopy.
- If a meniscal lesion that can be repaired is noted after thorough probing to ensure that no additional meniscal damage is present, exsanguinate the extremity and inflate the tourniquet.

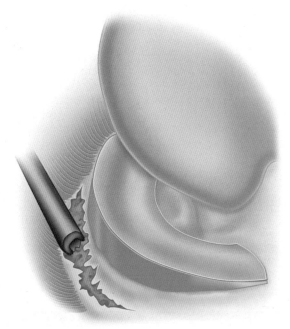

FIGURE 3.20 Preparation of meniscocapsular tear of medial meniscus through accessory posteromedial portal. **SEE TECHNIQUE 3.5.**

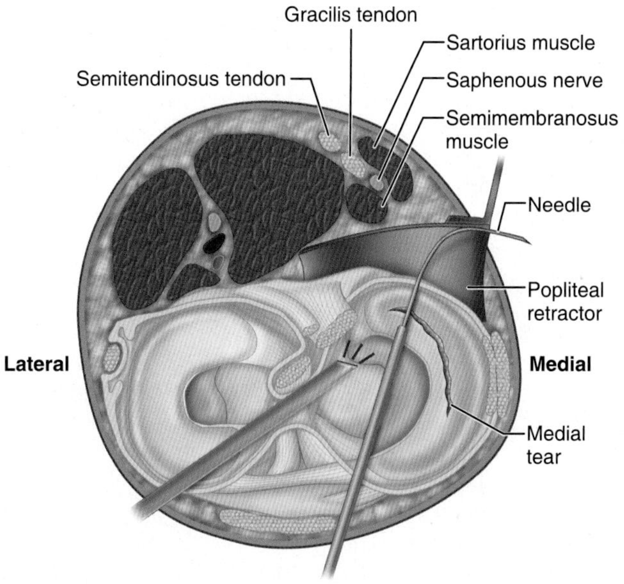

Gracilis tendon
Semitendinosus tendon
Sartorius muscle
Saphenous nerve
Semimembranosus muscle
Needle
Popliteal retractor
Lateral
Medial
Medial tear

FIGURE 3.21 Top view of joint with arthroscope, needle cannula, and popliteal retractor in place for medial meniscal repair. **SEE TECHNIQUE 3.5.**

- Have a leg holder in place for stressing the knee. This opens up the compartment to make viewing of the periphery of the meniscus possible.
- For repair of the medial meniscus, insert the 30-degree viewing arthroscope through the anterolateral portal and view and probe the extent of the tear.
- If the tear is acute and within the vascular red zone of the periphery of the meniscus, minimally prepare the rim before suturing. If the tear is clearly within the vascular red zone, do not resect that part peripheral to the tear. Resection of this material decompresses the meniscus from the peripheral side and has an effect similar to that of partial meniscectomy by narrowing the meniscus.
- If the tear is chronic, freshen and debride the torn surfaces, especially peripherally. Limit the excision to no more than about 0.5 mm of meniscal tissue if possible. This debridement and preparation of the torn surfaces can be accomplished with basket forceps, a shaver, curved meniscal knives, or small angled rasps introduced through the anteromedial, accessory medial, or posteromedial portal, while the tear is viewed with the arthroscope through the anterolateral portal. A small rasp is preferred for excoriating and abrading the meniscal surfaces (Fig. 3.20) and the superior and inferior parameniscal synovium.
- Specific cannulas are made to allow for the best approach to meniscal tears based on the location. Place the cannula in such a position to angle the needle away from the posterior midline structures and to place the needle perpendicular to the tear site.
- If a peripheral tear is beyond the posteromedial corner of the knee, use an all-inside meniscal fixation device or repair the meniscus using the inside-out technique.
- For the inside-out technique, first make a 5- to 7-cm incision over the posteromedial aspect of the knee, dissecting

through the subcutaneous tissue down to the posteromedial corner of the knee.
- Identify the interval between the medial head of the gastrocnemius and the posterior capsule of the joint and retract the medial head of the gastrocnemius posteriorly off the posterior capsule.
- Place a popliteal retractor in this interval to protect the popliteal vessels and to aid in capturing the needles (Fig. 3.21).
- Pass the cannula of the suturing instrumentation through the anterolateral portal and place its tip near the posterior limit of the tear.
- Remove the needle cradle and have an assistant load the cradle with the first needle.
- Pass the needle through the cannula to enter the meniscus 3 to 4 mm from the edge, aiming the needle in a slightly vertical direction so as to exit at or above the center of the torn edge. Observe the needle as it is advanced through the outer portion of the tear. Use the needle to align the meniscus anatomically before advancing through the outer rim. If good positioning is obtained, use the needle driver to advance the needle 1 cm more (Fig. 3.22).
- Pass the second needle to enter the meniscus or meniscosynovial junction peripheral to the first needle, forming a stacked vertical mattress or oblique mattress suture (Fig. 3.23).
- Pass the needles out through the capsule with the knee flexed 15 to 20 degrees while retracting the pes anserinus and saphenous nerve posteriorly.
- Clamp the paired sutures together with a hemostat.
- Vertical mattress sutures are placed from both surfaces of the meniscus in an alternating fashion every 3 to 4 mm. If it is difficult to maintain reduction of a bucket-handle tear, place the first mattress suture anteriorly to help hold the meniscus in place while subsequent sutures are passed.

- The choice of suture material has been varied. Some surgeons fear that all absorbable sutures would degrade before adequate healing and may cause an inflammatory reaction around the knot. Other surgeons are concerned that nonabsorbable sutures would remain as stress risers within the meniscus or cause abrasive wear to the articular surface of the femur or tibia or penetrate and capture the medial collateral ligament. To date, no studies have shown any deleterious effects of using absorbable sutures with a long tensile life or nonabsorbable sutures. We prefer nonabsorbable sutures for larger, more centrally located tears because of the prolonged healing time.
- If the tear involves mainly the middle third of the medial meniscus and the capsule has not been opened posteriorly to protect the neurovascular elements, make an incision over the medial joint line, before pushing the initial needle through the capsule and into the subcutaneous tissue.
- Expose the capsule parallel to the peripheral tear of the meniscus and throughout its length. Exposing this area before passing the sutures through the capsule lessens the likelihood of cutting the sutures in making the exposure.
- When all sutures are passed into this medial incision, tie them over the capsule. It is important to arthroscopically view the meniscus as the sutures are tied to ensure reduction of the tear site without deformation.
- The safest position of the knee for suture of lateral meniscal tears is near 90 degrees of flexion. The peroneal nerve drops more inferiorly with flexion and is protected.
- Make a 3-cm to 4-cm posterolateral skin incision, extending distally just anterior to the tip of the fibula with two thirds of the incision extending distal to the joint line.
- Develop the interval between the iliotibial band and biceps and retract the biceps posteriorly. Use careful dissection to reflect the lateral gastrocnemius head off the posterior capsule. Place a hip skid or needle deflector between the capsule and the gastrocnemius head.
- If the posterior extent of the tear is near the midline, protect the popliteal vessels before bringing the needles through the capsule by placing a wide metallic retractor between them and the posterior capsule. The common peroneal nerve lies slightly posterior to the posterior aspect of the biceps femoris tendon, so the needles must always exit anterior to the biceps tendon. It is much better, however, to make the posterior skin incision and expose the area of the posterior capsule and peroneal nerve before bringing the sutures through the posterior aspect of the capsule.
- If the posterior horn cannot be repaired from the contralateral portal, place the needle from the ipsilateral portal, directed away from the neurovascular bundle (Fig. 3.24A).

POSTOPERATIVE CARE There is no universally accepted method of immediate postoperative management of meniscal repairs. Currently, after an isolated meniscal repair, we place the extremity in an immobilizer for 7 to 10 days. Range-of-motion exercises (20 to 80 degrees) are begun immediately for 20 minutes four times daily. Touch-down weight bearing is allowed for the first 2 weeks, partial weight bearing for 2 to 4 weeks, and full weight bearing at 4 to 6 weeks. Jogging is allowed at 3 months, and squatting and return to sports are allowed at 4 to 6 months. If the meniscal repair is performed in conjunction with an anterior cruciate ligament reconstruction, we prefer to treat the ligament primarily. This involves placing the knee in full extension immediately and allowing early full range of motion. Touch-down weight bearing on crutches is continued for the first 6 weeks. When stable repair in the red-red zone has been obtained, we allow the patient to return to sports at approximately 3 months, provided that complete return of function has been obtained.

OUTSIDE-TO-INSIDE TECHNIQUE

With this technique, a suture is introduced through a spinal needle that is inserted from outside to inside. It has been recommended as a safe approach to the posterior meniscal horns. We have found this technique most appropriate and safest for tears located in the anterior aspect of either meniscus. Johnson used a suture retrieval technique in which the suture is passed through the spinal needle and a second needle is passed through the meniscus in a vertical mattress configuration. A wire loop is used to retrieve the first suture and pull it back through the meniscus, forming a mattress repair (Figs. 3.24 and 3.25).

Certain points for this technique must be emphasized. For posteromedial repairs, the knee should be flexed 10 to 20 degrees for the incision and for passing the needles to allow the sartorial nerve to lie anterior to the repair site. For anteromedial repairs, the knee should be in 40 to 50 degrees of flexion for the incision and repair to allow the sartorial nerve to lie posterior to the repair site. For lateral repairs, the knee should be flexed 90 degrees to allow the nerve to be posterior to the repair site. The meniscus and parameniscal tissue must be prepared with a rasp before the repair. A small, 5- to 6-mm working cannula should be placed in the ipsilateral side for suture management.

TECHNIQUE 3.6 *Figures 3.24 and 3.25*

- Make a small skin incision and extend it through the subcutaneous tissue down to the capsule opposite the site of the meniscal tear.
- Under arthroscopic observation, introduce an 18-gauge needle from outside to inside, penetrating the meniscal rim and the meniscal fragment.
- Remove the stylet and pass a doubled over 20-gauge wire or #0 PDS suture into the joint.

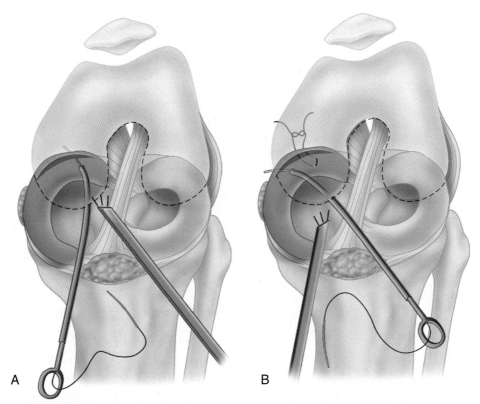

FIGURE 3.22   **A,** Most posterior sutures are placed with cannula in ipsilateral portal. **B,** Antero-lateral and midmedial sutures are inserted with cannula through contralateral portal. Stacked vertical or oblique mattress sutures provide better holding strength than depicted horizontal mattress sutures. **SEE TECHNIQUE 3.5.**

- Retrieve the doubled wire or suture through a 5-mm cannula in the ipsilateral portal.
- Use the wire or suture as a suture shuttle to pass one end of a nonabsorbable suture through the meniscus.
- Repeat the process, placing another needle 3 to 4 mm from the first one. Insert a doubled 20-gauge wire through the needle and retrieve it out the cannula to shuttle the second limb of the suture through the meniscus to form a vertical mattress suture.
- Tie down the suture over the capsule and repeat the process as often as necessary to stabilize the meniscal tear securely.
- For large peripheral lesions on the medial side, such as a displaced peripheral bucket-handle tear, a combination of inside-to-outside and outside-to-inside methods can be used.
- Place a single horizontal mattress suture, using a cannulated technique, into the midportion of the tear anterior to the posteromedial corner. This suture provides the necessary stability to the large bucket-handle fragment and prevents gross displacement when the spinal needle loaded with suture material is placed through the posterior and anterior horn regions of the fragment (Fig. 3.26).

POSTOPERATIVE CARE Postoperative care is the same as that described for Technique 3.5.

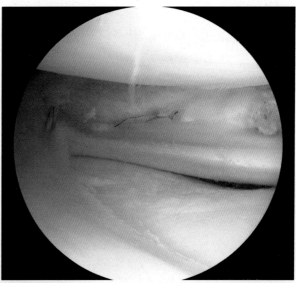

FIGURE 3.23   All-inside meniscal repair. **SEE TECHNIQUE 3.5.**

LATERAL MENISCAL SUTURING

TECHNIQUE 3.7

- The technique for suture placement on the lateral side is similar to that described for the medial side, with the common peroneal nerve most at risk when suturing the posterior horn of the lateral meniscus.

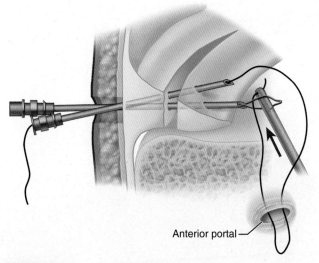

FIGURE 3.24 Johnson technique. Permanent suture brought in through anterior portal and placed into wire cable loop. **SEE TECHNIQUES 3.5 AND 3.6.**

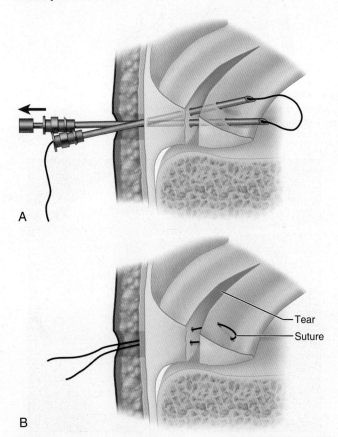

FIGURE 3.25 Johnson technique. **A,** Second suture is pulled through to complete suture attachment. **B,** Sutures are brought into place after needles and cable loops have been removed. **SEE TECHNIQUE 3.6.**

- Keep the knee near 90 degrees of flexion when suturing the posterior horn of the lateral meniscus because in this position the nerve falls well below the joint line posterolaterally. With the knee in nearly 90 degrees of flexion or in the figure-four position, posterior and posterolateral

suturing involves little risk of injury to the peroneal nerve if the needles enter and exit the capsule superior to the palpable biceps femoris tendon.
- Sutures can be placed inside-out or outside-in, in a stacked vertical mattress configuration. Place the sutures approximately 3 mm from the edge and space every 4 to 5 mm.
- If approximation and stability have been achieved, tie the sutures to each other over appropriate bridges of the posterolateral capsule. Tie the sutures with the knee in full extension.
- Immobilize the knee in a commercial knee immobilizer with the knee in extension.

POSTOPERATIVE CARE Postoperative partial weight bearing on crutches is maintained for 4 to 6 weeks, depending on the stability of the tear and the distance of the tear from the peripheral blood supply.

OUTSIDE-IN REPAIR OF COMPLETE RADIAL TEAR OF THE LATERAL MENISCUS

TECHNIQUE 3.8

(STEINER ET AL.)
- Position the patient supine with a well-padded pneumatic tourniquet placed on the upper thigh. Prepare and drape the operative leg in the usual sterile fashion. Exsanguinate the leg and inflate the tourniquet.
- Create a standard anterolateral portal, then an anteromedial portal under direct arthroscopic visualization.
- Conduct a diagnostic arthroscopy to ensure that there is no additional intraarticular pathology.
- Place the leg in a figure-four position and thoroughly examine the entire lateral meniscus for additional injury.
- Begin by debriding the central portion of the meniscus at the tear in the semilunar pattern (Fig. 3.27A).
- Place a PassPort cannula (Arthrex, Naples, FL) into the anterolateral portal, with the arthroscope in the anteromedial portal, and palpate and transilluminate the lateral joint line.
- Advance a Meniscus Mender II (Smith & Nephew, London, UK) needle through the lateral capsule and into the meniscus at an oblique angle to the tear, anterior-to-posterior, entering the posterior segment of the meniscus through the tear and exiting on the top surface (Fig. 3.27B).
- Make a 2- to 3-cm transverse incision directly on the joint line, and gently elevate skin flaps to expose the capsule.
- Introduce the loop of a Chia Percpasser (DePuy Synthes, Raynham, MA) into the knee joint through the needle and bring it out of the anterolateral portal with an atraumatic grasper.
- Pass a #0 nonabsorbable suture through the Chia loop and pull it through the meniscus and lateral capsule, leaving one limb of the suture remaining through the anterolateral cannula.

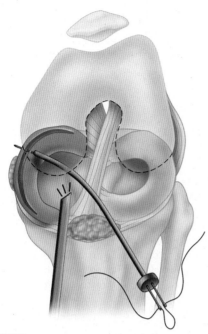

FIGURE 3.26   Suture placement in midportion of large bucket-handle tear using curved cannula technique. **SEE TECHNIQUE 3.6.**

- Make a second outside-in pass in the opposite direction to the first pass; this will have a starting point on the lateral capsule more posterior to the first pass.
- Advance the needle through the lateral capsule and into the anterior segment of the meniscus through the tear at an oblique angle, posterior-to-anterior, exiting on the top surface (see Fig. 3.27B).
- Repeat the insertion and retrieval of the suture passer, and pull the loop out of the anterolateral cannula.
- Insert the suture limb through the loop and bring it out of the lateral capsule. Gently pull on both limbs simultaneously, which should begin to reduce the meniscal tear. If not, an additional crossing suture may be needed. Tag both suture limbs for ease of identification.
- During needle insertion, stabilize the meniscus with a spinal needle introduced into the knee through the anterolateral portal.
- Insert a second suture in a standard horizontal mattress fashion. Insert the needle through the skin opening and into the meniscus, parallel and slightly posterior to the tear, exiting on the undersurface of the meniscus.
- Use the suture passer to pass a #0 nonabsorbable suture. Insert the needle parallel to the first, anterior to the tear, and exiting on the undersurface of the meniscus (Fig. 3.27C). Pass the suture limb and tag both limbs.
- Place the final suture in a standard horizontal mattress fashion, exiting on the top surface of the meniscus (Fig. 3.27D). This suture should be either slightly more central or peripheral than the first crossing suture depending on the placement of the first suture.
- Relax the knee to a neutral position, and tie the sutures over the lateral capsule in the order in which they were placed.
- Reinsert the arthroscope and inspect the repair.

POSTOPERATIVE CARE For the first 5 weeks after surgery, knee range of motion is limited to 90 degrees of flexion and weight-bearing is limited to 50%. A hinged knee brace is worn at all times. After 5 weeks, the brace is discontinued and full knee range of motion and full weight-bearing are allowed. Sport-specific drills are allowed at 3 months after surgery, with full return to sports involving pivoting, squatting, twisting, and running typically allowed at 5 months.

HIDDEN LESIONS: RIPS, RAMPS, AND ROOTS

A Wrisberg rip is a traumatic enlargement of the popliteal hiatus resulting in lateral meniscal mechanical popping during knee extension from a figure-four position that may not be identifiable on MRI (Fig. 3.28). Rips and ramp tears may be missed up to 50% of the time and root tears 70% of the time on MRI; thus a strong sense of suspicion for these lesions must be maintained if the symptoms and appropriate mechanism of injury are present.

A ramp tear of the posteromedial meniscal capsular attachment associated with an acute ACL tear may be missed 24% of the time if visual examination and probing are not carefully performed (Fig. 3.29). When symptoms warrant, a posteromedial portal may be necessary to find and repair this lesion. Using a posteromedial cannula and a curved spectrum, #0 sutures can be passed and tied with a knot pusher to secure the lesion. The Ultra Fast-Fix system (Smith & Nephew, Memphis, TN) also can be used to secure fixation in most cases.

Root tears may be visible on MRI (Box 3.3) and should be repaired when possible in patients younger than 50 years of age (Fig. 3.30). LaPrade et al. reported equal healing rates in patients younger than and older than 50 years of age if they had stable knees with normal alignment and grade 2 or lower chondral changes. Other studies have shown that patients with obesity, smoking, and extrusion of the meniscus of 3 mm or more have less satisfactory results. Meta-analyses have shown repair to be cost-effective compared to conservative treatment at 5- and 10-year follow-up. Partial meniscectomy is not beneficial.

LaPrade et al. described a classification system for meniscal root tears based on tear morphology (Fig. 3.31).

RADIAL TEARS AND MENISCAL ROOT TEARS

Radial tears that extend to the capsule may be repaired in young patients with otherwise healthy menisci. Synovial rasping followed by longitudinal repair, consisting of two longitudinal sutures on the superior surface and one on the inferior surface, is indicated in young patients willing to follow stringent postoperative protocol (Fig. 3.32).

Root tears of the lateral meniscus may do well by rasping and allowing them to heal in situ. Unstable root tears of the posterior horn of the medial or lateral meniscus may be repaired to a freshened posterior bony bed using an anterior cruciate ligament guide to drill from the anterolateral tibia to the base of the root footprint. A suture shuttle device is used to pass simple sutures through the meniscus and then out through the bone tunnel; the sutures are then tied anteriorly. The repair also may be accomplished using a 2.7 suture anchor placed through a high posteromedial portal.

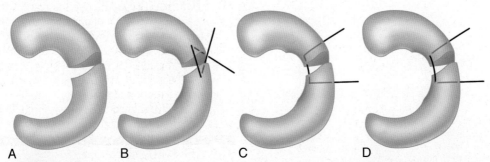

FIGURE 3.27 Outside-in repair of complete radial tear of left lateral meniscus. **A,** Debridement of central portion of the meniscus surrounding complete radial tear in semilunar pattern. **B,** First suture is crossing horizontal mattress stitch. This suture is essential for providing reduction vectors on tear without lateral displacement of meniscus. **C,** Second suture is non-crossing, horizontal mattress suture that enters peripheral body of meniscus and exits on undersurface. **D,** The third and final suture also is non-crossing horizontal mattress suture exiting on top surface of meniscus, more centrally located than first suture. (Redrawn from Steiner SR, Feeley SM, Ruland JR, et al: Outside-in repair technique for a complete radial tear of the lateral meniscus, *Arthroscopy Tech* 7:e285, 2018.) **SEE TECHNIQUE 3.8**.

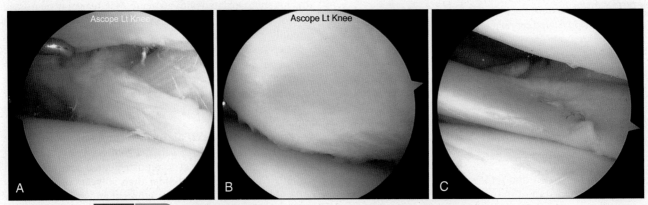

FIGURE 3.28 **A,** Meniscocapsular rip at the popliteal hiatus. **B,** Abrasion of undersurface of meniscus secondary to meniscal instability. **C,** Repaired rip.

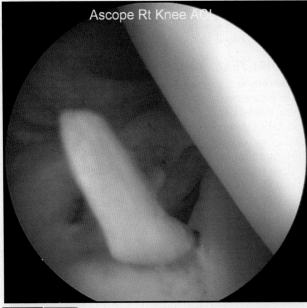

FIGURE 3.29 Posterior meniscal capsular ramp tear.

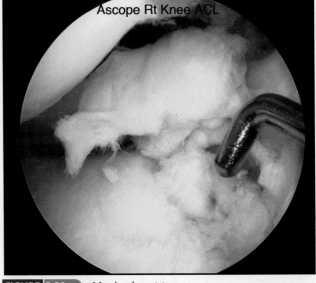

FIGURE 3.30 Meniscal root tear.

TRANSTIBIAL PULL-OUT REPAIR OF RADIAL OR MENISCAL ROOT TEAR

TECHNIQUE 3.9

(PHILLIPS)

- Make the initial arthroscopy portal in the compartment contralateral to the intended repair. Use a spinal needle to direct the intended working portal just off the edge of the patellar tendon, directed to the repair site. Insert a 5-mm cannula through which instruments will be inserted.
- Use a low-profile Arthrex guide to ream a 3-mm tunnel to the anatomic repair site. Make a 2-cm skin incision and clear soft tissues before reaming.
- After reaming to the anatomic repair site, withdraw the reamer 1 mm and rasp the repair site to stimulate healing.
- Pass a knee Scorpion repair device (Arthrex, Naples, FL) through the 5-mm plastic cannula, and pass a simple no. 0 FiberWire suture through the posterior part of the meniscus 3 mm from the tear site. Place the suture in the Scorpion with the tails equal in length. Retrieve the loop out the cannula, pass the tails through the loop, and tighten down the cinch knot.
- Pass a second suture through the anterior aspect of the meniscus and leave both pairs of sutures in the cannula.
- Push a nitinol loop up the reamer and retrieve the loop out the cannula. Shuttle the meniscal sutures down the 3-mm tunnel using the nitinol loop (Fig. 3.33).
- Pre-drill the cortex just distal to the tunnel and use a swivel-lock device to secure the sutures.

POSTOPERATIVE CARE Postoperative care is the same as that described for Technique 3.5.

ALL-INSIDE TECHNIQUE

There are numerous suture-based fixators on the market at this time. The holding strength and short-term follow-up healing rates using these devices approach that of inside-out suture fixation. We use these devices for most repairs. The advantages of these devices are the ease of use and elimination of accessory surgical incisions. The disadvantages are meniscal damage from deployment of the fixator, difficulty in obtaining a vertical repair, and the cost.

The same principles apply to use of all-inside devices as to inside-out techniques. Proper selection and preparation of meniscal tears and avoidance of vascular damage by aiming needles away from neurovascular structures and by setting the needle stop at 14 mm or 16 mm are necessary to penetrate the peripheral rim without over-penetrating and resulting in complications. Contralateral portals are made 1 cm above the joint line and predetermined with a spinal needle to allow best placement. Mattress sutures are passed through both superior and inferior sutures; use of curved needles makes this easier. Posterior sutures are placed first or, in the case of a bucket-handle meniscal tear, the meniscus is reduced with a mid-body suture first. Sutures must not be over-tightened to avoid their cutting through the tissues.

BOX 3.3

Clinical Pearls for the Diagnosis and Treatment of Meniscal Root Tears

Clinical Diagnosis
- Suspect in patients with posterior knee pain
- Evaluate for effusion and painful flexion

MRI Evaluation
- Evaluate for meniscal extrusion greater than 3 mm at level of the MCL
- Evaluate for ghost meniscal sign on sagittal MRI
- Evaluate for vertical linear defects on coronal MRI
- Differentiate true root tear from posterior horn radial tear
- Determine status of cartilage
- Evaluate for presence of bony edema or insufficiency fractures of ipsilateral tibiofemoral joint

Treatment
- Intimate knowledge of root insertional anatomy is essential for restoration of meniscal function
- Indications for surgical repair: young patients with traumatic tears and excellent chondral health
- Proper tensioning of root repair
- Proper anatomic placement of root repair on tibia

MCL, Medial collateral ligament; MRI, magnetic resonance imaging.
Modified from Bhatia S, LaPrade CM, Ellman MB, LaPrade RF: Meniscal root tears: significance, diagnosis, and treatment, *Am J Sports Med* 42:3016, 2014.

BIOLOGICS FOR HEALING

Although the exact role of fibrin clot, platelet-rich plasma, or stem cells in meniscal healing is unknown, many authors recommend its use when repairing isolated meniscal tears that are 3 to 5 mm from the periphery. Marrow stimulation can be accomplished when the medial wall of the intercondylar notch is reamed or drilled so as to protect the posterior cruciate ligament and create a channel to the cancellous bone. When anterior cruciate ligament reconstruction is done concomitantly, cell stimulation is unnecessary because of the hemarthrosis associated with the reconstruction.

Meniscal scaffolds have been used in Europe since the 1990s. Collagen scaffolds have been used the longest and have shown some evidence of decreasing symptoms after meniscectomy in some patients. More recently, polyurethane scaffolds have shown some evidence of ingrowth potential. These can be used in patients with more than 25% meniscal resection but stable peripheral rim and roots, stable, normally aligned knees, grade 1 to 3 cartilage changes, and post-meniscectomy syndrome. Currently, research into the functionality, effectiveness, and safety of these scaffolds is ongoing, and the devices have not been released for general use in the United States.

MENISCAL REPLACEMENT

Meniscal replacement continues to evolve using bone-plug techniques with better-defined indications and more asymptomatic results (> 90%). The question remains how much chondroprotective function a transplanted meniscus produces. In a meta-analysis evaluating meniscal transplants, lateral transplants performed better than medial transplants. At 5- to 10-year follow-up, approximately 85% of transplants survived; at longer than 10-year follow-up, survival rates of approximately 55% are reported.

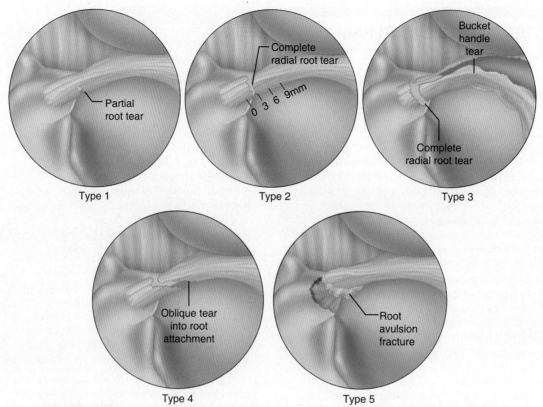

FIGURE 3.31   Classification of meniscal root tears based on tear morphology: partial stable root tear (type 1), complete radial tear within 9 mm from the bony root attachment (type 2), bucket-handle tear with complete root detachment (type 3), complex oblique or longitudinal tear with complete root detachment (type 4), and bony avulsion fracture of the root attachment (type 5). (Redrawn from LaPrade CM, James EW, Cram TR, et al: Meniscal root tears: a classification system based on tear morphology, *Am J Sports Med* 43:363, 2015.)

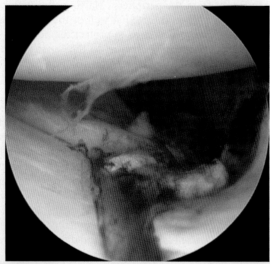

FIGURE 3.32   Repair of complete radial tear of lateral meniscus. Note that first vertical mattress suture approximates meniscal fragments. Later, more vertical mattress sutures are added to suture posterior aspect of capsule. At least two vertical mattress sutures are placed and often a third "stacked" vertical mattress suture is necessary.

The functional relief provided by meniscal transplant is clouded further by the fact that many of the patients had concomitant procedures for realignment, stabilization, or osteochondral transplant at the time of the meniscal transplant.

Cryopreserved menisci have been shown to perform similar to fresh frozen menisci with similar risks, in particular that of acquired immunodeficiency syndrome (AIDS; 1 in 1.6 million). Investigational studies of biologic tissue scaffolds for partial or complete meniscal replacement are in progress. These grafts may provide more acceptable replacements in the future, but at this time results are short term and limited in number.

Meniscal allograft is indicated in a patient who has had a previous meniscectomy, who is age 50 years or younger, and who has symptoms localized to the tibiofemoral compartment and no advanced arthrosis as evidenced by flattening of the condyles or excessive osteophyte formation. A joint space of 2 mm or greater on standing posteroanterior view is necessary. Contraindications include malalignment, instability that the patient does not wish to have corrected, chondromalacia greater than grade III, and previous joint infection.

In addition, the patient should be motivated, well informed, and willing to decrease impact-loading activities. When deciding whether a fresh frozen or a cryopreserved meniscus is to be used, one should be familiar with the allograft procurement and ensure that a quality, young, healthy graft is secured. Best results are obtained with a meniscal allograft that has a bone block or a bone bridge attached. Sizing is best done on anteroposterior radiographs, and MRI may be used to determine meniscal coverage.

A technique used at the University of Pittsburgh is described. The technique is divided into four parts: graft preparation, tunnel placement, graft insertion, and graft fixation.

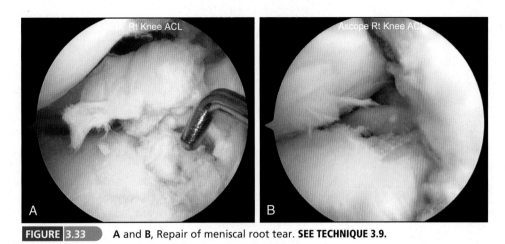

FIGURE 3.33   **A** and **B**, Repair of meniscal root tear. **SEE TECHNIQUE 3.9.**

MENISCAL REPLACEMENT

TECHNIQUE 3.10

GRAFT PREPARATION

- After patient positioning, diagnostic arthroscopy, and bed preparation, obtain a true lateral radiograph of the involved knee.
- Measure the anteroposterior diameter of the appropriate tibial plateau, taking into account any magnification factor.
- Thaw the fresh frozen meniscal allograft at a temperature of less than 40°F to prevent denaturing of the collagen.
- Prepare each meniscal horn bony insertion site to cylindrical 7-mm bone plugs (Fig. 3.34A).
- Place nonabsorbable sutures through the roots of each meniscal horn and respective bone plugs to allow for meniscal insertion, passage, and fixation into osseous tunnels (Fig. 3.34B).
- Demarcate the meniscus-bone interface with a sterile marking pen for accurate assessment of complete graft seating to the level of the bone-meniscal tunnel junction.

TUNNEL PLACEMENT

- Place the arthroscope and arthroscopic guide in the anterolateral and anteromedial portals to provide optimal exposure and tunnel placement for both lateral meniscal bony insertion sites. The anterior and posterior horn insertion sites of the medial meniscus are best seen with the arthroscope in the anteromedial and posteromedial portals. Placement of the arthroscopic guide in the contralateral anterior portal is optimal for each medial meniscal horn insertion site.
- After determining that the intraarticular placement of the arthroscopic guide is appropriate, place the extraarticular exit over the contralateral portion of the tibial metaphysis at the level of the fibular head midway between the tibial tubercle and the posteromedial or posterolateral border of the tibia. The advantage of drilling tunnels from the contralateral metaphysis is that tunnel divergence would be greater, providing a larger bony bridge between the two tunnels (i.e., less chance of tunnel "blowout").

- Make a 3-cm longitudinal incision in the skin and elevate the periosteal flaps. Enough exposure is needed for parallel placement of two 7-mm osseous tunnels with a 1-cm bone bridge between them.
- Drill the tibial tunnels under arthroscopic guidance.
- Insert a tibial drill guide through the appropriate anterior portal and seat it in the "footprint" of the meniscal horn bony insertion site.
- Drill a guidewire through the tibial jig.
- Remove the guide and confirm the position of the guidewire before creating the tibial tunnel.
- Overdrill the tibial guide pin with a 7-mm cannulated reamer.
- Debride the tibial tunnel of all soft tissue, chamfer and smooth with an arthroscopic rasp to facilitate bone plug insertion, and prevent graft abrasion at the plateau-tunnel interface.

GRAFT INSERTION

- Make an accessory 3-cm incision at the posteromedial or lateral corner as would be done if performing an inside-out meniscal repair.
- With careful dissection, expose the posterior border of the lateral collateral ligament laterally or the junction of the posterior border of the medial collateral ligament and the posterior oblique ligament medially.
- Make a 1.5-cm arthrotomy at the posterior border of the lateral collateral ligament and medial collateral ligament for lateral and medial meniscal allograft insertion.
- Using the arthroscope, pass a looped 18-gauge malleable wire retrograde through the posterior tibial tunnel to outside the knee through the vertical capsular incision located at the posterolateromedial border.
- Pull the sutures that were placed in the posterior horn and bone plug of the meniscal allograft through the posterior tibial tunnel with the use of the looped wire.
- Apply tension through these sutures to seat the posterior bone plug of the medial and lateral meniscal allograft.
- To avoid potential fracture of the anterior bone plug, a two-step process is used for anterior horn insertion and seating.

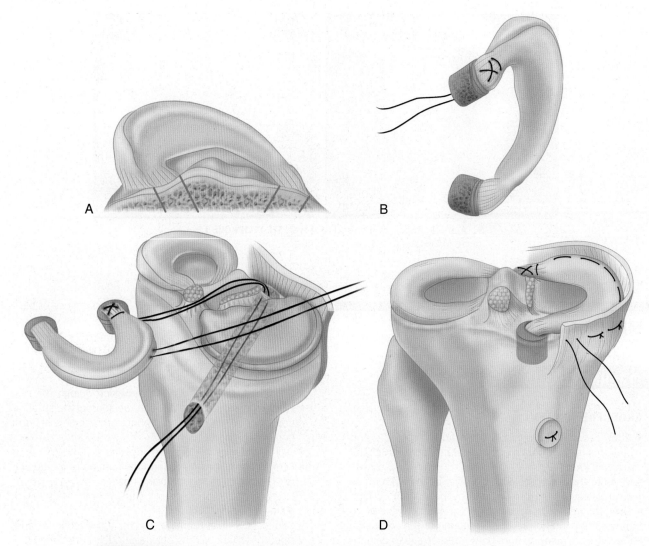

FIGURE 3.34 Double bone plug technique. **A** and **B,** Graft preparation. **C,** Insertion of graft, including reduction suture. **D,** Appearance on completion. **SEE TECHNIQUE 3.10.**

- Introduce the looped 18-gauge wire through the ipsilateral anterior portal and bring it outside the knee through the posterior capsular incision (Fig. 3.34C).
- Pull the sutures that anchor the anterior portion of the allograft out the ipsilateral anterior portal, guiding the anterior bone plug into the front half of the knee via the medial or lateral gutter.
- Carefully pass the anterior bone block along the gutter and take care to avoid fracturing the bone plug.
- Pass the malleable wire retrograde through the anterior tibial tunnel into the knee and bring it out of the ipsilateral anterior portal to accompany the sutures anchored to the anterior bone plug.
- Pass the sutures through the looped wire and guide them through the anterior tibial tunnel out the front of the knee.
- Reduce the anterior bone plug into the respective osseous tunnel under arthroscopy. This seats the meniscal allograft in its anatomic position with the anterior and posterior bone plugs in their respective osseous tunnels.

GRAFT FIXATION
- Place 2-0 Ethibond (Ethicon, Inc., Somerville, NJ) nonabsorbable sutures in a vertical or horizontal mattress fashion.
- Insert the sutures from the upper and lower meniscal surfaces to approximate the meniscus and capsule completely.
- When all the sutures have been passed, but before tying, apply tension to the peripheral, meniscal root, and bone plug-anchoring sutures while moving the knee through a complete range of motion.
- Closely observe meniscal kinematics while probing to assess stability and reduction. Tie the peripheral sutures over the capsule.
- Tie the sutures anchoring the tibial bone plugs over the bone bridge separating the tunnels (Fig. 3.34D).
- Perform a standard layered closure for each incision.

POSTOPERATIVE CARE The operated extremity is placed in a long leg hinged knee brace. Knee range of motion from 0 to 90 degrees is begun immediately postoperatively. The patient is permitted crutch-assisted partial weight bearing with the brace locked in full extension for the first 6 weeks. At 6 weeks, the brace is removed, and the patient is progressed to full weight bearing. Closed chain exercises are emphasized, and deep flexion is avoided for the first 6 months. Bicycling, swimming, and straight-ahead jogging at half speed are allowed at 3 to 6 months. Hard running, agility maneuvers, and full squats are prohibited until after 6 months. Competitive sports are prohibited until 9 to 12 months postoperatively.

ARTHROSCOPIC SURGERY FOR OTHER DISORDERS
■ LOOSE BODIES IN THE KNEE JOINT

Removal of loose bodies from the knee joint is especially suitable for arthroscopic techniques. A loose body may be a singular, isolated problem, or multiple loose bodies may indicate the presence of a more complex pathologic process, such as synovial chondromatosis. Every attempt should be made to identify the underlying process to manage the condition correctly.

Loose bodies can be classified into the following types:

1. *Osteocartilaginous.* These loose bodies are composed of bone and cartilage and are detectable radiographically. Osteocartilaginous loose bodies may originate from several sources, the most common being osteochondritis dissecans, osteochondral fractures, osteophytes, and synovial osteochondromatosis.
2. *Cartilaginous.* These radiolucent loose bodies usually are traumatic and originate from the articular surfaces of the patella or the femoral or tibial condyle.
3. *Fibrous.* These radiolucent loose bodies occur less frequently and result from hyalinized reactions originating usually from the synovium secondary to trauma or, more commonly, from chronic inflammatory conditions. Synovial villi become thickened and fibrotic, may become pedunculated, and may detach and fall into the joint as loose bodies. Chronic inflammations, such as tuberculosis, may produce multiple fibrinous loose bodies known as "rice bodies."
4. *Others.* Intraarticular tumors, such as lipomas, and localized nodular synovitis may be pedunculated and by palpation feel like loose bodies or, in rare instances, drop free into the joint. Bullets, needles, and broken arthroscopic instruments also may appear as foreign loose bodies within the knee.

REMOVAL OF LOOSE BODIES

TECHNIQUE 3.11

- Two techniques generally are used, based on the problem facing the surgeon: (1) small loose bodies are removed from the knee joint by suction and lavage of the joint, and (2) larger loose bodies are removed using triangulation techniques.

- Insert the 30-degree viewing arthroscope through the anterolateral portal. Rarely is bleeding a problem in loose body removal; inflating the tourniquet usually is unnecessary.
- Perform a complete systematic diagnostic arthroscopy, moving sequentially and systematically through the joint. If the loose body is large and radiopaque, preoperative radiographs give an indication of its location; however, it may have moved since the radiograph was taken.
- Search the joint systematically for additional loose bodies, including the suprapatellar pouch, the medial and lateral gutters, the medial and lateral compartments, the popliteal hiatus, the intercondylar notch, and the posterior compartments.
- If the loose body is in the suprapatellar pouch, it may float away from the arthroscope or grasping instrument. In addition, the slightest turbulence in the irrigation fluids or the slightest touching with the grasper frequently makes it move away. This can be reduced by turning off the outflow of irrigating solution and inserting a small suction tip. Frequently, the loose body is drawn to the suction tip, where it can be held until a third instrument is brought into the knee to grasp it.
- The loose body also can be trapped or stabilized by triangulating a spinal needle to it, piercing it with the needle, and holding it in place until a grasper is inserted, usually through a superolateral or superomedial portal (Fig. 3.35).
- When it is within the jaws of the grasper, slowly withdraw the loose body to the portal entrance.
- If necessary, enlarge the entrance so that the loose body can be extracted. It is better to enlarge the portal than to have the loose body slip from the grasper and become free again within the joint.
- If multiple loose bodies are present, remove the smaller ones first. Removal of the largest ones first may require enlargement of the portal and can result in significant leakage of irrigation solutions from the joint.
- When all loose bodies that can be seen have been removed, suction the joint, especially the posterior compartments and the intercondylar notch. Occasionally, this pulls small, previously unseen loose bodies into view.
- Try to identify, if possible, the pathologic process producing the loose bodies, and treat it appropriately (i.e., by biopsy, synovectomy, or chondroplasty).
- Loose bodies that gravitate into the posterior compartment can be seen with the viewing arthroscope through a posteromedial or a posterolateral portal or a central portal using a 70-degree oblique viewing arthroscope (Fig. 3.36).
- Triangulating a grasping instrument into the posteromedial or posterolateral compartment, with the arthroscope also through a posteromedial or posterolateral portal, can be difficult because of crowding and collision of instruments.
- Pass the 70-degree oblique viewing arthroscope through the intercondylar notch and into the appropriate posterior compartment, locate the loose body, and triangulate a grasping instrument through a posteromedial or posterolateral portal to remove it.
- Loose bodies also can be difficult to find in the anterior compartment around the fat pad under the anterior horns of the menisci. If it is difficult to find an anterior

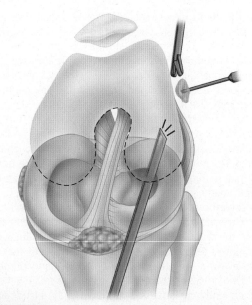

FIGURE 3.35 Removal of loose body. Loose body is impaled with needle, and grasper is inserted through superolateral portal. **SEE TECHNIQUE 3.11.**

loose body, add a midpatellar portal to view the area and allow instrumentation and probing through both of the anterior portals.

- Loose bodies large enough to require a major incision for removal can be removed in smaller fragments by morselization if desired. Do not use the delicate basket forceps or other arthroscopic instruments for this purpose, or severe damage to the instrument can result. It is better to use a Kerrison rongeur or an arthroscopic burr to break up larger loose bodies for removal.
- Remove pedunculated "loose bodies," caused by disorders such as nodular synovitis, using standard triangulation techniques after the restraining pedicle is cut with scissors.
- Instrument breakage during arthroscopic procedures may occur, and portions of broken instruments can drop into the joint. Under these circumstances, remain calm, turn off the irrigating solution, move the knee as little as possible, and always keep the fragment in view. Do not proceed with the intended surgical procedure until the instrument part is removed.

POSTOPERATIVE CARE Postoperative care is the same as that described for Technique 3.1.

■ SYNOVIAL PLICAE OF THE KNEE

Embryologically, the knee joint forms from three synovial compartments. Normally, these fuse into a single synovial cavity with the intervening synovial partitions resolving. The important synovial plicae of the knee represent unresolved remnants of these partitions. These plicae are synovial folds, usually classified according to their anatomic relationship to the patella: suprapatellar, infrapatellar, medial patellar, and lateral patellar plicae. They vary in frequency, size, thickness, and clinical significance. The term *plica* or *shelf* generally is used to describe a normal synovial fold; and if the plica

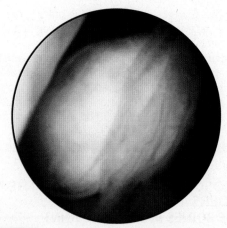

FIGURE 3.36 Loose body in posteromedial compartment. Complete knee arthroscopy should always include examination of posteromedial compartment. **SEE TECHNIQUE 3.11.**

is believed to be contributing to the patient's symptoms, it should be referred to as a *pathologic plica*.

The *infrapatellar plica*, or ligamentum mucosum, probably never produces symptoms but can make it difficult to pass the arthroscope from one compartment to the other; if it is prominent, viewing of the anterior cruciate ligament can be difficult. It can vary from a thin band of synovium running from the back side of the fat pad into the intercondylar notch to a nearly complete synovial partition separating the medial and lateral compartments. The *suprapatellar plica* is superior to the patella and partially divides the suprapatellar pouch into two compartments. Rarely does it cause symptoms in the knee. A *lateral patellar shelf* or *plica* has been described but is exceedingly rare.

The most common of these plicae to be of clinical significance is the *medial patellar plica*. Its incidence has been reported to range from 10% to more than 50% in normal knees. The frequency of the medial patellar plica and its possible role in the cause of anterior knee pain have been more greatly appreciated as diagnostic arthroscopy has developed.

The medial patellar plica begins just superior to the patella and sometimes continues with the distal extent of the suprapatellar plica, running distally along the medial side wall of the joint and over the medial femoral condyle to insert onto the fat pad. This structure causes symptoms only if it becomes thickened and inelastic from trauma or chronic inflammation. A common precipitating cause is a direct blow to the anteromedial knee region, traumatizing the plica. This results in swelling and inflammatory changes. Repetitive knee flexion and extension in such instances may cause thickening and hyalinization within the plica, leading to loss of elasticity. If this is accompanied by increased activities, the narrow, noncompliant structure may act as an abrasive band, rubbing across the medial femoral condyle instead of smoothly gliding over it. This abrasive action with time may result in chondromalacia of the medial femoral condyle. Pathologic medial patellar plica has a fairly thickened, rounded, fibrotic, and white inner border. As the knee is moved from extension to 90 degrees of flexion, this pathologic plica makes firm contact with the underlying femoral condyle at 30 to 40 degrees of flexion. Either a softened area of articular cartilage on the edge of the medial femoral condyle or a pannus of synovium growing over the edge of the condyle from the medial gutter is an additional clue that the plica may be pathologic and responsible for the patient's symptoms, provided that the examination and symptom complex are consistent.

Clinically, the patient usually describes striking the anteromedial aspect of the knee on a hard object, a fall on the anterior aspect of the knee, or some direct blow to this region. This is followed by a chronic, aching discomfort in the anterior aspect of the knee, which is made worse by activities. The patient also may sense a clicking sensation during flexion and extension of the joint. Effusion rarely is noted. On examination, a locally tender area well above the joint line on the anteromedial aspect of the knee usually is found. Occasionally, with active flexion and extension of the joint, a popping of the plica over the medial femoral condyle may be noted, more commonly at about 30 to 40 degrees of flexion. Sometimes this thickened fibrotic plica is palpable along the medial border of the patella.

The initial treatment of pathologic medial plica should be conservative. Modification of activities to reduce repetitive flexion and extension movements of the knee should be advised. The patient should avoid keeping the knee flexed for prolonged periods, and quadriceps exercises consisting of isometric and stiff-legged exercises are advised, along with a short course of antiinflammatory medications. Occasionally, immobilization of the knee in extension for a few days or a local injection may be beneficial. Progressive resistive exercises of the quadriceps should be avoided because these repetitive flexion and extension movements of the knee aggravate the plica. Conservative measures usually are beneficial in medial plica syndromes of short duration. If the symptoms are chronic and conservative measures have failed, arthroscopic examination of the knee and resection of the pathologic plica may be required. In a review of 135 adolescents (165 knees) with medial synovial plica, only 36% were pain free at an average 4-year follow-up; 46% had mild residual symptoms, and 18% had pain that was not improved by surgery. Most patients, however, were satisfied with their outcomes, and 87% were able to return to sports.

RESECTION OF PLICA

TECHNIQUE 3.12

- Perform a complete and systematic diagnostic arthroscopy to rule out other intraarticular pathologic conditions. If a thickened, inelastic, rounded, and whitish plica is noted, arthroscopic resection of the plica should relieve the symptoms.
- Examine the medial patellar plica with the 30-degree viewing arthroscope in the standard anterolateral portal.
- Confirm the pathologic nature of the plica further by viewing its superior aspect through a superolateral portal.
- If the plica is found to be pathologic, it is better to resect a large portion of it rather than simply to cut it. With the viewing arthroscope in the anterolateral portal, insert scissors or basket forceps through a superolateral portal (or side-biting baskets can be used through the anteromedial

portal), advance the scissors or forceps to the medial side wall, and, beginning at the superior aspect of the plica, excise 1 cm to 2 cm of it. A saucerization of the plica down to the synovial side wall should be the goal of treatment.
- Often, the initial division of the plica is accompanied by a snapping apart of the structure and a wide separation of its cut ends, indicating that the plica was under considerable tension. If necessary, insert the motorized shaver or synovial resector through the superolateral portal and remove the remaining tags of synovium and plica. Avoid overly aggressive synovial resection to reduce postoperative synovitis.
- Thoroughly lavage and suction the joint to remove any remaining debris.

OSTEOCHONDRITIS DISSECANS AND CHONDRAL DEFECTS OF THE FEMORAL CONDYLES AND PATELLA

Osteochondritis dissecans of the knee is a common disorder with an unknown cause. It is thought to result from ischemia of a localized area of subchondral bone, precipitated by infarction, trauma, or other causes. An area of subchondral bone becomes avascular, with subsequent changes occurring in the overlying articular cartilage. Osteochondritis dissecans must be differentiated from true osteochondral fractures and irregular ossification within the femoral condyles. Although it is well established that undisplaced lesions in skeletally immature children often heal if immobilized, surgery often is indicated for osteochondritis dissecans in mature or almost mature patients and for patients who have partially or completely detached fragments.

Osteochondritis dissecans of the femoral condyles has been classified radiographically, depending on the size and location of the lesion. Lesions of the medial femoral condyle have been described as central, laterocentral, and inferocentral (Fig. 3.37). Standard 45-degree posteroanterior, weight-bearing lateral views and patellofemoral joint views are helpful. Radiographs of the opposite knee also are necessary to evaluate for potential contralateral lesions. Bone age films to determine actual skeletal maturity are useful. MRI is an effective way to evaluate the size and integrity of osteochondritic lesions and may be necessary to determine healing of a lesion. MRI evidence of lesion instability is fluid under the lesion (in the crater) or subchondral edema.

Symptomatic lesions in skeletally immature patients are treated conservatively for 3 months, the duration being determined by the age of the patient, the size of the lesion, and whether it involves a weight-bearing area. Small lesions in non–weight-bearing areas can be treated with restriction of activities. For lesions 1 cm or larger in a weight-bearing area, the knee is immobilized, and partial weight bearing is allowed until some healing is noted on subsequent radiographs. Lesions destined to heal show some signs of healing over a 3-month period. The immobilizer is discarded after 4 to 6 weeks if symptoms permit. Partial weight bearing is progressed over the subsequent 4 to 8 weeks as healing progresses. Lesions showing no evidence of healing are considered for open or arthroscopic surgical treatment (Box 3.4). Early surgical intervention should be considered in

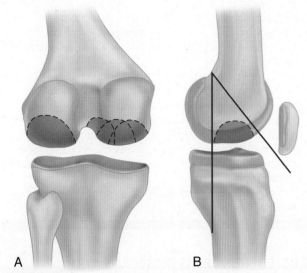

FIGURE 3.37 Locations of lesions of osteochondritis dissecans. **A,** Locations of lesions of medial femoral condyle (central, laterocentral, or inferocentral) and of lateral femoral condyle (inferocentral and often posterior). **B,** Lateral view of medial femoral condyle showing common location of lesions.

lesions that remain symptomatic (effusion and joint line pain) despite a conservative program. This is especially true in children approaching physeal closure. Incidental findings of an asymptomatic osteochondral lesion should be followed by repeat radiographs every 4 to 6 months until the lesion has healed or until skeletal maturity is reached. MRI is valuable in following the healing process. If after that time the lesion is still asymptomatic and radiographic findings are benign, follow-up should be on an as-needed basis.

Arthroscopic evaluation and treatment are indicated in all patients who are 12 years old or older as determined by bone age radiographs and who have lesions larger than 1 cm in diameter located primarily in a weight-bearing area. Lesions that are massive (>3 cm in diameter), lesions having large or multiple loose bodies that are thought to be replaceable, or lesions that are inaccessible to arthroscopic techniques are best treated by open arthrotomy. Treatment of the lesion is based on the arthroscopic examination. The lesions are classified into one of the following groups: (1) intact lesions, (2) lesions showing signs of early separation, (3) partially detached lesions, and (4) craters with loose bodies (salvageable or unsalvageable).

An intact lesion presents only a minor irregularity of the articular surface, with no break in the continuity of the surface. This is determined by careful arthroscopic probing. These lesions are treated by drilling multiple holes through the articular surface and into the subchondral fragment and underlying vascular bone. The use of imaging and retrograde drilling distal to the growth plate also may be used to preserve the articular surface. Because the articular surface viewed arthroscopically may show little or no surface irregularity, probing of the softened defect is the best means for identifying the lesion. Having preoperative images available and using an image intensifier during this process may assist in locating the site for drilling.

An early separated lesion presents an essentially intact smooth articular surface, but with greater irregularity than

---

BOX 3.4

Treatment of Chondral Lesions of the Knee (Least Effective to Most Effective)

- **Debridement**
  - Low demand
  - Low compliance
  - Mechanical symptoms
  - Minimal edema on T2-weighted MRI
- **Microfracture**
  - Contained lesion <2.5 cm, 8 mm deep
  - Moderate activity
  - Technique
    - Small 1- to 2-mm holes, 2-3 mm apart, varying depth
    - Prepare with sharp vertical walls and curettement of calcified basal layer
- **Cell transfer (ACI, MACI, JAC)**
  - Large lesion
  - Moderate activity
  - ACI: two operations required, third often necessary for mechanical symptoms
  - JAC: one operation, less cost, early results promising, insurance coverage?
- **OAT**
  - High demand
  - Lesion <2.5 cm
  - For best results, minimize cartilage trauma on insertion and maximize conformity of grafts to joint
  - Mini-open technique for two or more grafts
- **Fresh allograft**
  - Active
  - Lesion >2.5 cm
  - Moderate activity: 80%-90% success at 10 years
  - High activity: approximately 30% success at 4 years

ACI, Autologous chondrocyte implantation; *JAC,* juvenile articular cartilage; *MACI,* matrix-associated autologous chondrocyte implantation; *MRI,* magnetic resonance imaging; *OAT,* osteochondral allograft transplantation.

---

that of an intact lesion. The articular surface at some point shows a break in a small portion of the periphery of the lesion, and the fragment moves significantly when probed. These lesions should be treated by debridement and smoothing of the break in the articular surface followed by fragment stabilization. The fragment can be secured with bioabsorbable or metal screws. Screws have the advantage of fragment compression, which may be helpful in larger lesions. Non–weight bearing is necessary for approximately 6 weeks after surgery. Most metal screws need to be removed.

A partially detached lesion presents a greater disruption in the articular surface and, with probing, the lesion can be displaced or hinged on one edge. These lesions should be hinged open and the crater debrided to remove fibrous tissue and stimulate petechial bone bleeding. Occasionally, cancellous bone grafting in the crater base is required. When viewed arthroscopically, lesions that already have developed a loose body and a crater are treated by reconstruction of the crater, that is, by curettage and debridement to bleeding bone and by contouring and smoothing the edges and walls of the crater. If the loose body has detached recently, as indicated by hemorrhage or a little fibrous material within the crater, and the loose body can be replaced congruously, it is secured back

---

in the crater and stabilized. Displaced loose bodies with viable cartilage and some attached subchondral bone have been successfully reattached and have healed in more than 90% of patients in a study by Magnussen et al. The fragments were trimmed and cancellous bone graft added when necessary to fill the crater. When the fragment is not acceptable, the crater may be treated by microfracture or autogenous osteochondral transfer.

Osteochondritis dissecans of the patella may occur on the medial or lateral facet and the central ridge or the medial or lateral aspect of the trochlea. In the case of localized lesions, the first line of treatment is debridement and microfracture. For persistent mechanical symptoms with swelling and pain that does not respond to conservative treatment or microfracture, a second line of treatment in a mature individual with these lesions would be anterior medialization of the tibial tuberosity and autogenous osteochondral transplant as an open procedure if indicated. It is important to note that the condition of the surrounding cartilage, viability of the meniscus, stability of the knee, and alignment of the extremity weighs greatly on the long-term results of these lesions. Smoking and obesity negatively affect results as does age older than 30 to 45 years (Box 3.5).

in the continuity of the articular surface overlying the subchondral bone lesion.
- If the lesion is intact, perforate it with multiple holes using a 0.045-inch Kirschner wire. Position the Kirschner wire perpendicular to the articular surface, with the soft tissues protected by a sleeve or cannula over the wire (Fig. 3.38). Access for drilling inferocentral lesions of the medial femoral condyle usually is through the anteromedial portal; laterocentral lesions may be approached better by bringing the Kirschner wire through the anterolateral portal while viewing through the anteromedial portal. If the patient is not fully skeletally mature and the physis is open, take care not to penetrate too deeply and injure the physis. A radiographic image can be used to pass a 0.045-inch Kirschner wire starting distal to the physis and ending just proximal to the articular surface, thus preserving the cartilage. Passing one wire through the cartilage to exit laterally can act as a guide for the wires to be passed from proximal to the lesion.
- Thoroughly lavage and suction the joint and remove the instruments.

POSTOPERATIVE CARE Postoperative management consists of immobilization in a restricted motion brace, with the arc of motion controlled to prevent contact of the tibial articular surface with the lesion. Use of crutches with partial weight bearing is encouraged until early healing is noted radiographically. Four to 6 weeks of immobilization for young patients is common, whereas older patients with larger lesions should continue the immobilization and avoid weight bearing until definite radiographic evidence of healing is noted. Range-of-motion exercises should be performed for 15 to 20 minutes two to three times daily.

ARTHROSCOPIC DRILLING OF AN INTACT LESION OF THE FEMORAL CONDYLE

TECHNIQUE 3.13

- Perform a complete and systematic diagnostic arthroscopy with the 30-degree viewing arthroscope in the anterolateral portal.
- Inspect carefully the articular surface of the medial femoral condyle, varying the degree of flexion of the knee between 20 and 90 degrees to view the posterior extent of the lesion. The articular surfaces appear smooth except for a slightly raised irregularity at the borders of the lesion.
- Insert a probe through the anteromedial portal and carefully probe this irregular line to ensure there is no break

---

ARTHROSCOPIC SCREW FIXATION FOR OSTEOCHONDRITIS DISSECANS LESIONS IN THE MEDIAL FEMORAL CONDYLE

We generally prefer the use of an absorbable screw fixation technique for unstable fragments. For unstable fragments, metal screws provide greater security but must be removed. Bioabsorbable screws have less secure fixation, have variable absorption, and sometimes cause synovitis; however, removal may not be necessary.

TECHNIQUE 3.14

- Evaluate the defect and determine the best method of fixation. Displaced lesions that require contouring probably are best treated open through a parapatellar incision.

- For relatively stable lesions, debride the base and secure the lesion with cannulated bioabsorbable screws placed perpendicular to the lesion.
- If the defect is large, use cancellous bone obtained from the proximal tibia to fill the cavity.
- Secure the lesion with small 1.5- to 2.7-mm metal screws.

POSTOPERATIVE CARE Immediate range of motion is encouraged. Non–weight bearing with crutches for 12 weeks is necessary for healing and to protect the joint surfaces until the metal screws are removed arthroscopically if necessary.

OSTEOCHONDRITIC LOOSE BODIES

Osteochondritic loose bodies that are already completely detached and floating free within the joint usually are not suitable for reduction and fixation or bone grafting. Only a recently detached loose body with viable cartilage and bone and a fresh crater base is suitable for replacement and fixation. More often the loose body or bodies become rounded off and cannot be made to fit congruously back within the crater by either open or closed methods. In these instances, the loose bodies should be extracted from the joint, the base of the crater cleared of fibrous debris, the underlying eburnated and sclerotic bone perforated with multiple drill holes or abraded to bleeding cancellous bone, and the edges and walls of the crater contoured and smoothed without removing additional healthy articular cartilage.

Postoperatively, immediate motion and weight bearing are allowed. Prolonged protection in these circumstances does not seem to improve coverage of the base of the crater with fibrocartilaginous tissue. Constant passive motion for 6 weeks has proved effective.

Larger defects (1.0 to 2.5 cm) in a weight-bearing portion with a wall of intact cartilage surrounding the defect are preferably treated by use of an osteochondral autograft transfer (OATS) type of graft to plug the defect.

OSTEOCHONDRAL AUTOGRAFTS

The first reports of osteochondral autograft transfer were by Yamashita et al. in 1985 followed by Fabbriciani et al. in 1992.

The osteochondral transfer method for autogenous material has developed into two similar procedures. One method involves the use of individual donor cores 5 to 10 mm in size, whereas the other uses smaller plugs, ranging from 2.7 to 8.5 mm, which are believed to cause less trauma to the donor site and can be plugged into the recipient site to restore an area about 2 cm in diameter.

The larger graft, which proponents believe fills the recipient site with more cartilage, can be used in defects ranging from 1.0 to 2.5 cm. Many researchers think that the most advantageous size graft is 4.5 to 6.5 mm. When multiple grafts are used (mosaicplasty), an open technique is preferable to enable ideal restoration of the articular cartilage surface. When multiple grafts are taken, the defect is thought to fill with 60% to 80% of hyaline cartilage. To maximize cartilage transfer, a cartilage bone paste can be used to fill the small defects between the cartilage surfaces.

Osteochondral autograft transfer is indicated for patients who are younger than age 45 years and have a sharply defined defect with normal-appearing hyaline cartilage surrounding the borders of the defect. Lesions should be unipolar

and generally no more than 2.0 to 2.5 cm. Relative contraindications to the procedure are patients older than 45 years of age and obvious chondromalacia of the articular cartilage surrounding the defect. For best long-term results, normal mechanical alignment and a stable knee are necessary.

OSTEOCHONDRAL AUTOGRAFT TRANSFER

TECHNIQUE 3.15

- Inspect the osteochondral defect arthroscopically and measure the size of the lesion. Use a set of OATS sizer/tamps with heads of 5 to 10 mm to determine precisely the diameter of the defect. The color-coded tamps correspond in size with the diameter of the tube harvesters (Fig. 3.39A).
- Assemble the tube harvester driver/extractor.
- Load the donor tube harvester with the collared pin into the base of the driver and tighten the chuck. Screw a cartilage protector cap onto the back of the driver. When seated, the collared pin protrudes a few millimeters past the sharp cutting tip of the harvester to protect articular surfaces (Fig. 3.39B).
- When an acceptable position is established, drive the donor harvester with a mallet into subchondral bone or to a depth of approximately 15 mm. Avoid rotating the harvester during impaction.
- Remove the harvester and bone core by axially loading the harvester and rotating the driver 90 degrees clockwise and then 90 degrees counterclockwise (Fig. 3.39C).
- Fully insert the recipient harvester into the driver and insert the protector caps in a similar fashion. During socket creation, maintain a 90-degree angle to the articular surface to end up with a flush transfer. Rotate the harvester so that the depth markings are seen. Maintain a constant knee flexion angle during harvesting (Fig. 3.39D).
- After using a mallet to drive the tube harvester into subchondral bone to a depth of approximately 13 mm (2 mm less than the length of the donor core), extract the recipient bone core in the same manner as the donor bone core, and measure and record the depth of the core (Fig. 3.39E).
- Use the calibrated OATS alignment stick of the appropriate diameter to measure the recipient socket depth and align the angle of the recipient socket correctly in relation to the position of the insertion portal when using an arthroscopic approach (Fig. 3.39F).
- Reinsert the donor harvester, collared pin, and autograft core into the driver. Unscrew the cap and remove the T-handled midsection. This exposes the end of the collared pin that is used to advance the bone into the recipient socket.
- Insert the pin calibrator over the guide pin and press into the open back of the driver (Fig. 3.39G). Insert the donor tube harvester's beveled edge fully into the recipient socket. Stabilize the harvester during autograft impaction. Use a mallet to tap the end of the collared pin lightly and drive the bone core into the recipient socket (Fig. 3.39H).

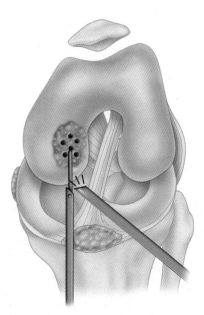

FIGURE 3.38 Technique for drilling intact lesion of osteochondritis dissecans. Multiple perforations of lesion of medial femoral condyle are made using Kirschner wire through anteromedial portal. **SEE TECHNIQUE 3.13.**

- Maintain a stable knee flexion angle and position of the harvester during this step. Carefully advance the collared pin until the end of the pin is flush with the pin calibrator on the back of the driver/extractor. This provides exact mechanical control to ensure proper bone core insertion depth. The predetermined length of the collared pin is designed to advance the bone core so that 1 mm of graft is exposed from the recipient socket when the pin is driven flush with the end of the pin calibrator. One can see the core insertion as it is occurring by viewing the core and the collared pin advancement through the slots in the side of the harvester.

- Alternatively, the core extruder is an option to using the mallet to insert the bone core into the recipient socket. Place the donor harvester into the chuck of the fully assembled tube harvester driver/extractor. As described previously, insert the beveled edge of the donor tube harvester into the recipient socket. While keeping the donor tube harvester firmly in position, slowly screw the core extruder into the rear of the fully assembled driver/extractor. Advance the core extruder by turning it in a clockwise motion, forcing the bone core from the donor tube harvester into the recipient socket. When the core extruder is fully seated, the bone core should remain slightly proud.

- Remove the donor tube harvester and position a sizer tamp, measuring at least 1 mm in diameter larger than the diameter of the bone core, over the bone core. Final seating of the bone core flush with surrounding cartilage is achieved by tapping the tamp lightly with the mallet (Fig. 3.39I).

- When multiple cores of various diameters are elected to be harvested and transferred into specific quadrants of the defect, each core transfer should be completed before proceeding with further recipient socket creation. This prevents potential recipient tunnel wall fracture and allows subsequent cores to be placed directly adjacent to previously inserted bone cores (Fig. 3.39J).

▌BONE GRAFTING

Cancellous bone grafts can be packed into the base of the crater in partially detached lesions before reduction and fixation to obliterate step-off. A cancellous graft can be obtained from the proximal tibia, using a trephine coring needle or similar device to obtain the harvest. This is placed arthroscopically or by open technique behind the osteochondritis dissecans lesion, packing it to a smooth surface before fixation with a cannulated screw. Autogenous chondrocyte implantation of the osteochondritis dissecans lesions should be contained and should have a depth of bone loss of less than 8 mm. Bone loss of more than 8 mm should be bone grafted, and a staged procedure should be performed 6 to 12 months later. These techniques are discussed further in other chapter.

Osteochondral defects larger than 2.5 cm are treated with allograft transfer or an autogenous chondrocyte implantation sandwich technique (Fig. 3.40). Osteochondritis dissecans treated with stacked "snowman" plugs have a reported short-term failure rate of 33%, and this procedure should not be routinely performed.

▌CRUCIATE LIGAMENT RECONSTRUCTION

The selection of grafts depends on the surgeon's preference and the tissues available. Among the autogenous tissues currently available, the most commonly used are central one third patellar tendon, quadrupled hamstrings of 8 mm or more, and, less commonly, quadriceps tendon grafts. Each of these grafts has been shown to have sufficient load-to-failure strength and stiffness to replace the cruciate ligament (Table 3.2). Another important consideration in selecting an appropriate graft is graft creep or stress relaxation of the graft over time, the occurrence of which may be more frequent with hamstring tendons than with ligaments, such as the patellar or quadriceps ligament. Fixation strength, including pull-out strength, graft slippage, and bony ingrowth, also is important. Fixation with interference screws, if performed properly, provides sufficient strength with bone–patellar tendon–bone grafts. Use of the BioScrew for fixation of soft-tissue grafts is enhanced by tunnel compaction and secondary fixation. The time of graft incorporation into bone varies considerably from study to study, ranging from 3 weeks for bone plugs to more than 3 months for soft tissues. Generally, bone plug graft incorporation into the tunnel occurs at around 6 weeks, with soft-tissue grafts taking 2 to 3 weeks longer. Aperture tunnel widening occurs to various degrees during the first 6 weeks and continues until 12 weeks, after which the tunnels begin to narrow somewhat.

Successful cruciate ligament reconstruction is best accomplished by secure anatomic graft placement and physiologic repair or reconstruction of all secondary stabilizers, including menisci. Failure rates for anterior cruciate ligament reconstruction have been shown to be significantly increased when preoperative 3+ pivot shift or hyperextension of more than 5 degrees is present. Anterior cruciate ligament plus anterolateral ligament reconstruction results in a less than 3% failure rate, 2.5 times lower than isolated anterior cruciate ligament reconstruction with bone–patellar tendon–bone graft, and 3.1 times lower than reconstruction with hamstring grafts. Failure of medial meniscal repair is 2 times lower with anterior cruciate and anterolateral ligament reconstructions combined. Abnormal varus alignment or tibial slope causes an increase in graft stress and failure. Double-bundle anterior cruciate or posterior

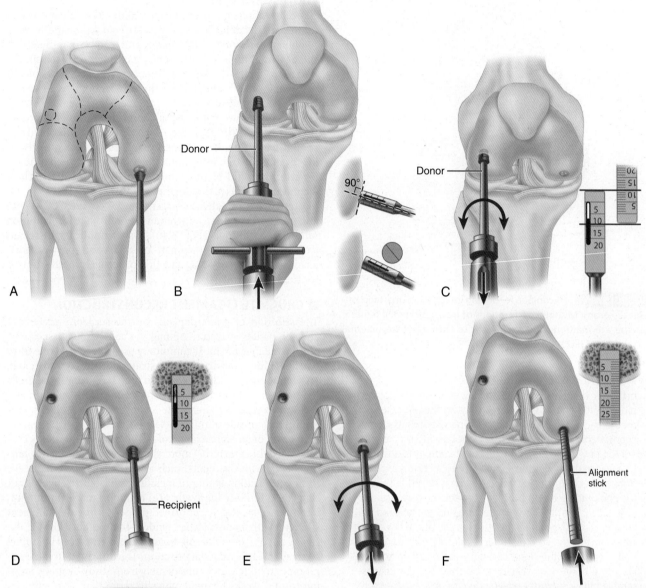

FIGURE 3.39 Osteochondral autograft transfer. **A,** Size of defect determined. **B,** Harvester driver extractor assembled with tube harvester and collared pin loaded. **C,** Harvester driven into subchondral bone. **D** and **E,** Harvesting of graft. **F,** Calibrated osteochondral allograft transplantation system (OATS) alignment stick of appropriate diameter used to measure recipient socket depth and align angle of recipient socket correctly to position of insertion portal.

cruciate ligament reconstruction has not shown clinically significant functional improvement. Likewise for posterior cruciate ligament reconstruction, no clinically significant improvements in functional results are obtained using inlay compared to transtibial or allograft compared to autografts. There is a clear difference in autograft superiority in anterior cruciate ligament reconstruction in young athletes and should be routinely used. Finally, snug suspension fixation allows more graft-to-bone contact and more complete healing for soft-tissue grafts.

Donor morbidity and cosmesis also must be considered when choosing a graft. Bone–patellar tendon–bone harvest is associated with increased risk for patellar tendinitis, especially if larger grafts are harvested. Acute and delayed stress fractures of the patella resulting from taking too deep of a

graft also have been reported. Properly harvested tendon and rehabilitation show no significant difference in arthritis. The weakness from harvesting two hamstrings approaches 20%. Injury to the saphenous nerve from graft harvest can be detrimental. The ideal graft and graft fixation techniques are still being developed. Currently, patellar tendon and hamstring grafts, when fixed at the joint line with secondary fixation on the tibia, have almost equal reported results, slightly favoring the patellar tendon for stability and lower failure rate. The ultimate goals of anterior cruciate ligament surgery are a graft with low morbidity; excellent cosmesis, strength, and stiffness; and secure early fixation and incorporation near the joint line.

At this time, there are over 100,000 anterior cruciate ligament reconstructions done yearly, with the number

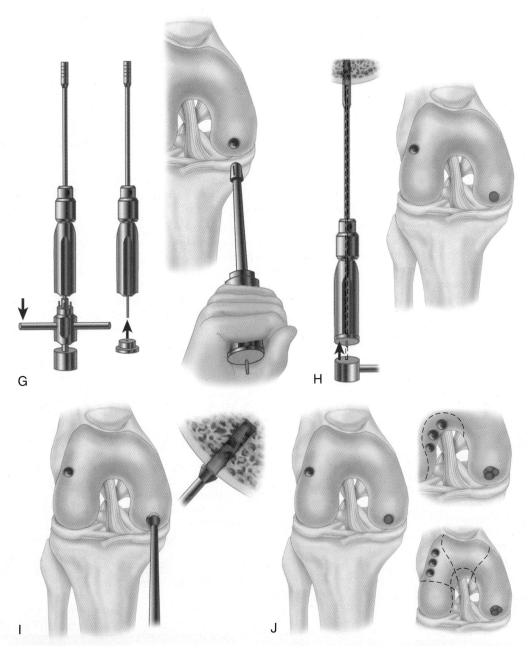

G

H

I

J

FIGURE 3.39, Cont'd **G,** Donor harvester, collared pin, and autograft core reinserted into driver. **H,** Donor tube harvester inserted into recipient socket. **I,** Sizer tamp, measuring 1 mm in diameter larger than bone core, positioned over bone core. **J,** Harvested and transferred cores. **SEE TECHNIQUE 3.15.**

increasing. Also, the number of allografts being used for primary and revision procedures is increasing. The advantages of using allografts are decreased postoperative morbidity, improved cosmesis, decreased operating time, and preservation of the extensor mechanism, which may eliminate some postoperative symptoms of tendinitis or chondromalacia. Arguments against using allografts are that the length of time for allograft maturation and the percentage of incorporation of the graft into the ligamentous structure vary. Studies have shown failure rates in athletes to be as much as two to four times that of autograft. The potential for infection is low, including bacterial infection and hepatitis. The possibility of AIDS transmission is approximately 1 in 1.5 million.

The cost and availability of good, young allografts of appropriate length also is an issue. The increased use of allografts in primary procedures is making it more difficult to obtain these for revision or for multiple ligament procedures. The use of allografts in our opinion is best reserved for revision surgery in patients who do not wish to have the patellar tendon harvested from the contralateral leg and for patients with multiple ligamentous injuries in whom morbidity may be increased from harvesting a graft in an already severely injured knee. Allografts also may be useful in athletes who are negatively affected by harvest site symptoms. In revision surgery, reported failure rates range from 27% to 46%. The best results are obtained with the use of autografts. The first

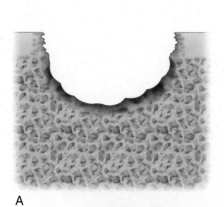
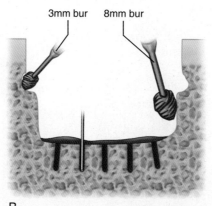
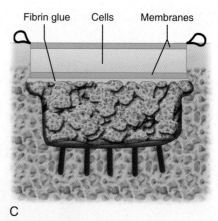

A B C

FIGURE 3.40 Technique for "sandwich" implantation of autologous chondrocytes. **A,** Osteochondral defect and bone defect are similar. **B,** High-speed burr, usually 8 mm in diameter, is used to remove all subchondral sclerotic bone back to healthy-appearing spongy bone. Base is drilled multiple times with a Kirschner wire to enhance the blood supply to the grafting site. A 3-mm burr is used to undermine the subchondral bone to secure the membrane when it is glued to graft with gentle pressure and covered by a neutral patty as the tourniquet is released and knee is brought into full extension. Neutral patty is removed, defect is separated and dry from underlying marrow space and bone graft. **C,** Second membrane is sutured to surface and sealed with fibrin glue. Cultured chondrocytes are then injected or "sandwiched" between two membranes. (Redrawn from Minas T, Oguar T, Headrick J, et al: Autologous chondrocyte implantation "sandwich" technique compared with autologous bone grafting for deep osteochondral lesions in the knee, *Am J Sports Med* 46:322, 2018.)

TABLE 3.2

Ultimate Load to Failure and Stiffness of Current Graft Selections in Cruciate Ligament Surgery

GRAFT SELECTION	ULTIMATE STRENGTH TO FAILURE (N)	STIFFNESS (N/MM)
Native ACL (Woo et al.)	2160	242
Native PCL (Race, Amis)	1867	—
Patellar tendon (Cooper et al.)	2977	455
Quadruple hamstring tendon (semitendinosus and gracilis) (Hamner et al.)	4140	807
Quadriceps tendon (Stäubli et al.)	2353	326

ACL, Anterior cruciate ligament; *PCL,* posterior cruciate ligament.
From Brand J, Weiler A, Caborn DNM, et al: Graft fixation in cruciate ligament reconstruction, *Am J Sports Med* 28:761, 2000.

attempt at anterior cruciate ligament reconstruction should be the best attempt.

The keys to surgical success are ample mental preparation, knowledge of recent literature, and proper patient evaluation, including assessment of potential stresses, ligamentous deficiencies (including the anterolateral ligament), and ultimate goals of the patient. This evaluation should help to determine what to correct and how and when to proceed with surgery. Finally, prioritizing the surgical approach is necessary as far as alignment, instability, articulation, and the meniscus are concerned. Preparation also includes knowledge of potential complications and the ability to recognize and resolve them (Figs. 3.41 and 3.42).

ANTERIOR CRUCIATE LIGAMENT RECONSTRUCTION

For pathologic laxity of the anterior cruciate ligament in an active, healthy individual who wishes to remain active, our preferred treatment is endoscopic anterior cruciate ligament reconstruction with patellar tendon autograft or a quadrupled hamstring graft of 8 mm or more. Surgery is performed as an outpatient or 23-hour admission after the acute inflammatory reaction has resolved. We use physical therapy to regain muscle tone and motion before the surgical procedure, which usually takes 10 to 21 days before surgery.

ANATOMIC SINGLE-BUNDLE ENDOSCOPIC ANTERIOR CRUCIATE LIGAMENT RECONSTRUCTION USING BONE–PATELLAR TENDON–BONE GRAFT

TECHNIQUE 3.16

- Place the patient supine on the operating table.
- After general endotracheal anesthesia has been administered, examine the uninjured knee to obtain a reference examination for ligamentous laxity. Examine the injured knee and record Lachman and pivot shift instability.

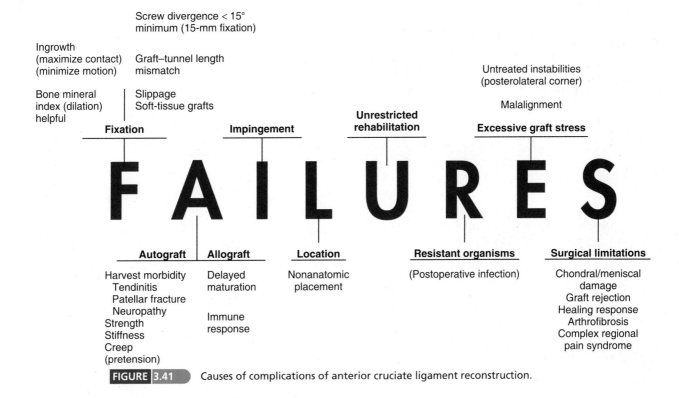

FIGURE 3.41 Causes of complications of anterior cruciate ligament reconstruction.

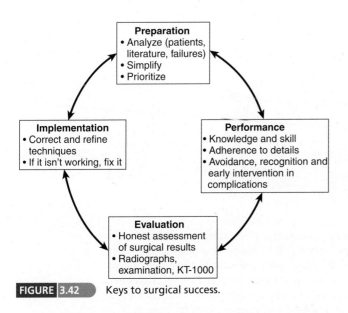

FIGURE 3.42 Keys to surgical success.

- Apply a tourniquet around the upper thigh and use a well-padded lateral post. Secure a 5-L intravenous saline bag to the table to act as a stop to maintain 90 degrees of knee flexion (Fig. 3.43A).
- Prepare and drape the extremity with standard arthroscopy drapes and use an Esmarch wrap for exsanguination. Inflate the tourniquet to 100 mm Hg above the patient's systolic pressure.
- If preoperative examination revealed significant laxity, proceed with patellar tendon harvesting.
- Arthroscopic joint portals can be made through this initial skin incision. If the status of the anterior cruciate ligament is in question (Fig. 3.44), or if more than 90 minutes

of tourniquet time is anticipated for completion of the procedure, arthroscopy portals should be made for joint evaluation and notch debridement before inflating the tourniquet and making the skin incision for harvest of the patellar tendon.

- Inject the portals with lidocaine and epinephrine to help control bleeding and maintain hypotensive anesthesia. An arthroscopy pump can be used to maintain proper joint distention and to reduce bone bleeding.
- Unless contraindicated, administer antibiotics and ketorolac (Toradol) before tourniquet inflation (30 mg intravenously in patients younger than 65 years; 15 mg in patients older than 65 years or in those weighing less than 50 kg). Two additional doses can be given postoperatively, not to exceed 120 mg or 60 mg, respectively.

GRAFT HARVEST

- With the knee held in 90 degrees of flexion, make a 4- to 6-cm medial parapatellar incision starting inferior to the patella and extending distally medial to the tibial tuberosity. The length of this incision depends on the size of the patient.
- Expose the patella and tendon by subcutaneous dissection.
- Make a straight midline incision through the peritenon and dissect the peritenon from the patellar tendon, taking the flaps medially and laterally.
- With the knee held flexed to maintain some tension on the patellar tendon, measure the width of the tendon.
- Harvest a 10-mm-wide graft or one third of the tendon, whichever is smaller, from the central portion of the tendon, extending distally from the palpable inferior tip of

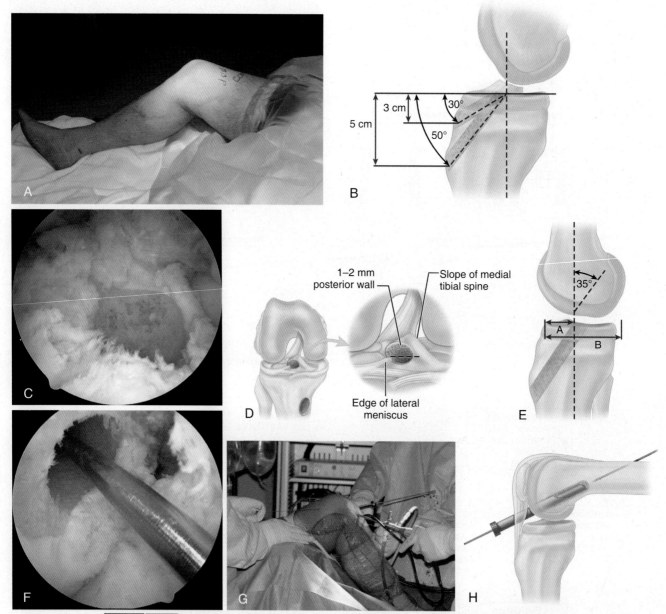

FIGURE 3.43 Anatomic single-bundle anterior cruciate ligament reconstruction. **A,** Saline arthroscopy bag is secured to table to assist in maintaining knee flexion. **B,** Increase in tibial guide angle. Length of tunnel can be increased. **C,** Tibial tunnel using inner edge of lateral meniscus and medial tibial spine as reference points. Tibial tunnel should be reamed into edge of medial spine and should be centered just slightly anterior to inner edge of lateral meniscus. **D,** Three reference points—inner edge of lateral meniscus, base of medial spine, and posterior cruciate ligament—are used for tibial guidewire. **E,** Tibial tunnel should be posterior to roof of altered intercondylar notch to prevent graft impingement in knee extension. **F,** Note position of femoral tunnel, about 4 to 5 mm off articular surface and 2 to 3 mm anterior to over-the-top spot. **G,** With knee flexed more than 100 degrees, guidewire is placed up femoral tunnel through middle cannula. Interference screw is passed, ensuring that guidewire and traction suture is straight line and ensuring minimal divergence between screw and bone plug. **H,** Use of sheath to protect graft and to assist in placing screw parallel to graft. **SEE TECHNIQUE 3.16.**

the patella. Maintain straight, single-fiber plane incisions while harvesting the tendon. The size of the graft is individualized. For a large football lineman, an 11-mm graft or double-bundle graft may be indicated. For a small patient, a 9-mm or possibly an 8-mm graft and tunnels may be indicated.

- Use an oscillating saw with a 1-cm-wide blade to make the bone cuts. Run the saw blade 15 degrees oblique to a line perpendicular to the anterior cortex of the patella, keeping 2 mm of the saw blade visible, to make a cut 8 mm in depth. This cut should be about 10 mm wide × 17 mm long measured from the bony tip of the patella.

- Make 25-mm-long cuts distally and free the tibial graft with a curved osteotome.
- Flip the plug and place it back into the harvest site. Drill a 2-mm hole, 3 mm from the distal tip of the plug, and pass a no. 5 Tevdek suture (Deknatel OSP, Fall River, MA). An assistant should hold this at all times to ensure that the graft is not contaminated.
- Complete the patellar cut with the saw placed at the inferior pole of the patella, 7 to 8 mm deep and parallel to the anterior cortex.

GRAFT PREPARATION

- Secure the graft to the top drape on a previously prepared table that holds appropriate-sized bone plug trials, rongeurs, a 2-mm drill bit, a Silastic block, a skin marker, no. 5 Tevdek sutures on Keith needles, and an 18-gauge steel wire.
- Commercially available graft preparation boards make tensioning and graft preparation much easier.
- Contour the graft with the rongeurs so that it fits through the 10-mm trial, ensuring that the complete graft would pass through the trial.
- Drill a single hole in the patellar plug about 3 mm from the end.
- Bullet the end of the bone plug to make passage easier.
- Drill a hole in the tibial bone plug. This plug should be 20 mm.
- Place a no. 5 nonabsorbable suture through the better bone plug to be placed into the femoral tunnel and an 18-gauge wire through the other plug, which is placed into the tibial tunnel. The use of a wire prevents cut-out before firm fixation is obtained.
- Mark the bone-tendon junction on the cancellous side of the graft at both ends with a methylene blue pencil and measure the total graft length. Wrap it in a sterile saline-soaked sponge and place it in a safe holding location.
- Use electrocautery to make an inverted L-shaped flap through the tibial periosteum, starting about 2.5 cm distal to the joint line and extending distally 1 cm medial to the tibial tuberosity.

- Reflect the flap medially with a periosteal elevator to expose the proximal tibia for later placement of the tibial tunnel.
- Make standard anteromedial and anterolateral arthroscopy portals, taking care not to damage the remaining portion of the patellar tendon.
- Systematically examine the knee and evaluate and treat any associated intraarticular pathologic condition.
- Perform meniscal suturing before securing the anterior cruciate ligament graft.
- With the arthroscope in the anterolateral portal and a 5.5-mm full-radius resector in the anteromedial portal, release the ligamentum mucosum and partially resect the fat pad to allow full exposure of the joint during the procedure.
- Resect the soft tissue from the intercondylar notch and from the tibial stump by sliding the resector between the remaining stump of the anterior cruciate ligament and the posterior cruciate ligament. The opening of the blade should always be pointed superiorly or laterally to avoid damage to the posterior cruciate ligament.
- Leave the outline of the tibial and femoral footprint intact as a reference guide (Figs. 3.45 and 3.46). Visualize the lateral intercondylar ridge, the lateral bifurcate ridge, and the extent of the footprint that covers the lower third of the notch wall. Use an awl to make a hole in the posterosuperior part of the footprint so that the tunnel will have a 2-mm posterior wall and be about 5 mm superior to the articular cartilage in the posterosuperior aspect of the footprint just below the intercondylar ridge. After properly marking the footprint while visualizing from the anteromedial portal, the scope can be changed to the anterolateral portal and a small internal notchplasty can be performed to aid with graft placement.
- With the knee in 30 degrees of flexion to expose the opening of the notch, evaluate the available space between the posterior cruciate ligament and lateral wall and the architecture of the roof. Use a 5.5-mm burr to enlarge the notch as indicated. The notch should be opened to look like an inverted U. Do not extend the notchplasty

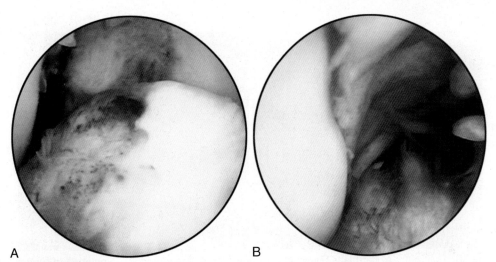

A   B

FIGURE 3.44   **A,** Calcified stump of anterior cruciate ligament after chronic tear. **B,** Empty lateral wall sign indicating anterior cruciate ligament-deficient knee; anterior cruciate ligament can be attached to posterior cruciate ligament, giving false indication of functional ligament. **SEE TECHNIQUE 3.16.**

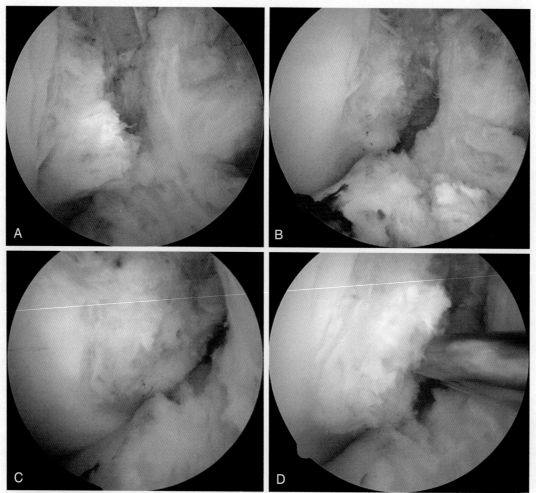

FIGURE 3.45   **A,** View of anterior cruciate ligament footprint using a 30-degree scope through a lateral parapatellar portal. Note proximity of anterior cruciate ligament footprint to articular surface of femoral condyle. **B,** Same footprint from medial parapatellar portal. Entire extent of footprint can be visualized more adequately through this view. **C,** Femoral footprint just posterior to center of anterior cruciate ligament footprint is marked with awl to use as reference point for reaming of femoral tunnel. **D,** Reamer. **SEE TECHNIQUE 3.16.**

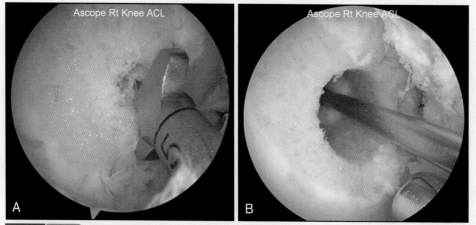

FIGURE 3.46   **A,** Flat-blade reamer for femoral tunnel preparation. **B,** Completion of tunnel preparation. **SEE TECHNIQUE 3.16.**

too far medially or superiorly, which would interfere with the patellofemoral articulation. Often, the opening needs to be enlarged only 2 to 3 mm superiorly and laterally. The burr can be placed in reverse to remove the articular fringe and smooth the initial notchplasty.

- As the notchplasty proceeds posteriorly, flex the knee from 45 to 60 degrees; when the notchplasty is complete, the knee should be at 90 degrees of flexion. Use controlled strokes with the burr from posterior to anterior. Posteriorly, open the notch enough to accommodate the 10-mm endoscopic reamer. Smooth the edges of the tunnel by placing the burr in reverse or by using an arthroscopic rasp.

TIBIAL TUNNEL PREPARATION AND DETERMINING APPROPRIATE LENGTH

- If transosseous drilling of the femoral tunnel is planned, the tibial tunnel will need to be placed at a 45-degree sagittal angle, starting just lateral to the medial collateral ligament. More acute angles tend to undercut the tibial articular suture and result in an oblique nonanatomic aperture. This does allow for a longer tibial tunnel, and the anatomic femoral footprint can be successfully reamed about 60% of the time through the tibial tunnel. A low medial portal may be preferable to independently ream the femur in the posterosuperior aspect of the direct fibers of the anterior cruciate ligament stump.
- When placing the tibial guide intraarticularly, be aware of the intended tunnel length and direction so that the graft can be secured in an anatomic, impingement-free position. Proper length and direction of the tunnel require a starting point approximately 1 cm proximal to the pes anserinus and about 1.5 cm medial to the tibial tuberosity to form a 30- to 40-degree angle with the shaft of the tibia. One should see this wire being directed to approach the femoral pilot hole (see Fig. 3.43B). Intraarticular reference points that can serve as guides include the anterior cruciate ligament stump, the inner edge of the anterior horn of the lateral meniscus, the medial tibial spine, and the posterior cruciate ligament (see Fig. 3.43C and D).
- When evaluating pin placement in a two-dimensional picture, in the anteroposterior plane, ensure that the guidewire exits just anterior to a reference line extended medially from the inner edge of the lateral meniscus. This point should be approximately 7 mm anterior to the posterior cruciate ligament and 2 to 3 mm anterior to the peak of the medial spine at the center of the anterior cruciate ligament footprint. In the mediolateral plane, ensure that the wire enters at the base of the medial spine or just slightly medial to the center of the anterior cruciate ligament footprint (see Fig. 3.43D).
- The unaltered roof of the intercondylar notch normally forms an angle of 35 to 40 degrees with the long axis of the femur (see Fig. 3.43E). To prevent impingement, an internal notchplasty, as previously described, may be necessary, as is appropriate tunnel placement. Use the tibial and femoral landmarks described earlier and place the guide at 55 to 60 degrees to the tibial plateau surface to obtain sufficient tunnel length and an angle that allows the graft angle to approximate that of the original. Measure the tibial tunnel length directly off the guide

calibrations and approximate the length of the tendinous portion of the graft. The tunnel length should be sufficient to allow at least 20 mm of bone to be secured in the tibial tunnel for stable fixation.

- If the tendinous portion of the graft is 50 mm long or less, increase the guide angle to produce a longer tibial tunnel. The tunnel can be easily increased to 45 to 50 mm long to accommodate the longer graft.
- Using the guide, advance the wire approximately 10 mm into the knee while observing through the arthroscope.
- Place a clamp over the intraarticular end of the Kirschner wire to prevent advancement. Ream over the wire with a reamer 2 mm smaller than the intended final tunnel.
- Leave the protruding end of the reamer in the tunnel and examine the tunnel for appropriate impingement-free position as the knee is moved through a full range of motion.
- Make necessary adjustments with the 8-mm reamer.
- Prevent bowstringing of the anterior cruciate ligament graft over the posterior cruciate ligament by leaving a 2-mm posterior wall between the tibial tunnel and the posterior cruciate ligament. By directing the tunnel just lateral to the posterior cruciate ligament, the graft lies on the posterior cruciate ligament without bowing around the ligament.
- Ream the tunnel with a reamer the size of the graft and use the full-radius resector to contour the edges of the tunnel and resect any remaining soft tissue that might block extension.
- Place a rasp through the tunnel to complete contouring and ensure that the external portion of the tunnel is free of soft tissue.

FEMORAL TUNNEL PREPARATION

- Visualize from a high anteromedial portal just medial to the tip of the patella.
- Use a spinal needle to identify the best position for a low medial portal about 2.5 cm medial to the patellar tendon and just above the meniscus. A guide is placed to ensure that the tunnel is just anterior to the anteromedial bundle; that is, leaving a 2-mm posterior wall and about 5 mm from the femoral articular surface (see Fig. 3.43F). Flex the knee 120 degrees and use a flat-blade reamer to avoid articular damage and to allow optimal visualization of tunnel placement (see Fig. 3.44). Advance the reamer 1 mm and recheck the tunnel location. If it is in the desired location, ream a 30-mm tunnel if possible.
- Carefully retract the reamer and remove it from the joint, being careful not to enlarge the tunnel and ream out the posterior wall of the femur.
- Smooth the edges of the femoral tunnel with a full-radius resector.
- Use the tunnel notcher to make a 25-mm-long slot per the guidewire.

GRAFT PASSAGE

- Use the eyelet guidewire to pass a suture loop with tails through the femoral tunnel and out through the lateral thigh. Retrieve the loop through the femoral tunnel. Use this loop to pass the graft up through the tibial tunnel and then guide it into the femoral tunnel using a probe. The cancellous surface of the femoral bone plug is positioned to face anteriorly.

- When the graft is in the femoral tunnel, pass a flexible guidewire through the medial portal, and with the wire parallel to the graft, advance both up into the tunnel. Ensure that at least 2 cm of bone plug remains in the tibial tunnel for later fixation; if necessary, recess the graft into the femoral tunnel and choose a longer interference screw to fix the graft at the femoral aperture.

GRAFT FIXATION

- Secure the graft with an interference screw with a sheath passed through the low medial portal to form a straight line with the tunnel (see Fig. 3.43G and H). The screw should firmly engage the bone and be flush with the femoral aperture. Visualization is aided by placing the scope into the top of the notch and looking down on the tunnel.
- Move the knee through a range of motion while holding tension distally on the graft to ensure that there is no impingement or pistoning of the graft. If the graft tightens more than 2 mm with knee flexion, remove the graft and move the femoral tunnel, or both tunnels, slightly posterior using a convex arthroscopic rasp. Slight tightening during knee extension is normal.
- Rotate the tibial bone plug counterclockwise (right knee) so that the cancellous plug faces laterally, thus replicating the anterior cruciate ligament fiber orientation.
- If no graft pistoning or impingement is evident, hold the tension on the graft for approximately 3 minutes while cycling the knee to allow for collagen fiber stress relaxation. If the graft tends to impinge in one direction, use the screw to push the bone graft in the opposite direction.
- Tension the graft with 8 to 10 lb of pull. Overtensioning of the graft can cause failure because of joint capture or graft necrosis.
- Secure the graft with a screw equal to the gap size plus 5 mm with the knee in full extension.
- If the tendon is so long that the bone plug is completely out of the tibial tunnel, as may be the case with an allograft mismatch, then a biocomposite or noncutting screw 1 mm smaller than the tunnel can be used for soft-tissue fixation of the patellar tendon and bone construct.
- Move the knee through a full range of motion and ensure there is no evidence of capture of the knee joint. Observe and probe the graft arthroscopically to ensure that it is taut. The graft should be slightly tighter than a normal anterior cruciate ligament. Also ensure that there is no impingement and that no bone or screw protrudes into the joint from the tibial or femoral tunnel.
- Check the stability of the knee by Lachman and pivot shift maneuvers. The knee should be just slightly tighter than the uninjured knee.
- If fixation is secure, remove the 18-gauge wire and the tension sutures.

CLOSURE

- Loosely approximate the patellar tendon with simple interrupted absorbable sutures through the anterior portion of the fiber of the tendon.
- Place bone saved from contouring of the bone plugs into the patellar defect and close the peritenon.

- Remove the sutures from the thigh proximally (femoral bone plug) and from the tibial bone plug distally.
- Remove any protruding bone, leaving a smooth surface distally.
- Close the periosteal flap back over the tunnel.
- Close the subcutaneous tissues with interrupted 2-0 Vicryl suture and approximate the skin with a running subcuticular 4-0 Monocryl suture.
- Apply adhesive strips loosely over the closure and apply a sterile dressing, a cooling sleeve, and an elastic wrap.

POSTOPERATIVE CARE For the anterior cruciate ligament rehabilitation protocol, see Box 3.6.

TWO-INCISION TECHNIQUE FOR ANTERIOR CRUCIATE LIGAMENT RECONSTRUCTION USING BONE–PATELLAR TENDON–BONE GRAFT

The two-incision technique can be used for revisions, for recovery of a posterior wall blowout, and for pediatric patients.

TECHNIQUE 3.17

- The basics for the two-incision technique are as described for the endoscopic technique except a lateral exposure is necessary.

LATERAL EXPOSURE

- Make a 4-cm lateral incision starting 1.5 cm proximal to the flare of the lateral condyle and centered directly over the iliotibial band. Carry the dissection down to the iliotibial band and expose it with wide subcutaneous dissection.
- Divide the iliotibial band in its midline and extend it proximally and distally from the skin incision. The lower edge of the distal portion of the vastus lateralis can be felt by sweeping a finger along the intermuscular septum.
- Slide a periosteal elevator under the edge of the vastus lateralis and lift the muscle anteriorly over the lateral part of the femur without injuring the muscle belly.
- Place a Z-retractor over the femur to hold the vastus lateralis superiorly.
- Use electrocautery to make a longitudinal incision through the periosteum just proximal to the flare of the condyle and extend it proximally for about 2.5 cm. Use a periosteal elevator to expose the bone and the over-the-top spot where the flare of the condyle and the metaphysis of the femur meet. Coagulate the lateral genicular vessels in this area.

BOX 3.6

Anterior Cruciate Ligament Rehabilitation Protocol

Stage I: 0-2 Weeks
- Patellar mobilizations (emphasize superior/inferior glides)
- MCB 0-90 degrees
- Quadriceps sets/SLR all planes (emphasize SLR without extension lag)
- Prone/standing hamstring curls
- Passive extension (emphasize full extension)
- Prone hangs
- Pillow under heel
- Passive, active, and active-assisted ROM knee flexion
- Wall slides
- Sitting slides
- Prone towel pulls
- Edema control—compression pump
- Electrical stimulation for muscle re-education if poor QS
- PWB 50%-75% with crutches or WBTT without crutches if MCB locked in full extension
- Sleep in brace locked in extension

Goals
- Full knee extension ROM
- 90-Degree knee flexion ROM
- Good QS
- Emphasize normal gait pattern

Stage II: 2-4 Weeks
- MCB full ROM
- Progress ROM to 120 degrees by week 4
- Progress SLR and prone/standing hamstring curls with weights
- Bike for ROM, begin low-resistance program when ROM adequate
- Stool scoots
- FWB with crutches; discontinue crutches when ambulating without limp
- Begin double-leg BAPS, progress to single leg
- Begin double-leg press with light weight/high repetitions
- Wall sits at 45-degree angle with tibia vertical, progress time
- Lateral step-ups (4 inches) when able to perform single-leg quarter squat
- Hip machine and hamstring machine when able to perform SLR with 10 lb
- Treadmill (forward and backward) with emphasis on normal gait
- Knee extension 90-60 degrees (submaximal) with manual resistance by therapist

Goals
- ROM 0-120 degrees
- FWB without crutches, no limp

Stage II: 4-6 Weeks
- Progress to full ROM by 6 weeks
- Begin Kin-Com isokinetic hamstring progression (isotonic/isokinetic)
- Begin Kin-Com dynamometer quadriceps work 90-40 degrees isotonics with antishear pad
- Stairmaster (forward and backward)
- Progress closed chain exercises
- At 6 weeks, begin Kin-Com dynamometer quadriceps work 90-40 degrees isokinetics (start with higher speed and work on endurance)
- Aquatic exercises

Stage II: 8-10 Weeks
- Progress above-listed exercises
- Slow-form running with sport cord (forward and backward)
- Isokinetic quadriceps work at different speeds (60, 90, 120 degrees per second)
- Begin lunges
- At 10 weeks, begin Fitter, slide board

Stage III: 12-16 Weeks
- Full-range isotonics on Kin-Com dynamometer (begin moving antishear pad down)
- Knee extension machine with low weight/high repetitions
- Lateral sport cord drills (slow, controlled)
- Kin-Com dynamometer test hamstrings, discontinue isokinetic hamstrings if 90%
- Progress isokinetic quadriceps to full extension by 16 weeks

Stage IV: 16-20 Weeks
- Kin-Com dynamometer test for quadriceps, retest hamstrings if necessary
- Begin plyometric program with shuttle, minitrampoline, jump rope if quadriceps strength 65%, no effusion, full ROM, stable knee
- Begin jogging program if quadriceps strength is 65%

Stage V: 20-36 Weeks
- Agility training
- Sport-specific drills (e.g., carioca, 45 cutting, figure-of-eight)
- Retest quadriceps if necessary

Stage VI: Agility Testing 36 Weeks
- Return to sport if:
- Motion > 130 degrees
- Hamstrings > 90%
- Quadriceps > 85%
- Sport-specific agility training completed and testing passed
- Maintenance exercises two to three times per week

BAPS, Biomechanical Ankle Platform System; *FWB*, full weight bearing; *MCB*, motion control brace; *PWB*, partial weight bearing; *QS*, quadriceps setting; *ROM*, range of motion; *SLR*, straight-leg raises; *WBTT*, weight bearing to tolerance.

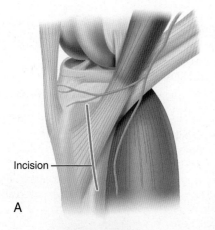 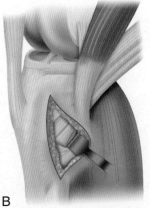 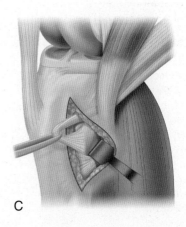

Incision

A   B   C

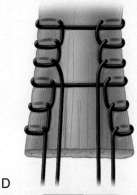

D

FIGURE 3.47   Endoscopic quadruple hamstring graft. **A,** A 3-cm incision is made over the pes anserinus tendon. **B,** Inferior retraction of the sartorius tendon, exposing the gracilis and semitendinosus tendons. **C,** Placement of Penrose drain around the hamstring tendon to be harvested. **D,** Two running, interlocking (Krackow) sutures. **SEE TECHNIQUE 3.18.**

ENDOSCOPIC QUADRUPLE HAMSTRING GRAFT

TECHNIQUE 3.18

GRAFT HARVEST

- Make a 4-cm incision anteromedially on the tibia starting approximately 4 cm distal to the joint line and 3 cm medial to the tibial tuberosity (Fig. 3.47A).
- Expose the pes anserinus insertion with subcutaneous dissection.
- Palpate the upper and lower borders of the sartorius tendon and identify the palpable gracilis and semitendinosus tendons 3 cm to 4 cm medial to the tendinous insertion (Fig. 3.47B).
- Make a short incision in line with the upper border of the gracilis tendon and carry the incision just through the first layer, taking care not to injure the underlying medial collateral ligament.
- With Metzenbaum scissors, carry the dissection proximally up the thigh. Stay in the same plane and maintain adequate exposure by using properly placed retractors. Careful observation of structures is necessary to avoid injuring the saphenous vein or nerve by straying from the plane of dissection.
- With a curved hemostat, dissect the gracilis and semitendinosus tendons from the surrounding soft tissues about 3 cm medial to their insertion onto the tibia.
- After carefully identifying each tendon, use a right-angle vascular clamp to pass a Penrose drain around the gracilis tendon and release its fibrous extensions to the gastrocnemius and semimembranosus muscles (Fig. 3.47C). These fibrous extensions come off the hamstring tendons at 6 cm to 7 cm proximal to their distal attachment. Subperiosteally dissect the tendons medially to the insertion and release them sharply. Do not damage or release the sartorius tendon. Place a nonabsorbable Krackow stitch on the tendon ends using different colored sutures to differentiate the two tendons (Fig. 3.47D). Use a tendon tube sizer to accurately measure the give of the quadrupled tendon.
- Palpate all sides of the tendon to ensure there are no fibrous extensions before releasing it with an open-end tendon stripper. If firm resistance is felt, redissect around the tendons with a periosteal elevator and Metzenbaum scissors. Release the tendon proximally by controlled tension on the tendon, while advancing the stripper proximally. The muscle should slide off the tendon as the stripper is advanced proximally.

- Use the same procedure to release the semitendinosus tendon.
- At a separate table, separate the muscle from the tendon with a no. 10 blade.
- Place a Krackow-type whipstitch in both ends of each tendon with no. 2 nonabsorbable sutures. Fold both tendons in half to form four strands of tendon.
- Perform a limited notchplasty and tunnel placement as described for the endoscopic bone–tendon–bone technique (see Technique 3.16).
- Ream the tibial tunnel at 50 degrees to the tibial articular surface. The tunnel is reamed 2 mm smaller than the graft size and serially dilated to produce a snug fit. Dilation of the tibial tunnel has been shown to significantly increase the pull-out strength. The tunnel length should be 30 to 35 mm to allow fixation near the articular surface.
- A low anteromedial portal is used for reaming the femoral tunnel. Use an EndoButton (Smith & Nephew, Memphis, TN) or similar type device to secure 20 to 25 mm of tendon in the femoral tunnel. After tensioning the graft for 3 minutes while cycling the knee, use a composite screw 1 mm smaller than the tunnel for tibial fixation and use secondary suture and post fixation. A screw sheath, soft-tissue fixation device may also be used to secure the tibial end of the graft.

POSTOPERATIVE CARE See Box 3.6 for postoperative anterior cruciate ligament rehabilitation. We generally proceed more slowly with rehabilitation when a hamstring graft has been used. The patient generally is allowed to return to full activity at around 9 to 12 months.

ALL-INSIDE QUADRUPLE HAMSTRING GRAFT ANTERIOR CRUCIATE LIGAMENT RECONSTRUCTION

A quadriceps graft can be harvested through a 4-cm vertical incision extending proximally from the superior patella. Instrumentation is available to simplify the harvest for primary or revision procedures.

TECHNIQUE 3.19

- After graft harvest, prepare the graft by folding it appropriately and then, using a "buried knot" technique, start from the inside of the graft and place the needle around two limbs. Wrap the suture around the graft, then place the needle through the second set of graft limbs from outside-in. Tension the suture and tie a knot to secure the stitch. Repeat on the other end of the graft for a total of two stitches in each end (Fig. 3.48A).
- Assuming a maximal intraarticular length of 30 mm, there will be approximately 20 mm of graft in the femoral and tibial

socket. Drill the femur 20 mm deep and the tibia approximately 30 mm deep to allow an extra 10 mm for tensioning.

FEMORAL SOCKET PREPARATION

- For medial portal drilling, use the TightRope Drill Pin, transportal ACL guides, and low profile reamers. Note the intraosseous length from the TightRope Drill Pin.
- After socket drilling, pass a suture with the TightRope Drill Pin for later graft passing (Fig. 3.48B).
- Using the FlipCutter drill, place the guide into the joint and push the drill sleeve down to bone and note the measurement where the drill sleeve meets the guide (Fig. 3.48C, inset).
- Drill the FlipCutter into the joint, remove the guide, and tap the stepped drill sleeve into bone. Flip the blade on the FlipCutter and ream until the desired socket depth is reached.
- Flip the FlipCutter blade straight and remove it from the joint while keeping the drill sleeve in place. Pass a FiberStick suture through the stepped drill sleeve and dock for later graft passage.

TIBIAL SOCKET PREPARATION

- Drill the FlipCutter reamer into the joint. Remove the marking hook and tap the stepped drill sleeve into the bone (Fig. 3.49A).
- Flip the blade and lock into cutting position. Drill on forward, with distal traction, to cut the socket. Use the rubber ring and 5-mm markings on the cutter to measure socket depth (Fig. 3.49B).

GRAFT PASSAGE

- Straighten the FlipCutter blade and remove from the joint. Pass a TigerStick suture into the joint and retrieve both the tibial TigerStick and the femoral FiberStick sutures out the medial portal together with a Suture Retriever (Fig. 3.50A). Retrieving both sutures at the same time helps avoid tissue interposition that can complicate graft passage.
- Pass the blue button suture and the white shortening strands through the femur. Remove slack from sutures and ensure equal tension. Clamp or hold both blue and white sutures and pull them together to advance the button out of the femur. Pull back on the graft to confirm that the button is seated (Fig. 3.50B).
- While holding slight tension on the graft, pull the shortening strands proximally, one at a time, to advance the graft. Pull on each strand in 2-cm increments (Fig. 3.50C). The graft can be fully seated into the femur or left partially inserted until tibial passing is complete, which allows fine tuning of graft depth in each socket.
- Cinch a suture around the end of the TightRope ABS loop to use for passing (Fig. 3.50D, inset). Load the cinch suture and the whipstitch tails from the graft into the tibial passing suture. Pull distally on the tibial passing suture to deliver both the TightRope ABS loop and the whipstitch sutures out of the tibial distally (Fig. 3.50D).
- Advance the graft into the tibia by pulling on the inside of the ABS loop and whipstitch sutures (Fig. 3.50E).
- Load the TightRope ABS button onto the loop. Pull on the white shortening strands to advance the button to bone and tension the graft (Fig. 3.50F). Ensure that the button has a clear path to bone so that no soft tissue is trapped underneath it.

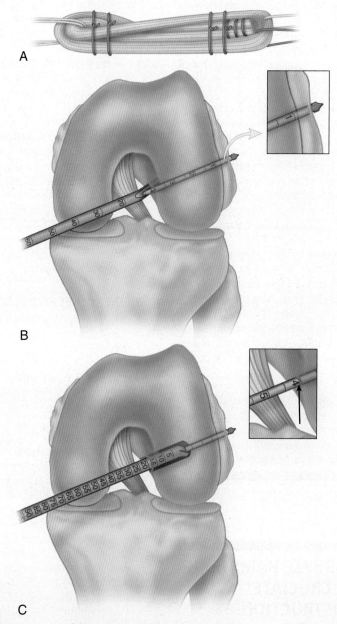

FIGURE 3.48 All-inside quadruple hamstring graft anterior cruciate ligament reconstruction. **A,** Graft preparation. **B** and **C,** Femoral socket drilling. Inset, Guide is placed into joint and drill sleeve is pushed down to bone. **SEE TECHNIQUE 3.19.**

■ Load the whipstitch sutures into the button and tie a knot for backup fixation (Fig. 3.50G). Alternatively, backup sutures can be fixed to the tibia using the Swivel Lock.

ANATOMIC DOUBLE-BUNDLE ANTERIOR CRUCIATE LIGAMENT RECONSTRUCTION

Anatomic double-bundle anterior cruciate ligament reconstruction places the femoral graft into the femoral footprint of the native anterior cruciate ligament, which has been shown to result in closer knee joint kinematics than the original isometric femoral position. A three-portal technique adds an accessory medial portal to create the femoral tunnel.

TECHNIQUE 3.20

(KARLSSON ET AL.)
■ A three-portal approach, using standard anterolateral and central medial portals and an accessory anteromedial portal, allows for a complete view of the entire ante-

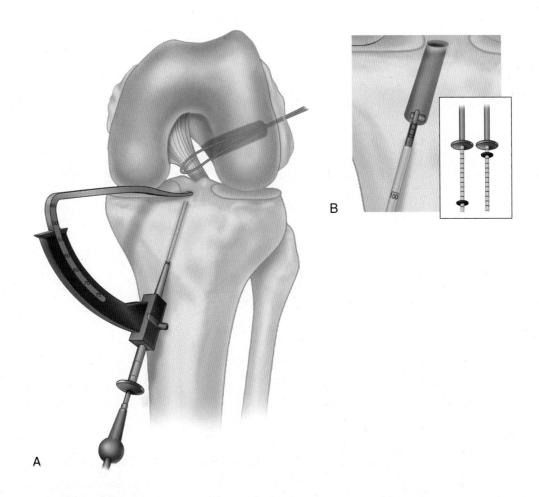

FIGURE 3.49 Tibial socket preparation. **A,** After reaming, stepped drill sleeve is tapped into bone. **B,** Measure socket depth using rubber ring and 5-mm markings on cutter. **SEE TECHNIQUE 3.19.**

rior cruciate ligament and its femoral and tibial insertion sites.

- Using a spinal needle, create the central portal while viewing through the lateral portal. The spinal needle should be in the center of the notch in a proximal to distal direction.
- Create the accessory anteromedial portal superior to the medial joint line, approximately 2 cm medial to the medial border of the patellar tendon. The femoral tunnels can be drilled through the accessory medial portal.
- Locate the ideal anterior cruciate ligament insertion sites for anatomic tunnel placement. Anterior cruciate ligament remnants can be used to determine this site. On the femoral side, the bony landmarks, such as the lateral intercondylar ridge and lateral bifurcate ridge, can be used, as well as posterior cartilage border. With the knee flexed 90 degrees, the femoral insertion site encompasses the lower 30% to 35% of the notch wall (Fig. 3.51).
- Mark the tibial and femoral insertion sites of the anterior cruciate ligament and measure to determine the tunnel location and size. If the insertion site is smaller than 14 mm in diameter, a double-bundle reconstruction may become challenging. The width of the notch entrance and

its shape will determine if a double-bundle technique can be used, but generally a notch width no smaller than 12 mm is the minimal size required.

- Create the femoral posterolateral tunnel first, through the accessory anteromedial portal, followed by the tibial anteromedial and posterolateral tunnels. Place the anteromedial and posterolateral tunnels in the center of the native anteromedial and posterolateral tibial and femoral insertion sites.
- Drill the femoral anteromedial tunnel through the accessory medial portal or through the tibial anteromedial or posterolateral tunnel if this allows for the native femoral insertion site to be reached.
- In determining the size of the tunnels, aim to restore as much of the native insertion site as possible while maintaining an approximately 2-mm bony bridge between the bundles.
- After the tunnels have been drilled, prepare the grafts. The graft size should be equal to the tunnel diameter. Tension the anteromedial and posterolateral grafts separately, with the anteromedial graft in approximately 45 degrees of knee flexion and the posterolateral graft in full knee extension.
- For fixation, use suspensory fixation on the femoral side to avoid disruption of the insertion site, which can occur

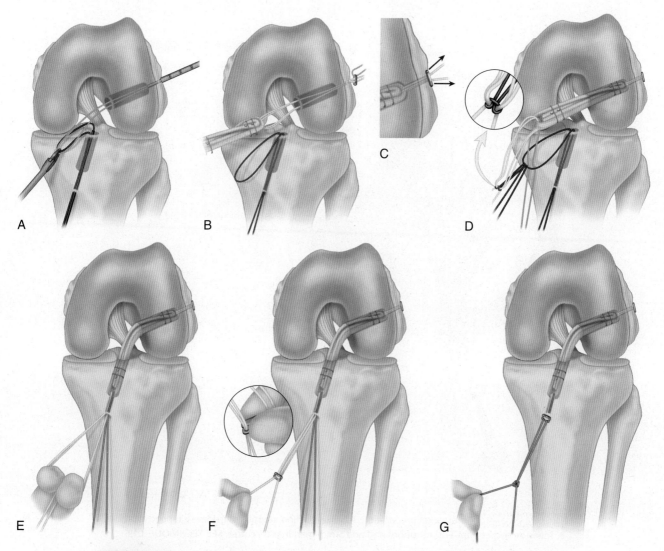

FIGURE 3.50 Graft passage. **A,** Femoral sutures are retrieved out medial portal. **B,** Blue and white sutures are passed through the femur and pulled together to advance the button out of femur. **C,** With slight tension on graft, the shortening strands are pulled proximally to advance graft; each strand is pulled in 2-cm increments. **D** and *inset,* Suture is cinched around end of Tight-Rope ABS loop to use for passing. Tibial passing suture is used to deliver TightRope ABS loop and whipstitch sutures out of distal distally. **E,** Graft is advanced into tibia. **F,** Button is advanced to bone and graft is tensioned. **G,** Whipstitch sutures are loaded into button and a knot is tied for backup fixation. **SEE TECHNIQUE 3.19.**

with aperture interference screw fixation. Use interference screw fixation on the cortical tibial side.

Quadriceps Tendon Graft. Use of a 10-mm-wide quadriceps tendon with an attached piece of patellar bone for anterior cruciate ligament reconstruction has been described. We have rarely used this as a revision technique, but it is an attractive alternative.

Anterior Cruciate Ligament Injuries in Skeletally Immature Individuals. With athletic activities becoming more competitive at a younger age, the incidence of anterior cruciate ligament injuries in skeletally immature individuals has rapidly increased over the past decades. These injuries present a particularly perplexing problem with the potential for physeal injury with reaming of tunnels that is

counterbalanced by the potential for meniscal damage from recurrent giving way in these individuals. Two principles must be followed: (1) preserve menisci if possible, and (2) prevent recurrent giving way. In some less active individuals with mild-to-moderate instability, reduction of activity level may be all that is necessary until they have had an appropriate growth spurt and maturing of the physes. In active, young boys, sometimes this is quite hard to accomplish. In these children when there is a meniscal tear or recurrent giving way, a physeal-preserving, soft-tissue graft procedure is best. A small central tunnel made in the tibia just above the physis with preservation of the physis in the femur seems to be a safe procedure. The benefit of stabilizing the knee seems to outweigh the small potential for growth disturbance if these procedures are done correctly. It is necessary to use a soft-tissue graft to avoid bone or fixation across the physis. The

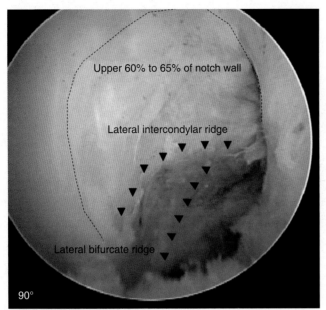

Upper 60% to 65% of notch wall

Lateral intercondylar ridge

Lateral bifurcate ridge

90°

FIGURE 3.51 Right knee in 90 degrees of flexion showing whole lateral wall of notch. Femoral anterior cruciate ligament (ACL) insertion site is clearly demarcated by lateral intercondylar ridge and lateral bifurcate ridge. It can be seen that anterior cruciate ligament attaches to lower 30% to 35% of lateral notch wall area when the knee is in operating position. (From Karlsson J, Irrgang JJ, van Eck, et al: Anatomic single- and double-bundle anterior cruciate ligament reconstruction, part 2, *Am J Sports Med* 39:2016, 2011.) **SEE TECHNIQUE 3.20.**

tunnel and the tibia can be drilled above the physis, or a small central tunnel through the physis probably is acceptable, particularly in Tanner stages II, III, and IV patients. In younger patients, a procedure going around the physis or an over-the-top procedure as described by Anderson and Kocher, Garg, and Micheli is recommended.

TRANSEPIPHYSEAL REPLACEMENT OF ANTERIOR CRUCIATE LIGAMENT USING QUADRUPLE HAMSTRING GRAFTS

The transepiphyseal replacement of anterior cruciate ligament using quadruple hamstring grafts procedure is indicated in patients in Tanner stage I, II, or III of development. The procedure is contraindicated in patients in Tanner stage IV of development, who can have conventional anterior cruciate ligament reconstruction. Pitfalls of this procedure are summarized in Box 3.7.

TECHNIQUE 3.21

(ANDERSON)

- Place the injured lower limb in an arthroscopic leg holder with the hip flexed to 20 degrees to facilitate C-arm fluoroscopic viewing of the knee in the lateral plane.
- Position the C-arm on the side of the table opposite the injured knee and place the monitor at the head of the table. View the tibial and femoral physes in the anteroposterior and lateral planes before the limb is prepared

---

BOX 3.7

Pitfalls of Transepiphyseal Replacement of the Anterior Cruciate Ligament Using Quadruple Hamstring Grafts in Skeletally Immature Patients

Suboptimal Graft Placement
- Optimal graft placement is essential to restore normal knee kinematics and avoid physeal injuries.
- Avoid placing the femoral or tibial drill hole anterior; correct positioning of the drill hole is crucial in preventing graft impingement.
- Surgery should not proceed without clearly seeing the physes on anteroposterior and lateral planes using C-arm.
- Guidewires should be inserted under real-time C-arm viewing.
- Confirm arthroscopically that the guidewires enter the joint in the center of the footprint of the anterior cruciate ligament on the femur and in the posterior footprint of the anterior cruciate ligament on the tibia.

Incorrect Diameter of Transepiphyseal Drill Holes
- A drill bit corresponding to the smallest size through which tendon would easily pass should be used to make transepiphyseal holes.
- A small-diameter drill bit is less likely to damage the physes, and a snug fit promotes healing of the graft to bone.
- Graft passage can be eased by chamfering the femoral hole and pushing the graft into the hole using a blunt instrument through an anteromedial portal while pulling a no. 5 FiberWire suture tied to an EndoButton.

Failure of Fixation
- Load to failure in this technique exceeds normal tensile loads on the anterior cruciate ligament.
- In the early phase of healing, failure can lead to instability.
- Check the femoral side fixation with C-arm to confirm that EndoButton washer is flush on lateral femoral condyle.

Graft Slippage Associated With Suture Post Fixation
- Minimize slippage by meticulous placement of whipstitches in tendon ends with tight loops placed in close proximity.
- Pretension graft using Graftmaster (Smith & Nephew Endoscopy, Andover, MA)
- When tendon graft extends through the tibial hole, augment the tibial fixation by suturing the tendons through the periosteum.

Data from Anderson AF: Transepiphyseal replacement of the anterior cruciate ligament using quadruple hamstring grafts in skeletally immature patients, *J Bone Joint Surg* 86A:201, 2004.

---

and draped. When the distal part of the femur is viewed, adjust the C-arm so that the medial and lateral femoral condyles line up perfectly with the lateral plane. Rotate the C-arm to see the extension of the tibial physis into the tibial tubercle on the lateral view of the tibia.
- Make an oblique 4-cm incision over the semitendinosus and gracilis tendons. Dissect these tendons free and transect at the musculotendinous junction with use of a standard tendon stripper and detach distally.
- Double the tendons and place a no. 5 FiberWire suture (Arthrex, Naples, FL) in the ends of the tendons with a whipstitch.

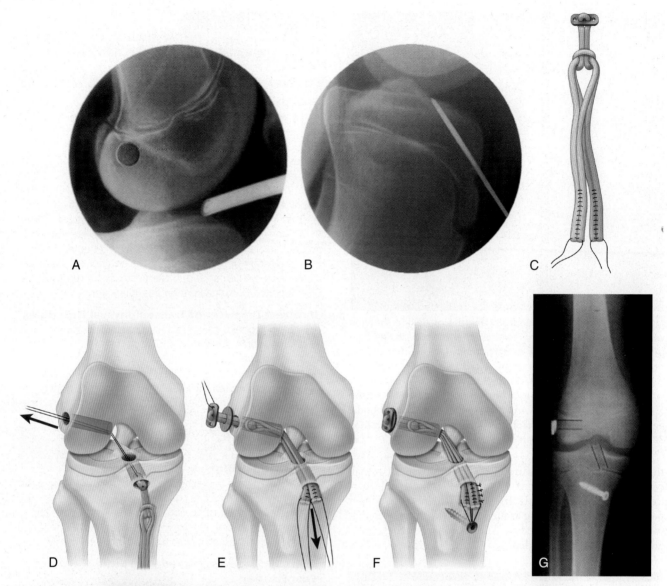

FIGURE 3.52 Anderson transepiphyseal replacement of anterior cruciate ligament using quadruple hamstring grafts. **A,** Graphically enhanced lateral view from C-arm after drilling of femoral hole. **B,** Lateral radiograph of tibia, showing correct position of tibial guidewire. Although guidewire appears to enter tibial tubercle in this view, it actually enters epiphysis medial to tibial tubercle. **C,** EndoButton continuous loop passed around middle of double tendons and looped on itself. **D,** Semitendinosus and gracilis tendons pulled up through tibia and out of lateral femoral condyle with use of no. 5 suture in EndoButton. **E,** EndoButton washer is placed over EndoButton, and washer is pulled back to surface of lateral femoral condyle. **F,** Quadruple hamstring grafts secured distally by tying no. 5 FiberWire sutures over tibial screw and post. **G,** Radiograph 4 months after surgery, showing properly placed transepiphyseal tibial and femoral holes. **SEE TECHNIQUE 3.21.**

- Place the doubled tendons under 4.5 kg (10 lb) of tension on the back table with the use of the Graftmaster device (Smith & Nephew Endoscopy, Andover, MA).
- Insert the arthroscope into the anterolateral portal and insert a probe through the anteromedial portal.
- Perform intraarticular examination in the usual manner.
- Remove debris in the intercondylar notch and perform a notchplasty to see the anatomic footprint of the anterior cruciate ligament on the femur.
- Repair any substantial meniscal tears found.
- With the C-arm in the lateral position, adjust the limb to show a perfect lateral view.

- Place the point of the guidewire over the lateral femoral condyle, corresponding with the location of the footprint of the anterior cruciate ligament on the femur. This point is approximately one fourth of the distance from posterior to anterior along the Blumensaat line and one fourth of the distance down from the Blumensaat line (Fig. 3.52A). Make a 2-cm lateral incision at this point.
- Incise the iliotibial tract longitudinally and strip the periosteum from a small area of the lateral femoral condyle.
- Use the C-arm to view the entry point of the guidewire in the anteroposterior and the lateral planes. With the C-arm in the lateral plane and with the use of a free-hand

technique, introduce the point of the guidewire 2 to 3 mm into the femoral epiphysis. Do not angulate the pin anteriorly or posteriorly, but rather keep it perpendicular to the femur in the coronal plane. Rotate the C-arm to the anteroposterior plane to ensure that the guidewire is not angulated superiorly or inferiorly.

- Drive the guidewire across the femoral epiphysis, perpendicular to the femur and distal to the physis (see Fig. 3.52A). Through the arthroscope, view the entrance of the guidewire into the intercondylar notch. The guidewire should enter the joint 1 mm posterior and superior to the center of the anatomic footprint of the anterior cruciate ligament on the femur.
- Leave the femoral guidewire in place and insert a second guidewire into the anteromedial aspect of the tibia, through the epiphysis, with the aid of a tibial drill guide. From the direct lateral position, rotate the C-arm externally approximately 30 degrees to show the physis clearly extending into the tibial tubercle. Drill the guidewire into the tibial epiphysis under real-time fluoroscopic imaging (Fig. 3.52B). The handle of the drill guide must be lifted for the wire to clear the anterior part of the tibial physis. The wire should enter the joint at the level of the free edge of the lateral meniscus and in the posterior footprint of the anterior cruciate ligament on the tibia.
- Arthroscopically confirm the appropriate position of both guidewires at this point.
- Use tendon sizers to measure the diameter of the quadruple tendon graft (which typically is 6 to 8 mm). A tight fit is important; consequently, use the smallest appropriate drill to ream over both guidewires.
- Chamfer the edge of the femoral hole intraarticularly and measure the width of the lateral femoral condyle. Choose the appropriate EndoButton continuous loop (2 to 3 cm) so that approximately 2 cm of the quadruple hamstring tendon graft remains within the lateral femoral condyle.
- Pass the EndoButton continuous loop around the middle of the double tendons and loop inside of itself to secure the tendons proximally (Fig. 3.52C). Alternatively, the tendons can be placed through the continuous loop before the tendon ends are sutured together. That requires drilling and measuring the length of the femoral hole before graft preparation, however. Otherwise, it is difficult to determine the appropriate length of the EndoButton continuous loop necessary to leave 2 cm of the tendon graft within the lateral femoral condyle.
- Place a no. 5 FiberWire suture in one end of the EndoButton and pass a suture passer from anterior to posterior through the tibia and out the lateral femoral condyle (Fig. 3.52D). Pull the EndoButton and tendons up through the tibia and out the femoral hole with the use of the no. 5 suture.
- Place an EndoButton washer, 3 to 4 mm larger than the femoral hole, over the EndoButton. Apply tension to the tendons distally, pulling the EndoButton and washer to the surface of the lateral femoral condyle (Fig. 3.52E). The washer is necessary to anchor the graft proximally because the hole in the femoral condyle is larger than the EndoButton.
- Place the graft under tension and extend the knee to determine arthroscopically if there is impingement of the graft on the intercondylar notch.
- An anterior notchplasty usually is unnecessary when this technique is used; however, if the anterior outlet of the in-

tercondylar notch touches or indents the graft in terminal extension, remove a small portion of the anterior outlet.
- With the knee in 10 degrees of flexion, secure the quadruple hamstring graft distally by tying the no. 5 FiberWire sutures over a tibial screw and post that is placed medial to the tibial tubercle apophysis and distal to the proximal tibial physis (Fig. 3.52F and G).
- If the tendon graft extends through the tibial drill hole, secure it to the periosteum of the anterior tibia with multiple no. 1 Ethibond sutures with use of figure-of-eight stitches (see Fig. 3.52F). Close the subcutaneous tissue and skin in a routine fashion and apply a hinged brace.

PHYSEAL-SPARING RECONSTRUCTION OF THE ANTERIOR CRUCIATE LIGAMENT

The procedure of Kocher, Garg, and Micheli consists of arthroscopically assisted, physeal-sparing, combined intraarticular and extraarticular reconstruction of the anterior cruciate ligament with use of an autogenous iliotibial band graft. It is a modification of the combined intraarticular and extraarticular reconstruction described by MacIntosh and Darby. Modifications include application in skeletally immature patients, arthroscopic assistance, graft fixation, and accelerated rehabilitation. Rehabilitation must be geared to the age of the young patient.

TECHNIQUE 3.22   Figure 3.53

(KOCHER, GARG, AND MICHELI)
- The procedure is done with the patient under general anesthesia as an overnight observation procedure.
- Position the child supine on the operating table with a pneumatic tourniquet around the proximal aspect of the thigh.
- With the patient under anesthesia, confirm anterior cruciate ligament insufficiency.
- Make an incision of approximately 6 cm obliquely from the lateral joint line to the superior border of the iliotibial band. Separate the iliotibial band proximally from the subcutaneous tissue with the use of a periosteal elevator under the skin of the lateral part of the thigh.
- Incise the anterior and posterior borders of the iliotibial band and carry the incisions proximally under the skin with the use of a curved meniscotome.
- Detach the iliotibial band proximally under the skin with the use of a curved meniscotome or an open tendon stripper.
- Leave the iliotibial band attached distally at Gerdy's tubercle.
- Dissect distally to separate the iliotibial band from the joint capsule and from the lateral patellar retinaculum.
- Tubularize the free proximal end of the iliotibial band with a whipstitch using a no. 5 Ethibond suture (Ethicon, Johnson & Johnson, Somerville, NJ).

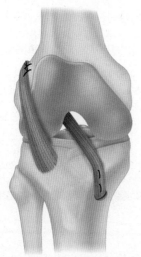

FIGURE 3.53   Technique of physeal-sparing, combined intraarticular and extraarticular reconstruction of anterior cruciate ligament. (Redrawn from Kocher MS, Garg S, Micheli LJ: Physeal sparing reconstruction of the anterior cruciate ligament in skeletally immature prepubescent children and adolescents, *J Bone Joint Surg* 87A:2371, 2005.) **SEE TECHNIQUE 3.22.**

- Examine the knee with the arthroscope through standard anterolateral and anteromedial portals, treat any meniscal injury or chondral injury, and excise the anterior cruciate ligament remnant.
- Identify the over-the-top position on the femur and the over-the-front position under the intermeniscal ligament.
- Perform a minimal notchplasty to avoid iatrogenic injury to the perichondrial ring of the distal femoral physis, which is in close proximity to the over-the-top position.
- Bring the free end of the iliotibial band graft through the over-the-top position with the use of a full-length clamp or a two-incision, rear-entry guide and out through the anteromedial portal.
- Make a second incision of approximately 4.5 cm over the proximal medial aspect of the tibia in the region of the pes anserinus. Carry the dissection through the subcutaneous tissue to the periosteum.
- Place a curved clamp from this incision into the joint under the intermeniscal ligament.
- Make a small groove in the anteromedial aspect of the proximal tibial epiphysis under the intermeniscal ligament with the use of a curved rat-tail rasp to bring the tibial graft placement more posterior.
- Bring the free end of the graft through the joint, under the intermeniscal ligament in the anteromedial epiphyseal groove, and out through the medial tibial incision.
- Place the knee in 90 degrees of flexion and 15 degrees of external rotation. For extraarticular reconstruction, fix the graft on the femoral side through the lateral incision using mattress sutures on the lateral femoral condyle at the insertion of the lateral intermuscular septum.
- Fix the tibial side through the medial incision with the knee flexed 20 degrees and tension applied to the graft.
- Make a periosteal incision distal to the proximal tibial physis as confirmed fluoroscopically.

- Make a trough in the proximal medial tibial metaphyseal cortex and suture the graft to the periosteum at the rough margins with mattress sutures.

POSTOPERATIVE CARE Postoperatively, the patient is permitted touch-down weight bearing for 6 weeks. Immediate mobilization from 0 to 90 degrees is allowed for the first 2 weeks, followed by progression to full range of motion. Continuous passive motion from 0 to 90 degrees is used for the first 2 weeks postoperatively to initiate motion and overcome the anxiety associated with postoperative movement in young children. A protective hinged knee brace is used for 6 weeks after surgery with motion limits of 0 to 90 degrees for the first 2 weeks. Progressive rehabilitation consists of range-of-motion exercises, patellar mobilization, electrical stimulation, pool therapy (if available), proprioception exercises, and closed chain strengthening exercises during the first 3 months postoperatively followed by straight-line jogging, plyometric exercises, sport cord exercises, and sport-specific exercises. Return to full activity, including sports that involve cutting, usually is allowed 6 months postoperatively. A custommade knee brace is used routinely during cutting and pivoting activities for the first 2 years after return to sports.

Azar and Miller developed a surgical technique of arthroscopic-assisted ACL reconstruction using a quadruple-looped hamstring graft with a synthetic graft extender and a distal femoral physeal-sparing technique. The graft extender allows a consistent quadrupled hamstring graft, allows the optimal portion of the graft to be delivered to the intraarticular position, and provides sufficient length for proximal and distal fixation. They reported that all 17 patients with this procedure had a stable Lachman test and were able to return to sporting activities.

PARTIAL TRANSEPIPHYSEAL ACL RECONSTRUCTION IN SKELETALLY IMMATURE ATHLETES

TECHNIQUE 3.23

(AZAR AND MILLER)

GRAFT HARVEST
- After induction of general anesthesia, confirm clinical instability of the knee with Lachman and pivot shift tests.
- Inflate a pneumatic tourniquet and perform diagnostic arthroscopy, with repair of any additional pathology as needed.
- Make a 3-cm longitudinal incision 6 cm below the anteromedial tibial plateau and 3-cm medial to the tibial tubercle and identify the gracilis and semitendinosus tendons.

- Carry dissection down to the sartorial fascia and elevate it off the superficial medial collateral ligament in an inverted-L fashion.
- Identify the hamstring tendons and use a right-angle clamp to separate the gracilis from the semitendinosus.
- Use a sharp No. 15 blade to peel the semitendinosus and gracilis off the sartorius at their insertion point and place a clamp on the end of the gracilis tendon.
- Clear attachments from the gracilis and use a tendon stripper to extract the tendon. Extract the semitendinosus in a similar manner.
- Repair the sartorial fascia.

GRAFT PREPARATION

- Place a whipstitch into the opposite ends of the tendons with a No. 2 nonabsorbable braided suture (Fig. 3.54A). Fold the tendons over a No. 10 French red rubber catheter that has been cut to 3 cm in length.
- Feed a braided nonabsorbable tape suture through the catheter to act as a graft extender (Fig. 3.54B).
- Trim and size the graft as necessary (Fig. 3.54C) and set it aside under a moistened sponge.
- Mark the optimal 3.5 cm of the graft with a blue marking pen to designate it as the intraarticular portion of the graft.

GRAFT FIXATION

- Use a motorized shaver to remove the remnant ACL and tissue from the intercondylar notch posterolaterally, taking care to protect the PCL.
- Place a tibial guide set at 60 degrees off the medial eminence and at the level of the posterior portion of the anterior horn of the lateral meniscus, just in front of the PCL insertion.
- Place a guide pin and drill a transtibial, transphyseal tunnel; ream the tunnel up to the graft size.
- Position the guide pin approximately 2.5 cm medial to the tibial tubercle apophysis to avoid damaging it. For patients younger than 10 years of age, we also typically avoid drilling the proximal tibial physis and instead groove the physis.
- Use a No. 11 blade to make an incision in the distal lateral thigh down to the fascial layer; incise the fascia and identify the iliotibial band.
- Palpate the posterior aspect of the iliotibial band and just anterior to this make a longitudinal incision with a No. 15 blade. Identify the lateral intermuscular septum.
- Use a periosteal elevator to elevate soft tissue, taking care to avoid the distal femoral physis.
- Pass an arthroscopic gaff through the lateral portal and around the lateral femoral condyle, taking care not to loop around the PCL in the intercondylar notch.
- Place the arthroscope into the medial portal, and place the gaff in the anterolateral portal and retrieve it in the lateral aspect of the femur in the area of the previous incision.
- Under direct observation, pass a No. 5 nonabsorbable braided suture through the end of the gaff and back into the joint. Then pass this suture out through the tibial tunnel for graft passage.
- Retrieve the prepared graft and use the suture-shuttle to pass it through the tibial tunnel and in an over-the-top

position around the back portion of the lateral femoral and out to the lateral cortex.
- Under direct fluoroscopic guidance, determine an entry point for a 6.5-mm fully threaded cancellous screw with washer on the distal femur proximal to the physis. Tie the nonabsorbable braided tape previously placed through the red rubber catheter over the 6.5-mm screw post (Fig. 3.54D).
- On the tibial side, place a second 6.5-mm fully threaded cancellous screw with a non-spiked washer distal to the tibial physis (Fig. 3.54E).
- Tension the graft with the leg in extension to avoid overtightening due to the over-the-top position and then tie it over the post (Fig. 3.54F). Assess stability with a Lachman maneuver.
- Reinsert the arthroscope to confirm appropriate graft placement and close the incision in standard fashion.

POSTOPERATIVE MANAGEMENT Patients are placed into a hinged knee brace locked in extension and are kept non–weight bearing on the involved extremity. Physical therapy begins within 1 week after surgery. At 3 weeks the knee brace is unlocked from 0 to 90 degrees. Weight bearing is advanced to partial weight bearing at 6 weeks when the brace is unlocked completely. At 6 weeks full weight bearing is allowed. At 4 months jogging and unrestricted strength training are allowed. Biodex dynamometer testing is obtained at 6 months' follow-up and as needed until release to full activity, which usually is between 9 and 12 months.

ANTERIOR CRUCIATE AND ANTEROLATERAL LIGAMENT RECONSTRUCTION (BOX 3.8)

TECHNIQUE 3.24

(PHILLIPS)
- Harvest the semitendinosus through the inferior portion of a medial parapatellar tendon incision or use a hamstring allograft.
- Make 1-cm incisions over the femoral and tibial insertions of the anterolateral ligament (ALL) as verified by imaging.
- Make a nick in the iliotibial band proximally and use Kelly forceps to spread the tissues, forming a tunnel between the iliotibial band and the underlying capsule.
- Secure the tendon graft distally with a 5.5-mm swivel lock (Fig. 3.55A).
- Pass the graft under the iliotibial band proximally to the insertion site (Fig. 3.55B).
- Place a femoral guidewire and verify its position with imaging, 5 mm proximal and posterior to the epicondyle.
- Taking care to prevent injury to the lateral collateral ligament or popliteus tendon, direct the wire proximally and anterior to avoid the femoral tunnel.

- Mark the graft and move the knee through a range of motion to evaluate isometry.
- Ream a 22-mm × 5-mm tunnel.
- Shorten the graft and place a Vicryl Krackow suture in the graft so as to seat 15 to 20 mm of the graft in the tunnel.
- Pull the guidewire out medially, seating the graft.
- Move the knee through a range of motion to check isometry.
- With the knee in 25 to 30 degrees of flexion, secure the graft with a polyetheretherketone (PEEK) interference screw equal to the tunnel size (Fig. 3.55C).

COMPLICATIONS OF ANTERIOR CRUCIATE LIGAMENT RECONSTRUCTION

Five-year follow-up studies of anterior cruciate ligament reconstruction using autograft bone–patellar tendon–bone grafts and hamstring grafts show similar results as far as stability and failure rates are concerned. Stiffness and strength tend to be slightly better with bone–patellar tendon–bone grafts, but overall results are comparable. Allograft studies at 5- and 7-year follow-up are similar to those with autograft, especially because the incidence of effusions and apparent graft rejection has decreased and graft procurement and

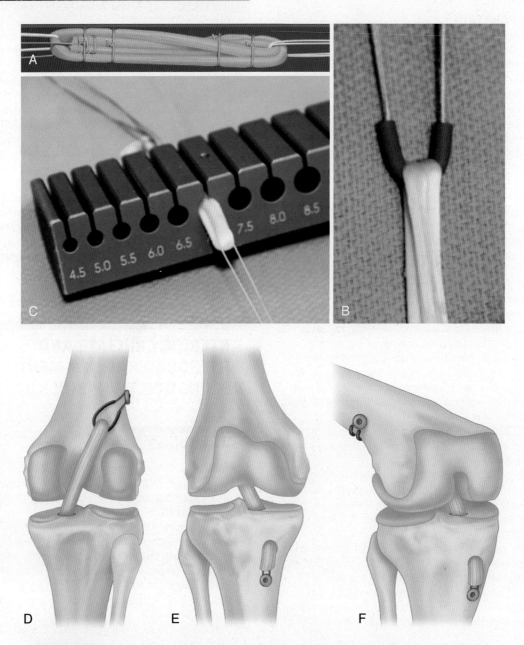

FIGURE 3.54 Technique for partial transphyseal anterior cruciate ligament reconstruction in skeletally immature athletes. **A,** Graft measurements. **B,** Graft with synthetic extender. **C,** Sizing of graft. **D,** Fixation of graft on the femoral side (blue lines represent physes). **E,** Fixation of graft on the tibial side. **F,** Final position of the graft. (From Bettin CC, Throckmorton TW, Miller RH, Azar FM: Technique for partial transphyseal ACL reconstruction in skeletally immature athletes: preliminary results, *Curr Orthop Prac* 30:19, 2019.) **SEE TECHNIQUE 3.23.**

sterilization techniques have improved. Failure rates seem to have stabilized at 7% to 8% at 5-year follow-up when graft failure is the cause of the poor outcome. Other studies measure failure by KT-1000 testing, giving way of the knee, or failure of the patient to return to a previous sporting activity. If these parameters are used to measure surgical failure, the percentage ranges from 5% to 52%. Although the failure rate has stabilized, the number of revision surgeries continues to increase, probably because of better follow-up protocols; higher patient demands, expectations, and activity levels; and the earlier age at which these procedures are being performed.

Economically, the cost of failure can be high. Additional procedures and rehabilitation, loss of work for the patient, and the potential loss of a college scholarship for a high school athlete can be financially burdensome.

Anterior cruciate ligament failure also may take an emotional toll on the patient. Psychologic trauma from additional surgery, frustration over prolonged rehabilitation, loss of motivation, and displaced anger may result. Physiologic consequences include additional surgical trauma from harvesting the graft, possible articular damage, and additional chondral or meniscal damage from chronic instability because many patients wait some time before revision surgery. Meniscal damage has been shown to occur in approximately 40% at 1 year, 60% at 5 years, and approximately 80% at 10 years, which is the same incidence as degenerative joint disease seen at 10 years.

The causes of anterior cruciate ligament reconstruction complications can be outlined by the failures as depicted in Figure 3.41. Most failures can be prevented by careful surgical planning and preparation, adherence to technique, attention to detail, and careful postoperative follow-up with early recognition and intervention for complications. Surgeons should be knowledgeable about the current literature and potential complications. If one is to advance on a surgical learning curve and decrease the number of complications, assessment of surgical results, radiographic evaluation of tunnels and screw placements, and careful, unbiased physical and KT-1000 examinations are necessary.

Complications can be divided into preoperative, intraoperative, and postoperative categories. Preoperative radiographic evaluation can eliminate most problems of excessive patellar tendon length, tuberosity ossicles, or aberrancy of the patella. Intraoperative complications can result from graft, fixation, or tunnel problems and are avoidable by attention to details. Methods for avoiding these complications are discussed subsequently. Less common or significant problems are noted in Figure 3.41.

Surgical failure can be caused by nonphysiometric tunnel placement, graft impingement, a weak graft, or weak graft fixation. Careful observation of the landmarks and correct placement of tunnels are essential to prevent excessive graft stress or impingement. We generally like to ream the tunnels initially with a reamer that is approximately 2 mm smaller than the definitive tunnel so that minor adjustments can be made easily. Use of a rasp or eccentric reaming to move a tunnel to an appropriate place is easily accomplished. Stress on the patella can be decreased greatly by carefully harvesting the patellar tendon graft. It is important to make straight cuts in line with the fibers and to ensure that the bone cuts are

---

BOX 3.8

Preferred Techniques for Anterior Cruciate Ligament Reconstruction in Athletes

- Primary reconstruction
  - Male—10-mm BPTB
  - Female—9 mm BPTB
- Chronic, revision, or 3+ pivot shift
  - BPTB + ALL reconstruction using semitendinosus harvested through same incision or Lemaire lateral extraarticular tenodesis

ALL, Anterolateral ligament; *BPTB*, bone–patellar tendon–bone.

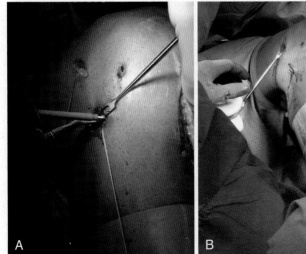
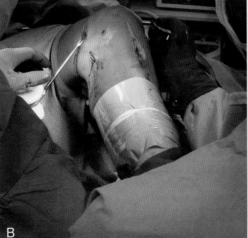
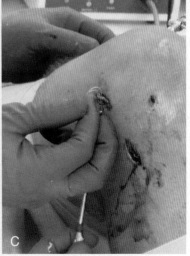

FIGURE 3.55 Reconstruction of the anterior cruciate and anterolateral ligaments. **A,** Graft is secured distally with a swivel lock. **B,** Graft is passed under the iliotibial band proximal to the insertion site. **C,** Graft is secured with a polyetheretherketone (PEEK) interference screw. **SEE TECHNIQUE 3.24.**

not too deep, especially in the patella, and that the length of the cut is 20 to 23 mm. Cuts should be slightly angled, and the patella should be bone grafted on completion to avoid late stress fractures.

At the time of the procedure, an internal notchplasty and careful viewing of the guidewire to ensure that it does not impinge on the roof or the wall of the tunnel with flexion and extension is essential. Also, one should ensure that it is not too far posterior, where it would impinge on the PCL. After placement and alterations have been made, the graft should be fully observed again, particularly in knee extension.

Postoperative problems include arthrofibrosis, which should be treated with nonsteroidal antiinflammatory drugs and supervised therapy. Therapy to rebuild muscular tone initially should be attempted to try to regain full knee extension. Supervised therapy is instituted three times a week with the patient working on range of motion three times daily, stressing prone hangs to regain full extension. If motion fails to progress over 4 to 6 weeks of therapy, and the patient has less than 90 degrees flexion after 6 weeks of supervised physical therapy, gentle manipulation and possibly arthroscopic evaluation should be considered. Postoperative radiographs are reviewed to ensure that the tunnels are correctly placed and that an obvious impingement is not demonstrable.

Loss of full extension, persistent effusion, anterior knee pain, or clicking or popping in the anterior part of the knee that is painful with terminal extension may indicate impingement. A lateral radiograph should be obtained with the knee in extension to ensure the tibial tunnel is posterior to the foot of the intercondylar notch and that screw placement in the femur is in the posterior aspect of the intercondylar notch.

Postoperative infections are uncommon with arthroscopic anterior cruciate ligament reconstructions, but persistence or recurrence of fever 5 to 6 days after the procedure with increased pain, loss of knee motion, and heat or erythema at the knee site may indicate early infection and must be treated appropriately and aggressively. If a knee aspiration shows a white blood cell count to be elevated (often ≥ 20,000/μL), arthroscopic irrigation and evaluation of the graft should be performed. If the graft is still intact and in good condition, it should be left in place, but the joint should be thoroughly irrigated, and repeat irrigation and debridement should be done at 48 to 72 hours if symptoms are not drastically improving. A combination of antibiotics intravenously for 2 to 3 weeks followed by oral antibiotics to complete a 6-week course of organism-specific antibiotic treatment is necessary.

In any postoperative infection, finding the source is crucial to prevent additional infections. Equipment sterilization procedures, preparation and draping techniques, handling of the graft by operating room personnel, and surgical techniques should be evaluated carefully. The surgical site of arthroscopy should always be prepared with a waterproof antibiotic solution and draped and sealed proximal and distal to the site of surgery.

The chance of deep venous thrombosis (DVT) is increased with smoking, obesity, and metabolic and hypercoagulable abnormalities. There is a 50% chance of DVT, 11% proximal, before arthroscopy in patients with high-energy trauma. Presurgery screening is indicated in these patients. Smoking

increases the failure rates of anterior cruciate ligament and meniscal repairs.

▌POSTERIOR CRUCIATE LIGAMENT RECONSTRUCTION

The PCL consists of three components: an anterolateral band, a posteromedial band, and the meniscofemoral ligaments. The larger anterolateral band is approximately 150% the strength and stiffness of the posteromedial band and tightens slightly with knee flexion. Structural properties of the two bundles are the same other than size, and they have co-functionality. The entire ligament has 1.5 to 2 times the strength of the anterior cruciate ligament, and the broadness of its femoral footprint is approximately 3 cm². The large insertion site of the dual ligaments makes physiometric reconstruction difficult.

Many PCL injuries have an associated ligamentous injury, most commonly the posterolateral corner. Hyperflexion is the most common cause for PCL injuries in athletes. Sometimes a partial PCL injury, with 1+ to 2+ posterior laxity, occurs. Shelbourne and Muthukaruppan reported good clinical outcomes when these injuries were treated conservatively initially, consisting of knee extension and a protective rehabilitation program with no active hamstring strengthening. Long-term results did not correlate with the initial degree of instability in isolated injuries. Subjective scores did not deteriorate with time.

PCL injuries in active, healthy athletes should be assessed with kneeling stress radiographs and MRI to evaluate associated injuries. Injuries of the posterolateral or medial corner should be repaired and augmented or reconstructed. PCL injuries with 3+ laxity (≥ 8 mm on stress radiographs) and symptomatic PCL injuries are reconstructed.

Double-bundle reconstructions have gained favor with many, but anatomic single-bundle techniques have good results, similar to those for transtibial and inlay techniques.

The two-tunnel technique has been shown in clinical studies to have increased stability and to better fill the large PCL footprint.

The single-tunnel technique, which we use mostly for reconstruction of multiple knee ligaments in knee dislocations, is described subsequently. The two-tunnel technique is used primarily in isolated PCL reconstruction. An Achilles tendon allograft is our preferred graft source for PCL reconstruction. Comparable results have been reported with allografts and autografts.

An all-arthroscopic inlay procedure, using a retrocutting reamer and a closed-ended tibial tunnel with suture fixation anteriorly, has been described by several authors; this, like aperture screw fixation, produces a shorter, stiffer graft construct and removes the "killer curve" that sometimes occurs in the transtibial technique, although a killer curve still remains on the femoral side.

Comparative studies show that anatomic single-tunnel and inlay procedures produce equal function and stability. Double-bundle techniques have been shown to be slightly better (2.5 mm of posterior displacement compared with 3.2 mm), with better IKDC scores, in most studies. The most important factors for long-term success are correction of associated instabilities and meniscal preservation. Slow, protected rehabilitation also increases the likelihood of knee stability and should emphasize early maintenance of knee extension, delayed weight bearing, and delayed return to sports. For multiligament instability, a simple single-tunnel procedure usually is effective; an isolated PCL double-tunnel procedure may be indicated.

LaPrade et al. showed that a decreased posterior tibial slope puts athletes at some increased risk of PCL injuries, but with double-bundle reconstruction there is no increased failure rate based on tibial slope.

SINGLE-TUNNEL POSTERIOR CRUCIATE LIGAMENT RECONSTRUCTION

TECHNIQUE 3.25

(PHILLIPS)
- Place the patient supine and apply a tourniquet high around the thigh. Use a padded lateral post to assist with valgus stress. Tape a 3-L saline bag to the table before draping to use as a foot bolster to help maintain 80 to 90 degrees of knee flexion during the procedure.
- Perform a routine systematic arthroscopic examination of the knee and repair any associated intraarticular abnormalities as necessary. If a meniscal repair is performed, the sutures should be tied after the ligament reconstruction is completed.
- Using standard anterolateral and anteromedial portals, debride the soft tissue and remaining cruciate ligament from the intercondylar notch.
- Perform an internal bony notchplasty as necessary.
- Viewing of the tibial attachment site of the posterior cruciate ligament (Fig. 3.56A) is improved by using a 70-degree viewing arthroscope in the anterolateral portal or by placing the 30-degree viewing arthroscope through a posteromedial portal.
- Using a full-radius resector, remove the remaining stump of the posterior cruciate ligament. Specially designed back-cutting knives, curets, and rasps also are available to assist in removing the remnants.
- Elevate the posterior capsule from its attachment to the posterior flat spot on the tibia using a curved curet or periosteal elevator passed through the intercondylar notch or the posteromedial portal.
- Contour an Achilles tendon allograft to make a bone plug 11 mm wide × 20 mm long.
- Place the tendinous part of the graft under tension and roll the graft with a running Vicryl suture. Place a no. 5 tension suture in the distal 5 cm of the graft, using a running interlocking suture. Place the graft on a graft tension board, maintained with 10 lb of tension for 15 minutes.
- If an autogenous patellar tendon is chosen as a graft, make a 7-cm midline incision, starting at the inferior patella and extending distally over the tibial tuberosity.
- Harvest the central third of the patellar tendon—10 to 11 mm wide and 25 mm long—with 8-mm-thick bone plugs.
- Contour the graft to pass through a 10- or 11-mm trial. The bone plug to be secured in the femoral tunnel should

be shortened to approximately 20 mm to make intraarticular passage easier.
- For making the tibial tunnel, we prefer to use the Arthrex drill guide system. With the 70-degree arthroscope in the anterolateral portal, insert the guide through the anteromedial portal and pass it through the notch.
- Place the guide tip 10 to 12 mm below the joint line in the posterior cruciate ligament facet.
- Orient the drill guide approximately 60 degrees to the articular surface of the tibia, starting just inferior and medial to the tibial tuberosity (Fig. 3.57A). A more perpendicular angle would create too much of an acute angle at the posterior tibia that may abrade the graft. A tibial tunnel that is started too distally may ream out the posterior tibial shelf. The simultaneous use of image intensification and arthroscopy aids in proper positioning of the drill guide before and during drilling. Calibrations on the tibial guide accurately measure the distance from the anterior tibial cortex to the tip of the guide.
- Adjust the guide pin so that it is protruding from the tip of the drill 1 cm less than the distance measured on the guide system to help prevent overdrilling (see Fig. 3.57A).
- The guide pin should exit posteriorly at the physeal scar area.
- Tap the pin in the final 1 cm to help prevent penetration. While tapping the pin in, place a curet through the posteromedial portal to protect the neurovascular structures from pin penetration during advancement and reaming. If adequate soft-tissue debridement has been performed, the guide pin can be observed arthroscopically as it exits the tibia. An image intensifier is used to confirm appropriate guidewire placement.
- The femoral physiometric point is 8 mm proximal to the articular cartilage at the 1-o'clock position on the right knee and at the 11-o'clock position on the left knee (Fig. 3.57B). Place the tip of the posterior cruciate ligament femoral guide through the anteromedial portal while viewing with the arthroscope in the anterolateral portal.
- Expose the femoral cortex through the 3-cm longitudinal incision and elevate the vastus medialis obliquus superiorly.
- Insert the guide pin midway between the articular margin of the medial femoral condyle and the medial epicondyle.
- Use the appropriate size reamer for the available graft, leaving 1 to 2 mm of distal bone at the articular margin.
- Pass a Gore smoother through the tibial tunnel into the joint and pull it through the central fat pad portal (Fig. 3.57C). The smoother is used to smooth and remove the posterior soft-tissue remnants. Do not enlarge the tibial tunnel excessively.
- When the smoother passes without undue resistance, attach the graft to the end of the smoother and pull the graft sutures and bone plug into the joint.
- Extreme flexion of the knee sometimes aids passage of the patellar bone plug from the posterior tibial aperture into the joint. Placing a switching stick through the posteromedial portal allows the guide sutures to be redirected over the stick to assist in passing the graft.
- Place a grasper through the femoral tunnel to grab the sutures. Use a probe or Allis clamp to assist the graft into the femoral tunnel.

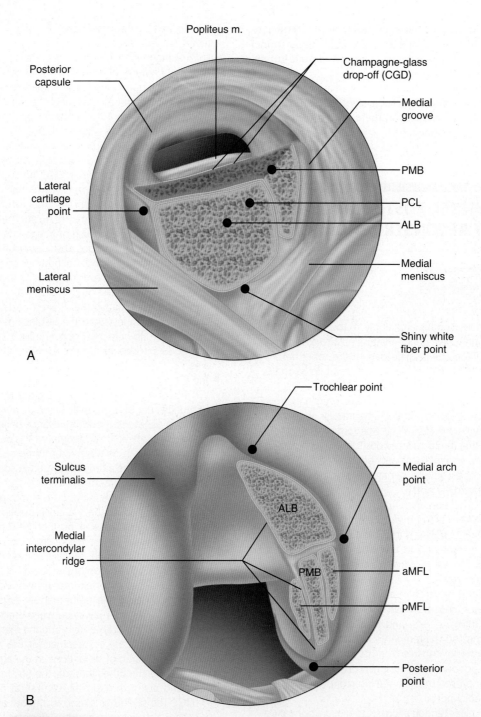

FIGURE 3.56 Arthroscopic view of the tibial attachment (**A**) and femoral attachment (**B**) of the posterior cruciate ligament (PCL) in a right knee, demonstrating pertinent landmarks. ALB, anterolateral bundle; aMFL, anterior meniscofemoral ligament; PMB, posteromedial bundle; pMFL, posterior meniscofemoral ligament. (Redrawn from Anderson CJ, Ziegler CG, Wijdicks CA, et al: Arthroscopically pertinent anatomy of the anterolateral and posteromedial bundles of the posterior cruciate ligament, *J Bone Joint Surg* 94:1936, 2012.) **SEE TECHNIQUE 3.56**

- Place the cancellous portion of the bone plug posteriorly to reduce graft abrasion.
- Before tibial fixation, ensure that the femoral bone plug would fit appropriately at the aperture of the femoral tunnel.
- Put the knee through a range of motion and ensure there is no more than 3 mm of graft pistoning through range

of motion from 0 to 100 degrees. If excessive pistoning is encountered, rasp the femoral tunnel proximal wall.
- Secure the femoral bone plug with a metal interference screw.
- Maintain graft tension and put the knee through a range of motion for 20 cycles to allow stress relaxation of the graft.

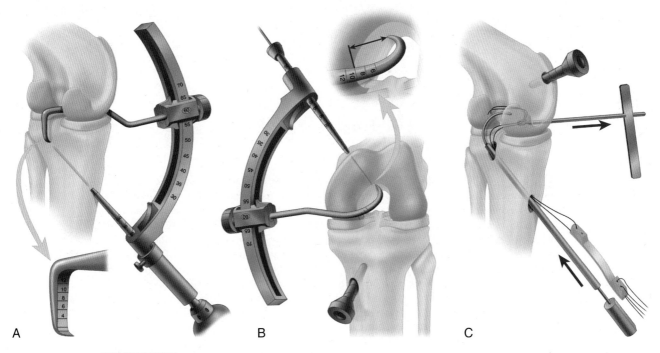

A   **B**   **C**

FIGURE 3.57   Posterior ligament reconstruction. **A,** Arthrex Popliteal Drill Stop prevents advancement of guide pin past the tip of the marking hook during drilling. **B,** Millimeter markings on Arthrex PCL Femoral Marking Hook allow determination of the distance of the femoral tunnel from the margin of the articular cartilage. **C,** Arthrex "Worm" Curving Suture Passer facilitates passing of graft sutures through tibial tunnel into intercondylar notch. **SEE TECHNIQUE 3.25.**

■ Secure the graft with an interference screw. If a soft-tissue graft is used, backup fixation over a post is indicated.

POSTOPERATIVE CARE Rehabilitation depends on the graft material selected, the size of the patient, and any other surgery done. After isolated posterior cruciate ligament reconstruction, the knee can be immobilized in extension in a removable knee immobilizer for 4 weeks. Early range-of-motion and quadriceps exercises are encouraged, but flexion is limited to 90 degrees for the first 4 weeks. Hamstring strengthening is begun at 3 months. During motion and strengthening therapy, care is taken to prevent posterior tibial stress. Return to sports is allowed at 9 months.

DOUBLE-TUNNEL POSTERIOR CRUCIATE LIGAMENT RECONSTRUCTION

TECHNIQUE 3.26

(LAPRADE ET AL.)
■ Prepare the anterolateral bundle graft from an Achilles tendon allograft with an 11-mm diameter and 20-mm

long calcaneal bone graft; tubularize the distal soft-tissue aspect of the graft.
■ Prepare the posteromedial bundle graft from a 7-mm diameter soft-tissue anterior tibial allograft by tubularizing each end of the graft.
■ Create standard anterolateral and anteromedial arthroscopic portals and identify the femoral attachments of the anterolateral and posteromedial bundles.
■ Outline the anterolateral bundle attachment between the trochlear point and medial arch point, adjoining the edge of the articular cartilage.
■ Mark the posteromedial bundle attachment approximately 5.8 mm proximal to the edge of the articular cartilage of the medial femoral condyle and slightly posterior to the anterolateral bundle tunnel.
■ Ream an 11-mm diameter closed socket tunnel to a depth of 25 mm for the anterolateral bundle and place a 7-mm reamer against the outlined posteromedial bundle to create the second tunnel of the same depth. Maintain a 2-mm bone bridge between the femoral tunnels (Fig. 3.58A-C).
■ Create a posteromedial portal to facilitate identification and preparation of the PCL attachment site. Drill a tibial guide pin, entering the anteromedial aspect of the tibial approximately 6 cm distal to the joint line and exiting posteriorly at the center of the PCL tibial attachment along the PCL bundle ridge (Fig. 3.59A, B).
■ Use a 12-mm acorn reamer to overream the tibial guide pin under direct posterior arthroscopic observation (Fig. 3.59C).
■ Insert a large smoother (Gore Smoother Crucial Tool, Smith & Nephew) up the tibial tunnel to facilitate graft

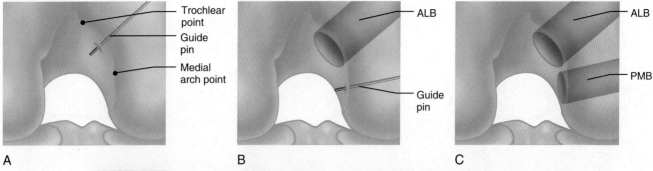

A

B

C

FIGURE 3.58 Medial aspect of femoral notch in right knee demonstrating sequence of double-bundle posterior cruciate ligament reconstruction. **A,** Guide pin is inserted (through an 11-mm reamer between trochlear point and medial arch point, adjacent to cartilage) to re-create anterolateral bundle (ALB). **B,** An 11-mm diameter closed socket tunnel is reamed to depth of 24 mm for ALB. Posteromedial bundle (PMB) attachment is reproduced next, approximately 5 mm posterior to edge of articular cartilage of medial femoral condyle and distal to medial arch point (also with help of 7-mm reamer placed in medial wall to assess for final position). **C,** Closed socket tunnel is reamed to depth of 25 mm for second tunnel (PMB). Of note, bone bridge of 2 mm should always be present between tunnels. (From LaPrade RF, Cinque ME, Dornan GJ, et al: Double-bundle posterior cruciate reconstruction in 100 patients at mean 3 years' follow-up. Outcomes were comparable to anterior cruciate ligament reconstructions, *Am H Sports Med* 46:1809, 2018.) **SEE TECHNIQUE 3.26.**

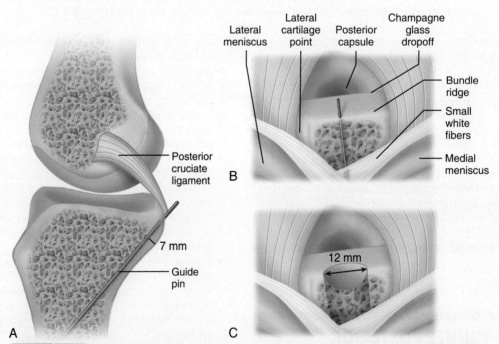

A

B

C

FIGURE 3.59 Tibial attachment of the posterior cruciate ligament (PCL) for double-bundle reconstruction. **A,** Guide pin is drilled, entering anteromedial aspect of tibia approximately 6 cm distal to joint line and exiting at center of the PCL tibial attachment along PCL bundle ridge. Positioning of guide pin should be assessed with fluoroscopy (7 mm anterior to the posterior cortex on lateral view and medial to lateral eminence on anteroposterior view.) **B,** Arthroscopically, pin should exit at center of bundle ridge, posterior to shiny white fibers and medial to lateral cartilage point. **C,** A 12-mm acorn reamer is used to overream tibial guide pin under direct posterior arthroscopic observation. CGD, champagne glass drop-off; LM, lateral meniscus; MM, medial meniscus. (From LaPrade RF, Cinque ME, Dornan GJ, et al: Double-bundle posterior cruciate reconstruction in 100 patients at mean 3 years' follow-up. Outcomes were comparable to anterior cruciate ligament reconstructions, *Am H Sports Med* 46:1809, 2018.) **SEE TECHNIQUE 3.26.**

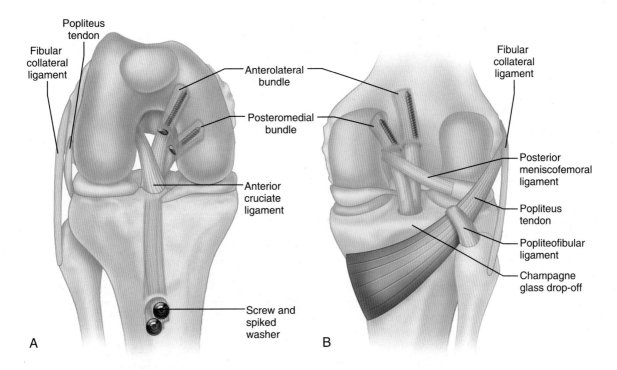

Fibular collateral ligament

Popliteus tendon

Anterolateral bundle

Posteromedial bundle

Anterior cruciate ligament

Screw and spiked washer

A

Fibular collateral ligament

Posterior meniscofemoral ligament

Popliteus tendon

Popliteofibular ligament

Champagne glass drop-off

B

FIGURE 3.60 Anterior (**A**) and posterior (**B**) views of anatomic double-bundle PCL reconstruction. Reconstructed ALB and PMB are shown, as well as size, shape, and location of their femoral and tibial tunnels. PMB enters the tibial tunnel posteromedial to ALB. PMB is posterior in transtibial tunnel, exits deep to ALB, and is fixed medially and distally to ALB. Femoral fixation of both bundles and champagne glass drop-off also are displayed. *ACL,* anterior cruciate ligament; *FCL,* fibular collateral ligament; *PFL,* popliteofibular ligament; *PLT,* popliteus tendon; *pMFL,* posterior meniscofemoral ligament (ligament of Wrisberg). (From LaPrade RF, Cinque ME, Dornan GJ, et al: Double-bundle posterior cruciate reconstruction in 100 patients at mean 3 years' follow-up. Outcomes were comparable to anterior cruciate ligament reconstructions, *Am H Sports Med* 46:1809, 2018.) **SEE TECHNIQUE 3.26.**

passage; pass the end of the smoother out the anterolateral arthroscopic portal.

- Fix the posteromedial bundle graft in the femoral tunnel with a 7- × 23-mm bioabsorbable interference screw and the anterolateral bundle graft with a 7- × 20-mm titanium interference screw.
- After the grafts are fixed in the femoral tunnels, pass the sutures in the ends of both grafts through the loop tip of the smoother and pull the smoother and the graft sutures in its eyelet tip distally down the tibial tunnel and out the anteromedial aspect of the tibia.
- Cycle the grafts and secure them individually with 6.5-mm cancellous bicortical screws and 18-mm spiked washers (Fig. 3.60). Suture the anterolateral bundle graft first at 90 degrees with an anterior drawer force to reproduce the normal tibiofemoral step off and then secure the posteromedial bundle graft at 0 degrees.

POSTOPERATIVE CARE Postoperatively, all patients remain non–weight bearing for 6 weeks. For the first 6 months, a dynamic posterior cruciate ligament brace is worn at all times except during bathing and dressing. Range of motion and edema control are begun the day after surgery. Prone knee flexion is limited to 90 degrees for the first 2 weeks; thereafter, knee motion is increased as tolerated. Weight bearing is initiated at 6 weeks with

low-resistance cycling on a stationary bike and leg presses performed to a maximum of 70 degrees of knee flexion. Progressive advancement into low-impact knee exercises is allowed as tolerated starting at 12 weeks.

Six months after surgery, patients are evaluated clinically and with kneeling posterior stress radiographs. Discontinuation of the brace for daily use is allowed if the side-to-side difference in kneeing stress radiographs was less than 2 mm, and jogging, side-to-side activities, and proprioceptive exercises are allowed. Functional testing (e.g., the Vail Sports Test) is done between 9 and 12 months after surgery to determine the patient's ability to return to full activity. A dynamic PCL brace is worn for sporting activities for the first year of athletic competition.

Inlay Technique. This technique, which allows direct fixation of a tibial bone plug to a tibial trough in the anatomic insertion of the PCL along the posterior tibia, has the advantages of eliminating acute graft angle changes and allows secure direct fixation to the posterior tibia, thus making a shorter, stiffer graft. The approach allows safe exposure of this area. The disadvantage of this technique is that access to the anterior and the posterior knee is necessary during the surgical procedure. The patient can be placed in the lateral decubitus position with the injured side up. The hip can be externally rotated for the arthroscopic part of the procedure, and then the knee can be straightened and placed on a padded Mayo stand for the posterior exposure. Conversely, an easier method for posterior exposure is made possible by placing a bump under the unaffected side and placing the affected side in a figure-of-four position. The surgeon starts on the opposite side of the table (i.e., the unaffected side). Tilting the table toward or away from the surgeon allows for better visualization during different parts of the procedure. Femoral tunnels are reamed at 1 o'clock and at 3 o'clock, 1 mm and 3 mm, respectively, off the articular surfaces before posterior exposure.

■ CHONDROMALACIA OF THE PATELLA SYNDROME

Chondromalacia, which means softening of the articular cartilage, has multiple causes. Cartilage changes can be classified from an arthroscopic standpoint based on the modified Outerbridge (Insall) classification: grade I, softening and swelling of the cartilage; grade II, fragmentation and fissuring in an area 0.5 inch or less in diameter; grade III, more severe fragmentation and fissuring involving an area of more than 0.5 inch in diameter; and grade IV, erosion of cartilage down to bone.

Chondromalacia can be treated conservatively in most patients with an emphasis on maximizing flexibility of the musculature and strengthening the vastus medialis obliquus muscle. Closed chain exercises are recommended, and some studies showed that taping and bracing were advantageous. Carefully evaluating lower extremity alignment, particularly for hyperpronation that can be corrected with orthotics, also can decrease patellofemoral stress.

If prolonged, conservative treatment fails, then surgical intervention may be necessary. Careful evaluation of the individual, including alignment, associated articular changes, ligamentous laxity, future goals, and rehabilitation potential, is necessary to obtain a good surgical result. In the case of chondromalacia with no significant malalignment and grade II or early grade III changes, arthroscopic debridement of the patellofemoral joint and reevaluation of the exercise program may be all that is necessary. Arthroscopic debridement of the articular surface can be done safely with mechanical instrumentation. For full-thickness chondral defects, realignment and cartilage cell transfer can give moderate to good relief.

Lateral release is indicated for excessive lateral pressure syndrome unresponsive to therapy and for lateral facet arthritis in combination with excision of a painful lateral facet osteophyte. Isolated lateral release for patellar instability has not been shown to be effective and may compound the problem caused by persistent quadriceps weakness. The most predictable criterion for success of a lateral release is a negative passive patellar tilt, a medial and lateral patellar glide of two quadrants or less, and a normal tubercle-sulcus angle with the knee at 90 degrees of flexion. The passive patellar tilt test is performed with the patient supine, the knee extended, and the quadriceps relaxed. The examiner lifts the lateral edge of the patella from the lateral femoral condyle. The patella should remain in the trochlea. An excessively tight lateral restraint is shown by a neutral or negative angle to the horizontal (Fig. 3.61A). The patellar glide test determines medial or lateral retinacular tightness (Fig. 3.61B). This test is performed with the knee flexed 20 to 30 degrees and the quadriceps relaxed. This position can be accomplished by placing a small pillow beneath

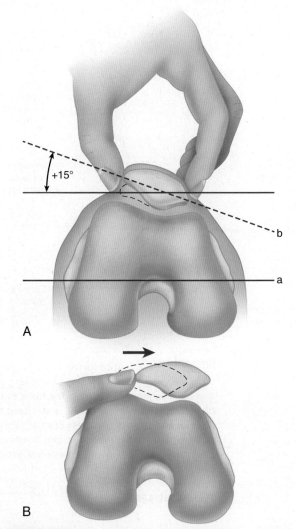

FIGURE 3.61 **A,** Passive patellar tilt test. Lateral edge of patella is lifted from lateral femoral condyle (b). Patella should remain in trochlea and not be allowed lateral subluxation. Excessively tight lateral restraint is shown by neutral or negative angle to horizontal (a). **B,** Patellar glide test in 30 degrees of flexion.

the knee. The patella is divided into longitudinal quadrants, and an attempt is made to displace the patella medially and laterally. A lateral patellar glide of three quadrants or more suggests an incompetent medial restraint. A medial glide of one quadrant is consistent with a tight lateral restraint, and a glide of three or more quadrants suggests a hypermobile patella. The tuberosity-sulcus angle is determined by measuring the Q angle with the knee at 90 degrees of flexion. The angle is formed by a line drawn from the center of the patella to the center of the tibial tuberosity and a line drawn from the center of the patella and passing perpendicular to the transepicondylar axis. This angle should be 0 degrees, and more than 10 degrees is definitely abnormal. The traditional Q angle measured from the tibial tuberosity to the center of the patella and extending to the anterior superior iliac spine likewise is a valuable measurement that should be evaluated when contemplating surgical procedures for the patella. Anteroposterior, 45-degree lateral, and 45-degree Merchant view radiographs are helpful in determining patellar tilt, subluxation, and Insall ratio,

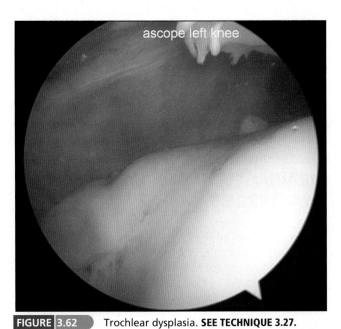

FIGURE 3.62   Trochlear dysplasia. **SEE TECHNIQUE 3.27.**

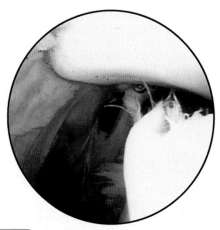

FIGURE 3.63   Patellofemoral joint viewed from superolateral portal; lateral subluxation of patella is evident. **SEE TECHNIQUE 3.27.**

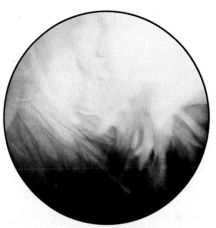

FIGURE 3.64   Grade III chondromalacia of patella involving central ridge and lateral facet. **SEE TECHNIQUE 3.27.**

as described in other chapter. Lateral release should extend only to the vastus lateralis and not include this structure.

LATERAL RETINACULAR RELEASE

TECHNIQUE 3.27

- View the patellofemoral joint with a 30-degree viewing arthroscope in the inferior or superior portal; either is adequate. With the arthroscope in the standard anterolateral portal and advanced into the patellofemoral joint, rotate the lens upward and downward alternately to view the articular surfaces of the patella and the trochlear groove of the distal femur (Fig. 3.62).
- Manually manipulate the patella with the thumb and index finger for complete viewing of the entire surface of the patella. The tracking of the patella and the dynamics of the patella and the patellofemoral joint can be viewed better from a superior portal (Fig. 3.63). The patella naturally rides laterally with the knee in extension, and observation of it in this position does not confirm that the patella is subluxable or riding laterally. As the knee is moved from full extension into 30 to 40 degrees of flexion, the patella enters the trochlear groove and should become congruous and centered at this degree of flexion. Persistent lateral tilt or overhang of the lateral facet over the edge of the lateral femoral condyle with the knee in this position suggests a lateral tracking phenomenon. Note the various degrees of chondromalacia of the patellar and trochlear articular surfaces and record them (Fig. 3.64).
- Before performing the lateral retinacular release, carry out a complete and systematic examination of the knee for other pathologic entities and trim and shave severe patellar articular surface chondromalacic changes where appropriate. Extensive shaving of chondromalacic areas on the patellar or trochlear surface probably has only short-term effects; shaving should be kept to a minimum, emphasizing removal of only degenerative fibrillated material. The objective is restoration of the proper dynamics of the extensor mechanism.
- When a complete arthroscopic examination has been done and any chondroplastic areas have been shaved, remove the arthroscopic instruments from the joint and evacuate the irrigating fluids.
- Attempt to palpate the inferior edge of the vastus lateralis tendon and mark this junction at its insertion into the patella with an 18-gauge spinal needle at the superior pole of the patella. If the edge of the tendon cannot be palpated, simply insert the needle at the superolateral corner of the patella.
- Insert the arthroscope through the superolateral or the anteromedial portal. Initially, insert the electrocautery into the anterolateral portal.
- Under arthroscopic guidance, divide the synovium and lateral retinaculum from the superolateral corner of the patella marked by the spinal needle to the inferior extent of the lateral border of the patellar tendon. Occasionally, the electrocautery must be placed in a superomedial or superolateral portal to complete the most inferior portion of the release. The release can

be extended proximally along the lateral border of the vastus lateralis tendon.

- Place a thick sponge pad over the superolateral aspect of the distal thigh just proximal to the patellar tendon to serve as a pressure pad over the cut superolateral geniculate vessels. This has reduced the incidence of troublesome hemarthrosis after release.
- A drain can be placed intraarticularly and removed after several hours.

POSTOPERATIVE CARE The knee is maintained in an immobile, extended position for 48 hours, and then gentle range-of-motion exercises are begun. Immobilization of the knee in extension for longer than 72 hours may allow the edges of the lateral retinacular release to adhere and become ineffective. Early range of motion tends to spread the release. Quadriceps isometric and stiff-leg exercises are encouraged. Weight bearing is allowed as tolerated.

▍ARTHROSCOPIC MEDIAL PARAPATELLAR PLICATION

Arthroscopic plication of the medial retinaculum has been described for patellar instability. The all-inside technique uses a 17-gauge Tuohy epidural needle to pass a no. 1 polydioxanone suture near the medial edge of the patella. The edge of the suture is retrieved out of a superolateral portal. The needle is backed up slightly to remain under the subcutaneous tissue and advanced posteriorly about 2 cm. The needle is passed back through the retinaculum, and the resulting loop of the suture is pulled out superiorly, taking both tails out superiorly. After passage of four to five sutures, they are tied arthroscopically through the anteromedial portal. An arthroscopic lateral release is performed. We do not do this procedure and believe that the same technique can be performed more adequately with nonabsorbable sutures and better imbrication through a small medial parapatellar incision.

SYNOVECTOMY

Arthroscopic synovectomy in rheumatoid disease and other chronic inflammatory conditions and in hemophilia has been reported to produce less morbidity, shorter hospitalization, and more rapid return of function to the joint.

TECHNIQUE 3.28

- Four or five portals, including the posteromedial and posterolateral portals, are used routinely. Approach the posterior compartment with a 70-degree viewing arthroscope placed through the intercondylar notch and place a full-radius resector through the corresponding posteromedial or posterolateral portal.
- Preserving the menisci, resect the synovial proliferation inferior to the menisci and around the cruciate ligaments, preserving the underlying structures.
- Carefully strip the synovial proliferation in the medial and lateral aspects of the knee off the junction of the synovium and the articular cartilage. Frequent repositioning of the arthroscope and motorized shavers is necessary to avoid damage to the articular cartilage and to reach all synovial recesses.

- After synovectomy, insert a drain in the knee and connect it to suction. Place the knee in a modified Jones dressing.

POSTOPERATIVE CARE Before discharge, the drain is removed. Weight bearing to tolerance with crutches is allowed, and range-of-motion and quadriceps-strengthening exercises are begun immediately.

DRAINAGE AND DEBRIDEMENT IN PYARTHROSIS

Arthroscopic debridement and lavage in pyarthrosis offer the advantages of reduced morbidity and shortened hospitalization. With the arthroscope, the knee can be lavaged with large volumes of fluid and any fibrinoid material and infected debris can be removed. With the advent of more resistant organisms, the use of appropriate cultures and initial use of broad-spectrum antibiotic coverage, including coverage for methicillin-resistant *Staphylococcus aureus,* are indicated. When the cultures are complete, antibiotics specific to the organism should be used.

TECHNIQUE 3.29

- The standard arthroscopic setup is used for arthroscopic debridement. Do not exsanguinate the extremity. Use a large-bore cannula or arthroscopic pump for irrigation.
- Make anteromedial and anterolateral portals to examine and debride fibrinoid exudate as indicated. Take appropriate bacterial cultures.
- Thoroughly lavage all compartments (anterior, posterior, and suprapatellar) and the medial and lateral gutters, using 9 to 10 L of fluid.
- Place suction drain tubes in the medial and lateral gutters through the arthroscopic cannula and then withdraw the cannula over the drain. Loosely approximate the portals with absorbable sutures.

POSTOPERATIVE CARE A Jones-type dressing is applied to immobilize the knee for 36 to 48 hours while appropriate antibiotics are administered. At 48 hours, the drains are removed and range of motion is begun. If the infection fails to respond to treatment, repeat debridement is considered at 72 hours.

OTHER APPLICATIONS OF ARTHROSCOPY OF THE KNEE

The following are additional, less frequent, applications for arthroscopy of the knee. Several are refinements of principles and techniques previously described in this chapter, and most should be attempted only by surgeons with considerable arthroscopic experience. Many of these techniques have not been sufficiently evaluated to determine the long-term results and are not described in detail.

▍ARTHROSCOPY IN FRACTURES AROUND THE KNEE

Arthroscopic techniques have been used to evaluate fractures of the anterior intercondylar eminence of the tibia, to reduce such fractures, and, after reduction, to fix the eminence with percutaneously inserted internal fixation. In addition, arthroscopy has been advocated to assess the degree of articular surface depression and the adequacy of reduction after tibial plateau fractures.

Good results have been reported with arthroscopically assisted fracture reduction and percutaneous fixation. Fracture patterns that are appropriate for arthroscopic management are those that can be internally fixed with a cancellous screw and do not require a major reduction or use of a buttress plate. Better fracture evaluation, reduced operative time and morbidity, shorter hospitalization, and quicker recovery have been cited as advantages to the arthroscopically assisted technique.

ARTHROSCOPICALLY ASSISTED FRACTURE REDUCTION AND PERCUTANEOUS FIXATION

TECHNIQUE 3.30

(CASPARI ET AL.)
- Make a small transverse incision in the skin 3 cm to 4 cm below the joint line and drill holes through the anterior cortex.
- With the use of an image intensifier and under arthroscopic guidance, insert a 0.25-inch osteotome through the cortical window and drive it under the fracture to elevate the fragments. By manipulating the osteotome and using the anterior cortex as a fulcrum, elevate the fragments under arthroscopic guidance. Caspari et al. termed this "indirect triangulation." They recommended over-elevation of the fragments.
- Remove the stress from the knee and move it through a range of motion. The femoral condyle serves to mold the surface of the tibial plateau back into its anatomic configuration. If necessary, insert a bone graft under the fracture through the cortical window.
- Obtain internal fixation by percutaneous or open technique.
- Use of an arthroscopic anterior cruciate ligament guide to place a guidewire into the fracture site also has been described. A reamer is used to make the cortical window and a tamp to elevate the fragments. A 15-mm Arthrex "coring" reamer can preserve local bone graft. Image intensification is used to place percutaneous cannulated screws.

POSTOPERATIVE CARE Postoperative management is tailored to the specific injury and the adequacy of reduction and fixation. If the fracture is stable, with rigid internal fixation, early controlled range of motion is begun.

■ **ARTHROFIBROSIS**

Arthroscopic techniques for lysis and excision of postoperative adhesions have been described. The arthroscopic procedure usually is combined with a gentle manipulation after the

release. If extensive infrapatellar contracture syndrome develops, as evidenced by peripatellar induration, restricted patellar mobility, and loss of knee motion, conservative means should be used to reduce inflammation and regain muscle tone and knee extension. An open technique, including lateral release and excision of the fat pad, may be necessary after the acute reaction has subsided.

ARTHROSCOPIC LYSIS AND EXCISION OF ADHESIONS

TECHNIQUE 3.31

(SPRAGUE)
- Insert an arthroscopic sheath and blunt trocar through standard anterolateral and anteromedial portals.
- Pass the blunt trocar carefully beneath the patella and into the suprapatellar pouch. Use the trocar to disrupt bluntly any adhesions in the suprapatellar pouch and in the medial and lateral gutters.
- Insert the arthroscope and inspect the joint in a routine manner. If the adhesions are dense, the patellofemoral joint usually is spared.
- Begin the debridement in the peripatellar region and extend it outward.
- When the suprapatellar pouch has been restored, insert an inflow cannula through a superior portal.
- Continue the dissection down into the medial and lateral gutters and compartments and finally into the intercondylar area. Avoid damage to the cruciate ligaments.
- Occasionally, proliferation of fibrous tissue is present within the intercondylar notch and anterior regions; this should be removed because it may limit extension. Some investigators recommend a lateral retinacular release as part of the procedure if patellar mobility is restricted after the arthroscopic release. Avoid iatrogenic fracture caused by excessive manipulation.
- After the systematic lysis of adhesions, perform a gentle manipulation. If any further adhesions are disrupted, debride these further arthroscopically.
- Thoroughly irrigate the joint, insert a suction drain, and apply a bulky compressive dressing.

POSTOPERATIVE CARE We have found it helpful to perform this procedure with the patient under continuous epidural anesthesia, which is maintained for 2 to 3 days after surgery. The patient is placed in a continuous passive motion machine immediately after surgery, and the suction drain is removed at 2 days.

COMPLICATIONS ASSOCIATED WITH KNEE ARTHROSCOPY

Large series on complications associated with knee arthroscopy published in the late 1980s reported overall complication rates for knee arthroscopy of less than 2%. More recent reports generally cite overall complication rates of less than 1%. Four large series with a combined total of 191,584 arthroscopic knee procedures reported complications in 1175 (0.6%), with the most common being infection and DVT or pulmonary embolism (PE). Data from the American Board of Orthopaedic Surgery from 2003 to 2009, however, showed an overall complication rate of almost 5%, with a range of 2.5% for meniscectomy to 20% for PCL reconstruction. Infection was the most common complication overall.

Complications increase with the difficulty of the case, and saphenous and peroneal nerve injuries are still being reported with arthroscopic repairs; however, with all-inside techniques the frequency of these injuries has decreased dramatically. The incidence of arthrofibrosis associated with anterior cruciate ligament reconstruction is increased when meniscal repair is performed. Likewise, the incidence of infection associated with anterior cruciate ligament reconstructions is slightly increased when the reconstruction is performed in conjunction with meniscal repair. Additional exposure, surgical time, and potential for joint contamination during the passing and retrieving of needles are probably the reasons.

Surgical complications related to ligamentous reconstruction are associated with multiple factors that have been reported (see Figs. 3.41 and 3.42). DVT is a real concern with long, complicated procedures, particularly in patients who are overweight, have a history of DVT, are taking birth control pills, or have been inactive as a result of injury. In patients with high-energy knee injuries in whom treatment is delayed for more than 2 weeks, preoperative ultrasound examination of the lower extremities usually should be done. When limited postoperative weight bearing is indicated in these patients, DVT prophylaxis with at least 81 mg of aspirin twice a day probably is warranted. The use of a sequential compression device (SCD) may be indicated for high-risk patients. Most of these causes of failures have been discussed in the technique section.

Careful attention to detail during surgery, including proper sterilization techniques, handling of the graft, and appropriate preparation and draping, can help to prevent postoperative infections. If a graft is contaminated by dropping it on the floor, the surgeon has two choices: change graft sources (i.e., a different autogenous graft source) or attempt sterilization of the dropped graft. Molina et al. reported the results of sterilization of dropped grafts in three solutions: (1) a 1-mL vial containing 40 mg of neomycin and polymyxin in 1000 mL of sterile saline, (2) 10% povidone-iodine solution, or (3) 4% chlorhexidine gluconate solution. Their results after a 90-second soak showed that one of 50 of the contaminated grafts that were soaked in chlorhexidine remained positive, three of 50 soaked in antibiotic remained positive, and 12 of 50 soaked in the povidone-iodine solution remained positive. Several more recent reports have confirmed the efficacy of 4% chlorhexidine for sterilizing contaminated grafts, including laboratory studies that included 495 graft samples. Bacitracin alone also was found effective (97%), as was a combination of neomycin and polymyxin B. With this in mind, it should be reasonable to retrieve the graft immediately from the floor, rinse it using sterile technique with a large volume of sterile saline, soak it in 4% chlorhexidine gluconate solution for at least 90 seconds (we recommend 10 minutes) and then in the neomycin

and polymyxin B solution for at least another 90 seconds (we recommend 10 minutes), and finally rinse it thoroughly. In a survey by Izquierdo et al., 196 sports-trained surgeons responded to a questionnaire on anterior cruciate ligament graft contamination (from a variety of sources). Forty-nine surgeons had experienced a total of 57 contaminations, 75% of which were treated with graft cleansing and proceeding with the reconstruction. In 18% of contaminations, the surgeon harvested a different graft, and in 7% an allograft was used. There were no reported infections. Sixty-five of the 147 surgeons with no graft contaminations responded with hypothetical treatments: 58% would cleanse the graft, 34% would harvest a different graft, and 8% would use an allograft.

When postoperative knee infections occur, early, thorough arthroscopic irrigation and debridement are indicated with repeat irrigation and debridement at 48 to 72 hours if the symptoms have not resolved. Anterior cruciate ligament grafts can be left in place, provided that no extensive deterioration of the graft is present at the time of initial irrigation. The appropriate intravenous antibiotics if susceptible generally are prescribed for 2 to 3 weeks, followed by oral antibiotics to complete a 6-week course of antibiotic treatment. A recent meta-analysis determined that approximately 85% of grafts could be salvaged with arthroscopic debridement and antibiotic therapy.

Abnormal healing reactions, arthrofibrosis, complex regional pain syndrome, and failure of graft incorporation fall under the category of surgical limitations, as do chondral or meniscal injuries. Surgical control over these conditions often is limited, but sometimes skill in surgical planning and timing can have an effect. Early surgical intervention for ligamentous injuries before regaining muscular tone and motion is associated with arthrofibrosis, as are surgical procedures such as medial collateral ligament repair on the femoral side and meniscal repair. Allowing motion and allowing the knee to calm before surgery has been shown to greatly decrease postoperative stiffness and arthrofibrosis.

Complex regional pain syndrome is a poorly understood condition that possibly could be decreased by better patient selection, decreased operating time, and early physical therapy. Early reports stated that overtightening of the anterior cruciate ligament graft might result in failure of graft maturation, but other studies have not supported this conclusion.

HIP

Arthroscopy of the hip continues to evolve and become more common with expanding indications. The number of hip arthroscopic procedures has grown significantly, increasing 600% between 2006 and 2010, as reported through the ABOS database. A recent database review showed the number of arthroscopic procedures in the hip increasing almost fivefold between 2008 and 2013, with the most common procedures being femoroplasty, labral repair, and acetabuloplasty.

Arthroscopy of the hip is a technically demanding procedure because of the sphericity of the femoral head and the dense capsule and musculature that surround the joint. Several papers have described a learning curve for hip arthroscopy, which may be as high as 60 cases before there is a decrease in major complications.

Arthroscopy of the hip gives the surgeon access to the central compartment and peripheral compartments of the hip. The central compartment includes the articular surfaces of the femoral head and acetabulum, the labrum, and the ligamentum teres. The peripheral compartment includes the femoral neck and the surrounding capsule and synovium. Numerous procedures involving the peritrochanteric space also have been described.

INDICATIONS/CONTRAINDICATIONS

The indications for hip arthroscopy continue to expand. Current indications include labral tears, removal of loose bodies, femoroacetabular impingement (FAI), chondral lesions, synovial disorders, ligamentum teres pathology, septic arthritis, psoas tendon disorders, extraarticular impingement (subspine and ischiofemoral), external snapping hip, greater trochanteric pain syndrome, proximal hamstring injuries, and sciatic nerve disorders. In addition, hip arthroscopy is used frequently in the setting of trauma. A systematic review by Niroopan et al. demonstrated good outcomes using hip arthroscopy for bullet extraction, loose body removal, femoral head fixation, acetabular fracture fixation, treatment of labral injuries, and debridement of ligamentum teres injuries. However, care must be taken in patients with acute trauma because the soft-tissue envelope of the hip may be disrupted, which can lead to excessive fluid extravasation into the abdomen and subsequent compartment syndrome.

Relative contraindications are obesity, hip dysplasia, and inability to distract the hip joint. Instrumentation may not be long enough to access the hip joint in obese patients. Hip arthroscopy may lead to chronic instability in patients with dysplasia; however, several authors have shown improvement in symptoms following hip arthroscopy in these patients. Domb et al. reported improvement of patient symptoms and no conversions to total hip arthroplasty in a 5-year follow-up of patients with borderline dysplasia treated arthroscopically.

In the evaluation of patients for hip arthroscopy, care needs to be taken to determine the radiographic level of osteoarthritis in the affected hip. Numerous studies have shown worse results in patients with preexisting osteoarthritis of the hip. Larson et al. found less symptomatic improvement after FAI correction in patients with osteoarthritis and no improvement in patients with advanced osteoarthritis compared to patients without radiographic signs of osteoarthritis. Chandrasekaran et al. showed a significantly higher rate of conversion to total hip arthroplasty in patients with Tönnis grade 2 arthritis (small cysts, moderate joint space narrowing, and moderate loss of femoral head sphericity).

GENERAL SETUP

Arthroscopy of the hip has been described with the patient supine or in the lateral position. Both positions offer some advantages, but the choice is surgeon dependent. The supine position offers ease of patient positioning, surgeon familiarity, and the ability to use a fracture table. The lateral position is often easier in obese patients. The lateral position does require distraction devices for the operating table.

Both techniques require the affected leg to be placed in traction for access to the joint, as well as for procedures involving the intraarticular portion or central compartment of the hip. Some commercially available distractors are available, but a regular fracture table can be used (Fig. 3.65A). Ten to 12 mm of distraction is needed for placement of 4.5- or 5.5-mm cannulas. With devices that have tensiometers, approximately 50 lb of force is needed. Traction time should be limited to less than 2 hours to decrease the chance of traction neurapraxias. A well-padded, often oversized perineal post is used. The post should be placed laterally. This improves the vector of the traction force and decreases the risk of neurapraxia (Fig. 3.65B). Often less traction is needed after the joint has been accessed, relieving the negative pressure. In both positions, image intensification is used extensively for portal placement.

After completion of the central compartment procedure, the leg is removed from traction and the hip is flexed, typically to 45 degrees. This relaxes the capsule and gives greater access to the peripheral compartment.

Both 30- and 70-degree arthroscopes are used for adequate visualization. The 70-degree arthroscopy is used for most central compartment procedures. Commercially available hip arthroscopy instruments are available. The instruments typically are longer than standard arthroscopy equipment. Various dilators and slotted cannulas are helpful for portal placement and exchanging instruments within portals, as well as minimizing soft-tissue trauma.

PORTALS

Supine position arthroscopy uses three standard portals: the anterolateral, anterior, and posterolateral (Figs. 3.66 and 3.67). The anterolateral portal typically is placed first with the aid of fluoroscopy. This portal is made approximately 1 cm superior and anterior to the anterior edge of the greater trochanter. The posterolateral portal is made 1 cm posterior and superior to the greater trochanter. The location of the anterior portal is determined by the intersection of a line drawn from the tip of the greater trochanter and a line extending inferiorly from the anterior superior iliac spine. The posterolateral and anterior portals are made under direct observation with the camera in the anterolateral portal. After establishing the additional portals, the camera is placed in the anterior portal to assess the placement of the anterolateral portal. Because the anterolateral portal is made without direct visualization, this portal needs to be inspected to be sure there has not been inadvertent penetration of the labrum. Numerous additional accessory portals can be placed under direct visualization depending on the procedure (Fig. 3.68).

The anterolateral portal pierces the gluteus medius muscle and then the hip capsule (Fig. 3.69A). The nearest neurovascular structures are the superior gluteal nerve and the sciatic nerve. The anterior portal passes through the sartorius and the rectus femoris muscles and then the hip capsule. This portal passes close to the lateral femoral cutaneous nerve and ascending branch of the lateral femoral circumflex artery (Fig. 3.69B). The posterolateral portal passes through the gluteus medius and minimus muscles. The closest neurovascular structure is the sciatic nerve (see Fig. 3.69C). A cadaver study determined the distances of the arthroscopic portals to neurovascular structures: the anterolateral portal is 6 cm from the superior gluteal nerve and 4 cm from the sciatic nerve, the posterolateral portal lies 2.2 cm from the sciatic nerve, and the anterior portal is 1.5 cm from the lateral femoral cutaneous nerve, although several branches of this nerve may be closer.

SUPINE POSITION ARTHROSCOPY

TECHNIQUE 3.32

(BYRD)
- Place the patient supine on the fracture table or on a regular operating table with a distraction device.
- Place a heavily padded perineal post, lateralizing it against the medial thigh of the operative leg (see Fig. 3.65B).
- Position the operative hip in neutral, slight abduction, and neutral rotation. Slight flexion may relax the capsule and facilitate distraction but can place more traction on the sciatic nerve and draw it closer to the joint, making it more vulnerable to injury.
- Apply traction to the operative extremity, and confirm distraction of the joint fluoroscopically.
- Three standard portals are used for this procedure: anterior, anterolateral, and posterolateral (Fig. 3.70A and B).

- Establish the anterolateral portal first, using a 6-inch, 17-gauge needle under fluoroscopy. The portal is in the safe zone.
- Take care that the labrum is not penetrated when establishing all arthroscopic portals. If excessive resistance is met during needle placement, redirect it under fluoroscopic control, aiming slightly more parallel to the femoral head and away from the edge of the acetabulum. Distend the joint with saline, pass the guidewire through the needle, and withdraw the needle. Pass the cannula operator assembly over the guidewire into the joint. Do not injure the articular surface of the head or penetrate the labrum when introducing the cannula.
- To make the anterior portal and the posterolateral portal, pass the spinal needle into the joint, observing the needle and its position with a 70-degree arthroscope. Verify correct placement with fluoroscopy.
- Place the anterior portal at the intersection of a line drawn from the anterior superior iliac spine and a transverse line drawn from the superior margin of the greater trochanter (see Fig. 3.67). The anterior portal penetrates the sartorius and rectus femoris before entering the anterior capsule (see Fig. 3.69). To avoid the lateral femoral cutaneous nerve, make the incision only through the skin.
- Rotate the 70-degree scope posteriorly, and make the posterolateral portal under arthroscopic and fluoroscopic control just superior to the margin of the greater trochan-

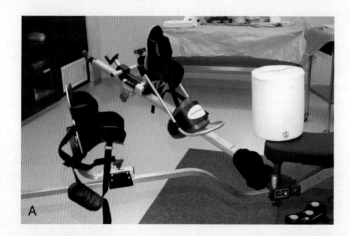

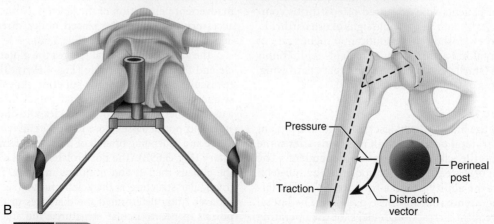

FIGURE 3.65 **A,** Commercially available distraction device. **B,** Perineal post for hip positioning of the operative leg. **SEE TECHNIQUE 3.29.**

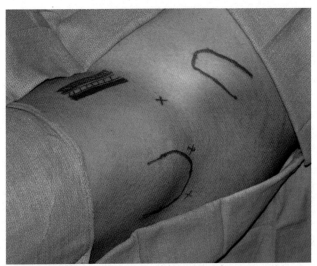

FIGURE 3.66   Landmarks outlined: femoral artery, vein, and nerve; greater trochanter; and anterosuperior iliac spine.

ter at its posterior border. The portal should be directed slightly cephalad and anteriorly, converging toward the anterolateral portal. It is important to have the hip in neutral rotation while making this portal to ensure that the sciatic nerve is not at risk.

- After establishing the three portals, place the outflow in the posterolateral portal.
- To view the acetabulum, labrum, and femoral head from each of the three portals, alternate the 70-degree scope and 30-degree scope between the anterolateral and anterior portals. Rotate the lens, and internally and externally rotate the hip. The 70-degree scope is best for viewing the labrum and the periphery of the acetabulum and femoral head, and the 30-degree scope is used for viewing of the central portion of the acetabulum, femoral head, and superior portion of the acetabular fossa (Fig. 3.71).
- Pass an arthroscopic knife through the cannula, and slightly incise the surrounding capsule transversely to allow greater maneuverability of the instruments (Fig. 3.72A and B).
- Use interchangeable, flexible cannulas with curved shaver blades to reach the greatest portion of the head and acetabulum and extra-length instrumentation for removal of labral or loose body fragments.
- Remove larger loose bodies piecemeal, carefully observing the retraction through the cannulas.
- After completing arthroscopy of the central compartment, the operative leg is released from traction and flexed 45 degrees. This allows relaxation of the capsule in order to proceed with examination of the peripheral compartment.
- The original anterior and anterolateral portals may be redirected onto the femoral neck. Alternatively, an ancillary portal may be established 4 to 5 cm distal to the anterolateral portal (Fig. 3.73). Fluoroscopy is used to guide placement onto the femoral neck.

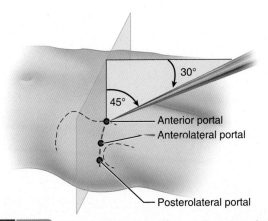

FIGURE 3.67   Three standard portals: anterior, anterolateral, and posterolateral. **SEE TECHNIQUE 3.29.**

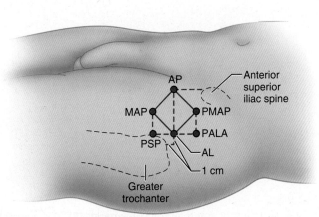

FIGURE 3.68   Additional accessory portals. *AL,* Anterolateral; *AP,* anterior; *MAP,* midanterior portal; *PMAP,* proximal midanterior portal; *PALA,* proximal accessory anterolateral portal; *PSP,* peritrochanteric space portal. (From Robertson WJ, Kelly BT: The safe zone for hip arthroscopy: a cadaveric assessment of central, peripheral, and lateral compartment portal placement, *Arthroscopy* 24:1019, 2008.)

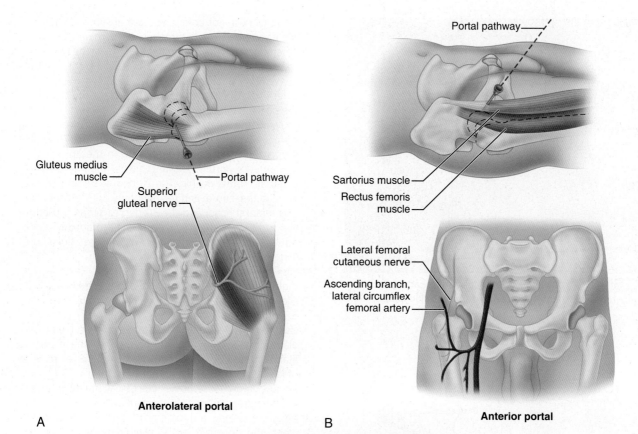

Gluteus medius muscle

Superior gluteal nerve

Portal pathway

Portal pathway

Sartorius muscle

Rectus femoris muscle

Lateral femoral cutaneous nerve

Ascending branch, lateral circumflex femoral artery

Anterolateral portal

A

Anterior portal

B

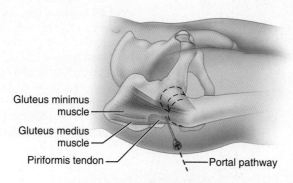

Gluteus minimus muscle

Gluteus medius muscle

Piriformis tendon

Portal pathway

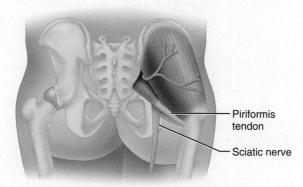

Piriformis tendon

Sciatic nerve

C

Posterolateral portal

FIGURE 3.69 Standard portals: anterolateral **(A)**, anterior **(B)**, and posterolateral **(C)**. SEE TECHNIQUE 3.32.

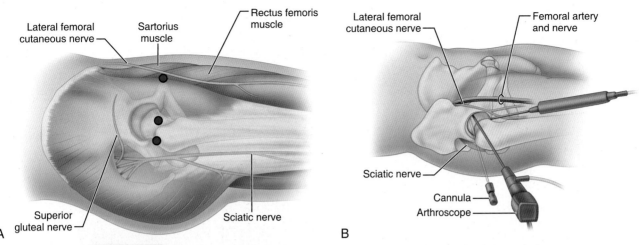

FIGURE 3.70 **A** and **B,** Diagrams of arthroscopic incisions around hip joint and their relationship to nerves in vicinity. **SEE TECHNIQUE 3.32.**

LATERAL POSITION ARTHROSCOPY

The lateral decubitus position for hip arthroscopy may be more familiar to surgeons who perform total hip arthroplasty with the patient in this position. In addition, in obese patients, the fat around the hip tends to fall away from the surgical site. In patients with large anterolateral bone spurs, the joint can be easily entered through the posterior peritrochanteric portal.

TECHNIQUE 3.33

(GLICK ET AL.)
- Place the anesthetized patient in the lateral decubitus position with the affected hip superior. A fracture table or a specialized distraction device may be used. A well-padded perineal post is placed. The post should be placed as lateral as possible on the surgical leg to protect the pudendal nerve and to improve the traction vector on the hip. The foot of the affected leg is placed in the foot holder to apply traction.
- Abduct the hip between 20 and 45 degrees, and extend it. The hip is placed in mild abduction, flexion, and external rotation. Use an image intensifier to evaluate traction and to guide instruments. Apply sufficient traction to create a space large enough to accommodate a 5-mm arthroscope and instruments.
- Prepare and drape the hip in a routine sterile manner to allow access as far anteriorly as the femoral artery and slightly past the posterior aspect of the greater trochanter.
- Place the affected leg in traction, and obtain a fluoroscopic image to ensure distraction of the joint 8 to 10 mm. If excessive force is required to distract the joint, a needle may be inserted into the joint under imaging. A small amount of air is then introduced into the joint, thereby breaking the vacuum seal of the hip. The required force needed for distraction will be reduced.
- Mark the anatomical landmarks, including the femoral artery anteriorly, the anterosuperior iliac spine, and the inguinal ligament, and outline the anterior, posterior, and superior portions of the greater trochanter.

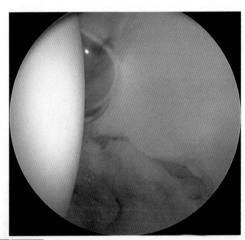

FIGURE 3.71 Arthroscopic view of the acetabular fossa. **SEE TECHNIQUE 3.32.**

- The lateral approach uses an anterior peritrochanteric, a posterior peritrochanteric, and a direct anterior portal. Additional portals can be made depending on the procedure.
- The anterior peritrochanteric portal is typically established first. Insert a 6-inch, 18-gauge spinal needle into the hip joint, under image intensifier guidance, starting just anterior to the anterior edge of the greater trochanter. Be sure not to penetrate the labrum.
- Air or fluid may then be injected into the joint for distension. A nitinol wire is then introduced through the spinal needle and into the hip joint. Image intensification is used to ensure placement.
- Make a skin incision at the needle site. The scope cannula is then placed over the wire and introduced into the joint. Again, an image intensifier is used. Avoid bending or breaking the nitinol wire.
- Establish an anterior portal for inflow. The anterior portal also is necessary for viewing of the anterior corners of the hip joint.
- Insert a spinal needle at a point where a sagittal line through the anterior iliac spine meets a horizontal line from the proximal tip of the greater trochanter. Angle the needle 45 degrees in the cephalad direction and 20

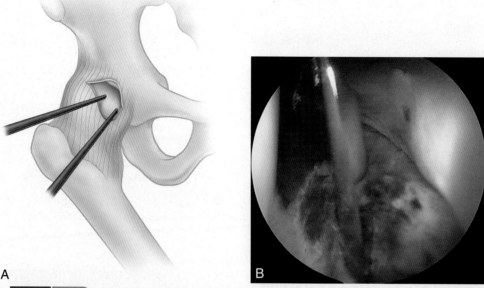

FIGURE 3.72 Capsulotomy. **A,** Anterolateral and anterior portals. **B,** View from anterior portal. **SEE TECHNIQUE 3.32.**

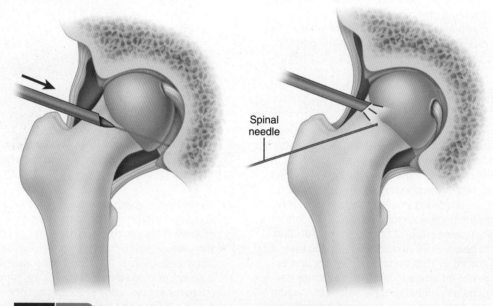

Spinal needle

FIGURE 3.73 Establishing an ancillary portal. **SEE TECHNIQUE 3.32.**

degrees medially, using the image intensifier and the arthroscope for guidance. The needle should enter the joint under direct visualization to ensure protection of the labrum and articular cartilage.

■ Make a small skin incision at the needle site, and insert a 5.25-inch inflow cannula. Branches of the lateral femoral cutaneous nerve are close to this portal; avoid them by incising only the skin and by bluntly dissecting through the subcutaneous tissues. The sheath and trocar push the nerve to the side as they are directed through the tissues.

■ Establish the posterior peritrochanteric portal in a similar fashion beginning at the posterior tip on the greater trochanter.

■ Make capsulotomies where each of the portals penetrate the capsule. This allows maneuverability and visualization by alternating the camera between the portals depending on the procedure being performed.

HIP CAPSULE

The capsule of the hip joint is composed of three ligaments: the iliofemoral, the ischiofemoral, and the pubofemoral ligaments. All of these ligaments are thickenings of the capsule and perform specific functions that contribute to hip stability. The iliofemoral ligament resists external rotation of the hip.

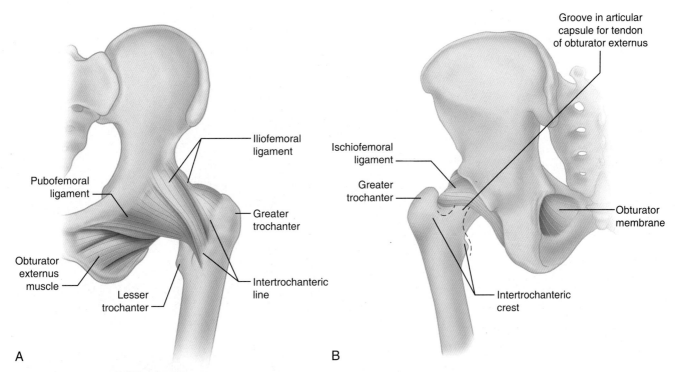

FIGURE 3.74 **A,** Anteroposterior view of the hip showing iliofemoral and pubofemoral ligaments. Note capsular insertion distally to intertrochanteric line. **B,** Posterior view of hip showing ischiofemoral ligament and relation to obturator externus tendon. (Redrawn from Bedi A, Galano G, Walsh C, Kelly BT: Capsular management during hip arthroscopy: from femoroacetabular impingement to instability, *Arthroscopy* 27:1720, 2011.)

The ischiofemoral ligament is a restraint to internal rotation. The pubofemoral ligament also helps to control external rotation (Fig. 3.74A and B).

During hip arthroscopy, the typical portals transverse the iliofemoral ligament. Because of the thickness of this ligament, various capsulotomies have been described to allow increased maneuverability and increased visualization of certain pathologies (Fig. 3.75A-C). Typically, for central compartment arthroscopy, an intraportal capsulotomy is made that connects the anterolateral and the anterior (or midanterior) portals (Fig. 3.75B). This capsulotomy runs parallel to the acetabulum. In cases of femoroacetabular impingement, this capsulotomy may not be adequate to visualize the full extent of the pathology. A T-shaped capsulotomy can be added to allow full visualization of the femoral neck (Fig. 3.75C).

Controversy exists in the repair of these capsulotomies. Some surgeons repair the entire capsulotomy, and others repair only the T-limb (vertical limb) of the capsulotomy (Fig. 3.75D and E). If instability is a concern, repair of the entire capsulotomy is recommended. Some studies show an increase in external rotation after capsulotomy, which returns to normal with repair. Another study showed improved patient outcomes when the entire T-capsulotomy was repaired compared to partial repair with only the vertical limb repaired. Domb et al. reported 5-year patient reported outcomes in repaired and unrepaired capsulotomies. Patients in both groups showed improvements, but the unrepaired group demonstrated a decrease in hip scores at 2- and 5-year follow-up and a higher conversion rate to arthroplasty. A recent systematic review of capsular management concluded that, based on current literature, there are not enough data to support the suggestion that routine capsular closure provides better functional outcomes.

ARTHROSCOPIC MANAGEMENT OF LABRAL TEARS

The acetabular labrum is a fibrocartilaginous structure that surrounds the periphery of the acetabulum and inserts on the transverse acetabular ligament. Blood supply to the acetabulum is primarily through the obturator artery, superior gluteal artery, and inferior gluteal artery. The periphery of the labrum is more vascularized than the articular region.

The labrum functions to increase the stability of the hip joint and to seal the hip joint and prevent escape of fluid. In the presence of a labral tear, this latter function is lost and may lead to increased contact pressure, which is thought to have a role in the development of degenerative disease of the hip. In a study of 436 patients, 73% of those with labral tears or fraying had articular damage, with most of the damage located in the same zone as the labral damage. Also, the severity of chondral damage was greater in patients with labral tears than in patients who had an intact labrum.

Seldes et al. described two types of labral injuries: a separation of the labrum from its articular attachment and tears in various planes within the substance of the labrum. A morphologic classification based on arthroscopic findings includes radial flap tears, radial fibrillated tears, longitudinal peripheral tears, and unstable tears. More recently, the majority of labral tears have been suggested to be related to abnormal joint morphology and function. Certain tears are seen with particular hip pathologies. Labral-chondral separation is more commonly seen with cam type impingement than with

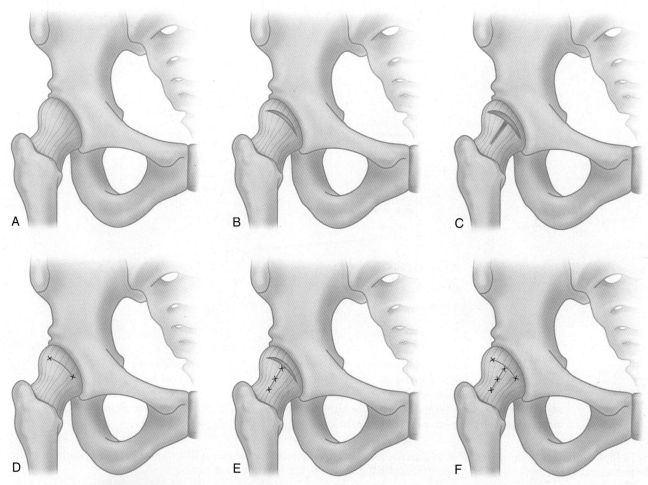

FIGURE **3.75**   Capsulotomy and capsular repair techniques. **A,** Hip joint. **B.** Interportal capsulotomy. **C.** T-capsulotomy. **D,** Repaired interportal capsulotomy. **E.** T-capsulotomy with partial repair. **F,** T-capsulotomy with complete repair. (From Ekhtiari S, de Sa D, Haldane CE, et al: Hip arthroscopic capsulotomy techniques and capsular management strategies: a systematic review, *Knee Surg Sports Traumatol Arthrosc* 25:9, 2017.)

femoroacetabular impingement, while intrasubstance tears are more typical of pincer impingement.

Patients with labral tears typically present with pain (usually groin pain) and mechanical symptoms. Byrd described the C-sign: when asked to localize the pain patients cup their hand, forming a C over the greater trochanter (Fig. 3.76). Pain may be positional, with symptoms increasing with sitting, driving, putting on shoes, or crossing the legs. Pain may be minimal with level walking. Evaluation should include radiographs of the pelvis and hip and advanced imaging when indicated. Associated conditions should be noted and treated at the time of surgery. CT scan offers greater detail in assessing bony architecture, while MRI and MRI-arthrogram are useful for identifying labral tears. Initial treatment is typically nonoperative, with rest, antiinflammatory agents, and physical therapy. Unresolved pain after nonoperative treatment is treated with labral debridement or repair.

In 2009, Byrd and Jones reported 10-year follow-up of patients with labral lesions treated with debridement. Hips that did not show any signs of arthritis had a significant increase in Harris Hip Scores, an improvement that remained

significant throughout the 10-year period. However, seven of eight patients with associated arthritis required total hip arthroplasty. Larson and Giveans compared the outcomes of labral debridement and labral repair in patients with femoral acetabular impingement and found that improvement in Harris Hip scores was greater in the labral refixation group.

Two main suture configurations are used when repairing labral tears. The suture can be looped around the entirety of the labrum for a circumferential repair. Alternatively, it can be passed through the substance of the labrum creating a labral base repair. The decision of which suture configuration to use is based on the quality of the labral tissue remaining. In patients with robust labral tissue, a labral base repair is typically used. When the labrum is significantly frayed, a circumferential repair is chosen to avoid the suture lacerating the remaining labrum. In either type of repair, it is essential to maintain the labral contact with the femoral head, reestablishing the suction seal. Anchors placed too far from the acetabular rim or sutures that are overtightened may evert the labral edge. Jackson et al. showed no difference in outcomes between the suture patterns in a retrospective study.

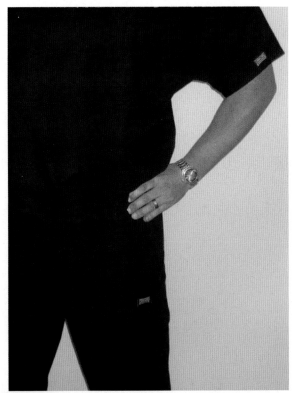

FIGURE 3.76   The "C" sign, which is indicative of a labral tear.

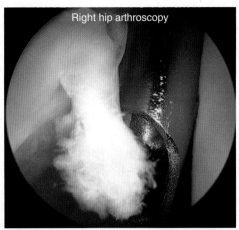

FIGURE 3.77   Labral tear. **SEE TECHNIQUE 3.34.**

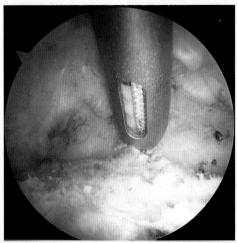

FIGURE 3.78   Placement of anchor in labral repair. **SEE TECHNIQUE 3.34.**

ARTHROSCOPIC REPAIR OF LABRAL TEARS

TECHNIQUE 3.34

(KELLY ET AL.)

- Establish anterior, anterolateral, and posterolateral portals in typical fashion, with the patient supine or in the lateral decubitus position. Often, a midanterior portal is established. This portal is helpful because it creates an easier angle to place anchors in the acetabular rim without penetrating the joint surface.
- Debride all torn tissue, leaving as much healthy labrum intact as possible (Fig. 3.77).
- When a labral tear is well identified, define the margins with a flexible probe. Controlled use of monopolar radiofrequency energy through the same flexible probe can contract the torn portion of the labrum and better define the edges.
- Use a flexible ligament chisel to detach the torn part of the labrum from the intact labrum, leaving only a small portion attached.
- Complete the débridement and remove the torn portion of the labrum with a motorized shaver.
- If the labrum is detached from the bone, stabilize the fibrocartilaginous tissue back to the rim of the acetabulum with a bioabsorbable suture anchor. Typically, the anchor should be placed on the acetabular rim, more on the capsular side than the articular side of the labrum, to achieve an appropriate angle that will not result in penetration of the anchor

into the joint. Ensure appropriate placement using fluoroscopy. Anchors can be placed through any portal (Fig. 3.78).
- After the sleeve for the anchor is placed in the appropriate position, tap the anchor while viewing the articular surface of the acetabulum to avoid iatrogenic chondral injury.
- When the anchor is placed, use a suture passer to deliver a limb of suture through a small portion of the substance of the labrum. Retrieve the suture and pass it through the labrum a second time, creating a vertical mattress suture. Pull the cannula back slightly to an extraarticular position and tie the suture down using standard arthroscopic knot-tying techniques.
- An intrasubstance split in the labrum can be repaired if it is well fixed to the acetabulum and has a stable outer rim. Fully define and débride the cleavage plane in the labrum of frayed, nonviable tissue.
- Use a spectrum to deliver a looped monofilament suture between the junction of the articular cartilage and the fibrocartilage labrum. Pull the working cannula back to the capsule and deliver a bird beak through the outer edge of the labrum peripheral to the tear.
- Grasp the loop and bring it out through the working cannula. Pass a bioabsorbable suture around the labral split using the looped monofilament as a suture lasso. Using tactile sensation, tie the knot in an extraarticular position

and use an automatic suture cutter to cut the remaining suture above the knot.

- After the labral repair, assess the capsule and the femoral head-neck junction by dynamic examination to determine if other pathologic processes are present that require capsular plication, thermal capsulorrhaphy, or osteoplasty for femoroacetabular impingement.

FEMOROACETABULAR IMPINGEMENT

Femoroacetabular impingement is abnormal contact between the proximal femur and the acetabulum during terminal motion. This abnormal contact leads to damage of the acetabular labrum and articular cartilage and may lead to what was previously thought of as idiopathic osteoarthritis of the hip.

Based on 600 surgical dislocations, Ganz et al. described two types of femoroacetabular impingement and the mechanisms by which this might lead to osteoarthritis: cam impingement, most common in young males, and pincer impingement, most common in middle-aged women. Cam impingement results from an abnormally shaped, nonspherical femoral head, with decreased head-neck offset, abutting against the acetabulum. The impingement typically occurs in flexion and results in a shearing of the articular surface and avulsion of the labrum (Fig. 3.79). Pincer impingement is abnormal contact between the acetabular rim and the femoral head-neck junction caused by acetabular overcoverage, which may be global, as in coxa profunda, or more focal in the anterosuperior acetabulum, as in acetabular retroversion (Fig. 3.80). This contact causes intrasubstance tears of the labrum. As pincer impingement worsens, the femoral head can be levered from the socket causing chondral damage in the posteroinferior acetabulum (contrecoup injury) (Figs. 3.81 and 3.82). In most cases, cam and pincer impingement exist together.

Patients with femoroacetabular impingement typically complain of pain in the groin with an insidious onset. Pain usually is exacerbated by exercise and may be positional. Patients may complain of pain with sitting, driving, or putting on socks and shoes.

Examination begins with observation of posture and gait. Palpation of the hip typically does not reproduce tenderness. Ranges of motion of both hips are checked, and asymmetrical range of motion is noted. The affected hip usually has decreased internal rotation. An impingement test may reproduce the patient's pain: with the patient supine and the hip flexed to 90 degrees, the hip is adducted and internally rotated (Fig. 3.83). A FABER (flexion, abduction, external rotation) test may show increased knee-to-table distance on the affected side in patients with femoroacetabular impingement.

Imaging evaluation begins with plain radiographs, which may include anteroposterior pelvic, false profile, cross-table lateral, frog-leg lateral, and Dunn views of the hip. The anteroposterior pelvic view should be well centered, with the tip of the coccyx pointing to the symphysis pubis. The distance between the coccyx and symphysis, on a well-centered view, should be 1 to 2 cm. The acetabulum is assessed for coxa profunda, acetabular protrusion, or acetabular retroversion. Coxa profunda is indicated when the acetabular teardrop lies medial to the ilioischial line. If the femoral head lies medial to the ilioischial line, acetabular protrusion is indicated. With

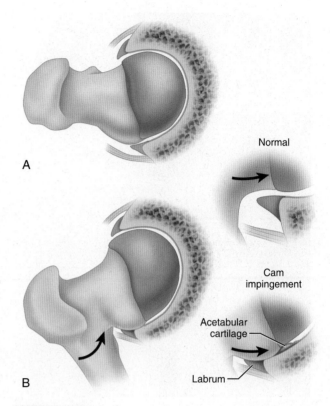

FIGURE 3.79 **A,** Cam impingement. **B,** With hip flexion, cam lesion glides under labrum, engaging edge of articular cartilage causing failure over time.

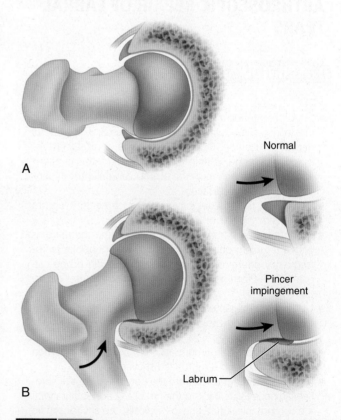

FIGURE 3.80 **A,** Pincer impingement from anterior acetabular prominence. **B,** Labrum is pushed against neck of femur causing failure over time.

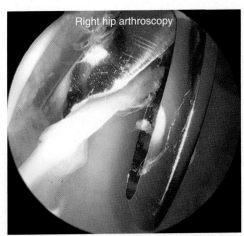

Right hip arthroscopy

FIGURE 3.81   Articular cartilage is sheared from the acetabulum.

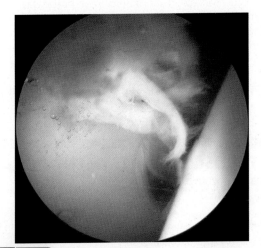

FIGURE 3.82   Labral tear.

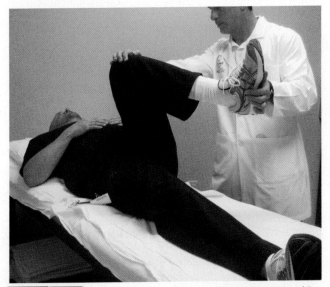

FIGURE 3.83   Impingement test is performed by provoking pain with flexion, adduction, and internal rotation of symptomatic hip.

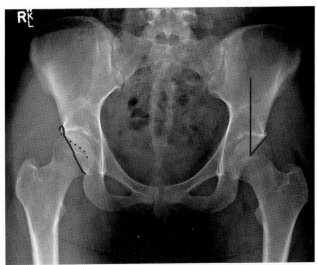

FIGURE 3.84   "Crossover sign" (left) is created when anterior wall crosses lateral to posterior wall in acetabular retropulsion. Center edge angle is created with line drawn perpendicular to horizontal axis of pelvis through center of femoral head and second line drawn to edge of sourcil.

acetabular retroversion, the anterior wall crosses lateral to the posterior wall, creating a "crossover sign" (Fig. 3.84). Certain measurements can be used to assess acetabular coverage. The center-edge angle is the angle formed between a line that is perpendicular to the transverse axis of the pelvis that passes through the center of the femoral head and a second line from the center of the femoral head to the lateral edge of the acetabular sourcil (see Fig. 3.84). Values of less than 20 to 25 degrees may indicate acetabular undercoverage. Any preoperative osteoarthritic changes of the hip are noted. On all views, femoral head sphericity and femoral head-neck offset are evaluated. The alpha angle is determined on the lateral radiographs. This angle is formed by a line through the center of the femoral head and neck and a second line from the center of the femoral head to the point where the femoral head radius exits a concentric circle drawn around the femoral head. An alpha angle of more than 50 degrees is typical in hips with loss of sphericity (Fig. 3.85). CT may help further define bony anatomy. MRI is used to assess labral and chondral injuries.

There is evidence to show that femoroacetabular impingement exists in asymptomatic patients. A review by Frank et al. documented a 37% occurrence of radiographic femoroacetabular impingement in asymptomatic individuals. The prevalence is even higher in the athletic population. There is no indication for operative treatment in asymptomatic individuals. These patients should be followed if symptoms do arise.

Treatment is initially nonoperative and includes activity modification, nonsteroidal antiinflammatory drugs, and physical therapy. Patients who do not respond to conservative treatment may be candidates for arthroscopic treatment. The goal of arthroscopic treatment is to treat labral pathology as well as chondral damage and to remove sites of bony impingement and reestablish the femoral head-neck offset. In a cadaver study, Mardones et al. showed that up to 30% of the femoral head-neck junction can be resected without producing a significant increase in the risk of femoral neck fracture.

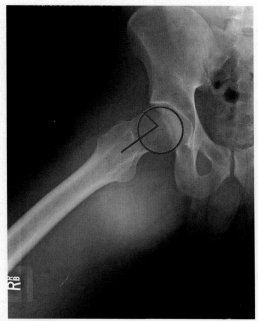

FIGURE **3.85** Alpha angle.

Mid-term results after femoroacetabular impingement correction continue to show improvement in pain and function. Menge et al. published survivorship and outcomes at 10 years after femoroacetabular impingement correction that included labral debridement or labral repair: 34% of patients had total hip arthroplasty within the 10-year period. Older age, less than 2 mm of joint space, and acetabular microfracture were more prominent in the group requiring total hip arthroplasty. Patients who did not require total hip arthroplasty had significant improvements in patient-reported outcomes and satisfaction, regardless of whether treatment was labral repair or debridement. Perets et al. showed statistically significant improvement in modified Harris Hip score and other hip scores at 5-year follow-up. In addition, 80% of patients returned to sports, with 71% returning to the same or higher level of ability compared to preoperative function. A systematic review showed that 87% of patients were able to return to sports. Reports of femoroacetabular impingement correction in professional athletes demonstrate return-to-play in basketball, hockey, and other sports.

ARTHROSCOPIC TREATMENT OF PINCER IMPINGEMENT

TECHNIQUE 3.35

(LARSON)
- Establish standard arthroscopic portals and examine the hip to confirm pincer impingement. A midanterior portal can be used to aid in anchor placement.
- If the pincer lesion can be seen (Fig. 3.86A), leave the labral-chondral junction intact and use a burr to resect the bony prominence (Fig. 3.86B).
- If exposure of the acetabular rim is needed to access the pincer lesion, place a banana blade through the anterior

portal and take down the labrum at the labral-chondral junction in the area of the lesion.
- Place a burr in the midanterior portal and position it on the anterior wall at the level of the acetabular overcoverage. Confirm with fluoroscopy that the burr is just distal to the crossover sign, resect the rim to the appropriate level, and confirm resection of the crossover with fluoroscopy. The camera can be switched to the anterior portal and the burr to the anterolateral portal to complete the more superior rim resection.
- Refix the labrum to the rim with suture anchors. Place the first anchor superiorly through the anterolateral portal, using fluoroscopy and direct observation to ensure that the joint is not penetrated. Pass one suture limb into the joint between the labrum and rim (Fig. 3.86C).
- Pass a bird beak or other penetrating grasper through the labrum, retrieve the suture, and tie it (Fig. 3.86D). Alternatively, loop the suture around the labrum instead of piercing the tissue.
- With the camera in the anterolateral portal, place the remaining anchors through the midanterior portal in a similar fashion.
- Remove traction from the leg, and move the hip through a range of motion to ensure there is no residual impingement.

ARTHROSCOPIC TREATMENT OF CAM IMPINGEMENT

TECHNIQUE 3.36

(MAURO ET AL.)
- After standard arthroscopic portal placement and examination, complete any needed central compartment procedures.
- Remove the leg from traction, and flex the hip approximately 45 degrees.
- With the camera in the midanterior portal, introduce an arthroscopic blade through a distal accessory anterolateral portal and make a T-shaped capsulotomy to allow inspection of the cam lesion. Flexion and external rotation will help expose inferior medial lesions, and extension and internal rotation will help expose superolateral lesions. Take care to avoid the retinacular vessels when treating lesions on the superolateral neck.
- Introduce a burr and resect the cam lesion to re-create a spherical femoral head. Use fluoroscopy to assist and confirm resection.
- Perform dynamic assessment of the hip. The hip is flexed and internally and externally rotated to ensure there is no residual impingement.
- Repair the limb of the capsulotomy that extends down the femoral neck in side-to-side fashion.

POSTOPERATIVE CARE Physical therapy and range of motion are begun in the first 24 to 48 hours. A stationary

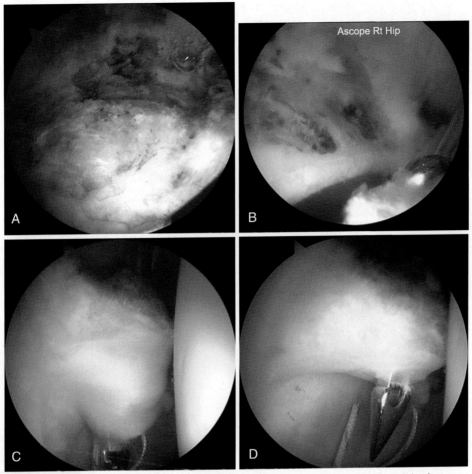

FIGURE 3.86 **A,** Pincer lesion. **B,** Pincer resection. **C,** Suture limb passed into joint between labrum and rim. **D,** Suture retrieved with bird beak grasper and tied. **SEE TECHNIQUE 3.35.**

bike may be used immediately. Patients are limited to touch-down weight bearing for 2 weeks. Extremes of motion are avoided for several weeks, particularly extension and external rotation. Some surgeons recommend bracing for the first few weeks. Impact activities are not recommended for 2 to 3 months. Return to sports may take 4 to 6 months.

LABRAL RECONSTRUCTION

The acetabular labrum provides several important protective roles in the hip. There are cases in which the labrum is too damaged to repair or may be absent. This may be seen in a primary or a revision setting. In young, active patients reconstruction of the labrum may help provide some protection to the joint. Several graft choices have been described, including IT band, gracilis, and ligamentum teres. The technique involves side-to-side repair with the native labrum and repair of the graft to the acetabular rim with anchors placed 1 cm apart. In a cadaver study, Lee et al. demonstrated an increase in joint contact forces with decreased contact areas after resection of the labrum. Reconstructing the labrum did produce a reversal of some of these changes. Short-term results have shown increased patient satisfaction and improved hip scores. Boykin et al. reported an average rate of return to sports of 85% after labral reconstruction in elite athletes. Improvements were seen in modified Harris Hip score and

patient satisfaction. In a 2-year follow-up, Domb et al. compared labral resection to labral reconstruction in similarly matched groups. Both groups showed improvement; however, in a few categories, patient-reported outcomes in the reconstruction group were significantly improved over the resection group. Perets et al. compared 2-year follow-up in patients requiring revision labral reconstruction to those with revision labral repair. Patients requiring labral reconstruction had lower preoperative patient-reported outcomes, but at follow-up both groups had similar increases in patient-reported outcomes, satisfaction, and VAS (visual analog scale) scores. There were no significant differences in the number of reoperation or major complications.

ARTHROSCOPIC LABRAL RECONSTRUCTION

TECHNIQUE 3.37

(MATSUDA)
- With the patient supine, confirm indications for labral reconstruction.

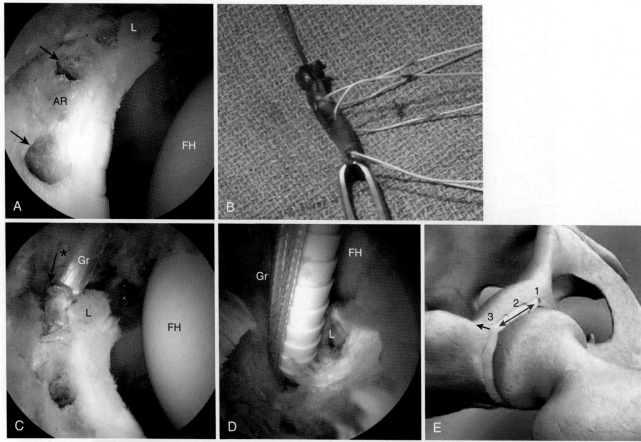

FIGURE 3.87   **A,** Supine arthroscopic view of right hip with 70-degree scope in anterolateral portal showing anterosuperior acetabulum after rim trimming and predrilling of suture anchor sites (black arrows). Red arrow indicates location of anterior suture anchor drill hole, which is hidden by stable labral margin (L); posterosuperior drill hole is not visible in field of view (AR, acetabular rim; FH, femoral head). **B,** Gracilis autograft after suture placement. Note simple midsubstance sutures and whip stitches at terminal ends of graft. **C,** Supine arthroscopic view of right hip during partial insertion of leading end of gracilis graft (Gr) into first suture anchor drill site with intimate contact and intentional overlap with labral margin (L). Arrow shows direction of suture anchor (asterisk) placement into acetabular rim (FH, femoral head). **D,** Supine arthroscopic view of right hip showing terminal end of gracilis autograft (Gr) being seated into final suture anchor site in overlapped position with posterosuperior labral remnant (L) permitting graft tensioning just before deployment of suture anchor (FH, femoral head). **E,** Image of right hip showing key steps of graft fixation to acetabular rim: 1, seating and fixation of leading autograft end into anterior suture anchor site; 2, labral graft fixation in intercalary section to anterosuperior rim; and 3, seating of "tail" end of graft into final suture anchor site in direction of black arrow with resultant tensioning of graft (red arrow) before final knotless suture anchor fixation to facilitate fluid seal. Yellow asterisk shows region of intentional overlap at labrum-graft junction.   (From Matsuda DK: Labral reconstruction with gracilis autograft, *Arthrosc Tech* 1:e15, 2012.) **SEE TECHNIQUE 3.36.**

- Establish a modified midanterior portal (MMAP), 3 cm anterior and 4.5 mm distal to the anterolateral portal.
- Debride the labrum to be reconstructed back to a stable rim.
- Drill the suture anchor sites on the acetabulum for later use with knotless anchors (Fig. 3.87A). Four or five anchors typically are used, spaced about 8 mm apart; the number of anchors used varies depending on the size of the labral defect.
- Remove the hip from traction, and flex the hip and knee (figure-of-four position).
- Harvest the ipsilateral gracilis tendon through a 2-cm vertical incision just medial and distal to the tibial tuberosity.

- Prepare the harvested tendon. Prepare the graft 2 cm longer than the defect to be grafted. Place a whipstitch in each end with No. 2 nonabsorbable suture. Place 2 or 3 simple midsubstance sutures (Fig. 3.87B).
- Pass the graft through the MMAP with an 8.25-mm cannula.
- Place the leading end of the graft partially in the most anterior drill hole, and fix it with the first anchor, achieving an interference fit (Fig. 3.87C).
- Fix the midsubstance sutures along the acetabular rim into the previously drilled holes, proceeding from anterior to posterior.

- Partially insert the end of the graft into the last drill hole, and fix it there (Figs. 3.87D and E).

■ ABDUCTOR TENDON TEARS

Lateral hip pain, or greater trochanteric pain syndrome, is a common complaint. Causes of greater trochanteric pain syndrome range from bursitis to partial or full-thickness tears of the abductor tendon. In patients with abductor tendon pathology, weakness may also be present. Initial treatment includes activity modification, physical therapy, nonsteroidal antiinflammatory medication, and trochanteric steroidal injections. In patients who do not respond, an MRI can determine the integrity of the abductor tendon. If pain and weakness persist, endoscopic tendon repair may be indicated. Short-term follow-up studies demonstrate improvement in symptoms, strength, and patient satisfaction. A systematic review showed similar results to open repair with fewer wound complications.

Endoscopic repair can be done with the patient supine or in the lateral position. If indicated, central and peripheral compartment arthroscopy are completed first.

Perets et al. reported 5-year outcomes in patients with endoscopic gluteus medius repairs with concomitant arthroscopy for labral tears. There was significant improvement in all measured hip scores, and no patients had clinical failure of the gluteus medius repair.

REPAIR OF THE ADDUCTOR TENDON

TECHNIQUE 3.38

(BYRD)
- Position the leg in slight extension and abduction; do not apply traction.
- Establish a distal anterior portal, anterior and distal to the vastus ridge, and insert a 30-degree arthroscope.
- Establish a proximal anterior portal under direct observation. Both portals should be aimed toward the vastus ridge, deep to the iliotibial band.
- Excise bursal tissue to expose the insertion of the abductor tendon, the vastus ridge, and the origin of the vastus lateralis.
- Establish a posterior portal at the posterior border of the vastus ridge.
- Mobilize the torn tendon edges, and use a burr to prepare the bony footprint.
- Place anchors in the footprint perpendicular to the cortical surface.
- Use mattress sutures to approximate the tendon edges to the prepared bed.

■ SNAPPING HIPS

There are a variety of causes of snapping hips. Intraarticular pathology such as labral tears, femoroacetabular impingement, or loose bodies may cause a sensation of snapping or popping in the hip. These causes are treated during hip arthroscopy when indicated. External snapping hip occurs when the iliotibial band snaps over the greater trochanter while the hip moves between flexion and extension. Patients often can reproduce this snapping, which can even be seen. In some patients, the snapping may be painless and no treatment is needed. Internal snapping hip occurs when the psoas tendon snaps over the iliopectineal eminence, femoral head, or a prominent acetabular component after total hip arthroplasty. Internal snapping is typically reproduced when the flexed, externally rotated hip is brought into extension and internal rotation.

For painful external or internal snapping hips, treatment typically is nonsurgical and consists of physical therapy, antiinflammatory medication, and steroid injection. For patients who do not respond to conservative management, surgical release may be indicated. For external snapping hips, an endoscopic release on the iliotibial band is performed by creating a diamond-shaped defect overlying the greater trochanter. Surgical treatment of internal snapping hips involves release of the psoas tendon at the lesser trochanter or at the level of the hip joint. At the level of the hip joint, the psoas tendon can be released through the central compartment with the leg in traction or through the peripheral compartment with the leg flexed. The psoas tendon typically is released at the end of the surgical procedure to prevent fluid extravasation into the retroperitoneal space. In a recent review, there were fewer complications and less postoperative pain associated with arthroscopic release compared to open procedures.

TREATMENT OF EXTERNAL SNAPPING HIP

TECHNIQUE 3.39

(ILIZALITURRI ET AL)
- Position the patient lateral, but do not place the leg in traction. The leg should have free range of motion in order to reproduce the snapping.
- Inject 40 to 50 mL of saline under the iliotibial band.
- Mark the location of the greater trochanter, and establish two portals in line with the femur, one proximal and one distal to the trochanter.
- Make the distal portal first and place a 30-degree arthroscope superficial to the iliotibial band.
- Make the proximal portal under direct observation and place a shaver through this portal.
- Use the shaver to create a plane superficial to the iliotibial band to expose the tendon.
- Place a radiofrequency probe in the proximal portal, and make a vertical cut in the iliotibial band starting at the level of the distal portal and extending proximally 4 to 6 cm.
- At the midportion of the vertical cut, make a 2-cm horizontal cut anteriorly and extend a similar cut posteriorly.
- Create the anterior and posterior flaps and resect them to create a diamond-shaped defect.
- Move the leg through a range of motion to ensure there is no residual snapping.

PSOAS RELEASE AT THE LESSER TROCHANTER

TECHNIQUE 3.40

- If indicated, complete a routine arthroscopic examination of the hip.
- Remove traction from the operative leg, flex the hip 15 to 20 degrees, and externally rotate it.
- Using fluoroscopic guidance, create a portal distal to the anterolateral portal in line with the lesser trochanter and insert a 30-degree arthroscope.
- Create a second, more distal portal for instrumentation.
- Identify the fibers of the psoas tendon within the psoas bursa. If needed for exposure, clear the bursa with a shaver.
- Use a radiofrequency device to divide the tendon.

PSOAS RELEASE AT THE JOINT LEVEL

TECHNIQUE 3.41

(WETTSTEIN ET AL.)
- After completion of central compartment hip arthroscopy, remove the hip from traction and flex it 30 degrees.
- Establish anterior and anterolateral portals. Insert a 30-degree arthroscope directed toward the anterior femoral neck through the anterolateral portal.
- Identify the medial synovial fold, zona orbicularis, and anterior hip capsule.
- Introduce a radiofrequency probe through the anterior portal and make an incision in the anterior capsule anterior to the medial synovial fold and proximal to the zona orbicularis. The psoas tendon lies directly anterior to the capsule at this level.
- Release the tendon.

■ REVISION HIP ARTHROSCOPY

As the number of arthroscopic hip procedures increases, so does the number of revision hip arthroscopies. The most common reason for revision hip arthroscopy is residual impingement, which may result from untreated or undertreated impingement at the initial procedure. Gwathmey, Jones, and Byrd reported that, in 190 consecutive revision hip arthroscopies, residual impingement was the most common finding at surgery. In most of the revision patients, there was no attempt at bony correction at the initial procedure. At a minimum of 2-years' follow-up after revision, 84.5% of patients had improvement in symptoms. Newman et al. compared 246 patients with revision hip arthroscopic surgeries to a matched control group with primary arthroscopy patients and found that revision patients did have significant improvements in postoperative outcome scores, but these scores were lower than in the primary group. Patients with more than two revisions have lower outcome scores.

COMPLICATIONS OF HIP ARTHROSCOPY

Reported complication rates for hip arthroscopy generally are low. A systematic review of 36,761 hip arthroscopies demonstrated a 3.3% complication rate. Traction neurapraxia affecting the femoral, sciatic, pudendal, or lateral femoral cutaneous nerves is the most commonly reported complication; these typically resolve spontaneously. Neurapraxia usually is caused by prolonged length of time the leg is placed in traction or excessive pressure from the perineal post. The lateral femoral cutaneous nerve also may be damaged if the anterior portal is placed too far medially. Excessive traction may also cause pressure damage to the perineal areas. Scuffing of the articular surfaces may occur, and this may be underreported. Iatrogenic damage to the labrum may occur during placement of the initial anterolateral portal, as this portal is not placed under direct visualization.

Other rare complications have been reported after hip arthroscopy, including abdominal compartment syndrome and hip instability. Abdominal compartment syndrome results from fluid extravasation into the retroperitoneal space. Fluid extravasation may track through the psoas tendon sheath; therefore a psoas release, if indicated, should be completed at the end of the procedure. In trauma patients, careful monitoring of the abdomen is required because of disruption of the soft-tissue envelope of the hip. Hip instability is a rare but serious complication of hip arthroscopy that may present as repetitive microinstability or a hip dislocation. A systematic review by Duplantier et al. looked at potential causes for instability and concluded that preoperative conditions such as dysplasia or ligamentous laxity may play a role. Postoperative conditions that may lead to instability include overresection of the acetabular rim, psoas tenotomy, unrepaired capsulotomy, and ligamentum teres debridement.

Arthroscopic treatment of femoroacetabular impingement may lead to complications because of bony overresection or underresection. Underresection of pincer or cam deformities can lead to incomplete relief and a need for further surgery. Overresection of a femoral neck cam lesion places the femoral neck at risk for fracture.

As with open hip surgery, there is a risk of heterotopic ossification after hip arthroscopy. A report of 300 cases had a 1.6% rate of heterotopic ossification, all of which occurred in a control group of 15 patients who did not receive prophylaxis. None of 285 patients who received nonsteroidal antiinflammatory drugs for 3 weeks developed heterotopic ossification.

REFERENCES

KNEE
General.

Balato G, Di Donato SL, Ascione T, et al.: Knee septic arthritis after arthroscopy: incidence, risk factors, functional outcome, and infection eradication rate, *Joints* 5:107, 2017.

Behery OA, Suchman KI, Paoli AR, et al.: What are the prevalence and risk factors for repeat ipsilateral knee arthroscopy?, *Knee Surg Sports Traumatol Arthrosc*, 2019 Jan 17, https://doi.org/10.1007/s00167-019-05348-y, [Epub ahead of print].

Bohensky MA, Ademi Z, deSteiger R, et al.: Quantifying the excess cost and resource utilisation for patients with complications associated with elective knee arthroscopy: a retrospective cohort study, *Knee* 21:491, 2014.

Bohensky MA, deSteiger R, Kondogiannis C, et al.: Adverse outcomes associated with elective knee arthroscopy: a population-based cohort study, *Arthroscopy* 29:716, 2013.

Burkhart SS, Miller MD, Sanders TG, et al.: *MRI-arthroscopy correlations of the shoulder, elbow, hip and knee: a case-based approach*, San Diego, CA, February 2011, AAOS Instructional Course Lecture, Annual Meeting of the American Academy of Orthopaedic Surgeons.

Hagino T, Ochiai S, Watanabe Y, et al.: Complications after arthroscopic knee surgery, *Arch Orthop Trauma Surg* 134:1561, 2014.

Hoshino Y, Rothrauff BB, Hensler D, et al.: Arthroscopic image distortion-part I: the effect of lens and viewing angles in a 2-dimensional in vitro model, *Knee Surg Sports Traumatol Arthrosc* 24:2065, 2016.

Karargyris O, Mandalia V: Arthroscopic treatment of patellar tendinopathy: use of 70° arthroscope and superolateral portal, *Arthrosc Tech* 5:e1083, 2016.

Kaye ID, Patel DN, Strauss EJ, et al.: Prevention of venous thromboembolism after arthroscopic knee surgery in a low-risk population with the use of aspirin. A randomized trial, *Bull Hosp Jt Dis* 73:243, 2015.

Lee DY, Park YJ, Song SY, et al.: Which technique is better for treating patellar dislocation? A systematic review and meta-analysis, *Arthroscopy*, 2018 Oct 6, pii: S0749-8063(18)30569-3, https://doi.org/10.1016/j.arthro.2018.06.052, [Epub ahead of print].

Martin CT, Pugely AJ, Gao Y, Wolf BR: Risk factors for thirty-day morbidity and mortality following knee arthroscopy: a review of 12,271 patients from the national surgical quality improvement program database, *J Bone Joint Surg* 95A:e98, 2013.

Matsushita T, Araki D, Hoshino Y, et al.: Analysis of graft length change patterns in medial patellofemoral ligament reconstruction via a fluoroscopic guidance method, *Am J Sports Med* 46:1150, 2018.

Nelson JD, Hogan MV, Miller MD: What's new in sports medicine, *J Bone Joint Surg* 92A:250, 2010.

Rong Z, Yao Y, Chen D, et al.: The incidence of deep venous thrombosis before arthroscopy among patients suffering from high-energy knee trauma, *Knee Surg Sports Traumatol Arthrosc* 24:1717, 2016.

Salzler MJ, Lin A, Miller CD, et al.: Complications after arthroscopic knee surgery, *Am J Sports Med* 42:292, 2014.

Sanchis-Alfonso V, Baydal-Bertomeu JM, Castelli A, et al.: Laboratory evaluation of the pivot-shift phenomenon with the use of kinetic analysis: a preliminary study, *J Bone Joint Surg* 93A:1256, 2011.

Thompson SR: Diagnostic knee arthroscopy and partial meniscectomy, *JBJS Essent Surg Tech* 6:e7, 2016.

Werner BC, Cancienne JM, Miller MD, Gwathmey FW: Incidence of manipulation under anesthesia or lysis of adhesions after arthroscopic knee surgery, *Am J Sports Med* 43:1656, 2015.

Westermann RW, Pugely AJ, Teis Z, et al.: Causes and predictors of 30-day readmission after shoulder and knee arthroscopy: an analysis of 15, 167 cases, *Arthroscopy* 31:1035, 2015.

Wyatt RWB, Maletis GB, Lyon LL, et al.: Efficacy of prophylactic antibiotics in simple knee arthroscopy, *Arthroscopy* 33:157, 2017.

MENISCUS

Bedi A, Kelly NH, Baad M, et al.: Dynamic contact mechanics of the medial meniscus as a function of radial tear, repair, and partial meniscectomy, *J Bone Joint Surg* 92A:1398, 2010.

Bhatia S, LaPrade CM, Ellman MB, et al.: Meniscal root tears. Significance, diagnosis, and treatment, *Am J Sports Med* 42:3016, 2014.

Blackwell R, Schmitt LC, Flanigan DC, Magnussen RA: Smoking increases the risk of early meniscus repair failure, *Knee Surg Sports Traumatol* 24:1540, 2016.

Brelin AM, Rue JP: Return to play following meniscus surgery, *Clin Sports Med* 35:669, 2016.

Bryceland JK, Powell AJ, Nunn T: Knee menisci, *Cartilage* 8:99, 2016.

Bin SI, Nha KW, Cheong JY, et al.: Midterm and long-term results of medial versus lateral meniscal allograft transplantation. A meta-analysis, *Am J Sports Med* 46:1243, 2018.

Chung KS, Ha JK, Ra HJ, et al.: A meta-analysis of clinical and radiographic outcomes of posterior horn medial meniscus root repairs, *Knee Surg Sports Traumatol Arthrosc* 24:1455, 2016.

Chung KS, Ha JK, Ra HJ, et al.: Prognostic factors in the midterm results of pullout fixation for posterior root tears of the medial meniscus, *Arthroscopy* 32:1319, 2016.

Ellis HB: Can a meniscus really regenerate so easily? A Level-I study says it can but not for everyone: Commentary on an article by Vangsness et al: Adult human mesenchymal stem cells delivered via intra-articular injection to the knee following partial medial meniscectomy: a randomized, double-blind, controlled study, *J Bone Joint Surg* 96:e14, 2014.

Eun SS, Lee SH, Sabal LA: Arthroscopic repair of the posterior root of the medial meniscus using knotless suture anchor: a technical note, *Knee* 23:740, 2016.

Faucett SC, Geisler BP, Chahla J, et al.: Meniscus root repair vs meniscectomy or nonoperative management to prevent knee osteoarthritis after medial meniscus root tears: clinical and economic effectiveness, *Am J Sports Med*, 2018 Mar 1:363546518755754, https://doi.org/10.1177/0363546518755754, [Epub ahead of print].

Feucht MJ, Grande E, Brunhuber J, et al.: Biomechanical evaluation of different suture techniques for arthroscopic transtibial pull-out repair of posterior medial meniscus root tears, *Am J Sports Med* 41:2784, 2013.

Fillingham YA, Riboh JC, Erickson BJ, et al.: Inside-out versus all-inside repair of isolated meniscal tears: an updated systematic review, *Am J Sports Med* 45:234, 2016.

Freymann U, Metzlaff S, Krüger JP, et al.: Effect of human serum and 2 different types of platelet concentrates on human meniscus cell migration, proliferation, and matrix formation, *Arthroscopy* 32:1106, 2016.

Hannon MG, Ryan MK, Strauss EJ: Meniscal allograft transplantation: a comprehensive historical and current review, *Bull Hosp Jt Dis* 73:100, 2015.

Harston A, Nyland J, Brand E, et al.: Collagen meniscus implantation: a systematic review including rehabilitation and return to sports activity, *Knee Surg Sports Traumatol Arthrosc* 20:135, 2011.

Haskel JD, Uppstrom TJ, Dare DM, et al.: Decline in clinical scores at long-term follow-up of arthroscopically treated discoid lateral meniscus in children, *Knee Surg Sports Traumatol Arthrosc* 26:2906, 2018.

Hendrix ST, Kwapisz A, Wyland DJ: All-inside arthroscopic meniscal repair technique using a midbody accessory portal, *Arthroscopy Tech* 6: e1885, 2017.

Herbort M, Siam S, Lenschow S, et al.: Strategies for repair of radial tears close to the meniscal rim—biomechanical analysis with a cyclic loading protocol, *Am J Sports Med* 38:2281, 2010.

Jacquet C, Erivan R, Argenson JN, et al.: Effect of 3 preservation methods (freezing, cryopreservation, and freezing + irradiation) on human menisci ultrastructure: an ex vivo comparative study with fresh tissue as a gold standard, *Am J Sports Med* 46:2899, 2018.

Jung YH, Choi NH, Oh JS, Victoroff BN: All-inside repair for a root tear of the medial meniscus using a suture anchor, *Am J Sports Med* 40:1406, 2012.

Keyhani S, Ahn JH, Verdonk R, et al.: Arthroscopic all-inside ramp lesion repair using the posterolateral transseptal portal view, *Knee Surg Sports Traumatol Arthrosc* 25:454, 2017.

Kim NK, Bin SI, Kim JM, Lee CR: Does medial meniscal allograft transplantation with the bone-plug technique restore the anatomic location of the native medial meniscus? *Am J Sports Med* 43:3045, 2015.

Konan S, McNicholas M, Vedonk P, et al.: Meniscal injuries: management and outcome. In Kerkhoffs GMMJ, Haddad F, Hirschman MT, et al, editors: *ESSKA Instructional Course Lecture Book, Glasgow 2018*, 2018. Berlin, Germany, 2018, Springer, pp 33–44.

Krych AJ, Pitts RT, Dajani KA, et al.: Surgical repair of meniscal tears with concomitant anterior cruciate ligament reconstruction in patients 18 years and younger, *Am J Sports Med* 38:976, 2010.

LaPrade CM, James EW, Cran TR, et al.: Meniscal root tears. A classification system based on tear morphology, *Am J Sports Med* 43:363, 2014.

LaPrade RF, LaPrade CM, James EW: Recent advances in posterior meniscal root repair techniques, *J Am Acad Orthop Surg* 23:71, 2015.

Lavender CD, Hanzlik SR, Caldwell 3rd PE, et al.: Transosseous medial meniscal root repair using a modified Mason-Allen suture configuration, *Arthrosc Tech* 4:e78, 2015.

Lind M, Nielsen T, Faunø P, et al.: Free rehabilitation is safe after isolated meniscus repair: a prospective randomized trial comparing free with restricted rehabilitation regimens, *Am J Sports Med* 41:2753, 2013.

McCulloch PC, Jones HL, Lue J, et al.: What is the optimal minimum penetration depth for "all-inside" meniscal repairs? *Arthroscopy* 32:1624, 2016.

Miller MD, Rodeo SL, Sgaglione NA, Noyes FR: *Meniscus repair and transplantation: update on surgical techniques and clinical outcomes, AAOS Instructional Course Lecture,* San Diego, California, February, 2011, Annual Meeting of the AAOS.

Moatshe G, Chahla J, Slette E, et al.: Posterior meniscal root injuries, *Acta Orthop* 87:452, 2016.

Moatshe G, Cinque ME, Godin JA, et al.: Comparable outcomes after bucket-handle meniscal repair and vertical meniscal repair can be achieved at a minimum 2 years' follow-up, *Am J Sports Med* 45:3104, 2017.

Moulton SG, Bhatia S, Civitarese DM, et al.: Surgical techniques and outcomes of repairing meniscal radial tears: a systematic review, *Arthroscopy* 32:1919, 2016.

Noyes FR, Barber-Westin SD: Repair of complex and avascular meniscal tears and meniscal transplantation, *J Bone Joint Surg* 92A:1012, 2010.

Rao AJ, Erickson BJ, Cvetanovich GL, et al.: The meniscus-deficient knee, *Orthop J Sports Med* 44:1724, 2016.

Rongen JJ, Govers TM, Buma P, et al.: Societal and economic effect of meniscus scaffold procedures for irreparable meniscus injuries, *Am J Sports Med* 44:1724, 2016.

Shieh AK, Edmonds EW, Pennock AT: Revision meniscal surgery in children and adolescents: risk factors and mechanisms for failure and subsequent management, *Am J Sports Med* 44:838, 2016.

Sihvonen R, Paavola M, Malmivaara A, et al.: Arthroscopic partial meniscectomy versus sham surgery for a degenerative meniscal tear, *N Engl J Med* 369:2515, 2013.

Sommerfeldt MF, Magnussen RA, Randall KL, et al.: The relationship between body mass index and risk of failure following meniscus repair, *J Knee Surg* 29:645, 2016.

Spencer SJ, Saitha A, Carmont MR, et al.: Meniscal scaffolds: early experience and review of the literature, *Knee* 19:760, 2012.

Steiner SR, Feeley SM, Ruland JR, et al.: Outside-in repair technique for a complete radial tear of the lateral meniscus, *Arthroscopy Tech* 7:e285, 2018.

Strauss EJ, Day MS, Ryan M, et al.: Evaluation, treatment, and outcomes of meniscal root tears: a critical analysis review, *JBJS Rev* 4, 2016, pii: 01874474-201608000-00004.

Thaunat M, Fayard JM, Guimaraes TM, et al.: Classification and surgical repair of ramp lesions of the medial meniscus, *Arthrosc Tech* 5, 2016:e871.

Thaunat M, Jan N, Fayard JM, et al.: Repair of meniscal ramp lesions through a posteromedial portal during anterior cruciate ligament reconstruction: outcome study with a minimum 2-year follow-up, *Arthroscopy* 32:2269, 2016.

Vangsness Jr CT, Farr 2nd J, Boyd J, et al.: Adult human mesenchymal stem cells delivered via intra-articular injection to the knee following partial medial meniscectomy: a randomized, double-blind, controlled study, *J Bone Joint Surg Am* 96:90, 2014.

Van Steyn MO, Mariscalco MW, Pedroza AD, et al.: The hypermobile lateral meniscus: a retrospective review of presentation, imaging, treatment, and results, *Knee Surg Sports Traumatol Arthrosc* 24:1555, 2016.

Verdonk R, Verdonk K, Huysse W, et al.: Tissue ingrowth after implantation of a novel, biodegradeable polyurethane scaffold for treatment of partial meniscal lesions, *Am J Sports Med* 39:774, 2011.

Vundelinckx B, Bellemans J, Vanlauwe J: Arthroscopically assisted meniscal allograft transplantation in the knee: a medium-term subjective, clinical, and radiografhical outcome evaluation, *Am J Sports Med* 38:2240, 2010.

OSTEOCHONDRAL DEFECTS

Bedi A, Feeley BT, Williams RJ: Current Concepts Review. Management of articular cartilage defects of the knee, *J Bone Joint Surg* 92A:994, 2010.

Boughanem J, Riaz R, Patel RM, Sarwark JF: Functional and radiographic outcomes of juvenile osteochondritis dissecans of the knee treated with extra-articular retrograde drilling, *Am J Sports Med* 39:2212, 2011.

Carey JL, Wall EJ, Grimm NL, et al.: Novel arthroscopic classification of osteochondritis dissecans of the knee: a multicentere reliability study, *Am J Sports Med* 44:1694, 2016.

Cotter EJ, Hannon CP, Christian DR, et al.: Clinical outcomes of multifocal osteochondral allograft transplantation of the knee: an analysis of overlapping grafts and multifocal lesions, *Am J Sports Med* 46:2884, 2018.

Gudas R, Gudaite A, Mickevicius T, et al.: Comparison of osteochondral autologous transplantation, microfracture, or debridement techniques in articular cartilage lesions associated with anterior cruciate ligament injury: a prospective study with a 3-year follow-up, *Arthroscopy* 29:89, 2013.

Harris JD, Siston RA, Pan X, Flanigan DC: Autologous chondrocyte implantation, *J Bone Joint Surg* 92A:2220, 2010.

Heir S, Nerhus TK, Rotterud JH, et al.: Focal cartilage defects in the knee impair quality of life as much as severe osteoarthritis: a comparison of knee injury and osteoarthritis outcome score in 4 patient categories scheduled for knee surgery, *Am J Sports Med* 38:231, 2010.

Jones MH, Williams AM: Osteochondritis dissecans of the knee: a practical guide for surgeons, *Bone Joint J* 98-B:723, 2016.

Kramer DE, Kalish LA, Abola MV, et al.: The effects of medial synovial plica excision with and with lateral retinacular release on adolescents with anterior knee pain, *J Child Orthop* 10:155, 2016.

Krych AJ, Robertson CM, Williams 3rd RJ, et al.: Return to athletic activity after osteochondral allograft transplantation in the knee, *Am J Sports Med* 40:1053, 2012.

Liu H, Zhao Z, Clarke RB, et al.: Enhanced tissue regeneration potential of juvenile articular cartilage, *Am J Sports Med* 41:2658, 2013.

Millington KL, Shah JP, Dahm DL, et al.: Bioabsorbable fixation of unstable osteochondritis dissecans lesions, *Am J Sports Med* 38:2065, 2010.

Minas T, Oguar T, Headrick J, et al.: Autologous chondrocyte implantation "sandwich" technique compared with autologous bone grafting for deep osteochondral lesions in the knee, *Am J Sports Med* 46:322, 2018.

Moseley JB, Anderson AF, Browne JE, et al.: Long-term durability of autologous chondrocyte implantation: a multicenter, observations study in US patients, *Am J Sports Med* 38:238, 2010.

Murphy RT, Pennock AT, Bugbee WD: Osteochondral allograft transplantation of the knee in the pediatric and adolescent population, *Am J Sports Med* 42:635, 2014.

Nishizawa Y, Matsumoto T, Araki D, et al.: Matching articular surfaces of selected donor and recipient sites for cylindrical osteochondral grafts of the femur: quantitative evaluation using a 3-dimensional laser scanner, *Am J Sports Med* 42:658, 2014.

Peterson L, Vasiliadis HS, Brittberg M, Lindahl A: Autologous chondrocyte implantation: a long-term follow-up, *Am J Sports Med* 38:1117, 2010.

Richmond J, Hunter D, Irrgang J, et al.: The treatment of osteoarthritis (OA) of the knee, *J Bone Joint Surg* 92A:990, 2010.

Safran MR, Seiber K: The evidence for surgical repair of articular cartilage in the knee, *J Am Acad Orthop Surg* 18:259, 2010.

Shaha JS, Cook JB, Rowles DJ, et al.: Return to an athletic lifestyle after osteochondral allograft transplantation of the knee, *Am J Sports Med* 41:2083, 2013.

Tompkins M, Hamann JC, Diduch DR, et al.: Preliminary results of a novel single-stage cartilage restoration technique: particulated juvenile articular cartilage allograft for chondral defects of the patella, *Arthroscopy* 29:1662, 2013.

Wong CC, Chen CH, Chan WP, et al.: Single-stage cartilage repair using platelet-rich fibrin scaffolds with autologous cartilaginous grafts, *Am J Sports Med* 45:3128, 2017.

ANTERIOR CRUCIATE LIGAMENT

Abouljoud MM, Everhart JS, Sigman BO, et al.: Risk of retear following anterior cruciate ligament reconstruction using hybrid graft of autograft augmented with allograft tissue: a systematic review and meta-analysis, *Arthroscopy* 34:2927, 2018.

Aga C, Riseberg MA, Fagerland MW, et al.: No difference in the KOOS Quality of Life subscore between anatomic double-bundle and anatomic single-bundle anterior cruciate ligament reconstruction of the knee: a prospective randomized controlled trial with 2 years' follow-up, *Am J Sports Med* 46:2341, 2018.

Akpinar B, Thorhauer E, Irrgang JJ, et al.: Alteration of knee kinematics after anatomic anterior cruciate ligament reconstruction is dependent on associated meniscal injury, *Am J Sports Med* 46:1158, 2018.

Anderson CN, Anderson AF: Management of the anterior cruciate ligament-injured knee in the skeletally immature athletes, *Clin Sports Med* 36:35, 2017.

Bettin CC, Throckmorton TW, Miller RH, Azar FM: Technique for partial transphyseal ACL reconstruction in skeletally immature athletes: preliminary results, *Curr Orthop Prac* 30:19, 2019.

Boden BP, Sheehan FT, Torg JS, Hewett TE: Noncontact anterior cruciate ligament injuries: mechanisms and risk factors, *J Am Acad Orthop Surg* 18:520, 2010.

Cancienne JM, Gwathmey FW, Miller MD, Werner BC: Tobacco use is associated with increased complications after anterior cruciate ligament reconstruction, *Am J Sports Med* 44:99, 2016.

Chen H, Chen B, Tie K, et al.: Single-bundle versus double-bundle autologous anterior cruciate ligament reconstruction: a meta-analysis of randomized controlled trials at 5-year minimum follow-up, *J Orthop Surg Res* 13:50, 2018.

Chen T, Zhang P, Chen J, et al.: Long-term outcomes of anterior cruciate ligament reconstruction using either synthetics with remnant preservation or hamstring autografts: a 10-year longitudinal study, *Am J Sports Med* 45:2739, 2017.

Colombet P, Saffarini M, Bouguennec N: Clinical and functional outcomes of anterior cruciate ligament reconstruction at a minimum of 2 years using adjustable suspensory fixation in both the femur and tibia: a prospective study, *Orthop J Sports Med* 6:232596711, 2018.

Delaloye JR, Murar J, Gonzalez M, et al.: Clinical outcomes after combined anterior cruciate ligament and anterolateral ligament reconstruction, *Tech Orthop* 33:225, 2018.

Desai VS, Anderson GR, Wu IT, et al.: Anterior cruciate ligament reconstruction with hamstring autograft: a matched cohort comparison of the all-inside and complete tibial tunnel techniques, *Orthop J Sports Med* 7: 2325967118820297, 2019.

Dhawan A, Gallo RA, Lynch SA: Anatomic tunnel placement in anterior cruciate ligament reconstruction, *J Am Acad Orthop Surg* 24:443, 2016.

El-Sherief FAH, Aldahshan WA, Wahd YE, et al.: Double-bundle anterior cruciate ligament reconstruction is better than single-bundle reconstruction in terms of objective assessment but no in terms of subjective score, *Knee Surg Sports Traumatol Arthrosc* 26:2395, 2018.

Forsythe B, Kopf S, Wong A, et al.: The location of femoral and tibial tunnels in anatomic double-bundle anterior cruciate ligament reconstruction analyzed by three-dimensional computed tomography models, *J Bone Joint Surg* 92A:1418, 2010.

Guenther D, Irarrázaval S, Bell KM, et al.: The role of extra-articular tenodesis in combined ACL and anterolateral capsular injury, *J Bone Joint Surg Am* 99:1654, 2017.

Häner M, Bierke S, Petersen W: Anterior cruciate ligament revision surgery: ipsilateral quadriceps versus contralateral semitendinosus-gracilis autografts, *Arthroscopy* 32:2308, 2016.

Iriuchishima T, Tajima G, Ingham SJN, et al.: Impingement pressure in the anatomical and nonanatomical anterior cruciate ligament reconstruction, *Am J Sports Med* 38:1611, 2010.

Joyce CD, Randall KL, Mariscalco MW, et al.: Bone-patellar tendon-bone versus soft-tissue allograft for anterior cruciate ligament reconstruction: a systematic review, *Arthroscopy* 32:394, 2016.

Karlsson J, Irrgang JJ, van Eck CF, et al.: Anatomic single- and double-bundle anterior cruciate ligament reconstruction, part 2, *Am J Sports Med* 39:2016, 2011.

Khan M, Rothrauff BB, Merali F, et al.: Management of the contaminated anterior cruciate ligament graft, *Arthroscopy* 30:236, 2014.

Kocher MS, Heyworth BE, Fabricant PD, et al.: Outcomes of physeal-sparing ACL reconstruction with iliotibial band autograft in skeletally immature prepubescent children, *J Bone Joint Surg Am* 100:1087, 2018.

Kopf S, Forsythe B, Wong AK, et al.: Nonanatomic tunnel position in traditional transtibial single-bundle anterior cruciate ligament reconstruction evaluated by three-dimensional computed tomography, *J Bone Joint Surg* 92A:1427, 2010.

Kopf S, Martin DE, Tashman S, Fu F: Effect of tibial drill angles on bone tunnel aperture during anterior cruciate ligament reconstruction, *J Bone Joint Surg* 92A:871, 2010.

Kursumovic K, Charalambous CP: Graft salvage following infected anterior cruciate ligament reconstruction: a systematic review and meta-analysis, *Bone Joint J* 98B:608, 2016.

Lecoq FA, Parienti JJ, Murison J, et al.: Graft choice and the incidence of osteoarthritis after anterior cruciate ligament reconstruction: a causal analysis from a cohort of 541 patients, *Am J Sports Med* 46:2842, 2018.

Leo BM, Krill M, Barksdale L, et al.: Failure rate and clinical outcomes of anterior cruciate ligament reconstruction using autograft hamstring versus a hybrid graft, *Arthroscopy* 32:2357, 2016.

Magnussen RA, Reinke eK, Huston LJ, et al.: Effect of high-grade preoperative knee laxity on 6-year anterior cruciate ligament reconstruction outcomes, *Am J Sports Med* 46:2865, 2018.

Marchant BG, Noyes FR, Barber-Westin SD, Fleckenstein C: Prevalence of nonanatomical graft placement in a series of failed anterior cruciate ligament reconstructions, *Am J Sports Med* 38:2010, 1987.

MARS group, Cooper DE, Dunn WR, et al.: Physiologic preoperative knee hyperextension is a predictor of failure in an anterior cruciate ligament revision cohort: a report from the MARS group, *Am J Sports Med* 46:2836, 2018.

Mayr HO, Bruder S, Hube R, et al.: Single-bundle versus double-bundle anterior cruciate ligament reconstruction—5-year results, *Arthroscopy* 34:2647, 2018.

Nawai DH, Tucker S, Schafer KA, et al.: ACL fibers near the lateral intercondylar ridge are the most load bearing during stability examinations and isometric through passive flexion, *Am J Sports Med* 44:2563, 2016.

Noyes FR, Huser LE, Levy MS: The effect of an ACL reconstruction in controlling rotational knee stability in knees with intact and physiologic laxity of secondary restraints as defined by tibiofemoral compartment translations and graft forces, *J Bone Joint Surg Am* 100:586, 2018.

Paci JM, Schweizer SK, Wilbur DM, et al.: Results of laboratory evaluation of acute knee effusion after anterior cruciate ligament reconstruction, *Am J Sports Med* 38:2267, 2010.

Pathare NP, Nicholas SJ, Colbrunn R, McHugh MP: Kinematic analysis of the indirect femoral insertion of the anterior cruciate ligament: implications for anatomic femoral tunnel placement, *Arthroscopy* 30:1430, 2014.

Pearle AD, McAllister D, Howell SM: Rationale for strategic graft placement in anterior cruciate ligament reconstruction: I.D.E.A.L. femoral tunnel position, *Am J Orthop (Belle Mead NJ)* 44:253, 2015.

Pfeiffer TR, Burnham JM, Hughes JD, et al.: An increased lateral femoral condyle ratio is a risk factor for anterior cruciate ligament injury, *J Bone Joint Surg Am* 100:857, 2018.

Plante MJ, Li X, Scully G, et al.: Evaluation of sterilization methods following contamination of hamstring autograft during anterior cruciate ligament reconstruction, *Knee Surg Sports Traumatol Arthrosc* 21:696, 2013.

Sasaki N, Ishibashi Y, Tsuda E, et al.: The femoral insertion of the anterior cruciate ligament: discrepancy between macroscopic and histological observations, *Arthroscopy* 28:1135, 2012.

Sernert N, Hansson E: Similar cost-utility for double- and single-bundle techniques in ACL reconstruction, *Knee Surg Sports Traumatol Arthrosc* 26:634, 2018.

Shimodaira H, Tensho K, Akaoka Y, et al.: Remnant-preserving tibial tunnel positioning using anatomic landmarks in double-bundle anterior cruciate ligament reconstruction, *Arthroscopy* 32:1822, 2016.

Sonnery-Cottet B, Saithna A, Cavalier M, et al.: Anterolateral ligament reconstruction is associated with significantly reduced ACL graft rupture rates at a minimum follow-up of 2 years: a prospective comparative study of 502 patients from the SANTI study group, *Am J Sports Med* 45:1547, 2017.

Southam BR, Colosimo AJ, Grawe B: Underappreciated factors to consider in revision anterior cruciate ligament reconstruction: a current concepts review, *Orthop J Sports Med* 6:1, 2018.

Tang X, Marshall B, Wang JH: Lateral meniscal posterior root repair with anterior cruciate ligament reconstruction better restores knee stability, *Am J Sports Med* Nov 19: 363546518808004. [Epub ahead of print]

Weber AE, Delos D, Oltean HN, et al.: Tibial and femoral tunnel changes after ACL reconstruction: a prospective 2-year longitudinal MRI study, *Am J Sports Med* 43:1147, 2015.

Webster KE, Feller JA, Kimp AJ, et al.: Revision anterior cruciate ligament reconstruction outcomes in younger patients: medial meniscal pathology and high rates of return to sport are associated with third ACL injuries, *Am J Sports Med* 46:1137, 2018.

Wiggins AJ, Grandhi RK, Schneider DK, et al.: Risk of secondary injury in younger athletes after anterior cruciate ligament reconstruction: a systematic review and meta-analysis, *Am J Sports Med* 44:1861, 2016.

Yamamoto Y, Tsuda E, Maeda S, et al.: Greater laxity in the anterior cruciate ligament-injured knee carries a higher risk of postreconstruction pivot shift: intraoperative measurements with a navigation system, *Am J Sports Med* 46:2859, 2018.

Yoon KH, Kim JS, Park SY, et al.: One-stage revision anterior cruciate ligament reconstruction: results according to preoperative bone tunnel diameter: five to fifteen-year follow-up, *J Bone Joint Surg Am* 100:993, 2018.

Zhang Y, Huang W, Yao Z, et al.: Anterior cruciate ligament injuries alter the kinematics of knees with or without meniscal deficiency, *Am J Sports Med* 44:3132, 2016.

ANTEROLATERAL LIGAMENT

Chahla J, Menge TJ, Mitchell JJ, et al.: Anterolateral ligament reconstruction technique: an anatomic-based approach, *Arthrosc Tech* 5:e453, 2016.

DePhillipo NN, Cinque ME, Chahla J, et al.: Anterolateral ligament reconstruction techniques, biomechanics, and clinical outcomes: a systematic review, *Arthroscopy* 33:1575, 2017.

Geeslin AG, Moatsche G, Chahla J, et al.: Anterolateral knee extra-articular stabilizers: a robotic study comparing anterolateral ligament reconstruction and modified Lemaire lateral extra-articular tenodesis, *Am J Sports Med* 46:607, 2018.

Kraeutler MJ, Welton L, Chahla J, et al.: Current concepts of the anterolateral ligament of the knee: anatomy, biomechanics, and reconstruction, *Am J Sports Med* 46:1235, 2018.

Schon JM, Moatshe G, Brady AW, et al.: Anatomic anterolateral ligament reconstruction of the knee leads to overconstraint at any fixation angle, *Am J Sports Med* 44:2546, 2016.

Smeets K, Bellemans J, Lamers G, et al.: High risk of tunnel convergence during combined anterior cruciate ligament and anterolateral ligament reconstruction, *Knee Surg Sports Traumatol Arthrosc*, 2018 Oct 8, https://doi.org/10.1007/s00167-018-5200-3, [Epub ahead of print].

POSTERIOR CRUCIATE LIGAMENT

Anderson CJ, Ziegler CG, Wijdicks CA, et al: Arthroscopically pertinent anatomy of the anterolateral and posteromedial bundles of the posterior cruciate ligament, *J Bone Joint Surg* 94:1936, 2012.

Bedi A, Musahl V, Cowan JB: Management of posterior cruciate ligament injuries: an evidence-based review, *J Am Acad Orthop Surg* 24:277, 2016.

Belk JW, Kraeutler MJ, Purcell JM, et al.: Autograft versus allograft for posterior cruciate ligament reconstruction: an updated systematic review and meta-analysis, *Am J Sports Med* 46:1752, 2018.

Bernhardson A, DePhillipo NN, Daney BT, et al.: Posterior tibial slope and risk of posterior cruciate ligament inury, *Am J Sports Med*, 2019 Jan 14 :363546518819176, https://doi.org/10.1177/0363546518819176, [Epub ahead of print].

Bernhardson AS, DePhillipo NN, Aman ZS, et al: Decreased posterior tibial slope does not affect postoperative posterior knee laxity after double-bundle posterior cruciate ligament reconstruction, *Am J Sports Med* Jan 18:363546518819786, https://doi.org/10.1177/0363546518819786. [Epub ahead of print]

Jang KM, Park SC, Lee DH: Graft bending angle at the intra-articular femoral tunnel aperture after single-bundle posterior cruciate ligament reconstruction: inside-out versus outside-in techniques, *Am J Sports Med* 44:1269, 2016.

LaPrade RF, Cinque ME, Dornan GJ, et al.: Double-bundle posterior cruciate ligament reconstruction in 100 patients at a mean 3 years' follow-up: outcomes were comparable to anterior cruciate ligament reconstructions, *Am J Sports Med* 46:1809, 2018.

Lee DY, Kim DH, Kim HJ, et al.: Biomechanical comparison of single-bundle and double-bundle posterior cruciate ligament reconstruction: a systematic review and meta-analysis, *JBJS Rev* 5:e6, 2017.

Lee DY, Kim DH, Kim HJ, et al.: Posterior cruciate ligament reconstruction with transtibial and tibial inlay techniques: a meta-analysis of biomechanical and clinical outcomes, *Am J Sports Med* 46: 27898, 2018.

Novaretti JV, Sheean AJ, Lian J, et al.: The role of osteotomy for the treatment of PCL injuries, *Curr Rev Musculoskelet Med* 11:298, 2018.

Pache S, Aman ZS, Kennedy M, et al.: Posterior cruciate ligament: current concepts review, *Arch Bone Jt Surg* 6:8, 2018.

Schuster P, Geßlein M, Mayer P, et al.: Septic arthritis after arthroscopic posterior cruciate ligament and multi-ligament reconstructions is rare and can be successfully treated with arthroscopic irrigation and debridement: analysis of 866 reconstructions, *Knee Surg Sports Traumatol Arthrosc* 26:3029, 2018.

Shin YS, Kim HJ, Lee DH: No clinically important difference in knee scores or instability between transtibial and inlay techniques for PCL reconstruction: a systematic review, *Clin Orthop Relat Res* 475:1239, 2017.

Spiridonov SI, Slinkard NJ, LaPrade RF: Isolated and combined grade III posterior cruciate ligament tears treated with double-bundle reconstruction with use of endoscopically placed femoral tunnels and grafts: operative technique and clinical outcomes, *J Bone Joint Surg* 93A:1773, 2011.

Wright JO, Skelley NW, Schur RP, et al.: Comparison of the anterolateral and posteromedial bundles, *J Bone Joint Surg* 98:1656, 2016.

OTHER ARTHROSCOPIC PROCEDURES OF THE KNEE

Bodendorfer BM, Kotler JA, Zelenty WD, et al.: Outcomes and predictors of success for arthroscopic lysis of adhesions for the stiff total knee arthroplasty, *Orthopedics* 40:e1062, 2017.

Cerciello S, Cote M, Lustig S, et al.: Arthroscopically assisted fixation is a reliable option for patellar fractures: a literature review, *Orthop Traumatol Surg Res* 103:1087, 2017.

Kampa J, Dunlay R, Sikka R, et al.: Arthroscopic-assisted fixation of tibial plateau fractures: patient-reported postoperative activity levels, *Orthopedics* 39:e486, 2016.

Le Baron M, Cermolacce M, Flecher X, et al.: Tibial plateau fracture management: ARIF versus ORIF—clinical and radiological comparison, *Orthop Traumatol Surg Res* 105:101, 2019.

Li J, Yu Y, Liu C, et al.: Arthroscopic fixation of tibial eminence fractures: a biomechanical comparative study of screw, suture, and suture anchor, *Arthroscopy* 34:1608, 2018.

Lipina M, Makarov M, Mukhanov V, et al.: Arthroscopic synovectomy of the knee joint for rheumatoid arthritis, *Int Orthop*, 2018 Oct 3, https://doi.org/10.1007/s00264-018-4160-z, [Epub ahead of print].

Liu TH: Complete arthroscopic synovectomy in management of recalcitrant septic arthritis of the knee joint, *Arthrosc Tech* 6:e475, 2017.

Song JG, Nha KW, Lee SW: Open posterior approach versus arthroscopic suture fixation for displaced posterior cruciate ligament avulsion fractures: systematic review, *Knee Surg Relat Res* 30:275, 2018.

Stiefel EC, McIntyre L: Arthroscopic lysis of adhesions for treatment of posttraumatic arthrofibrosis of the knee joint, *Arthrosc Tech* 6:e939, 2017.

Strauss EJ, Kaplan DJ, Weinbeg ME, et al.: Arthroscopic management of tibial spine avulsion fractures: principles and techniques, *J Am Acad Orthop Surg* 26:360, 2018.

Wang Z, Tang Z, Liu C, et al.: Comparison of outcome of ARIF and ORIF in the treatment of tibial plateau fractures, *Knee Surg Sports Traumatol Arthrosc* 25:578, 2017.

HIP

Abrams GD, Hart MA, Takami K, et al.: Biomechanical evaluation of capsulotomy, capsulectomy, and capsular repair on hip rotation, *Arthroscopy* 31:1511, 2015.

Adib F, Johnson AJ, Hennrikus WL, et al.: Iliopsoas tendonitis after hip arthroscopy: prevalence, risk factors and treatment algorithm, *J Hip Preserv Surg* 5:362, 2018.

Adler KL, Giordano BD: The utility of hip arthroscopy in the setting of acetabular dysplasia: a systematic review, *Arthroscopy* 35:237, 2019.

Alpaugh K, Chilelli BJ, Xu S, Martin DS: Outcomes after primary open or endoscopic abductor tendon repair in the hip: a systematic review of the literature, *Arthroscopy* 31:530, 2015.

Anthony CA, Pagely AJ, Gao Y, et al.: Complications and risk factors for morbidity in elective hip arthroscopy: a review of 1325 cases, *Am J Orthop (Belle Mead NJ)* 46:E1, 2017.

Ayeni OR, Alradwan H, de Sa D, Philippon MJ: The hip labrum reconstruction: indications and outcomes—a systematic review, *Knee Surg Sports Traumatol Arthrosc* 22:737, 2014.

Bayne CO, Stanley R, Simon P, et al.: Effect of capsulotomy on hip stability—a consideration during hip arthroscopy, *Am J Orthop (Belle Mead NJ)* 43:160, 2014.

Beckamnn JT, Wylie JD, Potter MQ, et al.: Effect of naproxen prophylaxis on heterotopic ossification following hip arthroscopy: a double-blind randomized placebo-controlled trial, *J Bone Joint Surg* 97A:2032, 2015.

Bedi A, Galano G, Walsh C, Kelly BT: Capsular management during hip arthroscopy: from femoroacetabular impingement to instability, *Arthroscopy* 27:1720, 2011.

Bedi A, Ross JR, Kelly BT, Larson CM: Avoiding complications and treating failures of arthroscopic femoroacetabular impingement correction, *Instr Course Lect* 64:197, 2015.

Begly JP, Buckley PS, Utsunomiya H, et al.: Femoroacetabular impingement in professional basketball players: return to play, career length, and performance after hip arthroscopy, *Am J Sports Med* 46:3090, 2018.

Begly JP, Robins B, Youm T: Arthroscopic treatment of traumatic hip dislocation, *J Am Acad Orthop Surg* 34:309, 2016.

Boden RA, Wall AP, Fehily MJ: Results of the learning curve for interventional hip arthroscopy: a prospective study, *Acta Orthop Belg* 80:39, 2014.

Botser IB, Smith Jr TW, Nasser R, Domb BG: Open surgical dislocation versus arthroscopy for femoroacetabular impingement and comparison of clinical outcomes, *Arthroscopy* 27:270, 2011.

Boykin RE, Patterson D, Briggs KK, et al.: Results of arthroscopic labral reconstruction of the hip in elite athletes, *Am J Sports Med* 41:2296, 2013.

Brandenburg JB, Kapron AL, Wylie JD, et al.: The functional and structural outcomes of arthroscopic iliopsoas release, *Am J Sports Med* 44:1286, 2016.

Byrd JW, Jones KS, Gwathmey FW: Arthroscopic management of femoroacetabular impingement in adolescents, *Arthroscopy* 32:1800, 2016.

Casartelli NC, Leunig M, Maffiuletti NA, Bizzini M: Return to sports after hip surgery for femoroacetabular impingement: a systematic review, *Br J Sports Med* 49:819, 2015.

Chahla J, Mikula JD, Schon JM, et al.: Hip capsular closure: a biomechanical analysis of failure torque, *Am J Sports Med* 45:434, 2017.

Chandrasekaran S, Darwish N, Gui C, et al.: Outcomes of hip arthroscopy in patients with Tönnis grade-2 osteoarthritis at a mean 2-year follow-up: evaluation using a matched-pair analysis with Tönnis grade-0 and grade-1 cohorts, *J Bone Joint Surg* 98A:973, 2016.

Chandrasekaran S, Lodhia P, Gui C, et al.: Outcomes of open versus endoscopic repair of abductor muscle tears of the hip: a systematic review, *Arthroscopy* 31:2057, 2015.

Chen WH, Lin CM, Huang CF, et al.: Functional recovery in osteoarthritic chondrocytes through hyaluronic acid and platelet-rich plasma-inhibited infrapatellar fat pad adipocytes, *Am J Sports Med* 44:2696, 2016.

Colvin AC, Harrast J, Harner C: Trends in hip arthroscopy, *J Bone Joint Surg* 94A:e23, 2012.

Cunningham DJ, Lewis BD, Hutyra CA, et al.: Early recovery after hip arthroscopy for femoroacetabular impingement syndrome: a prospective, observational study, *J Hip Preserv Surg* 4:299, 2017.

Cvetanovich GL, Weber AE, Kuhns BD, et al.: Hip arthroscopic surgery for femoroacetabular impingement with capsular management: factors associated with achieving clinically significant outcomes, *Am J Sports Med* 46:288, 2018.

Degen RM, Pan TJ, Chang B, et al.: Risk of failure of primary hip arthroscopy—a population-based study, *J Hip Preserv Surg* 4:214, 2017.

de Sa D, Cargnelli S, Catapano M, et al.: Femoroacetabular impingement in skeletally immature patients: a systematic review examining indications, outcomes, and complications of open and arthroscopic treatment, *Arthroscopy* 31:373, 2015.

Domb BG, El Bitar YF, Stake CE, et al.: Arthroscopic labral reconstruction is superior to segmental resection for irreparable labral tears in the hip: a matched-pair controlled study with minimum 2-year follow-up, *Am J Sports Med* 42:122, 2014.

Domb BG, Chaharbakhshi EO, Perets I, et al.: Hip arthroscopic surgery with labral preservation and capsular plication in patients with borderline hip dysplasia: minimum 5-year patient-reported outcomes, *Am J Sports Med* 46:305, 2018.

Domb BG, Gui C, Lodhia P: How much arthritis is too much for hip arthroscopy: a systematic review, *Arthroscopy* 31:510, 2015.

Domb BG, Philippon MJ, Giordano BD: Arthroscopic capsulotomy, capsular repair, and capsular plication of the hip: relation to atraumatic instability, *Arthroscopy* 29:162, 2013.

Domb BG, Rybalko D, Mu B, et al.: Acetabular microfracture in hip arthroscopy: clinical outcomes with minimum 5-year follow-up, *Hip Int* 28:649, 2018.

Domb BG, Stake CE, Botser IB, Jackson TJ: Surgical dislocation of the hip versus arthroscopic treatment of femoroacetabular impingement: a prospective matched-pair study with average 2-year follow-up, *Arthroscopy* 29:1506, 2013.

Domb BG, Yuen LC, Ortiz-Declet V, et al.: Arthroscopic labral base repair in the hip: 5-year minimum clinical outcomes, *Am J Sports Med* 45:2882, 2017.

Duplantier NL, McCulloch PC, Nho SJ, et al.: Hip dislocation or subluxation after hip arthroscopy: a systematic review, *Arthroscopy* 32(7):1428, 2016.

Ekhtiari S, de Sa D, Haldane CE, et al.: Hip arthroscopic capsulotomy techniques and capsular management strategies: a systematic review, *Knee Surg Sports Traumatol Arthrosc* 25:9, 2017.

Fowler J, Owens BD: Abdominal compartment syndrome after hip arthroscopy, *Arthroscopy* 26:128, 2010.

Frank JM, Harris JD, Erickson BJ, et al.: Prevalence of femoroacetabular impingement imaging findings in asymptomatic volunteers: a systematic review, *Arthroscopy* 31:1199, 2015.

Frank RM, Lee S, Bush-Joseph CA, et al.: Improved outcomes after hip arthroscopic surgery in patients undergoing T-capsulotomy with complete repair versus partial repair for femoroacetabular impingement: a comparative matched-pair analysis, *Am J Sports Med* 42:2634, 2014.

Frank RM, Lee S, Bush-Joseph CA, et al.: Outcomes for hip arthroscopy according to sex and age: a comparative matched-group analysis, *J Bone Joint Surg* 98A:797, 2016.

Geyer MR, Philippon MJ, Fagrelius TS, Briggs KK: Acetabular labral reconstruction with an iliotibial band autograft: outcomes and survivorship analysis at minimum 3-year follow-up, *Am J Sports Med* 41:1750, 2013.

Glick JM: Hip arthroscopy by the lateral approach, *Instr Course Lect* 55:317, 2006.

Gupta A, Redmond JM, Stake CE, et al.: Does primary hip arthroscopy result in improved clinical outcomes? 2-year clinical follow-up on a mixed group of 738 consecutive primary hip arthroscopies performed at a high-volume referral center, *Am J Sports Med* 44:74, 2016.

Gwathmey FW, Jones KS, Thomas Byrd JW: Revision hip arthroscopy: findings and outcomes, *J Hip Preserv Surg* 4:318, 2017.

Habib A, Haldane CE, Ekhtiari S, et al.: Pudendal nerve injury is a relatively common but transient complication of hip arthroscopy, *Knee Surg Sports Traumatol Arthrosc* 26:969, 2018.

Hanypsiak BT, Stoll MA, Gerhardt MB, DeLong JM: Intra-articular psoas tendon release alters fluid flow during hip arthroscopy, *Hip Int* 22:668, 2012.

Harris JD, McCormick FM, Abrams GD, et al.: Complications and reoperations during and after hip arthroscopy: a systematic review of 92 studies and more than 6,000 patients, *Arthroscopy* 29:589, 2013.

Hoppe D, de Sa D, Simunovic N, et al.: The learning curve for hip arthroscopy: a systematic review, *Arthroscopy* 30:389, 2014.

Horisberger M, Brunner A, Herzog RF: Arthroscopic treatment of femoral acetabular impingement in patients with preoperative generalized degenerative changes, *Arthroscopy* 26:623, 2010.

Ilizaliturri Jr VM, Camacho-Galindo J: Endoscopic treatment of snapping hips, iliotibial band, and iliopsoas tendon, *Sports Med Arthrosc* 18:120, 2010.

Jackson TJ, Hammarstedt JE, Vemula SP, Domb BG: Acetabular labral base repair versus circumferential suture repair: a matched-paired comparison of clinical outcomes, *Arthroscopy* 31:1716, 2015.

Javed A, O'Donnell JM: Arthroscopic femoral osteochondroplasty for cam femoroacetabular impingement in patients over 60 years of age, *J Bone Joint Surg* 93B:326, 2011.

Kemp JL, MacDonald D, Collins NJ, et al.: Hip arthroscopy in the setting of hip osteoarthritis: systematic review of outcomes and progression to hip arthroplasty, *Clin Orthop Relat Res* 473:1055, 2015.

Khan M, Adamich J, Simunovic N, et al.: Surgical management of internal snapping hip syndrome: a systematic review evaluating open and arthroscopic approaches, *Arthroscopy* 29:942, 2013.

Larson CM: Arthroscopic management of pincer-type impingement, *Sports Med Arthrosc* 18:100, 2010.

Larson CM, Clohisy JC, Beaulé PE, et al.: Intraoperative and early postoperative complications after hip arthroscopic surgery: a prospective multicenter trial utilizing a validated grading scheme, *Am J Sports Med* 44:2292, 2016.

Larson CM, Giveans MR, Taylor M: Does arthroscopic FAI correction improve function with radiographic arthritis? *Clin Orthop Relat Res* 469:1667, 2011.

Lee S, Kuhn A, Draovitch P, et al.: Return to play following hip arthroscopy, *Clin Sports Med* 35:637, 2016.

Leunig M, Ganz R: The evolution and concepts of joint-preserving surgery of the hip, *Bone Joint J* 96B:5, 2014.

Locks R, Chahla J, Frank JM, et al.: Arthroscopic hip labral augmentation technique with iliotibial band graft, *Arthrosc Tech* 6:e351, 2017.

Malviya A, Raza A, Jameson S, et al.: Complications and survival analyses of hip arthroscopies performed in the National Health Service in England: a review of 6,395 cases, *Arthroscopy* 31:836, 2015.

Márquez Arabia WH, Gómez-Hoyos J, Llano Serna JF, et al.: Regrowth of the psoas tendon after arthroscopic tenotomy: a magnetic resonance imaging study, *Arthroscopy* 29:1308, 2013.

Marquez-Lara A, Mannava S, Howse EA, et al.: Arthroscopic management of hip chondral defects: a systematic review of the literature, *Arthroscopy* 32:1435, 2016.

Matsuda DK: Labral reconstruction with gracilis autograft, *Arthrosc Tech* 1:e15, 2012.

Martin D, Tashman S: The biomechanics of femoroacetabular impingement, *Op Tech Orthop* 20:248, 2010.

Matsuda DK, Burchette RJ: Arthroscopic hip labral reconstruction with a gracilis autograft versus labral refixation: 2-year minimum outcomes, *Am J Sports Med* 41:980, 2013.

Mauro CS, Voos JE, Kelly BT: Femoroacetabular impingement surgical techniques, *Op Tech Orthop* 20:223, 2010.

McCormick F, Alpuagh K, Nwachukwu BU, et al.: Endoscopic repair of full-thickness abductor tendon tears: surgical technique and outcome at minimum of 1-year follow-up, *Arthroscopy* 29:1941, 2013.

McCormick F, Nwachukwu BU, Alpaugh K, Martin SD: Predictors of hip arthroscopy outcomes for labral tears at minimum 2-year follow-up: the influence of age and arthritis, *Arthroscopy* 28:1359, 2012.

Menge TJ, Briggs KK, Philippon MJ: Predictors of length of career after hip arthroscopy for femoroacetabular impingement in professional hockey players, *Am J Sports Med* 44:2286, 2016.

Menge TJ, Chacla J, Soares E, et al.: The Quebec City slider: a technique for capsular closure and plication in hip arthroscopy, *Arthroscopy* 32:2513, 2016.

Minkara AA, Westermann RW, Rosneck J, et al.: Systematic review and meta-analysis of outcomes after hip arthroscopy in femoroacetabular impingement, *Am J Sports Med*, 2018 Jan 1: 363546517749475, https://doi.org/10.1177/0363546517749475, [Epub ahead of print].

Mitchell JJ, Chahla J, Vap AR, et al.: Endoscopic trochanteric bursectomy and iliotibial band release for persistent trochanteric bursitis, *Arthrosc Tech* 5:e1185, 2016.

Murata Y, Uchida S, Utsunomiya H, et al.: A comparison of clinical outcomes between athletes and nonathletes undergoing hip arthroscopy for femoroacetabular impingement, *Clin J Sport Med* 27:349, 2017.

Nakano N, Lisenda L, Jones TL, et al.: Complications following arthroscopic surgery of the hip: a systematic review of 36 761 cases, *Bone Joint J* 99-B:1577, 2017.

Nepple JJ, Byrd JW, Siebenrock KA, et al.: Overview of treatment options, clinical results, and controversies in the management of femoroacetabular impingement, *J Am Acad Orthop Surg* 21(Suppl 1):S53, 2013.

Newman JT, Briggs KK, McNamara SC, et al.: Revision hip arthroscopy: a matched-cohort study comparing revision to primary arthroscopy patients, *Am J Sports Med* 44:2499, 2016.

Nho SJ, Magennis EM, Singh CK, Kelly BT: Outcomes of the arthroscopic treatment of femoroacetabular impingement in a mixed group of high-level athletes, *Am J Sports Med* 39(Suppl):14S, 2011.

Nielsen TG, Miller LL, Lund B, et al.: Outcome of arthroscopic treatment for symptomatic femoroacetabular impingement, *BMC Musculoskelet Disord* 15:394, 2014.

Niroopan G, de Sa D, MacDonald A, et al.: Hip arthroscopy in trauma: a systematic review of indications, efficacy, and complications, *Arthroscopy* 32:692, 2016.

O'Connor M, Minkara AA, Westermann RW, et al.: Return to play after hip arthroscopy: a systematic review and meta-analysis, *Am J Sports Med* 46:2780, 2018.

Pennock AT, Philippon MJ, Briggs KK: Acetabular labral preservation: surgical techniques, indications, and early outcomes, *Op Tech Orthop* 20:217, 2010.

Perets I, Craig MJ, Mu BH, et al.: Midterm outcomes and return to sports among athletes underling hip arthroscopy, *Am J Sports Med* 46:1661, 2019.

Perets I, Rybalko D, Mu BH, et al.: In revision hip arthroplasty, labral reconstruction can address a deficient labrum, but labral repair retains its role for the reparable labrum: a matched control study, *Am J Sports Med* 46:3437, 2018.

Philippon MJ, Briggs KK, Carlisle JC, Patterson DC: Joint space predicts THA after hip arthroscopy in patients 50 years and older, *Clin Orthop Relat Res* 471:2492, 2013.

Philippon MJ, Ejnisman L, Ellis HB, Briggs KK: Outcomes 2 to 5 years following hip arthroscopy for femoroacetabular impingement in the patient aged 11 to 16 years, *Arthroscopy* 28:1255, 2012.

Philippon MJ, Schroder e Souza BG, Briggs KK: Hip arthroscopy for femoroacetabular impingement in patients aged 50 years or older, *Arthroscopy* 28:59, 2012.

Philippon MJ, Schroder e Souza BG, Briggs KK: Labrum: resection, repair and reconstruction sports medicine and arthroscopy review, *Sports Med Arthrosc* 18:76, 2010.

Philippon MJ, Weiss DR, Kuppersmith DA, et al.: Arthroscopic labral repair and treatment of femoroacetabular impingement in professional hockey players, *Am J Sports Med* 38:99, 2010.

Piuzzi NS, Slullitel PA, Bertona A, et al.: hip arthroscopy in osteoarthritis: a systematic review of the literature, *Hip Int* 26:8, 2016.

Randelli F, Pierannunzil L, Banci L, et al.: Heterotopic ossifications after arthroscopic management of femoroacetabular impingement: the role of NSAID prophylaxis, *J Orthop Traumatol* 11:245, 2010.

Redmond JM, Gupta A, Dunne K, et al.: What factors predict conversion to THA after arthroscopy? *Clin Orthop Relat Res* 475:2538, 2017.

Rhee SM, Kang SY, Jang EC, et al.: Clinical outcomes after arthroscopic acetabular labral repair using knot-tying or knotless suture technique, *Arch Orthop Trauma Surg* 136:1411, 2016.

Riff SJ, Kunze KN, Movassaghi K, et al.: Systematic review of hip arthroscopy for femoroacetabular impingement: the importance of labral repair and capsular closure, *Arthroscopy* 35:646, 2019.

Ross JR, Larson CM, Bedi A: Indications for hip arthroscopy, *Sports Health* 9:402, 2017.

Scher DL, Belmont Jr PJ, Owens BD: Case report: osteonecrosis of the femoral head after hip arthroscopy, *Clin Orthop Relat Res* 468:3121, 2010.

Schüttler KF, Schramm R, El-Zayat BF, et al.: The effect of surgeon's learning curve: complications and outcome after hip arthroscopy, *Arch Orthop Trauma Surg* 138:1415, 2018.

Shin JJ, de Sa DL, Burnham JM, et al.: Refractory pain following hip arthroscopy: evaluation and management, *J Hip Preserv Surg* 5:3, 2018.

Shin JJ, McCrum CL, Mauro CS, et al.: Pain management after hip arthroscopy: systematic review of randomized controlled trials and cohort studies, *Am J Sports Med* 46:3288, 2018.

Shindle MK, Voos JE, Heyworth BE, Kelly BT: Arthroscopic management of labral tears in the hip, *J Bone Joint Surg* 90A(Suppl 4):2, 2008.

Skendzel JG, Philppon MJ, Briggs MJ, Goljan P: The effect of joint space on midterm outcomes after arthroscopic hip surgery for femoroacetabular impingement, *Am J Sports Med* 42:1127, 2014.

Spiker AM, Degen RM, Camp CL, et al.: Arthroscopic psoas management: techniques for psoas preservation and psoas tenotomy, *Arthrosc Tech* 5:e1487, 2016.

Stevens MS, Legray DA, Glazebrook MA, Amirault D: The evidence for hip arthroscopy: grading the current indications, *Arthroscopy* 26:1370, 2010.

Vaughn ZD, Safran MR: Arthroscopic femoral osteoplasty—cheilectomy for cam-type femoroacetabular impingement in the athlete, *Sports Med Arthrosc* 18:90, 2010.

Walters BL, Cooper JH, Rodriguez JA: New findings in hip capsular anatomy: dimensions of capsular thickness and pericapsular contributions, *Arthroscopy* 30:1235, 2014.

Watson JN, Bohnenkamp F, El-Bitar Y, et al.: Variability in locations of hip neurovascular structures and their proximity to hip arthroscopic portals, *Arthroscopy* 30:462, 2014.

Weber AE, Harris JD, Nho SJ: Complications in hip arthroscopy: a systematic review and strategies for prevention, *Sports Med Arthrosc* 23:187, 2015.

White BJ, Patterson J, Herzog MM: Revision arthroscopic acetabular labral treatment: repair or reconstruct? *Arthroscopy* 32:2513, 2016.

The complete list of references is available online at *expertconsult.inkling.com*.

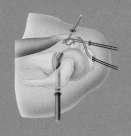

CHAPTER 4

ARTHROSCOPY OF THE UPPER EXTREMITY

Barry B. Phillips, Tyler J. Brolin

Diagnostic and surgical arthroscopy of the upper extremity has become much more common as surgeons have developed proficiency with the arthroscope and appropriate instrumentation has been developed. A thorough knowledge of the anatomy, disorders, arthroscopic variations, and pathologic findings of each joint is essential to perform the procedures successfully and to minimize complications. This chapter discusses indications for arthroscopic treatment, patient preparation, portal anatomy, specific arthroscopic techniques, and complications after arthroscopy of the shoulder, acromioclavicular, and elbow joints.

SHOULDER

Painful syndromes, altered function, and signs and symptoms of instability and internal derangement are frequent in the shoulder. The causes of such dysfunctions can be difficult to prove. The underlying cause often can be established by a careful history and physical examination combined with appropriate radiographic evaluation of the shoulder girdle, cervical spine, and thoracic cavity. Further workup

may include other diagnostic studies, including stress radiographs, CT with or without intraarticular contrast dye, MRI with or without intraarticular contrast dye, ultrasound, and electromyographic studies/nerve conduction studies.

Appropriate radiographs should be obtained and include anteroposterior view with arm in external rotation, true anteroposterior view (Grashey view) with arm in internal rotation, scapular outlet view, and axillary lateral view. In an adolescent athlete, with dominant-side pain during sports requiring overhead motion, anteroposterior views with the shoulder in internal and external rotation help to evaluate for physeal injury. Young adults with symptoms of instability may require further radiographs, including West Point, Bergeneau, and Stryker notch views, to evaluate for potential glenoid and humeral head bony defects.

MRI is useful to evaluate the soft-tissue structures surrounding the shoulder and is most useful in identifying rotator cuff pathology. Magnetic resonance arthrography (MRA) is most commonly used to identify capsulolabral pathology which can be difficult to visualize with standard MRI. In acute instability, hemarthrosis provides good contrast medium;

thus MRA may not be necessary. MRA is especially helpful in evaluation of biceps labral complex or superior labral anterior to posterior (SLAP) tears and better delineates humeral avulsion of the glenohumeral ligament. For chronic instability or if radiographs indicate bony defects from instability, three-dimensional CT is the best means of quantifying bone loss in deciding whether an arthroscopic or open reconstruction is warranted.

Careful thorough preoperative planning is essential for all arthroscopic surgical procedures. The surgeon also should consider potential unexpected findings and mentally prepare for an open procedure when necessary to obtain the best results.

INDICATIONS

For developmental, traumatic, degenerative, or inflammatory conditions of the shoulder resulting in pain, instability, or disability that cannot be controlled by conservative measures, arthroscopic treatment performed by a skilled surgeon results in a low-risk, high-reward reproducible procedure. Contraindications to shoulder arthroscopy include local skin conditions, remote infections that might spread to the joint, and increased medical risks. Surgeons considering arthroscopic procedures should adhere to appropriate indications for the technique and should advise patients about the possibility of an open procedure if arthroscopic findings warrant it.

PATIENT POSITIONING AND ANESTHESIA

Two basic positions for shoulder arthroscopy have been described: the lateral decubitus and the "beach-chair" positions. Both positions have potential advantages and disadvantages, and the decision between the two is largely dependent on the surgeon's training and comfort with each position. Advantages of the lateral decubitus position include better ability to apply traction to the arm, better access to the posterior shoulder, and ease and safety of position. Advantages of the beach-chair position include more anatomic orientation, greater ease of manipulating the arm with an arm positioner, less risk of traction neuropraxia, and ability to easily convert to an open procedure. There remain concerns over cerebral perfusion with the beach-chair position because complications of stroke and death have been reported from hypotensive episodes. Blood pressure at the brachium is lower than that in the cerebrum and potentially significantly lower if carotid artery disease is present. Because blood pressure measured in the calf of a patient in the beach-chair position can be easily 40 mm Hg higher than the accurate cerebral perfusion pressure, pressure should be monitored on the opposite brachium or with cerebral perfusion monitors when possible. Recent studies, however, have demonstrated safety with shoulder arthroscopy in the beach-chair position with no cognitive deficits and much lower frequency of clinical deoxygenation events.

■ LATERAL DECUBITUS POSITION

The patient is placed in the lateral decubitus position with the affected shoulder exposed and is supported by a vacuum bean-bag and kidney rest. A chest strap is used for additional support. The patient's head is supported by a foam rest, and care is taken to protect the eyes and the downside ear. An axillary roll often is requested by anesthesiologists to improve ventilation.

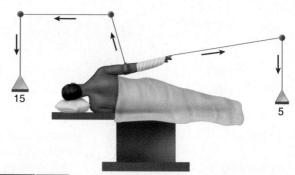

FIGURE 4.1   Traction for distraction of glenohumeral joint with minimal inferior subluxation. Wide 4-inch sling should be used; amount of traction and length of procedure should be monitored.

Peripheral pulses and pulse oximeter readings should be evaluated to ensure axillary structures are not compromised. All pressure points are padded, with a pillow beneath the down leg protecting the peroneal nerve and lateral malleolus and one or more pillows between the knees and ankles. This straight lateral decubitus position can be modified by tilting the patient 20 degrees posteriorly, so that the glenoid surface is placed parallel to the floor.

Using a commercially available sterile arm traction device, 10 to 13 lb of traction is applied. Overdistraction with excessive weight should be avoided. The principle is more one of balanced suspension. Only the amount of traction required for clear viewing should be used. Most arthroscopists use 30 to 60 degrees of abduction and 20 to 30 degrees of forward flexion and pay more attention to the amount of traction and the length of the procedure (Fig. 4.1). A small, soft bolster can be placed in the axillary area to provide lateral displacement of the humeral head.

The arm position for arthroscopy of the subacromial space and acromioclavicular joint is slightly different. The arm is brought down to 20 to 45 degrees of abduction and 0 degrees of flexion. This position permits mild inferior subluxation of the humeral head, opening up the subacromial space.

■ BEACH-CHAIR POSITION

The patient is placed supine on the operating room table with a commercially available beach-chair attachment. Pillows or commercially available pads are placed under the knees to take tension off the sciatic nerve. The patient's head is securely fastened to the headrest with a foam face-mask. Eye protection is ensured, and the endotracheal tube is placed to exit from the contralateral side of the mouth. The patient is carefully inclined so that the undersurface of the acromion is roughly parallel with the floor, generally 70 to 80 degrees of inclination after satisfactory blood pressure is obtained. If concerns over blood pressure are present the patient can be inclined halfway and repeat blood pressure measurement obtained. Once in position, special attention is paid to the alignment of the cervical spine to avoid cervical extension. The patient is secured to the bed with straps over the waist and lower extremity as well as kidney rests (Fig. 4.2).

Commercially available arm positioners with sterile attachments are valuable in allowing the surgeon to easily position the upper extremity during the surgical procedure and freeing up a surgical assistant who now does not have to hold the arm.

CONTROL OF BLEEDING DURING ARTHROSCOPY

Hemostasis is paramount during shoulder arthroscopy. Bleeding during shoulder arthroscopy decreases visualization and lengthens the surgical procedure. One method of controlling bleeding is to add 1 mL of 1:1000 epinephrine to each 3000-mL bag of irrigant, if the patient has a stable pressure and no cardiac contraindications. We have not experienced any anesthetic problems with this mixture. Another technique, and perhaps the most effective, is to use hypotensive anesthesia, with a systolic blood pressure of 90 to 100 mm Hg. A systolic-to-pump pressure gradient of approximately 40 mm Hg should be maintained when possible. Elevation of the fluid bags 3 feet above the level produces a similar pressure

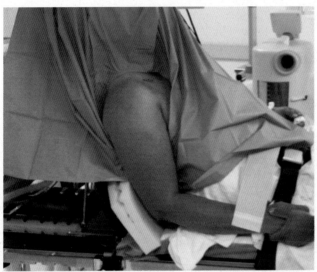

FIGURE 4.2 Beach-chair position for arthroscopic shoulder stabilization.

gradient of 66 mm fluid flow pressure. The surgeon also should be aware of locations that have a tendency to bleed, including the areas around the scapular spine, coracoacromial ligament, and coracoid base.

FLUID EXTRAVASATION

Fluid extravasation also is more of a problem during shoulder arthroscopy than during knee arthroscopy. The increased depth of tissue traversed makes reinsertion of cannulas difficult. Tissue is traumatized, or "new" portals are created with subsequent passes, and fluid extravasation is worsened. Established portals should be maintained by an interchangeable cannula system or by cannulas with rubber diaphragms that close while instruments are being exchanged. Procedures such as subacromial decompression are extraarticular, and fluid extravasation can be pronounced. Lo and Burkhart evaluated 53 patients immediately after shoulder arthroscopy and found an average fluid weight gain of 8.7 lb. Keeping arthroscopy portals with a tight fit, avoiding violation of the deltoid fascia, and increasing pump pressure only when necessary can help avoid fluid extravasation.

PORTAL PLACEMENT

The number of described arthroscopic portals for the shoulder has greatly increased as shoulder surgical procedures have become more complex. The nomenclature for various portals often is confusing because authors have used the same descriptive terms for anatomically different portal sites. Before making arthroscopic portals, a thorough understanding of the local anatomy is necessary to prevent damage to neurovascular structures (Fig. 4.3). The portal that passes closest to a neurovascular structure is the low anterior portal approximately 1 cm from the cephalic vein. Awareness of the axillary nerve is important in portal placement anteriorly, posteriorly, and laterally. Posteriorly, the suprascapular nerve and circumflex scapular artery are approximately 2 cm from the portal site. Later portals, which are used to work on the glenohumeral space, should be directed to enter medial to the rotator cable (Table 4.1).

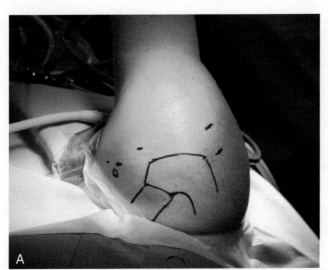

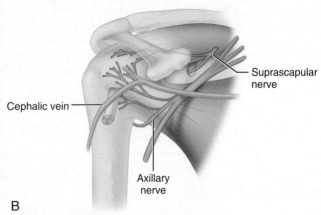

Suprascapular nerve

Cephalic vein

Axillary nerve

FIGURE 4.3 **A,** Bony landmarks outlined on skin. **B,** Anterior neurovascular structures. (**B** redrawn from Hulstyn MJ, Fadale PD: Arthroscopic anatomy of the shoulder, *Orthop Clin North Am* 26:597, 1995.)

	TABLE 4.1		
Description of Portals			
ANTERIOR	5-o'clock portal (Davidson)	The leading edge of the inferior glenohumeral ligament at the 5-o'clock position of the glenoid rim (right shoulder)	The arthroscope is placed through the posterior "soft point" portal, withdrawn, and replaced by a Wissinger rod, which is passed through the anterior capsule while the humerus is maximally adducted. Better with spinal needle outside-in technique. Percutaneous for better localization and angle to the glenoid. Percutaneous localization approximately 1 cm inferior and just lateral to coracoid 1 cm from cephalic vein entering joint just superior to the inferior glenohumeral ligament through junction of mid third and inferior third of subscapular tendon
	Anterior inferior (Wolf)	The arthroscope slides off the inferior edge of the coracoid tip	The arthroscope placed through the posterior "soft point" portal is withdrawn and replaced by a Wissinger rod, which is passed through the anterior capsule
	Anterior central (Matthews)	Skin point lateral to the coracoid	The space limited by the humeral head lateral, the glenoid rim medially, the long head of the biceps tendon superiorly, the subscapularis tendon inferiorly
	Anterior superior (Wolf)	Mid distance between the coracoid and the acromion	Enters the joint just anterior to the long head of the biceps tendon
	Superolateral (Laurencin)	Lateral to the acromion on a line drawn from the acromion to the coracoid	Enters the joint obliquely directly above the biceps tendon, where it pierces the rotator interval tissue
	Anterolateral (Ellman)	2 cm below the lateral edge of the acromion in the prolongation of its anterior edge	Medially to the subacromial bursa
POSTERIOR	Soft point	1.5 cm inferior and 2 cm medial to the posterolateral corner of the acromion	To the coracoid
	Central posterior (Wolf)	2 cm medial and 3 cm inferior to the posterolateral corner of the acromion	To the coracoid
	Posterolateral (Ellman)	2 cm below the lateral edge of the acromion in the prolongation of its posterior edge	Medially to the subacromial bursa, just medial to the ledge of the acromion
	7-o'clock portal (Davidson)	3–4 cm inferior and approximately 1 cm lateral to the posterolateral acromial edge	
LATERAL	Portal of Wilmington	1 cm anterior and 1 cm lateral to the posterolateral corner of the acromion	45-degree approach angle to the posterosuperior glenoid labrum
	Transrotator cuff (O'Brien)	1 cm posterior and 2 cm lateral to the anterolateral corner of the acromion	To the 11-o'clock position in the glenoid labrum (right shoulder) medial to the rotator arch
SUPERIOR	Neviaser portal	Superior "soft spot" surrounded by the clavicle anteriorly, the medial edge of the acromion 1 cm medially, and the spine of the scapula posteriorly	Down at 30 degrees laterally and slightly posteriorly into the glenohumeral joint
	Superior suprascapular nerve portal (Lafosse)	Percutaneous, approximately 7 cm medial to lateral border of acromion, approximately 2 cm medial to Neviaser portal. Approach to suprascapular notch.	

■ POSTERIOR PORTAL

The posterior portal is the primary entry portal for shoulder arthroscopy. It allows examination of most of the joint and assists in the placement of subsequent portals. Thus, before making the posterior portal, its purpose and functions should be known (Fig. 4.4). For visualization, the "soft spot" portal works well. This portal is located 1.5 to 3 cm inferior and 1 cm medial to the posterolateral tip of the acromion. Thus, the location attempts to pass through the posterior soft spot between the infraspinatus and teres minor muscles.

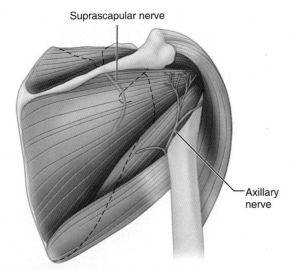

Suprascapular nerve

Axillary nerve

FIGURE 4.4 Posterior shoulder portal risks injury to suprascapular nerve if too medial and to axillary nerve if too inferior or lateral.

By placing the portal 1 cm medial to the posterolateral acromion, the portal can be made approximately parallel to the glenoid articular surface, making for easier passage of the arthroscopic instrumentation to the anterior part of the joint. To locate this spot, one places a hand on the top of the shoulder and palpates the coracoid process with the index or long finger and the posterior soft spot with the thumb. By rotating the humerus with the opposite hand, the posterior glenohumeral joint line often can be located with the thumb. If a posterior stabilization procedure is contemplated, or if two posterior portals are necessary, the portal is made 1.5 to 2 cm inferiorly in line with the acromial edge. For subacromial procedures, a portal 15 cm inferior and in line with the acromion works nicely. A second posterior portal can subsequently be made under direct vision. When a posterior procedure is the main focus, an anterior portal should be made first and then the posterior portals under direct vision.

ESTABLISHING A POSTERIOR PORTAL

TECHNIQUE 4.1

- Establish a posterior portal by inserting an 18-gauge spinal needle through the posterior soft spot into the joint. Place the index or long finger on the coracoid tip to direct the needle anteromedially toward the coracoid. The needle should meet little resistance entering the joint, but sometimes it abuts the humeral head.
- After the capsule has been entered, inject 30 to 40 mL of saline into the joint; far less fluid may be accepted if adhesive capsulitis is significant. There should be free flow into the joint and free backflow. Preinsufflation of the joint produces some distraction of the humeral head from the glenoid and makes entry into the joint with the cannulas easier. If the needle is extraarticular, however, the

initial fluid bolus is injected into the soft tissues, distorting the anatomy. Some authors prefer using a blunt trocar to enter the joint before joint distention because the glenoid neck and humeral head are more easily palpable without distention. The blunt trocar is used to palpate the neck and head area before entering into the triangle just superior to the glenohumeral articulation.

- After the skin site for the posterior portal is selected, inject this area and other planned arthroscopic portal areas with local anesthetic and epinephrine to decrease bleeding.
- Incise the superficial skin layer with a No. 11 knife blade. Avoid deeper penetration because it may precipitate excessive bleeding.
- Insert a cannula and blunt trocar along the path of the needle, anteriorly and medially toward the anterior joint line. Palpate the bony scapular neck and glenoid with the blunt tip of the trocar to determine the midpoint in a superoinferior direction. Slide the trocar laterally to locate the rim of the glenoid as a small ridge. Immediately lateral to this ridge is the entry site for the joint capsule. This position ensures that the entry site is as far medial as possible and that it passes through the muscular portions of the rotator cuff instead of damaging the tendinous portions.

■ POSTEROINFERIOR SEVEN-O'CLOCK PORTAL

Davidson and Rivenburgh described a 7-o'clock accessory posterior working portal for shoulder arthroscopy that allows direct access to the inferior glenohumeral capsule and avoids damage to the nearby structures. The inside-to-outside portal is created by using a switching stick passed through the 3-o'clock portal and directed posteroinferiorly. The switching stick is brought through a small skin incision and left in place. The outside-to-inside 7-o'clock portal is established by making a small skin incision 2 to 3 cm inferior and 1 cm anterior to the posterior acromial edge. A blunt-tipped rod is then inserted into the glenohumeral joint under direct vision.

■ ANTERIOR PORTAL

Multiple anterior portals have been described for diagnostic and surgical stabilization techniques. For complete diagnostic examination of the shoulder, an anterior portal is essential to allow observation of the posterior capsule and the rotator cuff and for an anterior view of the glenohumeral ligaments and the subscapularis tendon. The most commonly described anterior portal is made slightly lateral to a point halfway between the anterolateral tip of the acromion and the coracoid process. Other described portals are superior or inferior to this portal and lateral to a line drawn from the coracoid toward the anterolateral aspect of the acromion. The anteroinferior portal is made just lateral and slightly superior to the palpable coracoid process. The anterolateral portal is made approximately 1 cm lateral to the anterolateral tip of the acromion and enters the glenohumeral joint through the rotator interval. If this portal is made, a large inflow sheath should not be used to prevent damage to the rotator cuff musculature. When anterior stabilization procedures are contemplated, the anterior portals should be separated as much as is safely possible to allow easy placement of instruments without overcrowding and disrupting vision.

For repair of superior labral pathologic conditions, an accessory anterosuperior portal just anterior to the acromioclavicular joint may be needed.

The anterior portal is established after the posterior portal, and the posteriorly placed arthroscope is used to assist visually with its establishment. Two basic methods are used to establish the anterior portal: antegrade (outside-in) and retrograde (inside-out). With both methods, the cannula passes through the anterior soft spot, which corresponds to an intraarticular triangle bounded by the intraarticular portion of the biceps tendon superiorly, the superior intraarticular portion of the subscapularis tendon inferiorly, and the anterior edge of the glenoid at the base. Accessory portals are made by using a spinal needle to confirm appropriate placement of the portal that allows access to the pathologic process. The portal is made using an outside-in (antegrade) technique.

ANTEGRADE METHOD

TECHNIQUE 4.2

- Before joint distention, when anatomic landmarks can be palpated, mark on the skin the approximate sites for arthroscopic anterior portal placement.
- Push the arthroscope, which is already in the posterior portal, up into the anterior soft spot triangle formed by the glenoid articular surface, the biceps tendon, and the subscapularis tendon. Push the arthroscope up against the area of the joint capsule and, with the overhead lights off, transilluminate the area of intended portal placement.
- Back the arthroscope slightly away from this area and palpate externally from the intended portal site while observing arthroscopically the soft spot area. Pass a spinal needle from this spot into the joint. Manipulate the spinal needle within the joint to ensure ease of instrumentation.
- Withdraw the needle and, with a No. 11 blade, make a portal in this chosen spot.
- Pass a cannula with a blunt trocar into the joint capsule. Before penetrating the capsule, move the arthroscope superiorly so that the lens is not damaged as the trocar enters into the joint. Maintain careful control of the trocar to prevent damage to articular structures or to the arthroscope.
- If an accessory anterior portal is necessary, the decision about its location should be made before making the initial anterior portal. The accessory anterior portals should be separated by at least 2 to 3 cm. The appropriate position of an accessory portal also can be confirmed with a spinal needle.

RETROGRADE METHOD

TECHNIQUE 4.3

- "Drive" the arthroscope, which is in the posterior portal, directly into the soft spot. Then remove the arthroscope from its sheath, keeping the sheath against the anterior capsule.

- Pass a Wissinger rod or large blunted Steinmann pin into the cannula and advance it through the anterior capsular structures until the anterior skin is tented.
- Make a skin incision over the tip of the rod and advance the rod past the skin. Pass a cannula sheath over the Wissinger rod and advance it retrograde into the joint. Remove the rod to establish the anterior portal. This method is easier with larger shoulder joints but affords less flexibility in positioning.
- The anterior portal traverses the clavicular portion of the deltoid muscle and enters the rotator cuff interval of the anterior capsule. The structures at risk include the cephalic vein laterally and the musculocutaneous nerve, brachial plexus, and axillary artery and vein anteromedially. Generally, the musculocutaneous nerve passes 3 to 5 cm inferior to the tip of the coracoid, but several anatomic variations have been described, and staying lateral to the coracoid process is safer. Remaining superior to the leading edge of the subscapularis tendon avoids injury to the brachial plexus and vascular structures.

■ ANTEROINFERIOR FIVE-O'CLOCK PORTAL (USED WITH CAUTION)

The intraarticular starting point for establishing the retrograde anteroinferior portal is along the leading edge of the inferior glenohumeral ligament at the 5-o'clock position along the glenoid rim. The portal travels through the subscapularis and lateral to the conjoined tendon. Both the cephalic vein and the anterior humeral circumflex artery are in the path of this portal, but a blunt passer rod or cannula can effectively push these aside. The portal passes lateral to the musculocutaneous nerve and superolateral to the axillary nerve and approximately 1 cm from the cephalic vein. The distances between the portal and the musculocutaneous and axillary nerves have been measured at 22.9 + 4 mm (mean + SD) and 24.4 + 5.7 mm, respectively. The convexity of the humeral head should be moved away from the starting site, not only for visualization but also so that a Wissinger rod can be directed laterally. When the arm is unweighted, removed from traction, and placed alongside the body, the humeral head convexity moves superiorly. This allows appropriate access to the leading edge of the inferior glenohumeral ligament. Placing an object such as a rolled towel in the axilla distracts the joint and allows visualization of the starting site for the 5-o'clock portal. Conversely, using the outside-in 5-o'clock portal allows the portal to be created from a point lateral and inferior to the coracoid using spinal needle localization for best access to the inferior glenoid.

■ SUPERIOR PORTAL

Neviaser is credited with the description of the superior portal (supraclavicular or suprascapular portal). This portal is most useful for passage of suture retrieval devices for rotator cuff repair. It is bound anteriorly by the clavicle, laterally by the acromion, posteriorly by the base of the acromion and the scapular spine, and inferiorly by the posterosuperior rim of the glenoid. This portal penetrates the trapezius muscle and passes through the supraspinatus muscle belly. The suprascapular nerve and artery lie approximately 3 cm medial to the superior portal at its closest point.

ESTABLISHING THE SUPERIOR PORTAL

TECHNIQUE 4.4

(NEVIASER)
- The entry site is easily palpable as a soft spot. Introduce an 18-gauge spinal needle 1 cm medial to the medial acromion at an angle of 30 to 45 degrees to the skin and 10 degrees posteriorly to enter the joint at the superior margin of the glenoid just posterior to the attachment of the long head of the biceps tendon.
- Observe passage of the needle arthroscopically to confirm proper position before making a small skin incision.

■ SUPRASCAPULAR NERVE PORTAL AS DESCRIBED BY LAFOSSE

The suprascapular nerve portal is positioned between the clavicle and the scapular spine approximately 7 cm medial to the lateral border of the acromion. This portal is approximately 2 cm medial to the Neviaser portal.

■ LATERAL, POSTEROLATERAL, AND ANTEROLATERAL PORTALS

The lateral portal is the primary operative portal for the subacromial space. It is located 3 cm lateral to the lateral border of the acromion and passes through the deltoid muscle. One must ensure that instrumentation can be used and not be hindered by impingement on the lateral acromial edge. When advancing the cannula, it is initially directed downward and toward the tuberosity to enter the lateral extent of the bursa, allowing for a full view and ease of instrumentation. Accessory portals can be spaced anteriorly or posteriorly as necessary. The axillary nerve lies approximately 5 cm distal to the lateral border of the acromion.

Arthroscopy of the subacromial space usually can be accomplished through the initial posterior portal and the central anterior portal. The cannulas are easily redirected up into the bursa from the same skin incisions, after passing through the deltoid muscle.

When passing the anterior cannula, gentle palpation with the cannula tip can reveal the extent of the coracoacromial ligament, allowing redirection of the cannula just lateral to the ligament. In a very muscular individual or if the posterior portal has been placed too far inferiorly, a new portal, 1.5 cm inferior to the posterior acromion, may be required. Burkhart described two lateral portals for repair of SLAP lesions. Depending on the site of disruption, he used an anterolateral portal, 1 cm lateral and posterior to the anterolateral corner of the acromion, or a posterolateral portal, 1 cm anterior and lateral to the posterolateral corner of the acromion.

■ PORTAL OF WILMINGTON

This posterolateral accessory portal is used to approach posterior type II SLAP lesions, providing access to the glenoid and superior labrum. The location is 1 cm anterior and 1 cm lateral to the posterior acromial angle. Care should be taken when placing this portal so as not to damage the rotator cuff near its attachment to the greater tuberosity.

DIAGNOSTIC ARTHROSCOPY AND ARTHROSCOPIC ANATOMY

As with arthroscopy of other joints, a thorough knowledge of the major anatomic structures around the shoulder is necessary. The surgeon must be familiar with the normal anatomy to identify abnormal or pathologic processes.

The examination begins with identification of the soft spot between the biceps and subscapularis tendons (Fig. 4.5). The subscapularis is evaluated by having an assistant rotate and then lever the humerus posteriorly by placing a posterior force on the proximal humerus while pushing anteriorly at the elbow. The subscapularis recess is inspected for loose bodies. The examination consists of arthroscopically circling the joint, viewing the labral attachment at the biceps, and following the labral attachment to the glenoid and the capsular attachment to the humerus circumferentially around the shoulder back to the biceps superiorly. Capsular laxity is demonstrated by a drive-through sign and a rotator interval of more than 1.5 cm. A large sublabral hole or Buford complex variant where the middle glenohumeral ligament inserts at the base of the biceps must be distinguished from a true Bankart lesion, which extends inferiorly from the glenoid equator. Inferior glenohumeral ligament injuries may be off the glenoid, midsubstance, or off the humerus (humeral avulsion of the glenohumeral ligament [HAGL] lesions) or bipolar lesions and, when identified, should later be reexamined through an anterosuperior portal.

The biceps attachment to the superior labrum is thoroughly evaluated by applying traction to the biceps with a probe and by taking the arm out of traction to check for peel-back due to a SLAP lesion. The biceps tendon is followed to the bicipital arch while one evaluates for fraying, inflammation, instability, and chondromalacia where the tendon rubs against the humeral head.

Using the scope and looking superiorly, a circumferential examination in the reverse direction, starting at the biceps and progressing posteriorly, is undertaken to evaluate the rotator cuff insertion. The anterior footprint insertion of the rotator arch is just posterior to the biceps and is the key component of the supraspinatus insertion. The cuff is followed posteriorly; a healthy cuff attaches just off the articular surface of the humeral head. The posterior attachment of the rotator arch marks the overlap of the attachments of the supraspinatus and infraspinatus onto the humeral head and the start of the bare area. This area is evaluated for chondromalacia or a Hill-Sachs lesion. If a Hill-Sachs lesion is noted, the Hill-Sachs interval is measured from the posterior cuff insertion to the medial edge of the lesion. This loss of humeral articulation, as well as the amount of loss of anterior glenoid articulation (determined by using the glenoid bare area to measure the posterior radius compared with the anterior radius), is used to identify on-track or off-track lesions resulting from shoulder instability (described later).

The arthroscope is now moved to the anterosuperior portal, and the posterior portal can be used for probing. The arthroscope is inserted anteriorly to view the posterior articular surface, posterior labrum, posterior pouch, and posterior capsule for redundancy, synovitis, fraying from instability, or inflammatory processes (Fig. 4.5I). Although not as prevalent as the anterior band of the inferior glenohumeral ligament, the posterior band may be visible with internal rotation as it

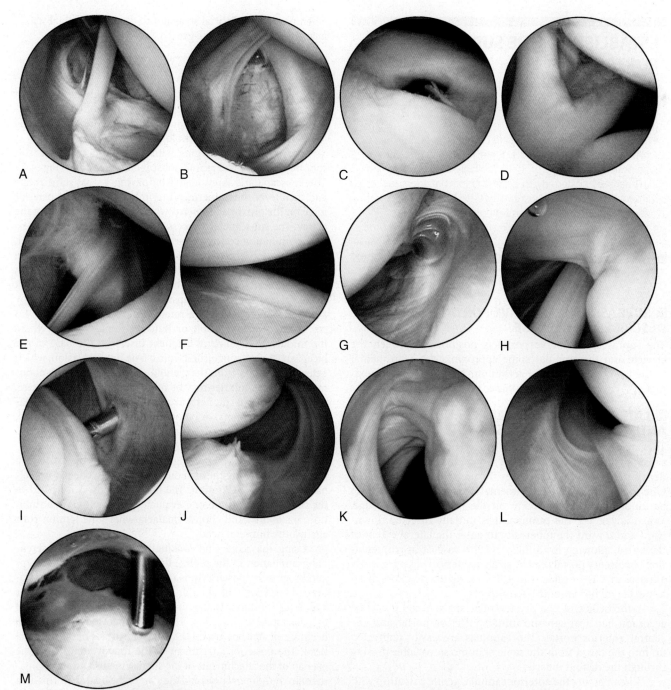

FIGURE 4.5 Patient is in lateral decubitus position, and glenoid is oriented horizontally. **A,** Superior part of shoulder joint with biceps tendon inserting into superior labrum. Humeral head is superior right, and glenoid is inferior. **B,** Superior glenohumeral ligament and subscapularis tendon on right with middle glenohumeral ligament inferiorly. **C,** Normal sublabral hole. **D,** Buford complex showing insertion of middle glenohumeral ligament directly into biceps anchor (see text). **E,** Middle cord variant of glenohumeral ligament crossing subscapularis tendon. **F,** Inferior pouch. Glenohumeral ligaments and labrum are seen. **G,** Capsular attachment to humeral head observed through inferior pouch. **H,** Rotator cuff evaluated for fraying, partial tears, or calcification. Supraspinatus tendon is seen superiorly with biceps tendon in center of picture. **I,** Posterior articular surface, posterior labrum, posterior pouch, and posterior capsule observed with arthroscope inserted anteriorly. **J,** Posterior band of inferior glenohumeral ligament. **K,** Anterior band of inferior glenohumeral ligament observed from anterior portal. Humeral insertion of ligament is superior. **L,** Capsulolabral attachment to glenoid observed through anterior portal. **M,** View of subacromial space with cuff below and acromion above.

approaches its insertion at the 7-o'clock to 9-o'clock positions posteriorly (Fig. 4.5J). After examination of the bare area in the humeral articular cartilage, the arthroscope is moved anteriorly to evaluate the rotator cuff by looking superiorly and the biceps-labral complex by looking inferiorly toward the glenoid. As the arthroscope is moved more anteriorly and directed back toward the inferior pouch, the glenohumeral ligaments can be seen from their humeral insertion down to the glenoid insertion. Careful observation for the ligamentous insertion to the humerus is indicated to rule out humeral avulsion of the glenohumeral ligament (HAGL). Figure 4.5K shows a normal glenohumeral ligament. By turning the arthroscope more inferiorly, the attachment of the anteroinferior glenohumeral ligament and the capsulolabral attachment can be seen (Fig. 4.5L). The middle glenohumeral ligament and subscapularis tendon and the subscapularis recess also can be observed, and the arthroscope can be moved inferiorly into the subscapular recess for evaluation of the subscapularis tendon and muscle. Loose bodies and loose implants in previously operated shoulders may be found in the subscapular recess. Glenoid bone loss is best evaluated by measuring the posterior radius of the bare area and comparing it with the radius of the anterior bare area through the anterosuperior portal.

To complete diagnostic arthroscopy of the shoulder for impingement, rotator cuff calcification, and inflammatory conditions, the subacromial bursa should be examined. The bursa extends from at least 2 cm anterior to the anterior edge of the acromion to approximately the midacromion posteriorly. To enter this space, all distention from the glenohumeral joint should be removed before removing any cannulas. The posterior cannula can be used to enter the subacromial space. The cannula is withdrawn from its previous placement and redirected so that the blunt edge of the trocar abuts the posterior edge of the acromion just medial to the posterolateral edge. It is redirected slightly inferior to the acromion so as to slide up under the acromion without probing into the soft tissue under the bone. At the tip of the acromion, the cannula is directed toward the surgeon's finger, which is placed at the anterolateral edge of the acromion. The cannula should not be aimed toward the acromioclavicular joint. The subacromial space can be increased, and the approach can be made easier by placing the arm in approximately 30 degrees of abduction. When the tip of the cannula is felt up under the anterolateral edge of the acromion, it is gently swept back and forth to free the area in the bursa.

The arthroscope is placed in the subacromial bursa, and contiguous structures are examined carefully. If the view is limited at this time, attempts can be made to reinsert the cannula or to sweep the cannula back and forth to open the bursa further. During this portion of the procedure, as in all arthroscopic shoulder procedures, maintaining a systolic blood pressure of no more than 30 mm Hg above the pump pressure is helpful. Initially, viewing superiorly, the undersurface of the acromion can be seen and evaluated for roughening or fraying, with an associated kissing lesion on the rotator cuff indicating impingement. The shoulder is rotated internally and externally, and increased abduction can be applied to evaluate the area for impingement. The arthroscope is turned to view medially the area of the acromioclavicular joint and the coracoacromial ligament as it ascends under the acromion. If the shoulder has impingement or inflammation, vision may be limited, and an anterolateral portal can be

made using an outside-in technique. A shaver is placed into the bursa under direct vision, and bursectomy is performed to allow better exposure of the rotator cuff. The rotator cuff and bursa should be cleaned from the area of the insertion to the tuberosity, which is the usual area of attrition, impingement, or calcification (Fig. 4.5M).

After rotation of the arm to evaluate the cuff through the posterior portal, the arthroscope can be placed in the lateral portal and directed toward the posterior bursal wall. The same procedure can be used to view directly the acromion superiorly and the clavicle for evidence of bony prominence or fraying indicating impingement.

The subacromial space should be examined thoroughly, which may require partial or subtotal bursectomy to see the rotator cuff and the undersurface of the acromion clearly. Any bony prominences of the acromion or the acromioclavicular joint should be evaluated and resected. The rotator cuff itself should be palpated for roughness, fraying, or calcifications. Although calcifications may be difficult to delineate, generally they can be palpated, or a slight bulge or vascular blush of the tendon can be seen.

The internal extent of the bursa is approximately 4 cm from the acromial edge with the axillary nerve always lateral to the bursa, on average 0.8 cm. The lateral extent of the bursa should not be violated arthroscopically. If an open repair technique is used, the palpable internal extent of the bursa can be used as the limit of safely splitting the deltoid.

General evaluation of the acromioclavicular joint can be accomplished through the subacromial portal. If an acromioclavicular spur is present, electrocautery and a shaver should be used to resect the soft tissue from the undersurface of the acromion; inferiorly directed pressure places the clavicle into the joint for better vision. The acromioclavicular joint also can be seen directly through the anterosuperior and posterosuperior portals by placing the spinal needles at approximately a 45-degree angle into the acromioclavicular joint from just anterior and posterior to the joint.

LOOSE BODIES

Loose bodies occasionally are encountered during shoulder arthroscopy. Small ones sometimes can be removed from the joint with suction applied to a large-caliber outflow cannula. Often by increasing the rate of inflow, the joint can be vacuumed without applying suction to the outflow.

ARTHROSCOPIC REMOVAL OF LOOSE BODY

TECHNIQUE 4.5

- Remove larger loose bodies with grasping forceps and triangulation techniques. Loose bodies tend to bob like apples, and turning off the inflow or outflow to decrease turbulence makes it easier to grasp the loose body. When securely grasped, extract the loose body with a slow, twisting movement to minimize the chance of its slipping from the jaws of the grasper. If necessary, enlarge the portal by spreading the joint capsule and soft tissues with the grasper or hemostat tips to prevent pulling the loose body from the jaws of the grasper.

- Extremely large loose bodies may have to be broken into smaller fragments by cutting them with a burr before they can be extracted through the portals. Keep the loose bodies contained to a localized accessible space when breaking the larger fragments. If the loose body floats away, insert a suction tip or apply suction to the outflow cannula to pull the loose body to the tip and stabilize it. Insert a grasping instrument to grasp it.

- Loose bodies tend to gravitate into the axillary pouch of the shoulder or occasionally into the subscapular recess. Loose implants likewise may be found in these areas. Other hiding places include the posterior recess behind the glenoid, the synovial folds behind the biceps tendon insertion on the glenoid, and at the site where the biceps tendon exits the joint. If a loose body is seen on a radiograph, but is not readily visible arthroscopically and is hidden within the subscapularis bursa, "milk" the loose body from the bursa by palpating in the subcoracoid area. From an anterior portal, drive the arthroscope into the subscapular bursa to examine this area fully.

- In addition to removing the loose body, determine its source because the underlying abnormality may need correction. Loose bodies may form from Hill-Sachs lesions or glenoid rim fractures in patients who have sustained dislocations. They also may be produced in shoulders with advanced arthritis or osteonecrosis where portions of the lesion have broken free.

SYNOVECTOMY

The arthroscope allows almost complete inspection of the shoulder joint and can be used successfully for selective biopsy of the synovium. A near-total synovectomy is possible using the arthroscope without the debilitating disruption of the deltoid or rotator cuff. The lateral decubitus position with the affected arm suspended in skin traction is preferred, and the three-portal (anterior, posterior, and superior) technique usually allows complete access. The superior and anterior portions of the joint are reached with operative instruments placed through the anterior portal and the arthroscope in the posterior or superior portal. The posterior and superior portions of the joint are reached with the operative instruments in the posterior portal and the arthroscope in the anterior or superior portal. For involvement of the inferior recess, accessory posterior and inferior operating portals may be necessary. Motorized synovial resectors are required for adequate arthroscopic synovectomy. Large-diameter (>5 mm) blades allow for more efficient resection of synovial tissue. Maintaining a systolic-to-joint distention pressure of 30 mm Hg or less and adding one ampule of epinephrine to the 3-L arthroscopy bag helps maintain clear vision.

DRAINAGE AND DEBRIDEMENT

As in the knee, the arthroscope has been recommended for drainage and debridement of a septic shoulder joint; however, few clinical studies have been reported. Arthroscopic debridement (1) improves inspection, irrigation, and debridement compared with multiple needle aspirations; (2) allows breaking up of intraarticular loculations; (3) decreases the potential for postoperative scarring and stiffness that occur after formal arthrotomies; and (4) can be done several times if necessary. A contraindication to arthroscopic debridement is an adjacent soft-tissue abscess.

LABRAL TEARS

The glenoid labrum consists of dense fibrocartilaginous tissues and some elastic fibers. On the inner side, the labrum is continuous with the hyaline cartilage of the glenoid, and on the outer side, it is continuous with the fibrous tissue of the capsule. The capsule and ligaments of the shoulder, including the biceps tendon, are attached to and become part of the glenoid labrum, which attaches to the glenoid. The labrum encircles the glenoid, increasing its depth around the humeral head, and provides increased stability. Saha has shown that adding the glenoid labrum increases the glenoid surface to 75% of the humeral head vertically and 57% in the horizontal direction. Karzel et al., in biomechanical testing of cadaver shoulder specimens, showed that the labrum affects the distribution of contact stresses when a compressive load is applied to the shoulder at 90 degrees of abduction.

The most common mechanisms of injury to the superior labrum (i.e., SLAP lesions) are extrinsic secondary to traction on the upper extremity and intrinsic during the throwing motion, which likewise produces traction on the biceps anchor. A second proposed mechanism of injury is torsional peel-back of the posterior superior labrum during the cocking phase of throwing. Compression, shear, and degenerative changes associated with decreased peripheral vascularity and age increase the likelihood of labral tears and decrease the likelihood of a successful repair.

To aid in localizing the site of labral injury, the glenoid labrum has been divided into six areas: (1) the superior labrum, (2) the anterior labrum above the midglenoid notch, (3) the anterior labrum below the midglenoid notch, (4) the inferior labrum, (5) the posteroinferior labrum, and (6) the posterosuperior labrum (Fig. 4.6). Lesions located above the equator of the glenoid (a line drawn between the 3-o'clock and 9-o'clock positions on the glenoid) often are associated with rotator cuff or biceps disease. Lesions located below the equator are highly suggestive of shoulder instability.

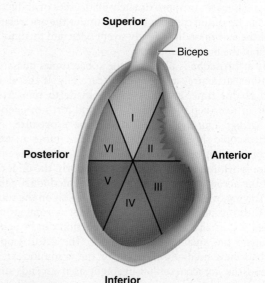

FIGURE 4.6 Glenoid labrum can be divided into six areas.

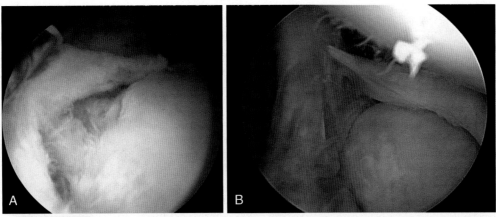

FIGURE 4.7 Labral tears. **A,** Type II. **B,** Type IV SLAP lesion with displaced labral fragment and tear extending into base of biceps. Biceps anchor was stable, and labrum was excised.

Snyder further classified superior labral anterior to posterior lesions and coined the term *SLAP lesions*. He categorized them into four basic varieties and a complex variety that involves a combination of two or more of the other SLAP lesions. These descriptive categorizations are used to determine treatment alternatives and to predict long-term results. Type I lesions, which can be treated with simple debridement, are described as fraying of the superior labrum with a solid biceps tendon anchor attachment. Type II lesions involve pathologic detachments of the labrum and biceps anchor from the superior part of the glenoid (Fig. 4.7A). These lesions most commonly progress posterior to the biceps but may progress anterior to or both anterior and posterior to the biceps attachment at the supraglenoid tubercle. Biceps-labral instability is evidenced by labral displacement of 5 mm or more with traction on the biceps tendon, hemorrhage, or fibrous granulation tissue at the insertion with long-standing lesions and superior articular cartilage changes. The peel-back test as described by Burkhart is used to evaluate for posterior extension of the lesion by removing the arm from traction and placing it in 90 degrees of abduction. The labrum is observed to displace medially on the scapular neck as the shoulder is externally rotated to 90 degrees.

Type III lesions, which occur with the meniscoid-type labrum, are vertical tears within the labrum that produce bucket-handle fragments. These can be excised, provided that the biceps anchor is securely fixed to the supraglenoid tubercle. Type IV lesions are bucket-handle type tears that extend up into the biceps tendon (Fig. 4.7B). These lesions also can be excised if less than 30% of the thickness of the biceps tendon is involved. Snyder suggested that if approximately one third of the biceps tendon is involved, suture repair of the segment should be considered. In older patients, if more than a third of the tendon is involved, he suggested performing biceps tenodesis or tenotomy after resection of the labral tear. Complex tears involving a combination of two or more of the previously described lesions should be treated with repair of the type II portion if present and resection of the other lesions, provided that there is a stable biceps anchor.

With multiple authors showing poor results with SLAP repairs in older individuals, the current thinking is that it is best to perform SLAP repairs in symptomatic athletes who do not respond to conservative therapy. Age is a determining factor: In general, for patients 40 years of age or younger, SLAP repair is recommended; 40 to 60 years, tenodesis; and over 60 years of age, tenodesis or tenotomy, depending on patient preference. Repairs must have low-profile knots or knotless constructs to prevent knot impingement. If a tenodesis is chosen and a component of shoulder instability is present, repair of the superior labrum probably is warranted.

ARTHROSCOPIC FIXATION OF TYPE II SLAP LESIONS

TECHNIQUE 4.6

(MODIFIED FROM BURKHART, MORGAN, AND KIBLER)

- Place the patient in the lateral decubitus position and place the arm in 30 to 45 degrees of abduction and 20 degrees of forward flexion with 5 to 10 lb of balanced suspension. Administer general anesthesia and place a warming blanket to prevent hypothermia. Use an arthroscopic pump to maintain intraarticular pressure at 50 to 60 mm Hg. Use serial compression devices on the lower extremities.
- Establish a viewing portal 2 cm below the posterolateral acromion and an anterior central working portal for routine diagnostic arthroscopy. Findings such as a superior sulcus of more than 5 mm in depth, a displaceable biceps root, a positive drive-through sign, and a positive peel-back sign are indicative of a SLAP lesion (Fig. 4.8).
- Use an arthroscopic probe to test the stability of the biceps-superior labral attachments to the glenoid. A normal superior sublabral sulcus covered with articular cartilage can be seen 5 mm medially beneath the labrum. If the sublabral sulcus is deeper than 5 mm, or if the labral attachments at the medial limit of the sulcus are tenuous, a SLAP lesion may be present.
- Assess whether the biceps root is easily displaceable with a probe. An unstable biceps root and superior labrum are easily displaced medially on the glenoid neck. Occasionally, the biceps root is unstable to probing, yet tenuous superior labral attachments are present. Such cases represent interstitial disruption of medially located attachments

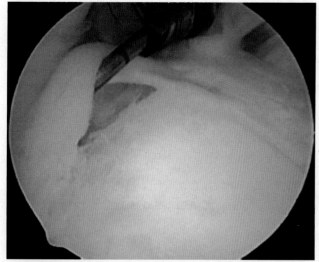

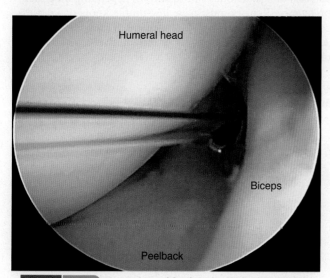

Humeral head

Biceps

Peelback

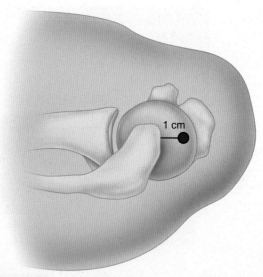

1 cm

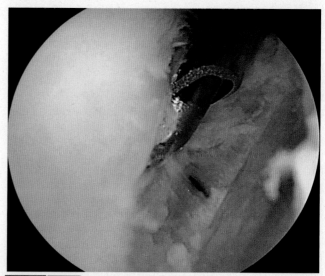

and require completion of the lesions, bone bed preparation, and repair.

- Sweep the arthroscope from superior to inferior between the glenoid and humeral head to see if the arthroscope can be easily "driven through" the joint. Although a positive drive-through sign indicates instability, "pseudolaxity" associated with SLAP lesions also may be the cause.
- The positive peel-back sign is diagnostic for a posterior SLAP lesion; however, isolated anterior SLAP lesions often have a negative peel-back test, but other arthroscopic signs, as described earlier, usually are positive. To perform the peel-back test, remove the arm from traction and observe the superior labrum arthroscopically as an assistant brings the arm to 90 degrees of abduction and 90 degrees of external rotation (Fig. 4.9). Performing this dynamic peel-back maneuver in a shoulder with a posterior SLAP lesion causes the entire biceps–superior labrum complex to drop medially over the edge of the glenoid.
- When the diagnosis of a SLAP lesion is made, repair the lesion immediately because swelling may occur that obliterates

the supralabral recess and obscures exposure. For the SLAP lesion repair, make three portals: a standard posterior viewing portal, an anterior portal located just above the lateral border of the subscapularis tendon, and an anterosuperior portal. The anterosuperior portal is located just lateral to the anterolateral corner of the acromion (Fig. 4.10). Use a spinal needle to locate this portal precisely so that it provides a 45-degree angle of approach to the anterosuperior corner of the glenoid for proper placement of the suture anchor. Alternatively, use a percutaneous shuttle through the superomedial (Neviaser) portal.

- Through the anterior portal, prepare the bone bed on the superior neck of the glenoid, beneath the detached labrum, using a motorized shaver (Fig. 4.11). Debride

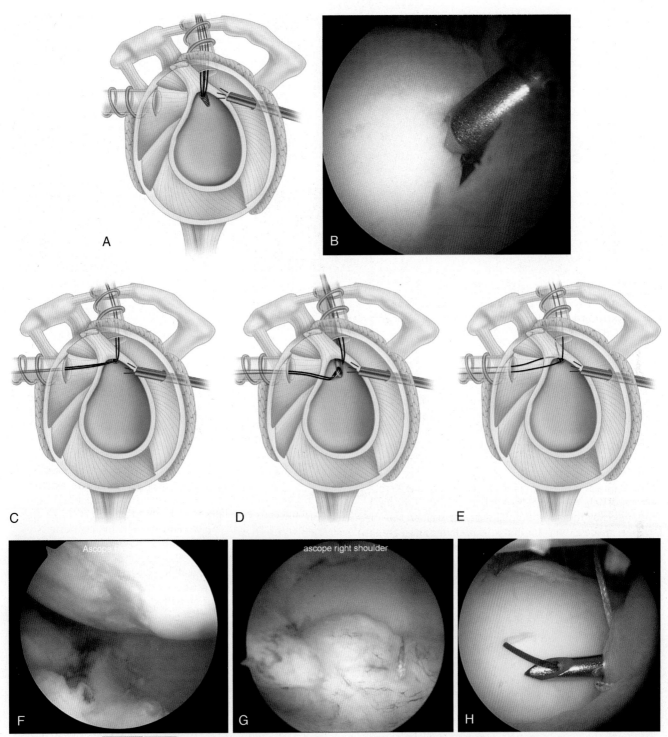

FIGURE 4.12   **A** and **B,** Anchor placement at base of biceps. **C** and **D,** Sutures passed through biceps anchor complex and retrieved posterior to biceps tendon. **E,** Suture retrieved anterior to biceps tendon. **F,** Humeral head erosion secondary to knot impingement. **G,** Knotless repair. **H,** Passage of suture shuttle at base of biceps. **SEE TECHNIQUE 4.6.**

the soft tissues carefully down to a bleeding base of bone, but do not remove bone.
- For fixation of SLAP lesions, use small-size suture anchors and simple translabral loop sutures, preferably small PEEK suture anchors (Fig. 4.12A). The most critical element to resisting peel-back forces in a mechanically effective manner

is to position a tight suture loop just posterior to the root of the biceps, with the loop attached to a suture anchor placed beneath the root of the biceps (Fig. 4.12B).
- To prevent suture or knot impingement, a vertical suture through the labrum or horizontal suture behind the biceps can be helpful in some cases (Fig. 4.12C to E). The strength

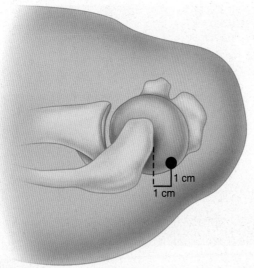

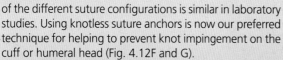

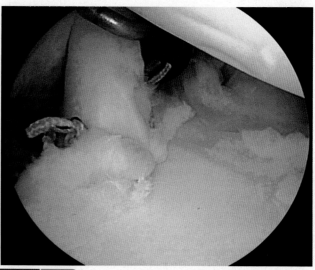

FIGURE 4.13 Posterolateral portal (portal of Wilmington) used to place suture anchor in posterosuperior quadrant of glenoid. Portal located 1 cm lateral and 1 cm anterior to posterior acromial angle. **SEE TECHNIQUE 4.6.**

FIGURE 4.14 Completed SLAP repair. **SEE TECHNIQUE 4.6.**

of the different suture configurations is similar in laboratory studies. Using knotless suture anchors is now our preferred technique for helping to prevent knot impingement on the cuff or humeral head (Fig. 4.12F and G).

- For superior labral lesions that extend posteriorly to overlie the posterosuperior quadrant, place a second anchor through a posterolateral portal (Fig. 4.13).
- Pass a Spear guide (Arthrex, Naples, FL) through the rotator cuff near the musculotendinous junction of the infraspinatus by this approach. Because the diameter of the Spear guide is only 3.5 mm, it is preferred over a standard 7-mm arthroscopy cannula for delivery of the suture anchor through the posterolateral portal. To minimize damage to the rotator cuff from portal placement, place only the 3.5-mm Spear guide through the posterolateral portal. This posterolateral portal is used for anchor placement only; suture passage and knot-tying for the posterior anchor are accomplished through the anterosuperior portal.
- Use the BirdBeak suture passers (Arthrex, Naples, FL) to pass the suture through the labrum. The 45-degree BirdBeak is ideal for passing sutures posterior to the biceps through the anterosuperior cannula, and the 22-degree BirdBeak is best for passing sutures anterior to the biceps through the anterior cannula. Penetrate the labrum with the BirdBeak from superior to inferior and grasp the suture; withdraw the BirdBeak to pull the suture out of the anterosuperior cannula. If the SLAP lesion extends anteriorly beyond the 1-o'clock position, place a separate suture anchor in that position for fixation of that portion of the labrum. A suture shuttle device through an anterior or a percutaneous Neviaser portal allows for less trauma and more accurate placement and is necessary for knotless anchors (Fig. 4.12H). The shuttle suture is placed before drilling to prevent inadvertent damage to the permanent sutures.

- After the repair, perform the peel-back and drive-through test again to be sure that they are negative, indicating that the pathologic process has been corrected (Fig. 4.14). If the drive-through sign remains positive, consider adjunctive measures for capsular tightening.

POSTOPERATIVE CARE The operated arm is placed at the side in a sling with a small pillow. Passive external rotation of the shoulder with the arm at the side (not in abduction) and flexion and extension of the elbow are emphasized immediately. Patients who require posteroinferior capsulotomy are started on posteroinferior capsular stretches (sleeper stretches) on the first postoperative day. The sling is discontinued after 3 weeks, and passive elevation is initiated. From weeks 3 to 6, progressive passive motion as tolerated is permitted in all planes, and sleeper stretches are begun in patients who did not have posteroinferior capsulotomy. From weeks 6 to 16, stretching and flexibility exercises are continued. Passive posteroinferior capsular stretching is continued, as is external rotation stretching in abduction. Strengthening exercises for the rotator cuff, scapular stabilizers, and deltoid are initiated at 6 weeks. Biceps strengthening is begun 8 weeks postoperatively.

At 4 months, athletes begin an interval throwing program on a level surface. They continue a stretching and strengthening program, with particular emphasis on posteroinferior capsular stretching. At 6 months, pitchers may begin throwing at full speed, and at 7 months they are allowed full-velocity throwing from the mound. All throwing athletes are instructed to continue posteroinferior capsular stretching indefinitely. A tight posteroinferior capsule probably initiates the pathologic cascade to a SLAP lesion, and recurrence of the tightness can be expected to place the repair at risk in a throwing athlete (Table 4.2).

TABLE 4.2

Rehabilitation Protocol for Superior Labral Anterior-Posterior Lesion

PHASE I—IMMEDIATE POSTSURGICAL

WEEKS 0–2 POSTOPERATIVE (TYPE II AND IV)	GOALS (BY END OF 2 WK)

1. P/AAROM with following restrictions
  FL <120 degrees
  ER/IR <30 degrees
2. Table slides in FL/pendulums
3. Scapular mobility exercises
4. Passive elbow FL
5. Active hand, wrist ROM and gripping exercises
6. Submaximal pain-free isometrics
  IR/ER
  ABD/ADD
  Scapular retraction/depression
	1. Independent with HEP
	2. PROM 120 degrees maximum FL/scaption
	3. PROM 30 degrees maximal ER/IR
	4. Full hand, wrist AROM
	5. Active elbow EXT to 30 degrees, full passive elbow FL
	Precautions
	1. Sling compliance
	2. No active biceps contraction
	3. Full active elbow EXT

PHASE II—GRADED AROM/STRENGTHENING

WEEKS 3–6 POSTOPERATIVE	GOALS (BY END OF 6 WK)
1. Glenohumeral joint mobilizations (grades I and II) 2. Progressing PROM to tolerance 3. Progress AAROM/AROM 4. Progress scapular mobility exercises (side lying) 5. Elbow FL—no resistance 6. UBE with low resistance 7. Initiate TheraBand ER/IR isometrics in neutral (sidestepping) 8. Rhythmic stabilization progression 9. PNF diagonals with light/moderate manual resistance	1. Independent with HEP 2. Gradually restore full PROM 3. Discontinue sling as pain decreases and proximal stability increases (wk 3–4) 4. Restore correct shoulder girdle mechanics (scapulohumeral rhythm) 5. Full active elbow FL (pain-free) 6. Full EXT by 4–6 WK depending on physician input 7. Able to comb hair (if dominant arm) 8. Sleep uninterrupted *Precautions* 1. No lifting 2. No ER with ABD >90 degrees
WEEKS 7–9 POSTOPERATIVE	GOALS (BY END OF 9 WK)
1. Continue progressing PROM—more aggressive mobilizations if needed (progress joint mobilizations grades III and IV as needed) 2. Elbow FL with light weights (1–5 lb) 3. UBE—increase intensity 4. Progress isotonics as able (TheraBand/light weight) 5. Progress rhythmic stabilization/PNF diagonals 6. Progress closed-chain exercises (especially wall push-ups)	1. Independent with HEP 2. AROM WNL 3. Able to reach behind back for wallet 4. Able to lift plate into eye-level cabinet *Precaution* No lifting >5 lb
WEEKS 10–11 POSTOPERATIVE	GOALS (BY END OF 11 WK)
1. Progress above exercises as tolerated 2. TheraBand ER/IR 45 to 90 degrees increase speed/intensity (must be pain-free and demonstrate correct mechanics) 3. Closed-chain scapular stability exercises (quadruped, tripod, side lying) 4. Progress proprioceptive training to include progressive weight-bearing exercises on unstable surfaces	1. MMT elbow FL 4/5 2. MMT shoulder FL 4/5 3. MMT shoulder ABD 4/5 4. MMT shoulder ER 4/5 5. MMT shoulder IR 4/5 6. Able to lift 3 lb into overhead cabinet 7. Maintain scapulohumeral rhythm with strengthening and functional activities 8. Able to tuck shirt and fasten bra *Precaution* No unilateral lifting overhead >5 lb

Continued

TABLE 4.2

Rehabilitation Protocol for Superior Labral Anterior-Posterior Lesion—cont'd

PHASE III—ADVANCED STRENGTHENING FOR RETURN TO SPORT

WEEKS 12–15 POSTOPERATIVE	GOALS (BY END OF 15 WK)
1. Progress isotonics increasing resistance/repetitions (exercises, throwing, lunges)	1. MMT shoulder musculature 5/5
2. Plyoball exercises if appropriate	2. Able to place ≥10 lb in overhead cabinet
Chest pass	
Overhead throw	
Sideway throw	
One-handed ball on wall	
3. Progress shoulder strengthening (lateral pull-downs, rows)	
4. Isokinetic strengthening as needed	
WEEKS 16 TO 24 POSTOPERATIVE	GOALS (BY END OF 6 MO)
1. Initiate interval throwing (per physician input)	1. Return to sport/activity of choice
2. Initiate sport-specific/functional training	2. Independent with exercise progression
3. Isokinetic testing if requested	

Protocol was developed for patients after SLAP lesion repair. Surgery and rehabilitation differ depending on type of lesion. Types I and III usually are treated with debridement. The biceps tendon is stable, so postoperative rehabilitation usually can progress as tolerated. Types II and IV indicate an unstable biceps tendon requiring repair. This protocol addresses range-of-motion limitations and limited active biceps work necessary for type II/IV repairs. This is a guideline and may be adjusted to the clinical presentation and physician's guidance.

ABD, Abduction; *ADD*, adduction; *AROM*, active range of motion; *ER*, external rotation; *EXT*, extension; *HEP*, home exercise programs; *FL*, flexion; *IR*, internal rotation; *MMT*, manual muscle testing; *P/AAROM*, passive or active-assisted range of motion; *PNF*, proprioceptive neuromuscular facilitation; *PROM*, passive range of motion; *ROM*, range of motion; *UBE*, upper body exercises; *WNL*, within normal limits.

BICEPS TENDON LESIONS

Biceps tendon lesions may be inflammatory, degenerative, or traumatic as a result of repetitive microtrauma or macrotrauma. The injury site or sites may include the attachment to the supraglenoid tubercle, SLAP, the tendon (intraarticular or extraarticular), and the bicipital arch. The bicipital arch consists of the conglomerate of the superior glenohumeral ligament and the coracohumeral ligament attachment at the superior bicipital groove. The ligaments are reinforced anteriorly by the subscapular tendon attachment and posteriorly by the supraspinatus attachment. In a study of 200 consecutive patients undergoing arthroscopic cuff repair, Lafosse et al. found 45% to have anterior, posterior, or both anterior and posterior biceps instability. Larger tears correlated with a higher incidence and degree of biceps instability. The researchers suggested internal and external rotation of the humerus in 0 to 30 degrees of abduction for dynamic evaluation of the biceps followed by probing to evaluate for static stability.

Boileau et al. described an hourglass-shaped biceps deformity that is associated with inflammation and triggering through the proximal pulley. Persistence of the triggering can result in pulley instability. The treatment is arthroscopic tendon debulking or tenodesis. In patients who have chronic impingement and persistent biceps tendinitis with more than 50% of the biceps tendon disrupted, or with biceps tendon subluxation as described by Lafosse et al., Habermeyer et al., and Bennett, an arthroscopic or mini–open tenodesis can be used (Fig. 4.15).

Tenodesis is favored over tenotomy in active patients for cosmesis and prevention of biceps cramping. Multiple articles support various fixation techniques, including interference screws, suture anchors, and soft-tissue fixation (percutaneous

intraarticular transtendon [PITT] procedure). The method of fixation seems to be less important than the quality of the tissue fixed.

Subpectoral tenodesis has been recommended to prevent the groove pain reported in some series. The potential for plexus and musculocutaneous nerve injury or humeral diaphyseal stress fractures has been reported with these techniques and must be considered.

Biceps tenodesis to treat type 2 SLAP tears has been reported to be successful in approximately two thirds of athletes, comparable to primary SLAP repair. Pitchers treated with tenodesis tend to have persistence of some anterior shoulder pain, as reported by Smith et al.

BICEPS TENDON RELEASE

TECHNIQUE 4.7

- Perform arthroscopy of the shoulder through standard anterior and posterior portals.
- Release the biceps tendon at its glenoid attachment with an arthroscopic electrode or arthroscopic scissors to allow for a thickened biceps tip, which should hang up in the bicipital sling, thus preventing a severe "Popeye" deformity.
- Debride any attached stump with a shaver.

POSTOPERATIVE CARE Patients are given a sling to wear for 3 to 5 days for comfort; a full range of motion is allowed. No resisted elbow flexion is allowed for 1 month.

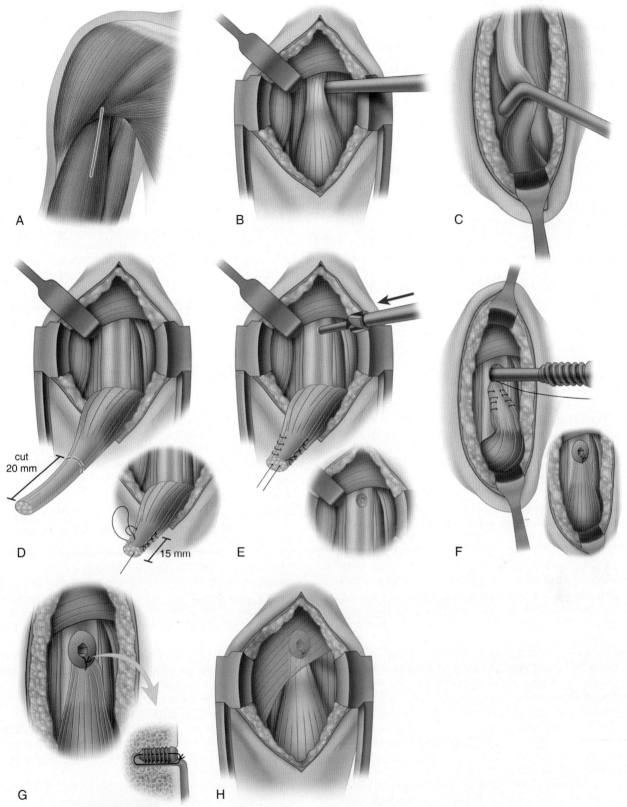

FIGURE 4.15 Mazzocca et al. subpectoral mini-open biceps tenodesis. **A,** Skin incision. **B,** Location of biceps tendon made by dissecting through superficial fascia using blunt dissection to palpate tendon. **C,** Probe is used to withdraw tendon from joint and out of incision. **D,** To ensure appropriate tensioning, 20 mm of diseased portion of tendon is excised. **E,** Guidewire is placed in center of bicipital groove, usually at junction of middle and distal thirds of intertubercular groove between lesser and greater tuberosities. A 7- or 8-mm acorn reamer is placed over this and reamed to 15 to 20 mm. **F,** Suture is placed through Arthrex Bio-Tenodesis driver, and one suture is left out. **G,** Bio-Tenodesis screw inserted into bone tunnel, and suture that was left out of driver is tied to suture that is in cannulated portion of tenodesis screw. **H,** Musculotendinous junction rests in its anatomic location underneath inferior border of pectoralis major tendon.

ARTHROSCOPIC BICEPS TENODESIS: PERCUTANEOUS INTRAARTICULAR TRANSTENDON TECHNIQUE

Sekiya et al. described a technique that should be used in middle-aged patients who are not participating in high-level sports or heavy lifting. Indications are as for other biceps tendon problems with chronic bicipital tendinitis and an associated tear, medial subluxation, or bicipital pain with an associated SLAP tear.

TECHNIQUE 4.8

(SEKIYA ET AL.)
- Place the patient in a beach-chair or lateral decubitus position.
- Insert a spinal needle from the anterior aspect of the shoulder into the bicipital groove and through the transverse humeral ligament and the lateral aspect of the internal capsule.
- Under direct view, pierce the biceps tendon with the spinal needle. Thread a No. 1 PDS (Ethicon, Somerville, NJ) through the spinal needle and pull it through the anterior portal with a grasper.
- Insert a second spinal needle through the transverse humeral ligament from the anterior shoulder and pierce the biceps tendon near the first suture. Thread a second No. 1 PDS through the spinal needle and pull it out of the anterior portal.
- These two sutures are used to pull a No. 2 braided, nonabsorbable suture through the biceps tendon. Tie the No. 2 suture to one strand of the PDS and pull it from the puncture wound in the anterior aspect of the shoulder through the biceps tendon and out of the anterior cannula. Tie the end of the suture that was pulled through the anterior cannula to the other PDS and pull it back through the anterior cannula, through the biceps tendon, and out of the anterior shoulder puncture wound. This creates a mattress suture, which secures the biceps tendon to the transverse humeral ligament in the bicipital groove.
- Repeat these steps to create a second mattress suture to secure the biceps tendon. Sutures of different colors can be used to simplify suture management.
- After the biceps tendon is adequately secured, use an arthroscopic scissors or biter to transect the biceps tendon proximal to the suture.
- Debride the stump of the biceps anchor down to a smooth, stable rim on the superior labrum.
- At this point, direct the arthroscope into the subacromial space. Establish a lateral portal and perform any concomitant procedures, such as a subacromial decompression or rotator cuff repair. Avoid transection of the previously passed sutures. We prefer to perform a subacromial bursectomy before passing tenodesis sutures.
- Locate the sutures securing the biceps tendon to the transverse humeral ligament in the bicipital groove in the subacromial space and pull through the lateral portal.

- Sequentially tie the sutures using standard arthroscopic knot-tying techniques or pass them through a swivel-lock device and secure them to the proximal groove.
- Remove all fluid and debris and close portals in the standard fashion. Dress the wound and place the shoulder in a sling.

POSTOPERATIVE CARE If an isolated arthroscopic biceps tenodesis was done, the patient is immediately started on passive pendulum exercises and active wrist and hand range-of-motion exercises. At 1 week after surgery, gentle passive elbow and shoulder range of motion is begun in all planes under the guidance of a physical therapist. The sling is used for 3 to 4 weeks. Active motion and gentle strengthening of the shoulder and elbow can begin 8 weeks after surgery. By 12 to 16 weeks after surgery, the patient is "weaned" from physical therapy to a home exercise program. Unrestricted use of the extremity is allowed 4 to 6 months after surgery.

ARTHROSCOPIC "LOOP 'N' TACK" TENODESIS

A suture "loop 'n' tack" tenodesis, performed by passing a FiberSnare (Arthrex) around and through the proximal biceps, is a quick and effective method for tenodesis. We have had good success with this technique.

TECHNIQUE 4.9

(DUERR ET AL.)
- With the patient in the beach-chair or lateral position, perform diagnostic arthroscopy through a standard posterior portal.
- After pathology of the long head of the biceps is identified, use an 18-gauge spinal needle to localize the anterior portal within the rotator interval directly over the biceps tendon; place a cannula for suture passing.
- Pass a looped nonabsorbable FiberSnare suture (Arthrex) around the biceps tendon (Fig. 4.16A); pass the free tail end through the looped end, and pull the tail to cinch the loop over the biceps tendon near its insertion at the superior labrum (Fig. 4.16B).
- Pass a tissue penetrator through the center of the biceps tendon, distal to the cinched loop, and grasp the free end and pull it through the tendon (Fig. 4.16C), tacking the loop in place (Fig. 4.16D).
- Cut the biceps tendon at its insertion.
- Load the free end of the suture into a PushLock suture anchor (Arthrex).
- Drill a pilot hole at the most distally visualized portion of the intraarticular bicipital groove, just above the subscapularis tendon.
- Seat the anchor with all slack taken out of the suture, allowing the tendon to translate distally with the bicipital groove, "tacking" the biceps in place.

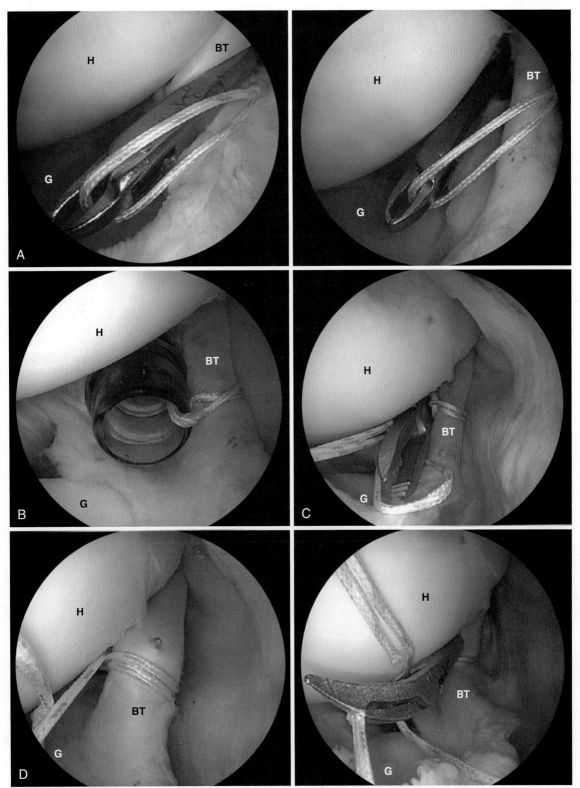

FIGURE 4.16 Loop 'n' tack tenodesis, as described by Duerr et al. Left shoulder in lateral decubitus position with a 30-degree arthroscope from the posterior portal (same orientation and position for all figures). **A** (left image). End of a looped suture is passed around biceps tendon (BT) from superior labrum to BT. Right image, suture is then pulled from inferior to BT to complete passage around it (G, glenoid; H, humerus). **B,** Free end of suture has been passed through looped end and is cinched to BT close to its insertion at superior labrum. **C,** Free end of suture is passed into the joint with excess slack. **D,** Tissue penetrator can be passed through the BT in a more distal position to secure the tendon without distalizing it. (From Duerr RA, Nye D, Paci JM, et al. Clinical evaluation of an arthroscopic knotless suprapectoral biceps tenodesis technique: loop 'n' tack tenodesis. *Orthop J Sports Med* 6:2325967118779786, 2018.) **SEE TECHNIQUE 4.9.**

POSTOPERATIVE CARE After isolated biceps tenodesis, patients are allowed immediate shoulder and elbow range of motion. A sling is worn for comfort for a week. When this procedure is combined with another procedure (e.g., rotator cuff repair), the other procedure typically dictates the rehabilitation protocol.

BICEPS TENODESIS: ARTHROSCOPIC OR MINI-OPEN TECHNIQUE WITH SCREW FIXATION

Tenodesis can be done with a PEEK tenodesis screw, with two suture anchors, or with the use of a FiberSnare. The resistance to cyclic loading is comparable in both techniques, whereas the ultimate pull-out strength of the biotenodesis screw is stronger than the suture anchors. Whether done arthroscopically or through a mini-open approach with a small anterior incision or a small subpectoral incision, long-term results are comparable, and the technique should be chosen based on the skills and experience of the operating surgeon.

TECHNIQUE 4.10

(ROMEO ET AL. MODIFIED)
- Place the patient in the lateral decubitus position, with the shoulder abducted 30 to 40 degrees and forward flexed 30 degrees.
- Pass an 18-gauge needle from the anterolateral corner of the acromion through the rotator cuff interval and into the biceps tendon.
- Pass a No. 1 monofilament suture through the 18-gauge needle, capture it with a grabber from the anterior portal and then extract it.
- Use a No. 11 blade along the same plane as the spinal needle to make a vertical incision in the lower portion of the visible biceps tendon sheath to aid in finding the tendon later in the subacromial space.
- After the tendon is marked with a suture, use an arthroscopic basket to release the tendon from its origin just lateral to the superior labrum. This completes the preparation for the biceps tenodesis during the glenohumeral joint arthroscopy.
- Make an anterolateral portal 2 to 3 cm below the palpable edge of the anterior acromion in the center of the anterior third of the acromion. Visualization is maintained through the lateral portal or with a 70-degree scope through the posterior portal; the anterior portal is the working portal.
- Place an arthroscopic shaver in the anterior portal and remove all adventitial tissue. Anatomic landmarks and the monofilament suture are used for localizing the tendon in the groove. The falciform ligament of the pectoralis tendon is a reproducible landmark. The biceps tendon is directly under this structure.
- Using an arthroscopic basket, identify the sheath and open it. Use electrocautery to clean surrounding tissues and use a probe to free the tendon. Extend the dissection

proximally to the lateral aspect of the rotator interval. Avoid proceeding too far medially. Otherwise, the dissection to expose the biceps tendon from the biceps sheath may lead to a partial displacement of the superficial attachment of the subscapularis tendon.
- Debride soft tissues to expose the bicipital groove.
- Pull the tendon directly out through the skin incision of the anterolateral portal.
- Place a hemostat on the tendon at the level of the skin to prevent it from retracting underneath the skin.
- The placement and tension of the tenodesis are important for anatomic repair. To approximate the intraarticular distance, remove 20 mm of tendon and place a Krackow stitch of No. 2 FiberWire.
- Allow the sutures to fall back into the subacromial space.
- Place cannulas into the anterior and anterolateral portals and shuttle the sutures into the anterior portal so that they are out of the way for the bone tunnel preparation.
- Use a lateral portal for exposure and identify the bicipital groove.
- For instrumentation, use an 8.25-mm clear cannula in the anterior portal to enhance exposure and minimize soft-tissue distention. Through the anterolateral portal, insert a tenodesis reamer into the center of the bicipital groove, 10 to 15 mm below the insertion of the supraspinatus lateral to the subscapularis insertion at the level of the transverse humeral ligament. The depth of insertion is 20 mm. For most men, an 8-mm reamer is used, and for most women, a 7-mm reamer. The tendon can be contoured slightly to make sure it fits easily. Ream to a depth of 25 mm.
- Retrieve the sutures out of the anterolateral portal and slide an 8-mm cannula over the sutures to align them over the tunnel.
- Pull the sutures through a swivel-lock tip and hold tension on the construct to push the biceps into the base of the tunnel.
- Insert the tenodesis screw flush with the cortex.
- Check for stability by rotating the humerus.

POSTOPERATIVE CARE Postoperative management depends largely on the types of procedures that were performed in conjunction with the biceps tenodesis. If only a biceps tenodesis was done, the postoperative procedure is the same as for arthroscopic acromioplasty (see Technique 4.17). Strengthening activities related to elbow flexion or forward elevation of the arm with the elbow extended should be restricted until 6 weeks after the biceps tenodesis.

SUBPECTORAL BICEPS TENODESIS

Successful arthroscopic subpectoral tenodesis has been described by several authors. Currently, mini-open or open subpectoral tenodesis with a small nonabsorbable screw is indicated in patients who are not athletes participating in contact sports or overhead throwing (see Fig. 4.15).

ANTERIOR INSTABILITY

Since Detrisac and Johnson first introduced the staple capsulorrhaphy in the 1970s, arthroscopic shoulder stabilization

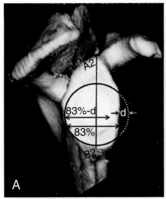 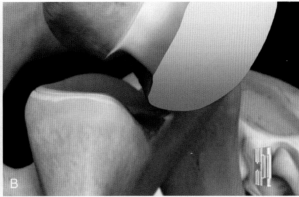

FIGURE 4.17 Off-track Hill-Sachs lesion. **A,** Three-dimensional CT showing glenoid face with bone loss of width *d*. In this case, the glenoid track is 83% of normal glenoid width *minus d*. A2-B2 is the long axis of glenoid. **B,** Relation of glenohumeral joint in abduction and external rotation. Note loss of contact of intact humeral articular surface with glenoid articular surface because of anteroinferior glenoid bone loss. Large Hill-Sachs interval (distance from posterior rotator cuff attachments to medial margin of Hill-Sachs lesion) is wider than glenoid track width of which has been reduced by glenoid bone loss. (From DiGiacomo G, Itoi E, Burkhart SS: Evolving concept of bipolar bone loss and the Hill-Sachs lesion: from "engaging/non-engaging" lesion to "on-track/off-track" lesion, *Arthroscopy* 30:90, 2014.)

procedures have evolved with continued development of technology and procedure modifications. Arthroscopic suture anchors, capsular plication, and interval closure repair techniques were developed, with a recurrence rate in appropriately selected patients being comparable to that of open techniques.

As the technique evolved, so did the indications and contraindications. In a study of 190 patients, Burkhart and DeBeer noted an increased recurrence rate (from 6.5% to 89%) in contact athletes when a 25% glenoid defect or an engaging Hill-Sachs lesion alone or in combination was present. Di Giacomo et al. developed the concept of "on-track" and "off-track" lesions based on evaluation of bipolar bone loss at the glenoid and humeral head (Fig. 4.17 and Box 4.1). Glenoid lesions involving more than 25% are treated with a Bankart-Bristow-Latarjet procedure. Glenoid lesions that involve less than 25% but are nonetheless off track are treated with an arthroscopic Bankart procedure with the addition of a remplissage procedure. This is especially important in contact athletes and has been shown to significantly decrease recurrence rates. Balg and Boileau developed an injury severity index (Table 4.3) and found a recurrence rate of 75% with glenoid bone loss and hyperlaxity. Shaha et al. showed that in the active military population, bone loss of 13.5% resulted in a significant decrease in functional outcomes. Likewise, Neviaser noted inferior results when treating anterior periosteal sleeve avulsions in young patients.

At this time, we believe that the arthroscopic procedure with plication and interval closure as indicated and repair of the capsulolabral defects produces comparable results to an open procedure. Surgeons should evaluate their skills and technical expertise and choose between an open and arthroscopic procedure based on the best procedure for their level of expertise and the pathologic process present.

Indications for shoulder stabilization procedures include primary dislocation in high-risk patients involved in contact or collision sports near the season's end or dislocation of the dominant shoulder in an athlete who uses an overhead

---

BOX 4.1

Determining If a Hill-Sachs Lesion Is "On Track" or "Off Track"

1. Measure the diameter *(D)* of the inferior glenoid, either by arthroscopy or from a three-dimensional CT scan or three-dimensional MRI.
2. Determine the width of the anterior glenoid bone loss *(d)*.
3. Calculate the width of the glenoid track (GT) by following the formula: $GT = 0.83\,D - d$.
4. Calculate the width of the HSI, which is the width of the Hill-Sachs lesion (HS) plus the width of the bone bridge (BB) between the rotator cuff attachments and the lateral aspect of the Hill-Sachs lesion: $HSI = HS + BB$.
5. If HSI > GT, the HS is off track, or engaging. If HSI < GT, the HS is on track, or nonengaging.

From DiGiacomo G, Itoi E, Burkhart SS: Evolving concept of bipolar bone loss and the Hill-Sachs lesion: from "engaging/non-engaging" lesion to "on-track/off-track" lesion, *Arthroscopy* 30:90, 2014.

motion. In-season instability treated aggressively with rehabilitation allows 75% of athletes to return to competition, though two thirds of those returning have additional instability episodes. Instability episodes produce bone loss and chondral damage of the glenoid and humeral head, as well as further soft-tissue damage. Long-term sequelae should be discussed with the patient. Recurrence of instability despite conservative treatment also is an indication for shoulder stabilization (Box 4.2). Contraindications include an uncooperative or medically unstable patient. Relative contraindications include glenoid bone loss of 25% (≈6 mm) and an off-track Hill-Sachs lesion and an anterior HAGL lesion.

The HAGL lesion was originally described by Nicola in 1942 and subsequently by Bach, Wolf, and Baker et al. Wolf described the HAGL lesion in 9.3% of patients with shoulder

TABLE 4.3

Instability Severity Index Score

PROGNOSTIC FACTORS	POINTS
Age at surgery (yr)	
≤ 20	2
>20	0
Degree of sport participation (preoperative)	
Competitive	2
Recreational or none	0
Type of sport (preoperative)	
Contact or forced overhead	1
Other	0
Shoulder hyperlaxity	
Shoulder hyperlaxity (anterior or inferior)	1
Normal laxity	0
Hill-Sachs on anteroposterior radiograph	
Visible in external rotation	2
Not visible in external rotation	0
Glenoid loss of contour on anteroposterior radiograph	
Loss of contour	2
No lesion	0
Total (points)	10

From Balg F, Boileau P: The instability severity index score, *J Bone Joint Surg* 89B:1470, 2007. Copyright British Editorial Society of Bone and Joint Surgery.

BOX 4.2

Indications for Shoulder Stabilization Modifiers

Bone loss >25% (6 mm) of glenoid—Latarjet procedure
Humeral head >6 mm deep or 18 mm wide—Consider remplissage for collision athletes
Soft-tissue multidirectional instability—Arthroscopic capsular shift
ALPSA—Restore anatomy anteriorly; consider plication
Anterior HAGL—Mini-open or arthroscopic repair
Posterior HAGL—Arthroscopic repair
SLAP lesion—Concomitant repair
Cuff lesion—Concomitant repair

ALPSA, Anterior labroligamentous periosteal sleeve avulsion; *HAGL,* humeral avulsion of glenohumeral ligament; *SLAP,* superior labral tear anterior to posterior.

instability. Both anterior and posterior humeral avulsions with and without a piece of bone and a floating inferior glenohumeral ligament both anteriorly and posteriorly have been reported. Preoperative MRI in the acute setting or MRA in the subacute setting as well as thorough arthroscopic examination are needed to identify and treat all points of damage (Fig. 4.18). Open and arthroscopic repairs of HAGL lesions have been described, and at this time most authors believe that an open procedure is the easiest and most reproducible way to repair anterior lesions.

Pertinent technical points for the success of arthroscopic Bankart repair include the following:
Realistic patient goals and time frames
Careful evaluation and identification of all significant pathologic conditions, including preoperative MRI or a three-dimensional CT scan to evaluate significant bone defects associated with recurrent instability. An arthroscopic examination through an anterosuperior portal is performed to evaluate glenoid bone loss forming the so-called inverted-pear defect.
Release of the capsular ligamentous complex to approximately the 6-o'clock position so that the underlying subscapularis muscle can be clearly seen to allow appropriate superior advancement of the capsule
Abrasion of the glenoid neck to promote bony bleeding for a well-vascularized bed for optimal capsular healing
Superior advancement of the glenohumeral complex to restore physiologic tension and eliminate any potential drive-through sign; an injury to the posterior inferior glenohumeral ligament is often present and should be repaired to restore normal tension; any appreciable Hill-Sachs lesion in a collision athlete is repaired with a remplissage procedure, except for a lesion of the dominant shoulder in a throwing athlete; secure anatomic fixation 1 to 2 mm over the articular surface with a minimum of three suture anchors and secure loop and knot fixation to compress the capsuloligamentous complex to the bone surface and provide adequate fixation during the early healing stage; placement of knots or knotless anchors to avoid impingement.
Repair of significant rotator interval, labral, and cuff defects
Supervised, goal-oriented rehabilitation

ARTHROSCOPIC BANKART REPAIR TECHNIQUE

TECHNIQUE 4.11

- Place the patient on the operating table in the lateral decubitus position with a beanbag and kidney rest. Carefully protect all bony prominences as well as the axillary area. Apply a heating blanket and serial compression devices around the lower extremities. Prepare and drape the patient so that there is wide exposure to the anterior, posterior, and superior aspects of the shoulder. Place the arm in 45 to 60 degrees of abduction and 20 degrees of forward flexion using 12 to 14 lb of traction.
- Outline the bony landmarks and mark the potential portals on the skin.
- Place the posterior portal 2 cm inferior and just medial to the posterolateral edge of the acromion.
- Before making additional portals, thoroughly examine the shoulder through the posterior portal to identify the most appropriate sites for placement of the anterior portals and for any additional posterior portals that may be necessary. Carefully visualize the entire labrum, 360 degrees of the shoulder joint, and the attachment of the glenohumeral ligament to the humerus from anterior to posterior.

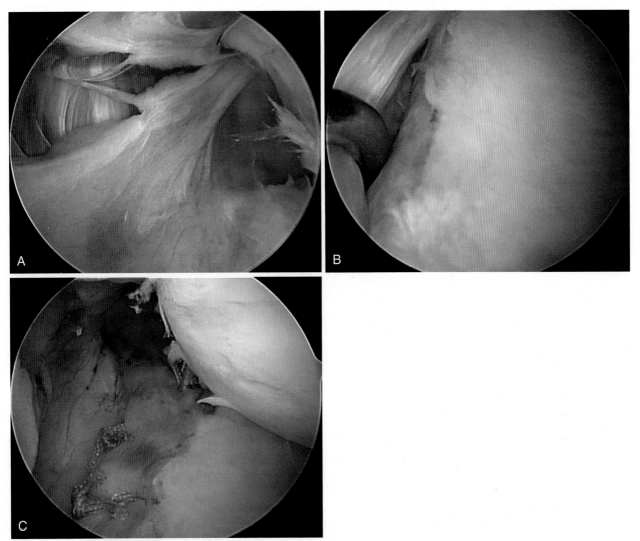

FIGURE 4.18   **A,** Humeral avulsion of glenohumeral ligament with exposure of posterior cuff. **B,** Posterior glenoid avulsion of glenohumeral ligament same patient. **C,** Repaired floating humeral avulsion of glenohumeral ligament.

Thoroughly evaluate the glenohumeral joint for bony loss of the glenoid or humeral head. Defects of the humeral head measured from the cuff to the medial edge of the lesion should be repaired by remplissage if the defect is more than 80% of the glenoid articular surface as measured anterior to posterior using a calibrated probe (see Technique 4.16). Glenoid bone loss greater than 6 mm should be restored with a Latarjet procedure. Proper preoperative planning eliminates surprises.

- After identifying the quadrant or quadrants of injury to the labrum, create the planned portals using spinal needle localization according to the quadrant approach as shown in Figure 4.19.
- Make an anterosuperior portal with the cannula entering the shoulder just posterior to the biceps tendon and anterior to the leading edge of the supraspinatus tendon. It is the best portal to visualize the full extent of the capsular ligamentous damage and bone loss (Fig. 4.20).

- Make an anterior central portal to place an 8.25-mm clear cannula just above the superior edge of the subscapularis tendon at an angle of approximately 45 degrees to the glenoid articular surface. This is used for placement of anchors and for instrumentation using a suture shuttle.
- If the lesion extends posterior, make a 7-o'clock portal posteriorly using spinal needle localization. Enter the joint at an appropriate angle for placement of a suture anchor in the inferior part of the glenoid if necessary or for placement of a shuttle for passing sutures along the capsular ligamentous complex.
- While viewing from the anterosuperior portal, use an elevator to free up the capsule down to the subscapularis muscle, which should be visible. Abrade the glenoid neck to stimulate healing (see Fig. 4.22A).
- While viewing from the anterosuperior portal if necessary, perform a capsular plication procedure posteriorly, extending along to the attachment of the posterior band of

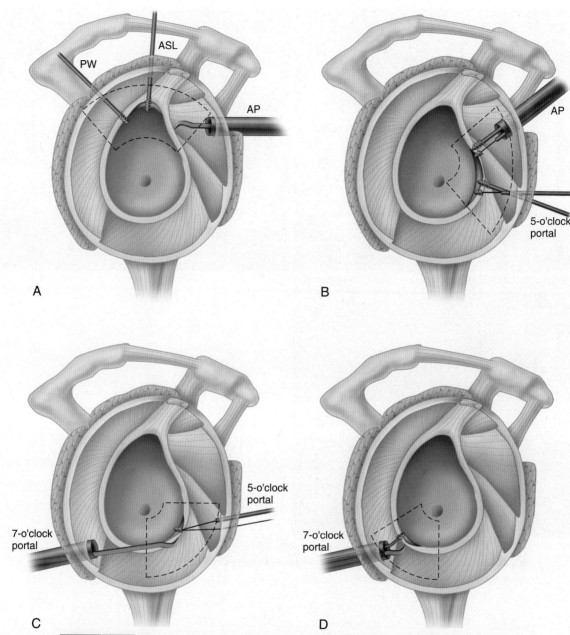

FIGURE 4.19 Four-quadrant approach by Seroyer et al. **A,** In superior quadrant, SLAP tears between 2 and 10 o'clock are accessible through anterior portal (AP), anterosuperior lateral (ASL), and portal of Wilmington (PW). **B,** In anterior quadrant, anteroinferior labral tears are accessible through anterior portal (AP) and 5-o'clock portal. **C,** In anteroinferior quadrant, anteroinferior capsulolabral tears are accessible through 5- and 7-o'clock portals. **D,** In posteroinferior quadrant, posterior labral tears can be accessed through 7-o'clock portal. **SEE TECHNIQUE 4.11.**

the inferior glenohumeral ligament. Using a rasp, freshen the soft tissue and the intended area of plication to incite some inflammation without damaging the tissue.

- Use a suture shuttle to pass PDS sutures, starting at about the 6-o'clock position and taking a bite of approximately 1 cm of capsule in a pinch-tuck technique, making sure that the needle comes out through the capsule and passes up under the labrum in its appropriate position. The

sutures can be tied at the time they are passed, but it may be easier to pass multiple sutures first, store them outside the cannula, and tie them later. Generally, three sutures are passed, with the upper extent being at the attachment of the posterior band of the inferior glenohumeral ligament.

- Now perform the anterior part of the Bankart procedure. Abrade the anterior neck and free up the capsule

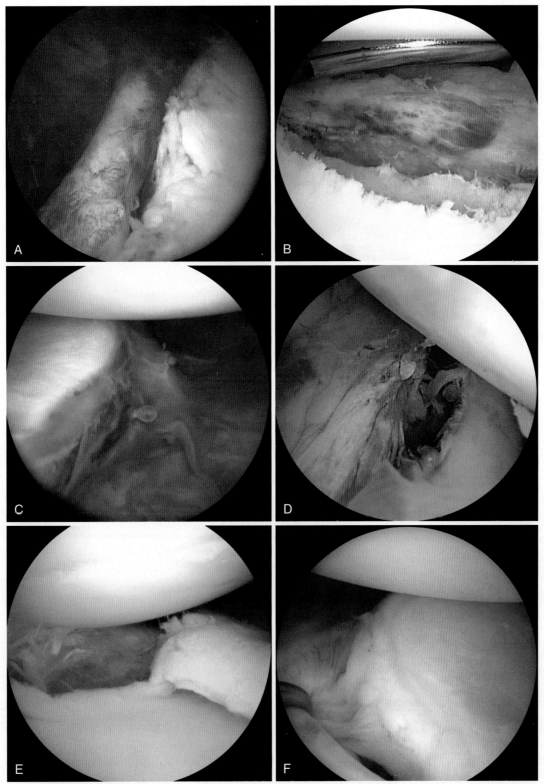

FIGURE 4.20   **A,** Bankart lesion. **B,** Bony Bankart lesion. **C,** Anterior labral periosteal sleeve avulsion. **D,** Glenoid avulsion of glenohumeral ligament. **E,** Glenoid labral articular disruption. **F,** Juvenile glenoid avulsion of the glenohumeral ligament. **SEE TECHNIQUE 4.11.**

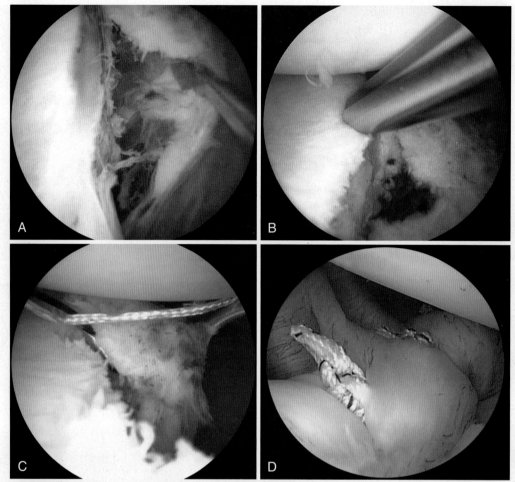

FIGURE 4.21 Bankart repair. **A,** Capsule and labral complex freed. **B,** Anchor inserted on articular edge. **C,** A 1-cm capsular bite taken with Spectrum suture passed distal to anchor. **D,** Knots tied recreating soft-tissue bumper. **SEE TECHNIQUE 4.11.**

and labral complex so it can be advanced superiorly (Fig. 4.21A). Plan the position of the suture anchors, trying to get three or four anchors placed below the 3-o'clock position.

- The most inferior anchor often is best placed using a 5-o'clock percutaneous portal made with the help of a spinal needle for localization. Place the spinal needle at a 45-degree angle to the articular surface. The Spear point guide can be placed at the 5:30 position on the neck, 1 to 2 mm on the articular surface for reaming and placement of the suture anchor. Note the exact position of the drill hole, observe the anchor as it is placed in the hole, use a mallet to tap the anchor down, and then check security by tugging on the sutures. To obtain the best area of bone for drilling at a lower level, an angled reamer and anchor inserter can be placed percutaneously. This provides excellent fixation in this position (Fig. 4.21B).
- The second and third anchors may be either single-loaded or double-loaded anchors and usually are PEEK double-loaded anchors. Recently, we have used knotless anchors to provide secure fixation without the risk of knot

impingement. When knots are used, use the cannula to direct the knot away from the articular surface as it is being seated. With this technique, take the most inferior suture out the posteroinferior cannula using a suture grasper. Obtain a good bite of the capsule and labrum just distal to the intended site of the anchor (Fig. 4.21C). Take the shuttle out of the posterior inferior cannula and secure it around the inferior suture limb of the anchor, and then retrieve it out the anterior cannula. Grasp the two sutures not involved in the first knot with a suture retrieval device from the posterior cannula, take them out the posterior cannula, and store them for later tying. The arthroscopic knot is then tied.

- Firmly secure the first suture that was passed through the labrum to the capsule and labrum up to the edge of the glenoid, creating an anterior bumper. Pass the superior of the two suture limbs that were passed out the posterior cannula back through the anterior cannula. Use the shuttle to pass the shuttle loop through the capsule and labrum. Carry this shuttle out the posterior cannula and shuttle the second suture through the capsule and out the

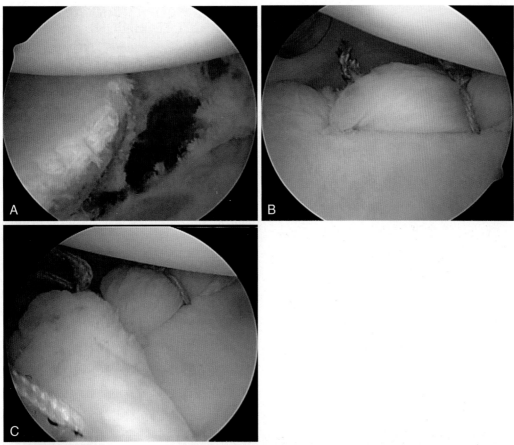

FIGURE 4.22 **A,** Abrasion of glenoid neck and capsular release to allow advancement of capsulolabral complex superiorly and laterally to restore anatomy and physiologic tension. Arthroscope is in anterosuperior portal. **B** and **C,** Restored anterior labral bumper. **SEE TECHNIQUE 4.11.**

anterior cannula. Use the cannula to direct the knot away from the joint surface as it is secured.

- Place a third anchor either single-loaded or double-loaded using the same technique. Sometimes, some of the lower sutures can be used in either a single simple repair or as a mattress suture, depending on the type of tear and tissue involved. This is determined at the time of surgery. Place three or four anchors, each separated by 5 to 7 mm. Tie the knots securely, re-creating a soft-tissue bumper (Figs. 4.21D and 4.22). At this time, if the plication sutures have not been tied, they should be tied posteriorly from the posterior cannula and secured. In our practice, we generally tie these earlier in the procedure when they are placed, but some authors prefer to tie them later.

- If the patient had hyperlaxity and significant sulcus associated with the Bankart lesion, perform a rotator interval closure at this time by withdrawing the anterior central cannula to just outside the capsule. Pass a crescent spectrum needle through the middle glenohumeral ligament several millimeters into the ligament and out into the joint. Maintain one limb outside the capsule while the limb in the joint is retrieved using a penetrator device through the anterior central cannula. Grasp the intraarticular limb

of the suture at the level of the superior glenohumeral ligament and retrieve it out of the cannula for extracapsular tying using an SMC (Samsung Medical Center, Seoul, South Korea)–type knot (see Fig. 4.57). Generally, two sutures are passed in securing the rotator interval if it is thought that the slight loss of external rotation is offset by the added stability of these additional sutures (Figs. 4.23 and 4.24).

- Upon completion, close the portals with subcuticular poliglecaprone 25 (Monocryl). Apply a sterile dressing and an UltraSling (DJO Global, Vista, CA).

POSTOPERATIVE CARE The sling is applied after surgery and worn for 4 to 6 weeks. Physical therapy is started 2 to 3 weeks after surgery. Active-assisted range of motion is performed from weeks 2 to 8, and isometric strengthening is performed from weeks 8 to 12. The athlete is allowed to return to preinjury conditioning programs and weight training at 12 weeks, and at 6 months he or she is allowed to participate in contact sports based on range-of-motion and strength guidelines dictated by the contralateral shoulder (Table 4.4).

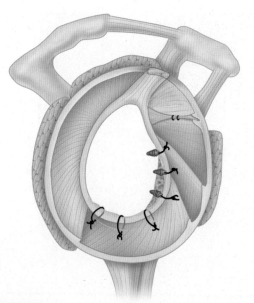

FIGURE 4.23 Completed Bankart repair with three anchors and capsule plicated inferiorly. Rotator interval is closed. **SEE TECHNIQUE 4.11.**

ARTHROSCOPIC BANKART-BRISTOW-LATARJET TECHNIQUE

Boileau, Mercier, and Olds proposed the combined technique as an alternative to capsulolabral repair in patients with anterior instability and significant glenoid bone loss. They reported a high rate of return to sports and a low rate of instability. Tasaki et al. reported 40 rugby players who had anterior dislocations treated with this procedure. All players returned to competitive rugby with no recurrent anterior dislocations at 2-year follow-up.

POSTERIOR INSTABILITY

Arthroscopic posterior shoulder stabilization has rapidly gained favor in recent years, with the results of open procedures having been less than adequate. Arthroscopic repairs have been shown to be effective in athletic and nonathletic patients. In a study by Bradley et al. reviewing 100 shoulder procedures for posterior recurrent shoulder instability, the American Shoulder and Elbow Surgeons score improved from 50.36 to 85.66 at a mean follow-up of 27 months. Overall, 89% of their patients were able to return to sports and 67% were able to return to the same level of sports

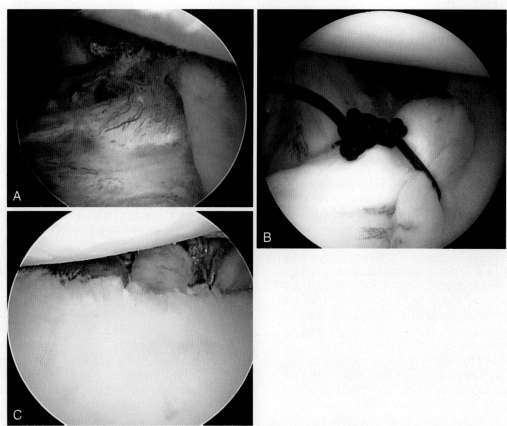

FIGURE 4.24 **A,** Repaired glenoid avulsion of glenohumeral ligament. **B,** Repaired juvenile glenoid avulsion. **C,** Completed bony Bankart repair. **SEE TECHNIQUE 4.11.**

TABLE 4.4	
Bankart Repair Rehabilitation Protocol	

PREOPERATIVE GOALS

1. Independent with postoperative exercise program
2. Independent with preoperative strengthening with isometrics and isotonics in pain-free, stable range

PHASE I

WEEKS 1–2 POSTOPERATIVE	**NO FORMAL PT IF PATIENT HAS ACHIEVED PREOPERATIVE GOALS**
1. Pendulum exercises 2. Elbow, forearm, wrist AROM 3. Wrist isotonics and grip exercises 4. Sling at all times	
WEEKS 3–4 POSTOPERATIVE (PT QIW-TIW)	**GOALS (BY END OF 4 WK)**
1. Initiate PT approximately 15 d postoperatively 2. PROM with the following restrictions 　FL <160 degrees 　Scaption to <150 degrees 　ER neutral to 30 degrees at 3 wk and 40 degrees at 4 wk 　IR in 45 degrees scaption <60 degrees 3. Gentle AAROM with cane 　FL <160 degrees 　ER neutral as above 4. Table slides in FL 5. Scapular mobility exercises 　Protraction/retraction 　Elevation/depression	1. Independent with HEP BID 2. PROM 150 degrees maximal FL 3. PROM 150 degrees maximal scaption 4. PROM 40 degrees maximal ER 5. PROM 60 degrees maximal IR in 45 degrees scaption 6. Full wrist, elbow AROM *Precautions* 1. Sling at all times except PT 2. No true ABD PROM 3. No ER with arm abducted from body
WEEKS 5–6 POSTOPERATIVE (PT QIW-TIW)	**GOALS (BY END OF 6 WK)**
1. PROM with the following restrictions: 　FL <170 degrees 　Scaption <160 degrees 　ER 45 degrees, scaption <60 degrees 　IR 45 degrees, scaption to 60 degrees 　Home ADD to WNL 2. AAROM—cane, pulley, wall walks 3. Submaximal (25%) isometrics at side for IR and ER, and ABD 4. Submaximal manual resistance scapular protraction/retraction and elevation/depression 5. AROM—prone EXT and rows, supine protraction and reverse Codman	1. Independent with HEP BID 2. PROM 170 degrees maximal FL 3. PROM 160 degrees maximal scaption 4. PROM 60 degrees maximal ER at 45 degrees scaption 5. PROM 60 degrees maximal IR at 45 degrees scaption 6. Home ADD to WNL *Precautions* 1. Use of sling during sleep and in crowds 2. No true ABD PROM 3. No ER with arm ABD from body >45 degrees

PHASE II—GRADED AROM AND STRENGTHENING

WEEKS 7–8 POSTOPERATIVE (PT BIW)	**GOALS (BY END OF 8 WK)**
1. PROM with the following restrictions 　FL to WNL 　Scaption to WNL 　ER 70 degrees, scaption to 70 degrees by end of wk 7 　ER 90 degrees, scaption to 70 degrees by end of wk 8 　IR to WNL 2. Continued AAROM activities as needed 3. AROM FL and scaption to 90 degrees 4. Isotonics when able 　FL and scaption with 1–2 lb 　ER and IR with 1–2 lb (side lying) or TheraBand (standing) 　Prone EXT, rows, and horizontal ABD <90 degrees 　Biceps curls; triceps EXT 5. UBE for endurance 6. Proprioceptive training (ball wall dribble, weighted reverse Codman, submaximal manual resistance PNF)	1. Independent with HEP QID 2. Discontinue sling at all times without increased pain 3. PROM FL to WNL 4. PROM scaption to WNL 5. PROM 70 degrees maximal ER at 90 degrees scaption 6. PROM IR to WNL 7. AROM FL and scaption at least 90 degrees with proper scapular mechanics 8. Able to lift 2 lb to eye-level cabinet 9. Able to perform all grooming and dressing activities independently and with normal mechanics 10. Able to retrieve wallet from back pocket 11. Able to open/close car door *Precautions* 1. Avoid terminal ER/ABD 2. Light-weight/high-repetition isotonics

Continued

TABLE 4.4

Bankart Repair Rehabilitation Protocol—cont'd

PREOPERATIVE GOALS

WEEKS 9–10 POSTOPERATIVE (PT BIW)	GOALS (BY END OF 10 WK)
1. PROM ER 90 degrees, scaption to WFL 2. Progress all AROM to WFL 3. Progress isotonic strengthening—Jobe rotator cuff program 4. Initiate isotonics—lateral pull-downs to chest, wall push-ups with elbows tight to side, step-ups, throwing lunges 5. Advance proprioceptive training to include progressive weight-bearing exercises on unstable surface 6. Advance endurance training for upper extremity and entire body	1. PROM WFL all directions 2. AROM WFL all directions 3. MMT 4/5 FL 4. MMT 4/5 scaption 5. MMT 4/5 ER 6. MMT 4+/5 IR 7. MMT 5/5 EXT 8. Able to place gallon milk in refrigerator 9. Able to lift 5 lb to eye-level cabinet 10. Able to lift 2 lb to overhead cabinet *Precaution* Evaluate for posterior capsular tightness; stretch if necessary
WEEKS 11–14 POSTOPERATIVE (PT BIM)	**GOALS (BY END OF 14 WK)**

1. Progress isotonics—increase resistance
2. Progress ER and IR isotonics toward 90 degrees ABD (TheraBand, weights)
3. Plyoball exercises if appropriate
   Chest pass
   Sideway throw
   Overhead throw
4. Isokinetic strengthening as needed
	1. Independent with isotonic HEP
	2. MMT 5/5 FL
	3. MMT scaption 5/5
	4. MMT ER 5/5
	5. MMT IR 5/5
	6. Able to lift 10 lb to eye-level cabinet
	7. Able to lift 5 lb to overhead cabinet
	8. Full return to strenuous work
	Precaution
	No bench press or flies until 6 months postoperatively

The Bankart repair is intended to stabilize the anterior portion of the shoulder capsule that has lost integrity owing to repetitive or traumatic insult. It is paramount to protect healing tissue of the anterior capsule during early stages of rehabilitation. Avoidance of terminal ABD/ER is crucial during this period. This protocol is a guideline and may be adjusted according to the clinical presentation and physician's guidance.

AAROM, Active-assisted range of motion; *ABD,* abduction; *ADD,* adduction; *AROM,* active range of motion; *BID,* twice a day; *BIW,* twice a week; *BIM,* twice a month; *ER,* external rotation; *EXT,* extension; *FL,* flexion; *HEP,* home exercise program; *IR,* internal rotation; *MMT,* manual muscle testing; *PNF,* proprioceptive neuromuscular facilitation; *PT,* physical therapy; *QID,* four times a day; *QIW,* four times a week; *TIW,* three times a week; *UBE,* upper body exercise; *WFL,* within functional limits; *WNL,* within normal limits.

as preoperatively. We likewise believe that arthroscopic repair allows full exposure and correction of intraarticular pathology of the shoulder, and it allows the surgeon to fully define hidden pathologic lesions that often are not evident on MRI. At this time, we use the procedure described by Kim et al. and often incorporate a rotator interval closure in contact athletes or in any patients who have an inferior component to their posterior instability. For traumatic posterior Bankart lesions, anatomic repair is performed with minimal plication to prevent over-constraint of the joint which results in anterior glenoid wear and arthritis from an eccentric humeral head. As with anterior instability, excessive bone loss of more than 25% of the glenoid, a large anterior Hill-Sachs lesion, excessive glenoid retroversion of more than 15%, or a pathologic collagen deficiency syndrome will result in inferior results; these conditions are relative contraindications to arthroscopic soft-tissue techniques.

POSTERIOR SHOULDER STABILIZATION

TECHNIQUE 4.12

(KIM ET AL.)

- Place the patient in the lateral decubitus position and prepare and drape the shoulder.
- Maintain the arm with lateral traction in 30 degrees of abduction and 10 degrees of forward flexion.
- Create a posterior portal 2 cm inferior to the posterolateral acromial angle. This position, which is about 1 cm lateral to a standard posterior glenohumeral portal, is used to improve access to the posteroinferior aspect of the glenoid labrum and capsule. We usually make the anterior-superior portal first to visually confirm the best angle for the posterior working portal.

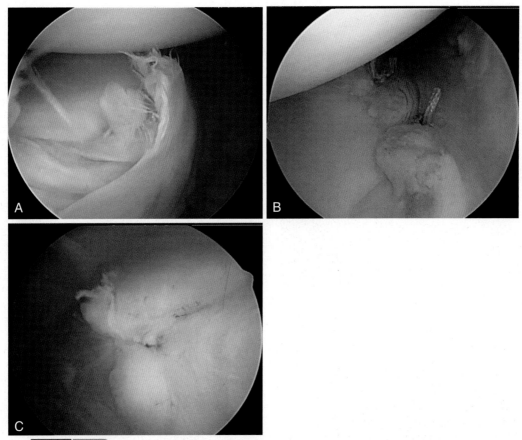

FIGURE 4.25   **A,** Posterior shoulder instability in pitcher resulting in capsulolabral detachment. **B,** Approximation of labrum with suture anchors. **C,** Closure of posterior arthroscopy portal by using shuttle relay to pass suture through one side of capsule and penetrate opposite side. Knot is tied extracapsularly and cut with knot cutter. **SEE TECHNIQUE 4.12.**

- Create two anterior portals, just distal to the acromioclavicular joint and proximal to the leading edge of the subscapularis, with at least 1 cm of distance maintained between them. If, while viewing through the anterosuperior portal, a loose flap of the posteroinferior aspect of the labrum is encountered, debride the labrum.
- Introduce a small meniscal rasp (CONMED, Utica, NY) through the posterior portal to abrade the incomplete tear of the posteroinferior aspect of the labrum and the corresponding glenoid wall. If the posteroinferior aspect of the labrum is detached from the inner surface, and the junction between the labrum and the glenoid articular cartilage is intact, completely detach the labrum with use of a Liberator knife (CONMED).
- Abrade the inferior and posterior aspects of the capsule to enhance healing.
- Place a suture anchor at the posteroinferior glenoid surface, within 2 mm of the margin of the glenoid, through the posterior portal. If a proper angle for suture anchor insertion cannot be achieved through the posterior portal, use an accessory posterior portal at about 1 cm inferior and lateral to the standard posterior portal under the guidance of a spinal needle to maintain a downward angle toward the posteroinferior aspect of the glenoid (Fig. 4.25).

- Retrieve one end of the suture through the anterior midglenoid portal.
- Introduce a 90-degree angle suture hook, loaded with a Shuttle Relay (CONMED), through the posterior portal to pierce the posterior band of the inferior glenohumeral ligament at the same level as the glenoid surface. The posterior band of the inferior glenohumeral ligament is always incorporated into the first suture.
- Shift the suture hook about 1 cm superiorly and pass it under the posteroinferior aspect of the labrum. Retrieve the Shuttle Relay through the anterior midglenoid portal.
- Load the suture into the Shuttle Relay and pull it back out of the posterior portal and tie an SMC knot. Use two or three suture anchors. Knotless anchors can be used and are our preference for posterior repairs (Fig. 4.26).

POSTOPERATIVE CARE The shoulder is immobilized in an abduction sling with an external rotation pillow for 6 weeks. The arm is maintained posterior to the longitudinal axis of the trunk. Pendulum and active-assisted range-of-motion exercises are initiated at 3 weeks. At that time, forward elevation in the scapular plane and external rotation exercises with the arm at the side are regularly executed. Internal rotation behind the back is started at 4 weeks postoperatively, but internal rotation with the arm

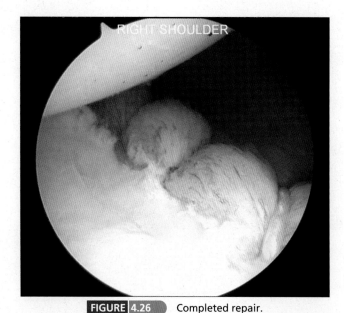

FIGURE 4.26   Completed repair.

elevated (the cross-body adduction position) is prohibited until 6 weeks postoperatively. At 6 weeks, internal rotation with the arm elevated and strengthening exercises are initiated. When the result of manual strength testing is 4+ or more, professional and collegiate-level athletes may perform more vigorous strengthening exercises. Sports activities are allowed after 4 to 6 months.

MULTIDIRECTIONAL INSTABILITY

Capsular laxity producing unidirectional and multidirectional instability can be successfully treated arthroscopically with plication or a shift procedure in one or more quadrants of the shoulder. Results of capsular volume reduction have been shown to be comparable with open techniques, although the capsular reinforcement by the open shifting of one leaf over the other is not replicated. We have had success arthroscopically comparable with open techniques but with much less morbidity. Bradley has shown that the use of anchors greatly increases the reliability and security of the shift. When posterior-inferior instability with a 2 to 3+ sulcus sign is present, a rotator interval closure is performed, and the capsule is shifted along the entire inferior glenohumeral ligament from the 3-o'clock to the 9-o'clock position. Overtightening of the capsule can result in eccentric wear and arthritis.

CAPSULAR SHIFT

TECHNIQUE 4.13

- After examining the anesthetized patient and determining the amount of hyperlaxity present, place the patient in a lateral decubitus position and maintain the position with a beanbag and kidney rest. Carefully pad bony prominences. Apply a heating blanket and serial compression

devices to the lower extremity. Place the arm in 45 degrees of abduction and 20 degrees of flexion with 10 lb of traction. During the procedure, it is helpful to have an assistant to position the shoulder to obtain the most advantageous view and to place gentle pressure anteriorly or posteriorly when slight traction is necessary.
- Outline bony landmarks and potential portal sites on the skin. Make a posterior portal is made about 3 cm distal and in line with the posterolateral acromial edge to evaluate the shoulder. The anterior portals are the anterosuperior lateral portal and the anterior central portal, which usually is about 1 cm lateral to the coracoid. Place working 8.25-mm cannulas later in the procedure in the posterior and anterior central portals. The anterosuperior portal is used for viewing.
- Use a small arthroscopic rasp to abrade the capsule and labrum around the area to be plicated, which generally extends from the length of the glenohumeral ligament attachment, starting posteriorly at the 9-o'clock position and extending anteriorly through the 3-o'clock position. Freshen the soft tissue.
- Starting on the side of the shoulder where the most instability is present, place 2-mm PEEK anchors at the articular edge spaced 3 cm or more apart. Use a shuttle to take 1-cm plication bites, using a combination of simple and mattress sutures to plicate the capsule. Advance the capsule superiorly and use the cannula to direct the knots away from the joint surface. Use a Spectrum suture passer (CONMED) to pass additional No. 0 PDS sutures to plicate as necessary.
- Carry the capsular plication around inferiorly, taking care not to get too deep or too far from the labrum so as to catch the axillary nerve. Extend the plication up to about the 9-o'clock position.
- Close the rotator interval. For significant multidirectional or posterior instability, this is done using a Spectrum suture after having withdrawn the anterior cannula to just anterior to the capsule. Pass a PDS through the superior portion of the middle glenohumeral ligament and then retrieve it with a penetrator-type grasper just superior to the superior glenohumeral ligament. Close the interval with two sutures anteriorly. On completion, close the posterior capsule similarly by passing a suture on each side of the rent and closing it with the cannula just outside the capsule. These techniques can be done most easily by viewing the anterior interval closure from the posterior portal and then moving the scope to the anterosuperior portal to view the posterior capsular closure.
- Close the arthroscopic portals with subcuticular Monocryl sutures and place sterile dressings.

POSTOPERATIVE CARE An UltraSling (DJO Global) is applied with the arm in neutral rotation. The arm is kept in the sling postoperatively for 6 weeks.

HUMERAL AND/OR GLENOID AVULSION OF THE INFERIOR GLENOHUMERAL LIGAMENT

Humeral avulsion of the inferior glenohumeral ligament can be most easily repaired with a mini-open technique for anterior lesions. Posterior lesions can be repaired using dual posterior portals. The glenoid avulsion of the anterior inferior glenohumeral ligament must be visualized and repaired back to the labrum, which usually is stable (see Fig. 4.18). The glenoid avulsion of the glenohumeral ligament is repaired back to a stable labrum using a Spectrum to pass a No. 1 PDS through the capsule. Repair the capsule to the labrum similar to the plication procedure. Repair of the posterior glenohumeral ligament is as described in Technique 4.14.

ARTHROSCOPIC REPAIR OF POSTERIOR HUMERAL AVULSION OF THE GLENOHUMERAL LIGAMENT

TECHNIQUE 4.14

- Place the patient in the lateral decubitus position, maintained with a beanbag and kidney rest. Place the arm in 60 degrees of abduction and 20 degrees of forward flexion maintained with 10 to 12 lb of traction.
- Three portals are used for posterior repair. A posterior portal, an anterosuperior portal, and a posterior 7-o'clock portal are normally necessary.
- Fully evaluate the shoulder for all pathologic entities. If it is determined that it is an isolated posterior avulsion of the glenohumeral ligament and capsular attachment and that the attachment to the glenoid is stable, then a humeral repair is undertaken. With the arthroscope in the anterosuperior portal, create two posterior portals and place a 6-mm plastic cannula in each portal. The posteroinferior portal is used for placement of an inferior suture anchor. Abrade the neck area. Place the anchor and retrieve the sutures through the posterosuperior portal. With a grasping instrument maintained in the superior portal to put tension on the capsule, visualize the approximate location of the anatomic attachment. Maintain tension on the capsule and place a penetrating retrieval device through the posteroinferior portal and through the capsule about 7 mm from its edge. Grasp the inferiormost suture and carry it into the inferior cannula. Use of a hand-off technique with an instrument from the superior portal can make this technique easier.
- Use the same technique to grab the more superior of the sutures, once again separating it from the previously retrieved suture by about 7 mm. Place the penetrator through the capsule about 7 mm from its torn edge and retrieve the second suture and take it back out the inferior capsule. Once again, the superior portal is used to keep tension on the capsule and a hand-off technique is used to aid in retrieving the suture and pulling it back through the capsule. Tie the mattress sutures down snugly, securing the inferior portion of the tear to the neck. Use the inferior cannula to tie the arthroscopic SMC knots.
- Place a second anchor in the more superior part of the anatomic attachment of the capsule in the posterior part of the neck. Place the penetrating device through the capsule and grab the inferior suture and pass it back out through the cannula. Grab the superior suture and again

pass it back out through the cannula. Tie the arthroscopic mattress suture through the superior portal to obtain excellent compression of the capsule to the neck to ensure adequate healing. If a side-to-side repair of the vertical component of the tear is achievable, a Spectrum with a crescent hook can be used to pass through the superior leaf of the tear. The suture can be retrieved with a penetrating device passed through the inferior leaf of the tear and then tied extracapsularly.
- On completion, check the stability and close the portals with Monocryl sutures.

POSTOPERATIVE CARE The patient is placed in an UltraSling with the arm in slight external rotation for 5 to 6 weeks.

HILL-SACHS LESION

REMPLISSAGE

The Hill-Sachs remplissage technique is similar to an arthroscopic repair of a partial-thickness, articular-surface rotator cuff tear. It consists of fixation of the infraspinatus tendon and posterior capsule to the abraded surface of the Hill-Sachs lesion (Fig. 4.27A). The addition of a remplissage procedure significantly reduces recurrence rates in contact athletes with Hill-Sachs lesions.

TECHNIQUE 4.15

(PURCHASE ET AL. [WOLF] TECHNIQUE)
- Place the patient in the lateral decubitus position and leaned back approximately 30 degrees. Place with the shoulder in 30 degrees of abduction and 15 degrees of forward flexion. Suspend the arm with 14 lb of distal traction.
- Enter the glenohumeral joint through a posterior portal that is placed at the lateral aspect of the convexity of the humeral head so that it is centered directly over the Hill-Sachs lesion (Fig. 4.27B). This remplissage posterior portal will allow initial visualization and evaluation of the joint as well as working access to the Hill-Sachs lesion. Create an anteroinferior portal in the rotator interval, which will be the primary working portal for the anterior labral repair. Establish an anterosuperior portal at the anterior margin of the acromion. This portal should enter immediately behind the biceps tendon. Switch the arthroscope from the posterior portal to the anterosuperior portal and place the cannula into the posterior portal.
- While viewing from the anterosuperior portal, assess the Hill-Sachs lesion, glenoid bone loss, and anterior labral lesion, as well as the location of the posterior portal. The posterior portal placement is correct if it is located directly over the Hill-Sachs lesion and at an angle that will allow the placement of two anchors. If the posterior portal is not in the correct position, optimize its location with the assistance of a spinal needle at this time.

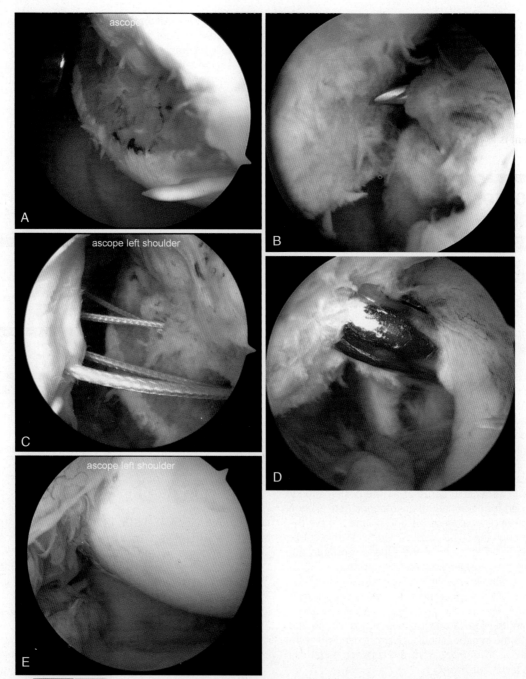

FIGURE 4.27   **A,** Hill-Sachs lesion. **B,** Remplissage needle localization. **C,** First anchor placed. **D,** Second anchor placed. **E,** Completed remplissage. **SEE TECHNIQUE 4.15.**

- Gently freshen the surface of the engaging Hill-Sachs lesion with a burr in reverse mode, taking care to remove a minimal amount of surface bone. Also freshen the surface of the entire posterior and inferior capsule with a whisker blade. In anticipation of a Bankart repair, the anterior labrum and glenoid neck must be prepared before one proceeds with the remplissage.
- While maintaining the camera in the anterosuperior portal, carefully withdraw the cannula in the posterior portal from the posterior capsule and infraspinatus tendon but not through the deltoid. The mouth of the cannula will be

in the subdeltoid space. Through the preexisting portal, pass the anchor cannula with the obturator through the infraspinatus tendon and posterior capsule. Place the first anchor in the inferior aspect of the Hill-Sachs lesion (Fig. 4.27C). Pass a penetrating grasper through the tendon and posterior capsule to grasp and pull one suture limb 1 cm inferior to the initial portal entry site. Place a second anchor in the superior aspect of the Hill-Sachs lesion. Use a grasper penetrator in the same fashion to pass one suture limb 1 cm superior to the initial portal entry site (Fig. 4.27D). Tie the inferior suture first with the knots remaining extraarticular in the subdeltoid space. Tie the superior suture to complete the remplissage. The knots can be visualized by opening the posterior wall of the subacromial bursa. These mattress sutures draw the infraspinatus and posterior capsule to the abraded bony surfaces, thus filling the Hill-Sachs lesion. A Bankart repair can now be completed (Fig. 4.27E).

- We generally use the remplissage sutures as the last step in the completion of a Bankart repair.
- Knotless techniques have been described and have the added benefit of avoiding arthroscopic knots in the subacromial space.

POSTOPERATIVE CARE Postoperative care and immobilization are individualized and based on the patient's history and pathologic findings. In general, an immobilizer is used for 6 weeks. Patients are allowed to remove the immobilizer for controlled activities of daily living such as eating, showering, and computer use within 1 to 2 days. They can remove it for these activities as long as the arm is not abducted and does not externally rotate beyond neutral. Active and resistive range of motion is started at 6 weeks. No at-risk work activities or contact sports are allowed for 6 months.

BONY BANKART LESIONS AND GLENOID FRACTURES

TRANSOSSEOUS BONY BANKART REPAIR

Simple fractures involving 25% of the glenoid surface can be reduced and secured using a percutaneous 5-o'clock portal and the Arthrex nesting guide system (Fig. 4.28A to C). Placement and fixation are confirmed with radiography. Most bony lesions are not of the size or bone quality for screw fixation and are best repaired with suture anchor fixation (Fig. 4.29A and B).

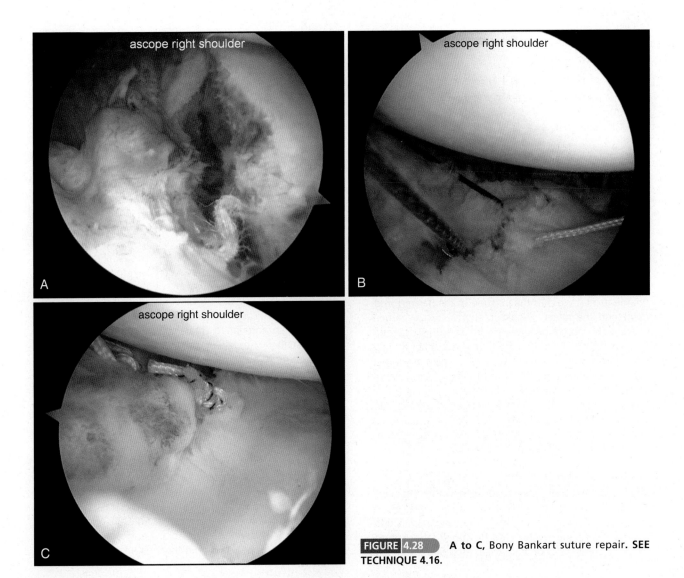

FIGURE 4.28 A to C, Bony Bankart suture repair. **SEE TECHNIQUE 4.16.**

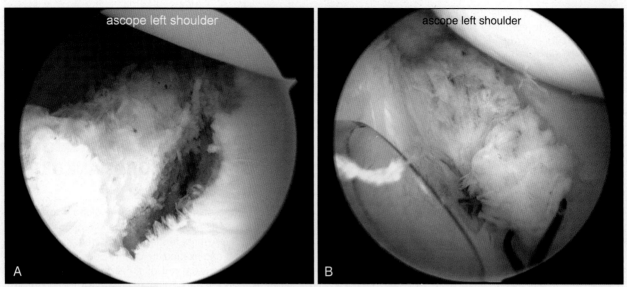

FIGURE 4.29 **A,** Larger bony fragment before screw fixation. **B,** After screw fixation. **SEE TECHNIQUE 4.16.**

TECHNIQUE 4.16

(DRISCOLL, BURNS, AND SNYDER)

- Place the patient in the lateral decubitus position with 10 lb of traction.
- Establish anterosuperior, anteroinferior, and posterior portals.
- Looking through the anterosuperior portal and working through the anterior midglenoid portal, remove clots and scar tissue interposed between the fracture fragment and intact glenoid using an arthroscopic grasper and shaver.
- Use a Liberator knife (CONMED) to free the bony fragments from the intact glenoid until subscapularis fibers can be seen and the bony fragment can be easily manipulated to an anatomic position with minimal tension.
- Pass a curved Spectrum suture passer (CONMED) loaded with No. 1 PDS through the capsulolabral tissues at the "hinge point," which is the junction of the Bankart fragment and the intact glenoid inferiorly. Circumferential fibers of the labrum generally are intact at this location.
- Retrieve both limbs of the PDS from the anterior midglenoid portal and place them outside the cannula, where they can serve as traction sutures to aid in manipulation of the fracture fragment (Fig. 4.30A).
- Use an electrofrequency device to clear soft tissue from the anterior surface fragment, medial to the capsule and labrum, to improve visualization of transosseous tunnels and suture passage later in the procedure.

BONY BANKART REPAIR

- The repair construct typically consists of three anchors: one at the inferior hinge point, one in the center of the intact side of the fracture defect, and one at the superior border of the fracture. As described later, sutures from the central anchor are passed through transosseous tunnels for bony fixation, and those from the anchors at the superior and inferior margins of the fracture site are used for soft-tissue repair and augmentation of the transosseous repair construct.
- Before the anchors are placed, drill two tunnels from posterior to anterior through the fracture fragment. Introduce the previously placed traction suture and a grasper through the anterior midglenoid portal, and use them to manipulate the fracture fragment laterally, exposing the subchondral bone of the fragment for tunnel drilling.
- Introduce a 14-gauge, 8-inch arthroscopy needle through the posterior portal (Fig. 4.30B) and into the subchondral bone of the fracture fragment slightly inferior to its center. If a 14-gauge needle is not available, a 2-mm drill bit used for meniscal root repair can be used to drill the holes, and a suture shuttle can be passed down the hole in the drill bit.
- Pass a 0.062-inch (1.6-mm) Kirschner wire through the needle and drill across the fracture fragment from posterior to anterior to create the first tunnel. Remove the Kirschner wire, taking care to leave the needle in position within the bony fragment.
- Pass a No. 1 PDS through the needle and across the fracture fragment from posterior to anterior and retrieve both limbs of the suture from the anterior cannula.
- Repeat these steps, creating a second tunnel and passing a second No. 1 PDS approximately 4 to 5 mm superior to the first tunnel (Fig. 4.30B). Store these sutures outside the anterior midglenoid cannula for later shuttling.
- Place the first suture anchor inferiorly at the edge of the intact articular cartilage adjacent to the hinge point. Use the posterior limb of the previously placed traction suture to shuttle one high-strength suture from the anchor around the anteroinferior capsulolabral tissue, and secure it with a sliding-locking knot and three alternating half-stitches.

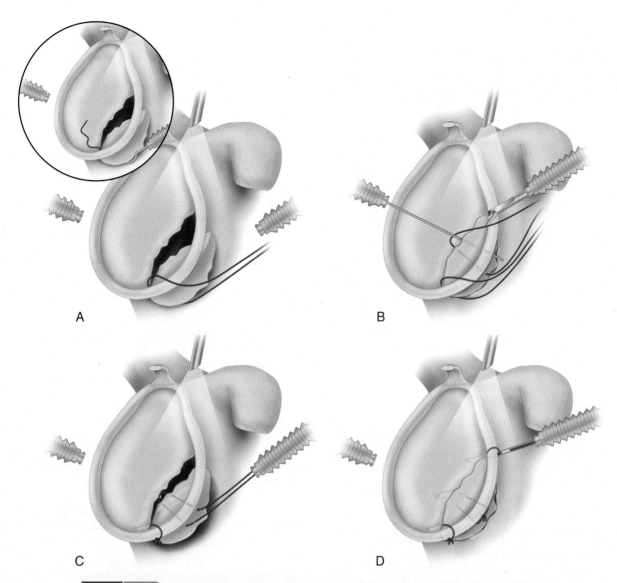

A

B

C

D

FIGURE **4.30**   Driscoll et al. arthroscopic transosseous bony Bankart repair. **A,** Both limbs of suture retrieved from midglenoid portal and placed outside cannula to serve as traction sutures. **B,** Sutures placed 4 to 5 mm superior to first tunnel and stored outside anterior midglenoid cannula to be used for shuttling. **C,** After inferior labrum is secured, a second anchor is placed, the suture ends of which are shuttled through tunnels and out anteriorly, where they are tied over the bony fragment as a mattress stitch. **D,** Final repair consists of three suture anchors, with inferior and superior sutures passing around labrum and capsule and middle suture passing through osseous fragment being tied over bone anteriorly. (From Driscoll MD, Burns JP, Snyder SJ: Arthroscopic transosseous bony Bankart repair, *Arthroscopy Tech* 4(1):e47, 2015.) **SEE TECHNIQUE 4.16.**

This results in good approximation of the fracture fragment and aids in subsequent final reduction.
- Place the second anchor in the center of the intact side of the fracture bed, between the two transosseous tunnels, at the osteochondral junction, not on the face of the glenoid. Retrieve the anterior and posterior limbs of the PDS in the inferior tunnel into the anterior midglenoid and posterior cannulas, respectively, and use them to shuttle one suture limb from the anchor through the posterior portal through the inferior tunnel from posterior to anterior.

- Shuttle the other limb of the suture through the more superior tunnel in a similar fashion, resulting in a mattress stitch capturing the bony fragment (Fig. 4.30C). Secure this stitch with a sliding-locking knot and three alternating half-hitches, taking care to adequately reduce the bony fragment before locking the initial knot.
- Place the third anchor at the superior margin of the fracture site and perform soft-tissue repair with one to two additional simple stitches using a curved suture passer and standard shuttling (Fig. 4.30D).

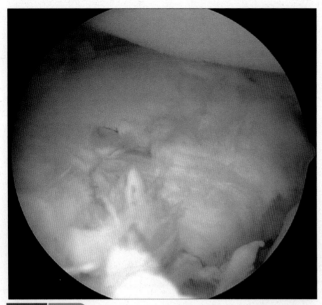

FIGURE 4.31 Arthroscopic view of completed Latarjet procedure.

■ LATARJET PROCEDURE

Lafosse and Boyle described arthroscopic Latarjet procedures, with which they have had good results and minimal complications (Fig. 4.31). These are procedures that should be performed only by advanced arthroscopists and after extensive training in a laboratory setting to see if one can safely reproduce results comparable to the excellent open Latarjet procedure results.

SUBACROMIAL IMPINGEMENT SYNDROME

Subacromial impingement syndrome is a common cause of anterolateral shoulder pain and pain with primarily overhead activities. The pain attributed to subacromial impingement can vary and includes subacromial bursitis, rotator cuff tendinopathy, and partial- and full-thickness rotator cuff tears. Extrinsic compression from the anterior acromion, coracoacromial ligament, and acromioclavicular joint have been implicated in rotator cuff pathology. There continues to be debate as to the relative importance extrinsic compression has in rotator cuff degeneration compared to intrinsic tendon degeneration from aging and hypovascularity. Both likely play a role and further studies are needed to clarify their respective contributions to subacromial impingement syndrome.

Imaging for subacromial impingement syndrome starts with standard radiographs. A true anteroposterior (Grashey) view is useful in measuring the critical shoulder angle and evaluating for acromioclavicular osteoarthritis with inferior osteophyte formation. The axillary lateral demonstrates the presence of an os acromiale. The scapular outlet view depicts acromial morphology. Bigliani et al. classified the acromial architecture into three types: type I is basically flat, type II is curved similar to the curvature of the humeral head, and type III has a hook on the anterior portion of the acromion potentially resulting in impingement. It is important to make the distinction between acquired acromial bone spurs attributed to CA ligament ossification and native acromial

morphology. Nicholson et al. found that the incidence of acromial bone spurs increases with age, whereas the acromial morphology does not change. Moor et al. were the first to describe the term "critical shoulder angle" (CSA). The CSA is measured as the angle between a line from the superior and inferior bony margins of the glenoid and an intersecting line from the inferior bony margin of the glenoid to the most inferolateral acromion on a true anteroposterior view of the shoulder. This measurement takes into account two independent components: glenoid inclination and lateral acromion extension. CSAs of more than 35 degrees have been shown to increase shear joint reaction forces, causing increased strain on the rotator cuff tendons, and correlate with presence of a degenerative rotator cuff tear. MRI allows further evaluation of subacromial impingement syndrome, especially allowing the surgeon to characterize potential sources of mechanical impingement and the status of the rotator cuff including severity of tendinosis as well as location and size of partial-thickness or full-thickness rotator cuff tears.

Surgical management of subacromial impingement syndrome includes subacromial bursectomy, release of the CA ligament, possible bony resection including acromioplasty or removal of distal clavicle osteophytes, and debridement or repair of any associated rotator cuff tears. The efficacy of arthroscopic acromioplasty is debated in the literature, and the decision is made based on preoperative imaging and correlated with these images at the time of surgery. Recently, Gerber et al. described a lateral acromioplasty in an attempt to correct for a high CSA to prevent retears after rotator cuff repairs. We have no experience with this technique, and further research is needed to determine efficacy.

Subacromial decompression with or without acromioplasty is indicated in patients with continued pain attributed to subacromial pathology despite an extensive trial of nonoperative treatment.

ARTHROSCOPIC SUBACROMIAL DECOMPRESSION AND ACROMIOPLASTY

TECHNIQUE 4.17

- After general anesthesia is administered, evaluate the shoulder for range of motion; gently regain any lost motion.
- Place the patient in the standard beach-chair position or lateral decubitus position using a beanbag and kidney rest under the torso, which is angled approximately 20 degrees posteriorly. The arm is maintained in 20 to 40 degrees of abduction in a balanced skeletal suspension device.
- Carefully outline the bony landmarks, including the acromion, distal clavicle, acromioclavicular joint, and coracoid process.
- Inspect the glenohumeral joint first for evidence of any labral or articular cartilage damage, biceps pathology, and undersurface rotator cuff tearing.

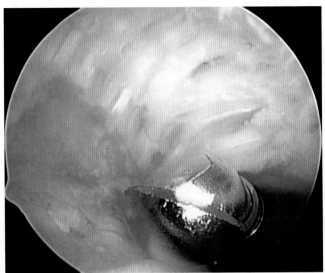

FIGURE 4.32 Thickness of cuff tear can be judged by distance of attached cuff fibers from articular surface. In this case, tear is about 8 mm when using 5.5-mm shaver as reference scale. **SEE TECHNIQUE 4.17.**

- If a rotator cuff partial tear is identified, debride the area of the tear with the full-radius resector to leave a smooth surface and to incite some petechial bleeding in the area. Gauge the depth of the tear, comparing it with the size of the shaver (Fig. 4.32). Normally, the supraspinatus insertion extends from the biceps to the bare area posteriorly and from the articular surface medially to approximately 17 mm laterally onto the tuberosity. If a high-grade articular surface tear is encountered, a No. 0 PDS suture is introduced through the tear with an 18-gauge spinal needle placed percutaneously just lateral to the acromion in line with the tear. The suture is retrieved from the anterior cannula, and a hemostat is placed on both limbs of the suture until the tear can be inspected from the bursal surface.
- Using a large 6-mm or 6.2-mm cannula, enter the subacromial space from the posterior portal.
- Advance a blunt trocar to touch the posterior aspect of the spine and advance it anteriorly to just beneath the anterolateral aspect of the acromion.
- Break up adhesions in the subacromial space with a sweep of the cannula medially and laterally.
- Palpate the undersurface of the acromion and coracoacromial ligament to ensure correct trocar placement and to palpate the area of impingement.
- Bring the arthroscope with the inflow connected through the posterior portal. Orient the camera in an upright position and direct the arthroscopic lens to view laterally where a spinal needle is being brought in through the area of the potential midlateral portal about 3 cm distal to the acromion in line with the posterior aspect of the acromioclavicular joint. Move the spinal needle in and evaluate its orientation to ensure that movement in the subacromial space would not be blocked by passing too close to the acromion.

- After establishing the midlateral portal, perform a complete subacromial bursectomy with the full-radius resector and electrocautery to view the superior surface of the cuff out to its attachment to the greater tuberosity and to view the undersurface of the acromioclavicular joint. It is best to start laterally and progress medially where bleeding can be anticipated.
- Place a spinal needle in through the acromioclavicular joint and place another spinal needle just at the anterolateral aspect of the acromion to identify these landmarks clearly.
- Use a thermal probe to morcellate the periosteum and the undersurface of the acromion, releasing the coracoacromial ligament. Maintain hemostasis at all times by using electrocautery and 1 mL of epinephrine per 3-L bag of fluid and by maintaining a systolic blood pressure to a pump pressure differential of 30 to 40 mm Hg.
- After morcellating the soft tissues of the undersurface of the acromion, place a 5.5-mm full-radius resector through the lateral portal to remove the soft tissues from the undersurface of the acromion after carefully identifying the anterior, medial, and lateral edges of the acromion for a distance of approximately 1.5 cm posterior (approximately the position of the shaver when it is in a direct perpendicular position to the acromion).
- Place a 5.5-mm acromionizer burr through the lateral portal and resect the lateral edge of the acromion just medial to the portal, starting at a depth of about 5 mm anterior and tapering posteriorly.
- After resecting the lateral aspect of the acromion, begin the anterior cut from anteromedial to the acromioclavicular joint, working anterolaterally. Deepen the cut through the anterior edge of the acromion to about 5 mm to try to resect the anterior aspect of the acromion back with the clavicle (Fig. 4.33A). Leave the periosteal sleeve attached and use it as a means to gauge the amount of resection of the anterior acromion and to protect the deltoid. Using strokes from anterior to posterior, taper the acromioplasty posteriorly, resecting about 5 mm of acromion anteriorly and tapering and smoothing the section posteriorly, removing only minimal bone. Working medially, the acromioclavicular joint can be located by the previously placed spinal needle and the fatty tissue over the acromioclavicular joint. Because of the vascularity and potential for bleeding, this area is resected at the end of the procedure.
- After completing the acromioplasty, use an acromionizer, a full-radius resector, or a small arthroscopic rasp to smooth the undersurface only if preoperative symptoms and radiographs indicate a significant pathologic process of the acromioclavicular joint.
- Evaluate the acromioclavicular joint area.
- Use a thermal device again to strip the soft tissue from the undersurface of the clavicle, which is identified by the spinal needle and by superior palpation of the clavicle. After resecting the soft tissue, compare the amount of acromial undersurface that has been resected with the undersurface of the clavicle as a reference for the amount of acromion resected.
- If preoperative radiographs show a bony spur of the acromioclavicular joint, use a burr to resect the undersurface of the clavicle for approximately 8 mm medial to the

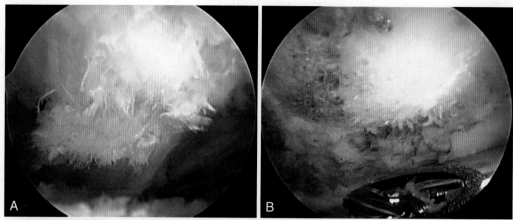

FIGURE 4.33　**A,** Subacromial impingement. **B,** Completed acromioplasty with resection of anterior hook. **SEE TECHNIQUE 4.17.**

joint, making this flush with the acromion. Do not resect the clavicle excessively, unless a Mumford-type procedure (see Technique 4.25) is considered.

■ View the completed procedure by placing the arthroscope in the anterolateral portal and viewing the cut anteriorly to evaluate the depth of the cut of the acromion and to ensure the undersurface of the acromioclavicular joint is smooth (Fig. 4.33B).

CHOCK-BLOCK METHOD FOR ACROMIOPLASTY

TECHNIQUE 4.18

■ Sampson et al. used a burr in the posterior portal to make a smooth undersurface acromioplasty. Place the arthroscope in the lateral portal and the burr in the posterior portal that was made 2 to 3 cm distal to the undersurface of the acromion. Pass the burr into the subacromial space parallel to the undersurface of the acromion. Pass the burr up under the anterior edge of the acromion into the space between the sheath and the concavity of the acromion to determine the amount of bone to be removed. Bring the burr back to the posterior edge of the apex over the curvature and, sweeping medial to lateral, resect the bone from the posterior part of the curve to the anterior aspect, keeping the burr flat to the acromion. By using a 4-mm burr, one can gauge the amount of acromion to be resected.

■ We have had excellent success by starting the procedure with the acromionizer in the lateral portal to resect the anterior and lateral edges of the acromion. The acromionizer is placed in the posterior portal to complete the procedure as above.

POSTOPERATIVE CARE　The arm is placed in a sling, and Codman pendulum exercises are begun on the first day.

The sling is discarded as soon as comfort permits, unless a cuff repair has been performed. Active-assisted range-of-motion exercises and isometric strengthening exercises for the deltoid and rotator cuff are begun within the first week. Light resistance exercises using elastic tubing are started the second week. Most patients have a full range of motion by 3 weeks, and supervised progressive exercises against resistance are instituted and continued for 3 months. Activities of daily living are resumed as soon as symptoms allow, and return to sports is delayed until full strength and endurance and pain-free motion are obtained.

PARTIAL-THICKNESS ROTATOR CUFF TEARS

Partial-thickness rotator cuff tears are common in the general population, with an increased incidence with increasing age. Sher et al. showed an overall prevalence of asymptomatic partial-thickness rotator cuff tears of 20%, which increased to 26% in patients older than 60 years. Partial-thickness rotator cuff tears can be classified as articular-sided, bursal-sided, or intratendinous tears (see Fig. 4.32). Ellman described a classification of partial-thickness rotator cuff tears based on location and depth of tearing noted at the time of shoulder arthroscopy. Currently, tears are classified as articular-sided (A), bursal-sided (B), or intratendinous (C) and are grade 1 if involving 3 mm or less, grade 2 if 3 to 6 mm, and grade 3 if more than 6 mm of tendon is torn (Fig 4.34). This is based on previous studies noting the width of the supraspinatus footprint, where grade 3 tears represent tears of more than 50% of tendon width. Generally, with MRI evaluation these tears are classified as low grade or high grade depending on whether they involve less than or more than 50% of the tendon width.

Partial-thickness tears have a limited ability to spontaneously heal as shown by histological and radiographic studies. A substantial portion of partial-thickness rotator cuff

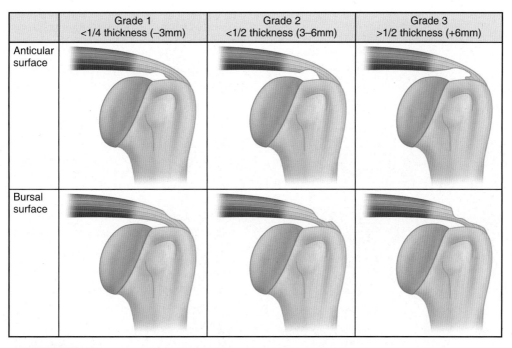

	Grade 1 <1/4 thickness (–3mm)	Grade 2 <1/2 thickness (3–6mm)	Grade 3 >1/2 thickness (+6mm)
Anticular surface			
Bursal surface			

FIGURE 4.34 Ellman classification of partial-thickness rotator cuff tears based on depth of defect.

tears will progress in tear size, as many as 53% in one study, and a portion of these will progress to full-thickness rotator cuff tears. Even with the risk of tear progression, most partial-thickness rotator cuff tears are best initially managed with nonoperative treatment. Surgical treatment with either rotator cuff repair or debridement is indicated for patients in whom nonoperative treatment fails. Most surgeons agree that tears involving more than 50% of tendon width are best treated with repair and those involving less than 50% with debridement and potential decompression. This treatment strategy has been validated by systematic reviews that have shown that most patients can achieve good to excellent functional results. A higher failure rate of debridement has been suggested for partial-thickness bursal-sided rotator cuff tears compared to articular-sided rotator cuff tears, leading some surgeons to favor repair of even low-grade bursal-sided tears.

The decision for in situ rotator cuff repair or completion to a full-thickness rotator cuff tear with subsequent repair is based on surgeon preference. The current literature supports both techniques, with no difference in functional outcome scores or re-tear rates between the two. Generally, in our practice this depends on the proportion and quality of the intact tendon. For tears with poor-quality tendon remaining and involving more than 80% of tendon thickness, we favor debridement.

Delamination-type tears of the articular side, which commonly occur in athletes involved in throwing and in sports requiring overhead motion, should be recognized. If delamination of the tear is present, a transtendinous repair is indicated. Finally, intratendinous tears that can be identified on MRI must be localized through preoperative planning and use of a spinal needle to identify the tear site. The tear can be opened using an arthroscopic knife and the edge debrided back slightly to promote local healing. Goodmurphy et al. showed that extensive debridement is unnecessary. These tears are repaired side-to-side using arthroscopic technique.

DEBRIDEMENT OF PARTIAL-THICKNESS ROTATOR CUFF TEARS

TECHNIQUE 4.19

- Place the patient in the standard beach-chair position or lateral decubitus position with a suspension device holding the arm in 45 degrees abduction and 0 degrees forward flexion.
- Arthroscopic working portals are as shown in Figure 4.35. We occasionally use an anterosuperior portal depending on the side and location of the tear. For simple debridement, usually three portals are sufficient. Identify the partial cuff tear, and if it is less than 50% thickness, debride to remove the damaged tissue and incite petechial bleeding of the area debrided. This can be done with a full-radius resector. Excessive tissue should not be removed.
- Carefully probe the tear to ensure that a delaminating type of tear is not present, which would require a transtendinous repair.
- Perform acromioplasty as necessary.

POSTOPERATIVE CARE Postoperative care is the same as for acromioplasty, with early range of motion and strengthening as tolerated.

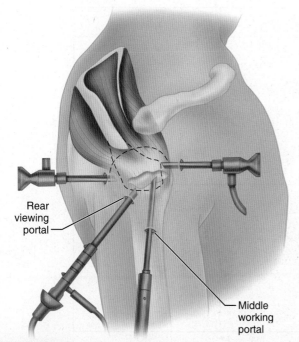

FIGURE 4.35 Relative location of portals. Middle working portal is located at center of rotator cuff tear and 3 cm lateral from lateral margin of acromion. Rear viewing portal is placed at posterior lip of tear and 1 cm lateral from lateral margin of acromion. Portal should be placed at least 2 cm from middle working portal to prevent overcrowding. **SEE TECHNIQUE 4.19.**

- Approximate delamination tears under physiologic tension using an arthroscopic suture grasper.
- Insert a spinal needle from lateral just off the edge of the acromion, through the normal tendon, and through the tear site. Pass a No. 1 PDS through the spinal needle and retrieve it out the anterior portal. Pass a second No. 1 PDS through a spinal needle in the opposite side of the tear site so that the two sutures are separated about 1 cm. Retrieve both sutures out the anterior portal and use them as suture shuttles.
- Tie a No. 2 nonabsorbable suture to each tail of the PDS pulled out of the anterior cannula. Using the percutaneous tails, pull the suture into the joint while carefully making sure that it does not tangle. Clip the suture ends with a hemostat.
- Repeat this procedure until secure side-to-side approximation can be obtained.
- Pass the arthroscope back into the subacromial space and identify the suture ends. Place a 7-mm clear plastic cannula through the midlateral portal, retrieve the sutures individually, and tie them in the subacromial space to approximate the undersurface, delamination, or transverse tear.
- On completion, pass the arthroscope intraarticularly to reevaluate the repair.

POSTOPERATIVE CARE The patient's arm is placed in a sling for 3 weeks, following which an accelerated program of small cuff tear rehabilitation is used (Tables 4.5 to 4.7).

REPAIR OF DELAMINATION AND LOCALIZED, ARTICULAR-SIDE PARTIAL-THICKNESS CUFF TEARS

TECHNIQUE 4.20

- Place the patient in the standard beach-chair position or lateral decubitus position for arthroscopic examination. If a significant delamination tear or a localized undersurface partial cuff tear involving 50% thickness is present, a transtendinous repair may be necessary.
- Lightly debride the area of the tear site and identify the extent of the tear. The depth of the tear can be determined by measuring the distance from the articular surface of the humerus to the healthy attached tendon on the tuberosity. A tear of more than 6 mm in depth would indicate a 50% thickness tear. Use the 4.5-mm shaver tip as a reference.
- After debridement of the tear site, view the subacromial space and perform a subacromial bursectomy using a combination of posterior and lateral portals made 2 to 3 cm lateral and posterior to the anterior acromial edge. Perform an acromioplasty if indicated.
- Place the arthroscope back into the glenohumeral joint through the posterior portal for visualization.

TRANSTENDINOUS REPAIR OF A PARTIAL ARTICULAR-SIDE SUPRASPINATUS TENDON AVULSION LESION

TECHNIQUE 4.21

- Place the patient in the standard beach-chair or lateral decubitus position and perform acromioplasty if indicated. Placing the arm in about 30 degrees of abduction is helpful for performing acromioplasty and bursectomy. For a transtendinous repair, move the arm gently to about 70 degrees of abduction. An assistant may position the arm to provide the best position to place the suture anchor.
- Use anterior midglenoid, anterolateral, and posterior portals for repair of the defect.
- Debride the tear to stimulate inflammation of the soft tissue and to remove the devitalized cuff. Abrade the tuberosity with a shaver or small burr to incite bone healing. This is started at the articular surface and extended laterally, but make sure not to disrupt the lateral attachment of the cuff. By leaving the lateral attachment intact, a suture anchor can be placed more medial to obtain a double-row type of fixation (Fig. 4.36A).

TABLE 4.5

Rotator Cuff Repair Rehabilitation Protocol (Minor Tear <2 cm)

PREOPERATIVE GOALS

1. PROM WFL (i.e., no frozen shoulder)
2. Independent in postoperative exercise program
3. Understands realistic postoperative goals and time frame

PHASE I—PROTECTION AND PROGRESSIVE PROM

IMMEDIATELY POSTOPERATIVELY

1. Sling at all times for 3 wk, then as needed for comfort
2. Stitches removed at 7–10 days (at physician's visit)
3. Begin pendulum exercises
4. AROM wrist and hand
5. Perform home exercise program two to three times a day

WEEK 1–3 POSTOPERATIVE (PT QIW-TIW)	**GOALS (BY 3 WK)**
1. Continue above exercises	1. Independent with HEP BID
2. PROM—FL, scaption, ER, ER in available scaption	2. PROM >150 degrees FL
3. Table slides—FL, scaption	3. PROM >50 degrees ER (neutral)
4. AROM—elbow, wrist, and hand	4. PROM >140 degrees ABD scaption
5. Begin scapular PNF	*Precautions*
6. Ice, E-stim for pain control, edema reduction	1. Sling at all times except during exercises (3 wk)
	2. No A/AAROM—would jeopardize repair
WEEKS 4–6 POSTOPERATIVE (PT QIW-TIW)	**GOALS (BY 6 WK)**
1. Wean from sling	1. PROM ≥160 degrees FL
2. PROM as above. Initiate true ABD stretch and gentle IR stretch	2. PROM ≥65 degrees ER
3. AROM <90 degrees (5 wk)	3. PROM ≥160 degrees scaption
4. Supine TheraBand ER stretch (as needed)	4. PROM 50 degrees maximum for IR
5. Cane exercises in supine—FL, scaption, ER neutral, ER in 90 degrees scaption	5. Able to comb hair—if dominant arm
6. Shoulder pulley—FL scaption	6. Able to open or close car door
7. Grades II–III capsular mobilizations	7. Able to reach behind back for wallet
8. Wall walks—FL, scaption	*Precautions*
9. Submaximal (25%) isometrics with arm at side—ER, IR, FL, ABD, EXT	1. Lifts nothing heavier than coffee cup
	2. No aggressive IR stretching

PHASE II—PROGRESSIVE AROM AND STRENGTHENING

WEEKS 7–8 POSTOPERATIVE (PT QIW-BIW)	**GOALS (BY 8 WK)**
1. Progress AROM to full by wk 8	1. A/PROM WNL FL
2. Isotonics (light weight/high repetition)—biceps curls, triceps EXT, shoulder shrugs, supine scapular protraction, reverse Codman	2. A/PROM WNL ABD
3. Supine manual resistance PNF patterns	3. A/PROM WNL ER
4. Clothespin, cupboard placing	4. PROM ≥60 degrees IR
5. UBE with minimal resistance	5. Able to lift plate into eye-level cupboard
6. Functional exercises according to patient's postoperative activity goals	6. Able to dress with normal mechanics
	Precautions
	1. Unilateral lifting limited to ≤3 lb
	2. Prevent posterior capsular tightness
	Throwing lunges
	Standing PNF
WEEKS 9–10 POSTOPERATIVE (PT 1×/2–3 WK)	**GOALS (BY 10 WK)**
1. Isotonics (light weight/high repetition)	1. MMT ≥4/5 FL
Standing—FL and ABD to 90 degrees, ER and IR with tubing	2. MMT ≥4/5 ABD
Prone—rows, horizontal ABD 90 and 120 degrees, EXT	3. MMT ≥4/5 ER
Side lying—IR and ER with towel roll under axilla	4. MMT ≥4+/5 IR
2. Increased resistance with UBE	5. Functional reach behind back to allow tucking in shirt
3. Begin wall push-ups with a plus, gradually progress toward lower levels (table, chair, bench, floor)	6. Able to place 2 lb into overhead cabinet
4. Weighted PNF patterns D1 and D2	7. Able to place gallon of milk in refrigerator
	Precaution
	Unilateral lifting limited to ≤10 lb

Continued

TABLE 4.5

Rotator Cuff Repair Rehabilitation Protocol (Minor Tear <2 cm)—cont'd

PHASE III—ADVANCED STRENGTHENING FOR PATIENTS RETURNING TO SPORT

WEEKS 11–16 POSTOPERATIVE (PT AS NEEDED)	GOALS (BY 16 WK)
1. Progress isotonic exercises	1. MMT 5/5 FL
2. Additional isotonics (wk 12)	2. MMT 5/5 ABD
Bench press (light weight, short range)	3. MMT 5/5 ER
Lateral pull-downs to chest	4. MMT 5/5 IR
Incline chest press	5. MMT 5/5 EXT
Short arc, high TheraBand ER and IR at 90 degrees ABD	6. Able to place ≥10 lb in overhead cabinet
3. Plyometrics (3 mo)—chest pass, Plyoball chop toss, overhead throw	7. Sport-specific goals
4. Return to throwing/racquet sports at 3 mo with normal strength, normal glenohumeral mechanics, and no pain	
5. Isokinetic evaluation if necessary	

Postoperative rehabilitation of a rotator cuff repair is guided largely by the size of the repair. Allowing the repair to heal adequately before stressing the tissue is paramount to successful rehabilitation.

A/AAROM, Active/active-assisted range of motion; *ABD*, abduction; *AROM*, active range of motion; *BID*, twice a day; *BIW*, twice a week; *ER*, external rotation; *E-stim*, electrical stimulation; *EXT*, extension; *FL*, flexion; *HEP*, home exercise program; *IR*, internal rotation; *MMT*, manual muscle testing; *PNF*, proprioceptive neuromuscular facilitation; *PROM*, passive range of motion; *PT*, physical therapy; *QIW*, four times a week; *TIW*, three times a week; *UBE*, upper body exercise; *WFL*, within functional limits; *WNL*, within normal limits.

TABLE 4.6

Rotator Cuff Repair Rehabilitation Protocol (Moderate Tear 2–5 cm)

PREOPERATIVE GOALS

1. PROM WFL (i.e., no frozen shoulder)
2. Independent in postoperative exercise program
3. Understands realistic postoperative goals and time frame

PHASE I—PROTECTION AND PROGRESSIVE PROM

IMMEDIATELY POSTOPERATIVELY

1. Sling at all times for 3 wk, then as needed for comfort
2. Stitches removed at 7–10 days (at physician's visit)
3. Begin pendulum exercises
4. AROM wrist and hand
5. Perform HEP two to three times a day

WEEK 1–3 POSTOPERATIVE (PT QIW-TIW)	GOALS (BY 3 WK)
1. Continue above exercises	1. Independent with HEP BID
2. PROM—FL, scaption, ER, ER in available scaption	2. PROM >130 degrees FL
3. Table slides—FL, scaption	3. PROM >40 degrees ER (neutral)
4. AROM—elbow, wrist, and hand	4. PROM >130 degrees ABD scaption
5. Begin scapular PNF	*Precautions*
6. Ice, E-stim for pain control, edema reduction	1. Sling at all times except during exercises (3 weeks)
	2. No A/AAROM—would jeopardize repair

WEEKS 4–6 POSTOPERATIVE (PT QIW-TIW)	GOALS (BY 6 WK)
1. Wean from sling	1. PROM ≥150 degrees FL
2. PROM as above. Initiate true ABD stretch and IR without overpressure	2. PROM ≥65 degrees ER
3. AROM <90 degrees (6 weeks)	3. PROM ≥160 degrees scaption
4. Supine TheraBand ER stretch (as needed)	4. PROM 50 degrees maximum for IR
5. Cane exercises in supine—FL, scaption, ER neutral, ER in 90 degrees scaption	5. Able to comb hair—if dominant arm
6. Shoulder pulley—FL scaption	6. Able to open or close car door
7. Grades II–III capsular mobilizations	*Precautions*
8. Wall walks—FL, scaption	1. Lifts ≤1 lb until 6 wk postoperatively
9. Submaximal (25%) isometrics with arm at side—ER, IR, FL, ABD, EXT	2. No aggressive IR stretching

Continued

TABLE 4.6

Rotator Cuff Repair Rehabilitation Protocol (Moderate Tear 2–5 cm)—cont'd

PHASE II—PROGRESSIVE AROM AND STRENGTHENING

WEEKS 7–8 POSTOPERATIVE (PT QIW-BIW)

1. Progress AA/AROM
2. Isotonics (light weight/high repetition)—biceps curls, triceps EXT, shoulder shrugs, supine scapular protraction, reverse Codman
3. Supine manual resistance PNF patterns
4. Clothespin, cupboard placing
5. UBE with minimal resistance

GOALS (BY 8 WK)

1. AROM ≥140 degrees FL
2. AROM ≥130 degrees ABD
3. AROM ≥60 degrees ER
4. PROM FL WNL
5. PROM ABD WNL
6. PROM ER WNL
7. PROM ≥60 degrees IR
8. Able to lift plate into eye-level cupboard
9. Able to reach behind back for wallet
Precautions
1. Unilateral lifting limited to ≤2 lb
2. Prevent posterior capsular tightness

WEEKS 9–12 POSTOPERATIVE (PT 1×2–3 WK)

1. Isotonics (light weight/high repetition)
   Standing—FL and ABD to 90 degrees, ER and IR with tubing
   Prone—rows, horizontal ABD 90 and 120 degrees, EXT
   Side lying—IR and ER with towel roll under axilla
2. Increased resistance with UBE
3. Begin wall push-ups with a plus, gradually progress toward lower levels (table, chair, bench, floor)
4. Weighted PNF patterns D1 and D2
5. Functional exercises according to patient's postoperative activity goals
   Throwing lunges
   Standing PNF patterns

GOALS (BY 12 WEEKS)

1. AROM WFL for FL
2. AROM WFL for ABD
3. AROM WFL for ER
4. MMT ≥4/5 FL
5. MMT ≥4/5 ABD
6. MMT ≥4/5 ER
7. MMT ≥4+/5 IR
8. Functional reach behind back to allow tucking in shirt
9. Able to place 2 lb into overhead cabinet
10. Able to lift gallon of milk into refrigerator
Precaution
Unilateral lifting limited to ≤10 lb

PHASE III—ADVANCED STRENGTHENING FOR PATIENTS RETURNING TO SPORT

WEEKS 11–16 POSTOPERATIVE (PT AS NEEDED)

1. Progress isotonic exercises
2. Additional isotonics (3 mo)
   Bench press (light weight, short range)
   Lateral pull-downs to chest
   Incline chest press
   Short arc, high TheraBand ER and IR at 90 degrees ABD
3. Plyometrics (4 mo)—chest pass, Plyoball chop toss, overhead throw
4. Return to throw/racquet sports progress at 4 mo with normal strength, normal glenohumeral mechanics, and no pain
5. Isokinetic evaluation if necessary

GOALS (BY 16 WK)

1. MMT 5/5 FL
2. MMT 5/5 ABD
3. MMT 5/5 ER
4. MMT 5/5 IR
5. MMT 5/5 EXT
6. Able to place ≥10 lb in overhead cabinet
7. Sport-specific goals

A/AAROM, Active/active-assisted range of motion; ABD, abduction; AROM, active range of motion; BID, twice a day; BIW, twice a week; ER, external rotation; E-stim, electrical stimulation; EXT, extension; FL, flexion; HEP, home exercise program; IR, internal rotation; MMT, manual muscle testing; PNF, proprioceptive neuromuscular facilitation; PROM, passive range of motion; PT, physical therapy; QIW, four times a week; TIW, three times a week; UBE, upper body exercise; WFL, within functional limits; WNL, within normal limits.

TABLE 4.7

Rotator Cuff Repair Rehabilitation Protocol (Massive Tear >5 cm)

PREOPERATIVE GOALS

1. PROM WFL (i.e., no frozen shoulder)
2. Independent in postoperative exercise program
3. Understands realistic postoperative goals and time frame

Continued

TABLE 4.7

Rotator Cuff Repair Rehabilitation Protocol (Massive Tear >5 cm)—cont'd

PHASE I—PROTECTION AND PROGRESSIVE PROM

IMMEDIATELY POSTOPERATIVELY

1. Sling and ABD pillow at all times for 4–6 wk, then as needed for comfort
2. Stitches removed at 7–10 days (at physician's visit)
3. Begin pendulum exercises
4. AROM wrist and hand
5. Perform home exercise program two to three times a day

WEEKS 1–4 POSTOPERATIVE (PT QIW-TIW)	GOALS (BY 4 WK)
1. Continue above exercises	1. Independent with HEP BID
2. PROM—FL, scaption, ER, ER in ≤45 degrees scaption	2. PROM ≥110 degrees FL
3. AROM—elbow, wrist, and hand	3. PROM ≥30 degrees ER (neutral)
4. Begin scapular PNF	4. PROM ≥110 degrees scaption
5. Ice and E-stim for pain control, edema reduction	*Precautions*
6. Grades II–III posterior and inferior capsular mobiliza-tions (begin wk 3, continue as needed throughout rehabilitation)	1. Sling at all times except when exercising
	2. No A/AAROM—would jeopardize repair
	3. Do *not* stretch IR

WEEKS 5–8 POSTOPERATIVE (PT QIW-TIW)	GOALS (BY 8 WK)
1. Wean from sling after 6 wk	1. PROM ≥150 degrees FL
2. AROM <60 degrees elevation after sling removal	2. PROM ≥65 degrees ER
3. PROM as above. Initiate IR without overpressure	3. PROM ≥160 degrees scaption
4. Supine TheraBand ER stretch (as needed)	4. PROM 50 degrees maximum for IR
5. Cane exercises in supine—FL, scaption, ER neutral, ER in 60 degrees scaption	5. Able to comb hair—if dominant arm
6. Shoulder pulley—FL, scaption	6. Able to open/close car door
7. Submaximal (25%) isometrics with arm at side—IR, FL, ABD, EXT	*Precautions*
	1. Lifts ≤1 lb until 8 wk postoperatively
	2. No aggressive IR stretching

PHASE II—PROGRESSIVE AROM AND STRENGTHENING

WEEKS 9–10 POSTOPERATIVE (PT QIW-BIW)	GOALS (BY 10 WK)
1. AROM ≤120 degrees elevation	1. AROM ≥110 degrees FL
2. Isotonics (light weight/high repetitions)—biceps curls, triceps EXT, shoulder shrugs, supine scapular protraction, reverse Codman	2. AROM ≥110 degrees scaption
	3. AROM ≥60 degrees ER
3. Clothespin, cupboard placing	4. PROM ≥160 degrees FL
4. UBE with minimal resistance	5. PROM ≥80 degrees ER
	6. PROM to 60 degrees IR
	7. Able to lift plate into eye-level cabinet
	8. Able to reach behind back for wallet
	Precautions
	1. Unilateral lifting limited to ≤2 lb
	2. Prevent posterior capsular tightness

WEEKS 11–14 POSTOPERATIVE (PT QIW)	GOALS (BY 14 WK)
1. Isotonics (light weight/high repetition)	1. AROM WFL for FL
Standing—FL and ABD to 90 degrees, ER and IR with tubing	2. AROM WFL for ABD
Prone—rows, horizontal ABD 90 and 120 degrees, EXT	3. AROM WFL for ER
Side lying—IR and ER with towel roll under axilla	4. MMT ≥4/5 FL
2. Increased resistance with UBE	5. MMT ≥4/5 ABD
3. Begin wall push-ups with a plus, gradually progress toward lower levels (table, chair)	6. MMT ≥4/5 ER
4. Supine manual resistance PNF patterns	7. MMT ≥4+/5 IR
	8. Functional reach behind back to allow tucking in shirt
	9. Able to place 2 lb into overhead cabinet
	10. Able to lift ½ gallon of milk into refrigerator
	Precaution
	Unilateral lifting limited to ≥5 lb

Continued

TABLE 4.7

Rotator Cuff Repair Rehabilitation Protocol (Massive Tear >5 cm)—cont'd

PHASE III—ADVANCED STRENGTHENING FOR PATIENTS RETURNING TO SPORTS

MONTHS 3–6 POSTOPERATIVE (PT AS NEEDED)	GOALS (BY 20 WEEKS)

1. Progress isotonic exercises
2. Progress wall push-ups to floor
3. Additional isometrics (3–4 mo)
    Bench press (light weight, short range)
    Lateral pull-downs to chest
    Incline chest press
    Short arc, high-speed TheraBand ER and IR at 90 degrees ABD
4. Weighted PNF patterns D1 and D2
5. Plyometrics (4 mo)—chest pass, Plyoball chop toss, overhead throw
6. Return to throw/racquet sport progression at 4 months with normal strength, normal glenohumeral mechanics, and no pain
7. Isokinetic evaluation if necessary
	1. MMT 5/5 FL
	2. MMT 5/5 ABD
	3. MMT 5/5 ER
	4. MMT 5/5 IR
	5. MMT 5/5 EXT
	6. Able to place ≥10 lb in overhead cabinet
	7. Sport-specific goals

It is important to stress to the patient that after a massive tear repair, AROM and strength are limited.

A/AAROM, Active/active-assisted range of motion; *ABD,* abduction; *AROM,* active range of motion; *BID,* twice a day; *BIW,* twice a week; *ER,* external rotation; *E-stim,* electrical stimulation; *EXT,* extension; *FL,* flexion; *HEP,* home exercise program; *IR,* internal rotation; *MMT,* manual muscle testing; *PNF,* proprioceptive neuromuscular facilitation; *PROM,* passive range of motion; *PT,* physical therapy; *QIW,* four times a week; *TIW,* three times a week; *UBE,* upper body exercise; *WFL,* within functional limits.

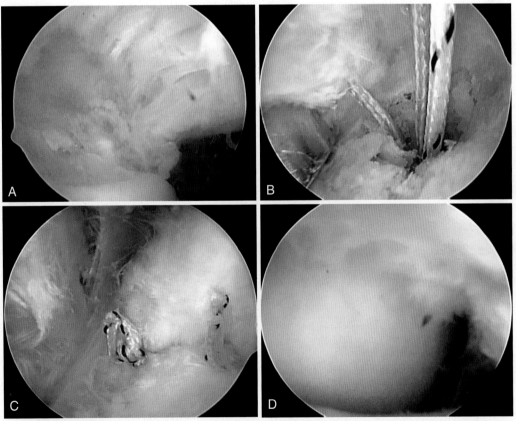

FIGURE 4.36 **A,** Eight-millimeter partial-thickness cuff tear with tuberosity abraded and lateral fibers left attached. **B,** Transtendinous placement of suture anchor just lateral to articular surface. **C,** Completed repair with knots tied in subacromial space. **D,** Intraarticular view of completed repair with footprint covered over to articular edge. **SEE TECHNIQUE 4.21.**

- Insert a spinal needle just lateral to the edge of the acromion to identify the site for anchor insertion. Place the transtendinous spinal needle just lateral to the anterior third of the acromion to visualize an appropriate angle to place a screw just lateral to the articular surface and angled away from the surface so as not to damage the articular surface (Fig. 4.36B).
- For suture anchor placement, make a small skin incision. Make a nick in the cuff in the plane of the fibers using an arthroscopic knife. Use a punch to make a small starting hole just lateral to the articular surface, ensuring that the angle is appropriate. Pass the suture anchor through the slit and into the hole. Under direct view, screw the suture anchor down securely. Ensure that the suture threads are subcortical.
- Pass a spinal needle from lateral just posterior to the previously placed suture anchor and pass a No. 1 PDS through the needle and out the anterior cannula to use as a suture shuttle. Using a suture grasper, pull one of the passed sutures out the anterior cannula. Place a simple throw from the PDS around this tail and pull the suture back up through the capsule just posterior to the suture anchor and out through the skin lateral to the acromion.
- Pass a second spinal needle just anterior to the anchor and pass a PDS from lateral, retrieve it anteriorly, and use it as a suture retriever. Using a grasper, retrieve one end of the second set of sutures out the anterior portal.
- Tie the PDS shuttle around the retrieved anterior limb of the second set of sutures and pull it back up into the subacromial space to form the second mattress suture. If necessary, the arthroscope may be placed anteriorly and a second suture anchored posteriorly in a similar fashion.
- Enter the subacromial space and place a 7-mm plastic cannula using a switching stick. Retrieve the paired sutures into the cannula. Starting posteriorly and working anteriorly, tie arthroscopic knots to secure the cuff back down to the tuberosity (Fig. 4.36C).
- On completion, view the intraarticular area to ensure that there is good approximation of the cuff to the tuberosity (Fig. 4.36D).

POSTOPERATIVE CARE The postoperative care is the same as that of a small rotator cuff repair (see Table 4.5).

FULL-THICKNESS ROTATOR CUFF TEARS

Rotator cuff tears are a significant cause of shoulder pain and morbidity. The overall prevalence of full-thickness rotator cuff tears is approximately 25% in patients over 60 years of age and increases to 50% in patients over 80 years of age. If a patient has a symptomatic full-thickness rotator cuff tear in one shoulder, they have a 50% chance of an asymptomatic full-thickness rotator cuff tear in the contralateral shoulder. Given the high number of asymptomatic full-thickness rotator cuff tears, re-tear rates after rotator cuff repair, and success of nonoperative treatment, there is much debate over the

TABLE 4.8

Stages of Fatty Degeneration of the Infraspinatus According to Time Elapsed Between the Onset of Functional Impairment and Operation

TIME	STAGE 0–1	STAGE 1.5–2	STAGE 2.5–4
<6 mo	1	2	
6 mo to 1 yr	2	1	2
1–2 yr		4	2
>2 yr		2	5

From Goutallier D, Postel JM, Bernageau J, et al: Fat muscle degeneration in cuff ruptures: pre- and postoperative evaluation by CT scan, *Clin Orthop Relat Res* 304:78, 1994.

optimal strategy for the treatment of symptomatic full-thickness rotator cuff tear.

Patients with symptomatic full-thickness rotator cuff tears typically complain of anterolateral shoulder pain that radiates into the subdeltoid location. Complaints of pain with overhead activity and lifting objects with an outstretched arm are common. Frequent night pain and sleep disturbance also are reported. In the evaluation of a potential rotator cuff tear, an MRI is obtained if the patient has no contraindications. MRI allows the surgeon to characterize the location, size, and amount of retraction of the rotator cuff tear, as well as the degree of atrophy and fatty infiltration of the rotator cuff musculature. The quality of the rotator cuff musculature is classified according to the degree of fatty infiltration originally described by Goutallier et al. for CT evaluation and modified by Fuchs et al. for MRI evaluation (Table 4.8). In this classification, grade 0 is normal muscle, grade 1 has some fatty streaks, grade 2 has more muscle than fat, grade 3 has equal amounts of muscle and fat, and grade 4 has more fat than muscle. Grades 3 and 4 are indications of a long-term chronic rotator cuff tear, which has a higher potential for failure when surgery is undertaken and likely is deemed irreparable. Another important consideration on MRI evaluation is whether any tendon stump remains attached to the greater tuberosity, which decreases the length of tendon for repair. Generally, an MRI is indicated in younger, active patients with acute rotator cuff tears and in patients with chronic rotator cuff tears in whom a trial of nonoperative treatment has failed.

The optimal treatment strategy remains a matter of debate in the literature. Nonoperative treatment leads to a successful outcome in 60% of patients, and is generally initiated in chronic full-thickness tears, especially in patients over 65 years of age. With nonoperative treatment, the patient and surgeon must understand the risk of tear progression, which is approximately 50% at 2 years. With long-standing rotator cuff tears the size, retraction, and degree of fatty infiltration can increase and can compromise the structural integrity and functional outcomes after rotator cuff repair. In patients with acute, full-thickness rotator cuff tears or chronic, full-thickness rotator cuff tears after failure of nonoperative treatment, rotator cuff repair is indicated. The timing of fixation of acute rotator cuff tears is debated, and generally we try to repair these within 3 months, given the report by Petersen and Murphy, which showed inferior outcomes after repair done more than 4 months after injury.

When surgery is contemplated, a risk-to-benefit ratio should be evaluated, with the probability of good-to-excellent results being quantified for the individual patient. This involves not only the tear characteristics (e.g., size, retraction, Goutallier grade), but also patient characteristics including smoking status, medical comorbidities, age, and compliance. Factors associated with failure after rotator cuff repair include larger tears, greater retraction, advanced Goutallier grade, older age, smoking status, osteoporosis, diabetes mellitus, hypercholesterolemia, and more aggressive rehabilitation protocols. Evaluation of the literature found that the best potential for healing was in patients younger than 70 years with acute, small tears (<3 cm) and a healthy tendon-bone interface who are compliant with sling wear and are able to undergo an extended rehabilitation program of 6 to 9 months. Studies have found that carefully selected patients older than 70 years did well after rotator cuff repair and functionally improved as much as younger patients. Once again, individualization of treatment is necessary, and thorough evaluation of potential healing and risks is needed to obtain the best long-term results. Determining which rotator cuff tears are repairable is important to avoid the morbidity of surgery that accompanies a prolonged rehabilitation period in patients with an unacceptably high risk of failure. Goutallier stages III and IV tears, if accompanied by a tendinous stump of less than 15 mm and a positive tangent sign, have a 90% failure rate. Given this, tears with significant retraction and advanced Goutallier grades III and IV usually are deemed irreparable and are treated with alternative strategies such as debridement, tendon transfer, superior capsular reconstruction, or reverse shoulder arthroplasty.

Intraoperative prognostic healing factors for rotator cuff repairs include tendon and bone quality and the ability to anatomically reduce and repair the tendon to its normal footprint on the tuberosity without undue tension. If anatomic repair cannot be achieved without significant tension, medialized repair can be performed. Strong fixation of the repair is essential to prevent gapping of the tendon during cyclic or rotational loading. The advantages of various fixation methods, including single-row, double-row, and transosseous equivalent repair techniques, have been investigated in clinical and biomechanical studies. In the laboratory, the single-row repair covers approximately 50% of the footprint of the original cuff attachment, whereas double-row repair has been shown in several studies to cover nearly 100% of the footprint. Biomechanically, the double-row repair has been shown to be superior in ultimate load-to-failure, compression, and resistance to gapping with rotation and cyclic loading, most important, along the anterior edge of the repair where the rotator cable attaches. Radiographic studies with MRI follow-up of double-row and transosseous equivalent repairs have shown higher healing rates compared to single-row repair. Clinically, there is no significant difference in healing in small- or medium-sized tears using single-row or double-row fixation. Large-to-massive tears tend to have superior results with transosseous equivalent or double-row repair, with greater healing noted; however, Trantalis et al. reported several disruptions of the repair at the muscle-tendon junction from overconstraint, described as type 2 failures.

The final issue is the cost of the repairs. Studies have shown that the lowest direct surgical costs are with single-row repair, with the transosseous equivalent repair having the second highest cost, and the double-row repair

with the highest cost because of increased operating room time and increased number of implants used. The greatest cost to the patient is failure from inadequate fixation and the need for revision surgery because of the repeat direct surgical costs and added indirect costs of time away from work. Thus, when determining fixation techniques, the best available technique for a particular patient with a particular pathologic process is still the one that should be used. Recent studies have shown double-row fixation to be more cost-effective than single-row repair because of lower re-tear risks.

Special techniques have been used to aid in the repair of retracted rotator cuff tears. Lo and Burkhart classified rotator cuff tears as crescent-shaped, U-shaped, and L-shaped (Fig. 4.37). Repair of retracted U- and L-shaped tears that cannot be adequately mobilized involves margin convergence with sutures starting medially and extending laterally along the tear to decrease the size, allowing easier approximation of the edges to the tuberosity using a double-row technique (Figs. 4.38 and 4.39). Chronic tears, such as chronic L-shaped tears (Fig. 4.40), and chronic massive contracted tears (Figs. 4.41 and 4.42), such as crescent cuff tears with retraction, require releases and interval slides before repair. The use of structural graft supplementation may be required for repair of these tears. Fixation usually is a single row just lateral to the articular surface to prevent tension overload and failure at the muscle-tendon interface.

Local stimulants, such as protein-rich plasma and mesenchymal stem cells, have been tried, but at present there are no significant scientific data showing that these substances are cost-effective or produce superior clinical results. Local bone marrow stimulation, as described by Snyder, allows the bone marrow elements to become involved in the repair and has shown some potential for increasing healing and should be considered.

Careful preparation is necessary before starting any technique. Being familiar with the procedure, understanding the known pathologic process, and being prepared to treat other presenting pathologic processes are critical. Given the available data, we prefer arthroscopic double-row or transosseous equivalent rotator cuff repair, with the number of medial and lateral row anchors dependent on tear size.

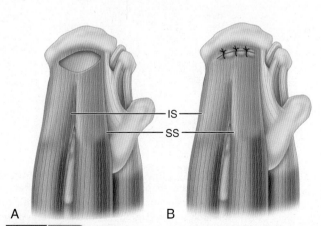

FIGURE 4.37 Crescent-shaped rotator cuff tear. **A,** Superior view of crescent-shaped rotator cuff tear involving supraspinatus (SS) and infraspinatus (IS) tendons. **B,** Repaired tear.

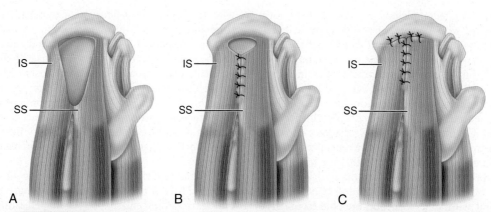

FIGURE 4.38 U-shaped rotator cuff tear. **A,** Superior view of U-shaped rotator cuff tear involving supraspinatus (SS) and infraspinatus (IS) tendons. **B,** U-shaped tears show excellent mobility from anterior-to-posterior direction and are initially repaired with side-to-side sutures using principle of margin convergence. **C,** Repaired margin is repaired to bone in tension-free manner.

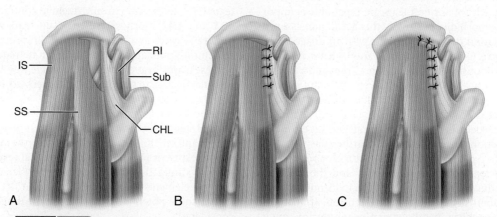

FIGURE 4.39 Acute L-shaped rotator cuff tear. **A,** Superior view of acute L-shaped rotator cuff tear involving supraspinatus (SS) and rotator interval (RI). **B,** Tears should be initially repaired along longitudinal split. **C,** Converged margin is repaired to bone. CHL, coracohumeral ligament; IS, infraspinatus tendon; Sub, subscapularis tendon.

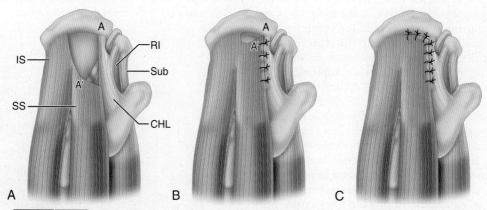

FIGURE 4.40 Chronic L-shaped tear. **A,** Superior view of chronic L-shaped tear, which has assumed U-shaped configuration. **B,** L-shaped tears show excellent mobility from anterior-to-posterior direction; however, one tear margin (usually posterior leaf) is more mobile. Tears should be initially repaired using side-to-side sutures by using principle of margin convergence. **C,** Converged margin is repaired to bone in tension-free manner. A, anatomic insertion site of supraspinatus tendon (A1); *CHL,* Coracohumeral ligament; *IS,* infraspinatus tendon; *RI,* rotator interval; *SS,* supraspinatus tendon; *Sub,* subscapularis tendon.

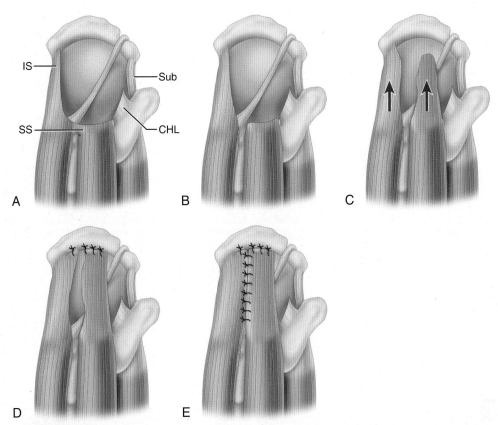

FIGURE 4.41   Massive, contracted crescentic rotator cuff tear. **A,** Superior view. **B,** Double-interval slide is performed by first doing anterior interval slide, then posterior interval slide releasing interval between supraspinatus (SS) and infraspinatus (IS). **C,** After release, improved mobility *(arrows)* of supraspinatus tendon and infraspinatus and teres minor tendons posteriorly. **D,** Supraspinatus tendon repaired to lateral bone bed in tension-free manner, and infraspinatus and teres minor tendons advanced laterally. **E,** Residual defect closed with side-to-side sutures. *CHL,* Coracohumeral ligament; *Sub,* subscapularis tendon.

ROTATOR CUFF REPAIR

TECHNIQUE 4.22

- Place the patient in a standard beach-chair position with the use of an articulating arm holder or in the lateral decubitus position while maintaining the extremity in 30 degrees of abduction and 10 degrees of forward flexion using sterile balanced suspension. Apply serial compression devices to the lower extremities to help avoid deep vein thrombosis.
- Carefully outline the bony landmarks and potential portals on the skin (see Fig. 4.35). Generally, four portals are used for arthroscopic rotator cuff repair: posterior portal, anterior portal, lateral portal, and posterolateral viewing portal. The anterior and posterior portals are used for retrieving and storing sutures, the posterolateral portal is used for viewing, and lateral portal is the working portal. The suture anchors will be placed just off the lateral edge of the acromion using spinal needle localization and percutaneous insertion.

- Through a standard posterior portal, perform a diagnostic arthroscopy. Treat any pathology of the long head of the biceps, subscapularis tendon, labrum, and cartilage surface at this time. Once complete, place the arthroscope in the subacromial space from the posterior portal. Identify the site and configuration of the tear. Create a lateral working portal in the center of the tear after spinal needle localization (Fig. 4.43A).
- Perform a complete subacromial bursectomy using a combination of an arthroscopic shaver and electrocautery, starting lateral and moving medially. Pay special attention to ensure visualization of the posterior extent of the tear to facilitate suture passage and retrieval. Perform acromioplasty as indicated.
- Carefully define the depth of the tear and determine the type of tear (crescent, U-shaped, or L-shaped configuration) (see Figs. 4.37 to 4.41). Determine the amount of retraction and mobility of the tendon with the aid of an arthroscopic grasper. If the tendon is retracted with poor mobility, perform standard releases of the articular surface with an elevator and, if needed, releases around the scapular spine and coracoid base to allow mobilization.

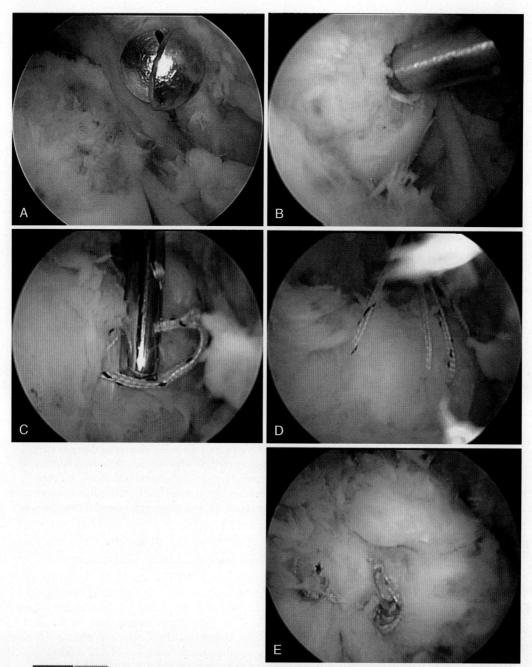

FIGURE 4.42 **A,** Arthroscopic subacromial view of massive retracted cuff tear and biceps in lower corner. Humeral tuberosity is to right. **B,** Placement of starting hole for medial anchor. Note 45-degree angle to shaft and placement 2 mm off articular edge. **C,** Use of Scorpion to place mattress suture 16 mm medial to torn edge. **D,** Completion of medial mattress suture placement and storage in cannula. Sutures can be used to pull tendon to its tuberosity to help identify appropriate placement of lateral anchors and sutures. **E,** Completed double-row repair with cuff securely repaired to anatomic footprint.

At that point, traction determines whether the tendon is repairable and if an anatomic repair can be achieved.

- Use a spinal needle to localize the location of a posterolateral viewing portal. Move the arthroscope to the posterolateral viewing portal for further characterization of the rotator cuff tear.

- Prepare the footprint with an arthroscopic burr or shaver to lightly decorticate the surface. Lightly abrade the undersurface of the rotator cuff as well to aid tendon-to-bone healing.

- Define the potential location of the anchors, separating the insertion points by 1 cm to prevent tuberosity

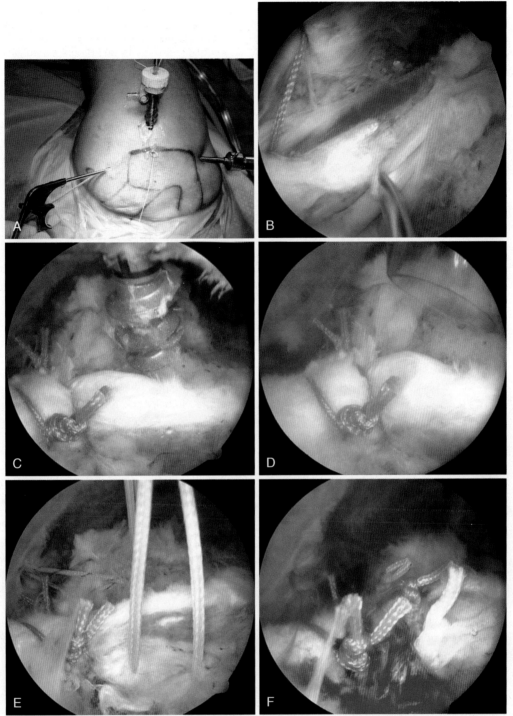

FIGURE 4.43 **A,** Portals for rotator cuff repair. **B,** Margin convergence and releases to reduce tension on repairs. **C,** Insertion of double-loaded anchor for mattress sutures 3 mm lateral to articular surface. **D-F,** Convergence is started at apex of tear, working from medial to lateral. **SEE TECHNIQUE 4.22.**

fracture. The type of repair—single-row, double-row, or transosseous equivalent—is at the discretion of the surgeon. Generally, for large rotator cuff tears, we favor double-row or transosseous equivalent repairs for their better biomechanical characteristics and lower re-tear rates. Percutaneously insert the desired number of medial row anchors just off the articular surface (Fig. 4.44). Make sure all anchors are inserted flush with the bony surface. For the double-row technique we use double-loaded screw-in type anchors, and for transosseous equivalent repairs we use knotless anchors preloaded with tape-type suture.

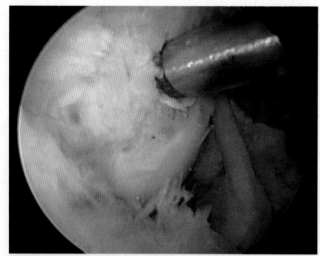

FIGURE 4.44 Anchors inserted just off edge of acromion through individual stab wounds. **SEE TECHNIQUE 4.22.**

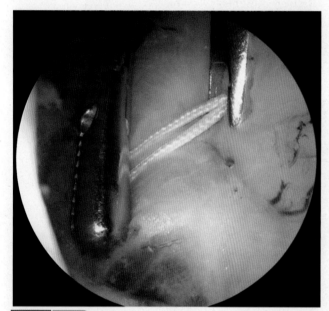

FIGURE 4.45 Placement of mattress sutures for cuff repair. **SEE TECHNIQUE 4.22.**

- Place an 8.25-mm notched cannula in the lateral portal for suture passage, starting anteriorly and progressing posteriorly. A retrievable suture passer is helpful in the passage of suture. Starting anteriorly, retrieve each limb of suture from the anterior medial row anchor out of the lateral cannula passed through the tendon. Pass the mattress sutures through the tendon about 4 mm lateral to the musculotendinous junction and separate by 7 mm (approximate width of the retrievable suture passer) (Fig. 4.45). Retrieve the suture limbs out the anterior portal.
- Once all sutures from the anterior-medial row anchor have been passed, start with the posterior-most suture from the posterior-medial row anchor and progress anteriorly.

Retrieve these sutures out the posterior portal. Pass all sutures in a horizontal mattress type configuration.
- If double-row fixation is planned, start with arthroscopic knot tying posteriorly and progress anteriorly. The choice of which suture is to be the post is determined by the characteristics of the tear, and the choice of arthroscopic knot is at the discretion of the surgeon. Once knots are tied, retrieve the sutures out their respective anterior and posterior cannulas. For transosseous equivalent repair, the sutures are passed and not tied.
- Bring one limb from each suture grouping out the lateral cannula. Determine the desired location of the posterior lateral row anchor by placing tension on all of the retrieved suture limbs. Use electrocautery to debride the lateral cortex of soft tissue. Load the suture limbs in the knotless lateral anchor, and insert it at the desired location while placing tension on each suture limb. Cut the excess suture. Repeat the process for the anterior lateral row anchor (Figs. 4.46 and 4.47).
- Move the arm through a range of motion to make sure there is no gapping of the anterior repair or impingement of the cuff on the acromion.
- Margin convergence and releases to reduce tension on the repairs should be performed if the rotator cuff cannot be anatomically repaired. (Fig. 4.43B and C).
- For margin convergence of a U-shaped tear or medial extension of an L-shaped tear, use a large crescent-type suture shuttle device, passing it through both leaves, and then retrieve a No. 2 nonabsorbable suture back through the two leaves, storing them for later tying.
- Begin the convergence at the apex of the tear, working from medial to lateral. Make sure to visually line up the tear in its normal anatomy (Fig. 4.43D to F).

See Video 4.1.

POSTOPERATIVE CARE The postoperative course is critical in obtaining excellent results. Use of a sling is encouraged for 6 weeks after almost all repairs. Strengthening exercises usually are not performed until 10 weeks after the repair to prevent overstrain on the cuff during the early healing phase.

MASSIVE CONTRACTED ROTATOR CUFF TEARS

REPAIR OF LARGE OR MASSIVE CONTRACTED TEARS USING THE INTERVAL SLIDE TECHNIQUE

TECHNIQUE 4.23

(TAURO ET AL.)
- Perform routine diagnostic arthroscopy first in the glenohumeral joint to assess the size and shape of the tear.

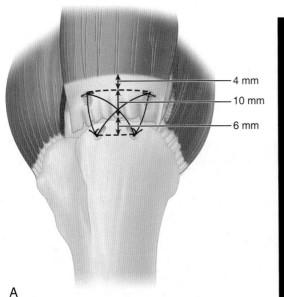

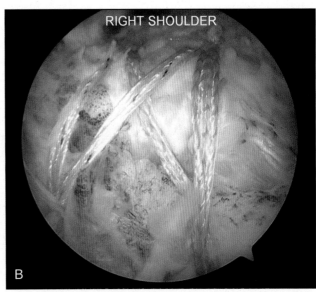

FIGURE 4.46   **A** and **B,** Transosseous equivalent repair. **SEE TECHNIQUE 4.22.**

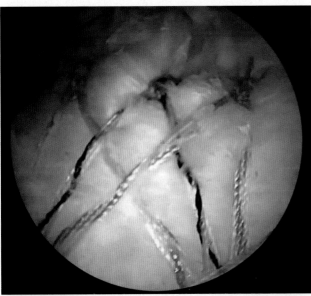

FIGURE 4.47   Completed rotator cuff repair. **SEE TECHNIQUE 4.22.**

is simply an arthroscopic adaptation of the open interval slide.

- While viewing from the posterior intraarticular portal, insert a narrow basket punch into the lateral subacromial portal, through the tear in the cuff, and into the joint (Fig. 4.48A). Divide the interval between the anterior border of the supraspinatus and the superior capsule (rotator interval) from lateral to medial. This also releases the tendon from the contracted coracohumeral ligament on the bursal side. With the biceps intact, make the release just caudad to the tendon. If the biceps is not intact, the release is started approximately at the anterosuperior pole of the glenoid. The release also can be judged by the character of the tissue being cut. In most cases, establishing a small percutaneous portal just adjacent to the lateral subacromial portal and using a grasper to help pull laterally on the tendon as it is released may be helpful.
- After the release is completed, repair the cuff down to the tuberosity using suture anchors, or repair it side to side with margin convergence, followed by repair to the tuberosity (Fig. 4.48B and C).

- Insert an atraumatic grasper through the lateral subacromial portal and assess cuff mobility from the articular side. If supraspinatus tendon mobility is poor, release the superior capsule at this time, with an arthroscopic elevator or electrosurgical cutting device inserted through the lateral subacromial portal. The release is accomplished by cutting through the capsule between the cuff tendon and glenoid rim from the rotator interval anteriorly to the scapular spine posteriorly.
- If a crescent-shaped tear does not reduce to bone or a longitudinal tear does not close from side to side, perform an arthroscopic interval slide. This soft-tissue release

SUPERIOR CAPSULE RECONSTRUCTION

Superior capsule reconstruction (SCR) was originally described by Mihata et al. in 2012 to restore superior stability in patients with massive irreparable posterior-superior rotator cuff tears. Biomechanical studies have shown that SCR can restore superior translation and decrease subacromial contact pressures seen with irreparable supraspinatus tears. This procedure was originally described with the use of fascia lata autograft but has evolved to most surgeons using acellular dermal matrix. Fascia lata allograft has been

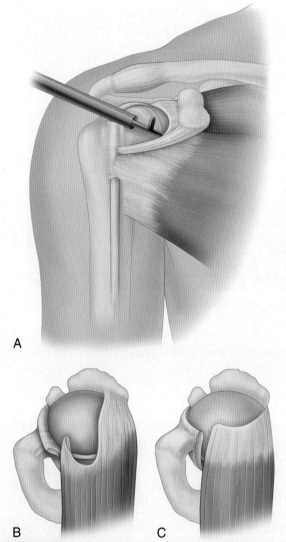

A

B   C

FIGURE 4.48   Tauro et al. interval slide technique for repair of large rotator cuff tear. **A,** Basket punch inserted through lateral subacromial portal to begin interval release. **B,** Completed interval slide release for crescentic tear. **C,** Completed interval slide release for longitudinal tear. **SEE TECHNIQUE 4.23.**

shown to have less elongation and better ability to restore shoulder biomechanics than acellular dermal matrix, but the widespread availability and ease of use has kept acellular dermal matrix a viable option. The addition of posterior interval side-to-side sutures from the infraspinatus remnant to the graft has also been shown to increase superior stability. Currently, only short-term clinical follow-up exists, with most studies showing a significant improvement in ASES and Constant outcomes scores, range of motion, and pain. SCR has been touted as a viable option for younger, more active patients, and a recent study by Mihata et al. showed that most of their patients were able to return to sport or physical work. Currently, there are multiple treatment options for massive irreparable rotator cuff tears, including reverse total shoulder arthroplasty, tendon transfers, arthroscopic debridement, and SCR, making the choice complex and

debated among shoulder surgeons. SCR has been reported to reverse pseudoparalysis in patients with massive irreparable rotator cuff tears. Two recent studies have shown success, but further research is needed to validate these studies with small numbers and short-term follow-up. Our current indication for SCR is a patient with an irreparable superior rotator cuff tear and an intact or repairable subscapularis tendon with preserved overhead function and a primary complaint of pain.

TECHNIQUE 4.24

- Place the patient in the standard beach-chair or lateral decubitus position as previously described.
- Establish a standard posterior portal and perform diagnostic arthroscopy.
- Pay special attention to the status of the subscapularis and biceps tendons. Place an 8.25-mm clear cannula anteriorly through the lateral aspect of the rotator interval. If a biceps tenodesis is indicated, perform this first using the "loop 'n' tack" method (see Technique 4.9). If the subscapularis tendon is torn, perform standard releases to allow tendon mobilization.
- Once mobilization is complete, using a combination of FiberTape (Arthrex) and Suture Tape, pass suture limbs through the subscapularis tendon with a retrievable suture passer (Arthrex Scorpion) starting inferiorly. Fix the suture limbs to the lesser tuberosity with 1 or 2 Arthrex 4.75-mm Swivel-Lock suture anchors, with the goal of placing one set of FiberTape and SutureTape into each anchor.
- Place the arthroscope into the subacromial space, and create a standard lateral portal at the midpoint of the superior rotator cuff tear. Perform a complete subacromial bursectomy using an arthroscopic shaver and electrocautery. It is important to be able to visualize the posterior extent of the rotator cuff tear. Perform an acromioplasty as indicated.
- Establish a posterolateral viewing portal halfway between the posterior and lateral portals, just off the acromial border. Place a switching stick and move the arthroscope to this portal.
- Mobilize the rotator cuff and, if deemed irreparable, perform superior capsule reconstruction.
- Using an arthroscopic shaver and electrocautery, clear the superior aspect of the glenoid and greater tuberosity of soft tissue and lightly decorticate them to aid in graft healing (4.49A). Leave the superior labrum intact because it may aid in superior stability.
- Place 3 Arthrex 2.6-mm FiberTak suture anchors percutaneously into the superior glenoid, 5 mm off of the articular margin after spinal needle localization (4.49B). Insert the anterior anchor just anterior to the acromioclavicular joint, the middle anchor through Neviaser portal, and the posterior anchor medial to the standard posterior portal.
- Place 2 Arthrex 4.75-mm SwiveLock suture anchors preloaded with FiberTape just off the articular surface in the greater tuberosity (1 anterior and 1 posterior) (4.49C).
- To obtain graft measurements, measure the distance between the medial row humeral anchors and the glenoid

approximately 30 degrees and support the torso with an inflatable beanbag.

- If using the lateral decubitus position use a sterile foam-padded traction device (STaR Sleeve; Arthrex, Naples, FL), to suspend the arm in 70 degrees of abduction and 15 degrees of forward flexion with 10 lb of traction.
- Make standard posterior and anterior portals and perform a complete 15-point anatomic review of the glenohumeral joint.
- Evaluate and repair any intraarticular pathologic process involving the biceps tendon, labrum, and articular surface of the rotator cuff.
- If using the lateral decubitus position, change the shoulder position to 20 degrees of abduction and 5 degrees of forward flexion in preparation for subacromial bursoscopy.
- Using the standard anterior and posterior portals, examine the subacromial bursa and the undersurface of the acromion, coracoacromial ligament, bursal surface of the rotator cuff, and acromioclavicular joint. Perform a selective subacromial decompression. If no impingement lesion is present, limit this to beveling the acromial facet of the acromioclavicular joint and removing the coracoacromial ligament beneath the acromion. Bevel the acromial facet to expose the tight or medially inclined acromioclavicular joint through the posterior subacromial portal.
- Resect the distal clavicle after subacromial bursoscopy and subacromial decompression. The decision to proceed with a complete distal clavicle resection should be made before beginning the surgical procedure.
- Begin the resection with the arthroscope in the posterior subacromial portal. Insert a 6-mm internal diameter outflow cannula connected to gravity drainage in the anterior subacromial portal and insert the electrosurgical tool with a subacromial electrode through an insulated cannula in the lateral portal. Use the electrode to transect and morcellize the inferior capsule and periosteum from the undersurface of the acromioclavicular joint and distal end of the clavicle.

- Insert a mechanical shaver through the lateral portal cannula to excise the soft-tissue debris created with the electrosurgical tool. When a large spur is present, it may be easier to start with the arthroscope lateral and the instrumentation posterior.
- Insert a 4-mm or 5.5-mm burr through the posterior portal to remove the posterior facet and spurs on the clavicle. Clear the bony debris from the burring by gravity drainage through the outflow cannula in the anterior subacromial portal.
- Insert the 4-mm or 5.5-mm burr with the hooded acromionizer sheath through the anterior portal into the acromioclavicular joint. Start the clavicular resection anteriorly and work to the posterior extent of the acromioclavicular joint capsule. Carefully observe and preserve the capsule. Use the burr to resect the remaining superior margin of the distal clavicle, avoiding injury to the superior capsule (Fig. 4.53A). Resect the superior aspect of the clavicle and any associated cyst, leaving a resection symmetrical to that of the inferior clavicle.
- Insert the arthroscope into the anterior portal to view the space of the resected acromioclavicular joint. Resect any remaining spurs or irregularities around the margins from either a lateral or a posterior portal. Bevel the undersurface of the clavicle slightly to remove any sharp edges. Estimate the width of resection of the acromioclavicular space using a two-pin technique. With the arthroscope in the anterior portal, place a pin vertically through the skin parallel to and at the midsection of the distal end of the clavicle. Place a second pin perpendicular to the medial border of the acromion and parallel to the central portion of the acromial facet (Fig. 4.53B). The distance between these two pins measured at skin level corresponds to the width of resection. The resection should be 6 to 8 mm.

POSTOPERATIVE CARE The patient is placed in an UltraSling. General passive range-of-motion and pendulum exercises are begun immediately. Exercises of the forearm, wrist, and hand are begun on the first postoperative day

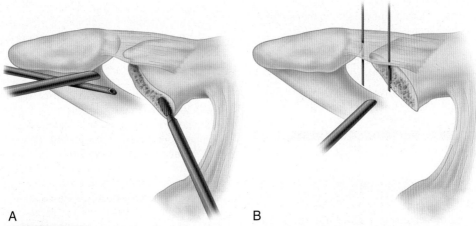

A   B

FIGURE 4.53 Tolin and Snyder arthroscopic resection of distal head of clavicle. **A,** Superior cortical rim of clavicle is removed. **B,** Two-pin technique used to measure width of resection. **SEE TECHNIQUE 4.26.**

with the aid of therapy putty. Overhead lifting, pulling, and pushing activities are restricted for 1 to 2 weeks, with a return to heavy labor and sporting activities allowed 2 to 3 months postoperatively.

SUPERIOR APPROACH

TECHNIQUE 4.27

(FLATOW ET AL.)
- Place the patient in the beach-chair position and administer a scalene block.
- Use needles to determine the location and orientation of the joint before introducing the instruments.
- Inject several milliliters of normal saline solution with an 18-gauge needle.
- Make two portal sites, one anterior and one posterior to the joint line. Use a 2.7-mm wrist arthroscopy unit until adequate space is present for a standard 4-mm arthroscope. Use electrocautery to coagulate small bleeders. Glycine or normal saline with 1:300,000 epinephrine and a shielded cautery unit can be used for irrigation.
- Using a full-radius resector, perform a complete synovectomy and clean soft tissue and any remaining cartilage from the articular surface of the outer end of the clavicle with a curet.
- Using the electrocautery unit, shell out the outer end of the clavicle so that the tube of soft tissue containing the acromioclavicular ligament and capsule is preserved.
- Begin bone resection with a small (2-mm) burr followed by larger (3.5- to 4.5-mm) burrs. Switch the burr from the anterior to the posterior portal to remove bone adequately under direct vision. Perform final beveling using rasps.
- Carefully examine the joint with the arthroscope from the anterior and posterior portals to ensure adequate removal of bone and check for loose fragments of bone or cartilage. Probe the edges to confirm that no overhanging ridges remain. The direct approach affords excellent exposure for final "sculpturing."
- After withdrawing the instruments, inject 0.25% bupivacaine (Marcaine) without epinephrine into the joint for postoperative comfort. Close the portal sites with resorbable sutures in a subcuticular fashion.

POSTOPERATIVE CARE Passive motion is allowed on the first postoperative day. Active exercises are allowed as soon as postoperative discomfort resolves, usually in 3 to 5 days. A sling is worn for comfort for 1 to 2 days postoperatively.

ACROMIOCLAVICULAR JOINT SEPARATION

Acromioclavicular joint separations are common shoulder injuries. Most low-grade injuries, including Rockwood types I and II, can be treated successfully nonoperatively, whereas high-grade injuries, types IV, V, and VI, generally are considered operative lesions. The treatment of type III acromioclavicular joint injuries remains controversial, with most treated nonoperatively; however, treatment must be tailored to each patient. Traditionally, acromioclavicular joint stabilization was performed strictly as an open procedure; however, with advanced arthroscopic techniques, more of these procedures are being done with an arthroscopically assisted technique. Arthroscopic techniques have the advantage of allowing evaluation and treatment of any concomitant glenohumeral pathology. Associated glenohumeral injuries have been shown to occur with as many as 53% of high-grade acromioclavicular joint separations. Most of these lesions involve articular-sided rotator cuff tears and SLAP tears, with advancing age being the most dominant predictor.

A variety of techniques for acromioclavicular joint stabilization have been described. The heterogeneity of the techniques has led to difficulty interpreting the available literature, with no clear consensus between nonanatomic and anatomic reconstruction or when and if allograft augmentation is needed. Despite the multitude of techniques, reported failure rates and overall complication rates remain relatively high, 21.8% and 14.2%, respectively, in a recent meta-analysis. We prefer to minimize the number and diameter of drill holes in the distal clavicle and coracoid process to decrease the postoperative fracture risk. Injuries more than 2 weeks old receive supplemental anterior tibialis graft augmentation to avoid the risk of loss of reduction and implant-related complications.

ARTHROSCOPICALLY ASSISTED AC JOINT RECONSTRUCTION

TECHNIQUE 4.28

- With the patient in the standard beach-chair position, examine the stability of the acromioclavicular joint and assess ease of reduction. Check to confirm that imaging of the affected extremity is possible.
- Create a standard posterior portal and use a 30-degree arthroscope to perform a diagnostic arthroscopy and treat any associated pathology if indicated.
- Create a standard anterior portal high and slightly lateral in the rotator interval. Using an arthroscopic shaver and electrocautery, take down the rotator interval with care to preserve the superior and middle glenohumeral ligaments. This allows visualization of the underlying coracoacromial ligament and coracoid process.
- Create a low accessory anterolateral portal in line with the upper border of the subscapularis, taking care to allow for preparation of the undersurface of the coracoid. Place a clear 8.25-mm cannula, and use a 70-degree arthroscope for the remainder of the case.
- Clear the undersurface of the coracoid process of soft tissue with electrocautery and lightly decorticate it with an arthroscopic shaver, taking care to reach the medial extent of the coracoid process where the pectoralis minor inserts.

- Once completed, use fluoroscopy to confirm placement of the superior incision overlying the clavicle, roughly 3 cm medial to the acromioclavicular joint.
- With a No. 15 blade scalpel, make a 3 to 4 cm vertical incision though skin and subcutaneous tissue overlying the clavicle. Use Bovie electrocautery to make full-thickness skin flaps both medially and laterally. Incise the clavipectoral fascia in full-thickness fashion in line with the clavicle. Free the clavicle of soft tissue attachment both anteriorly and posteriorly to allow graft passage. Mobilize the clavicle to ensure ease of reduction of the acromioclavicular joint. Resect the distal 5 to 8 mm of the clavicle with a microsagittal saw while protecting soft-tissue structures.
- With the arm supported in an arm positioner, reduce the acromioclavicular joint. Introduce an Arthrex AC Joint Reconstruction guide into the anterior portal and seat it at the base of the coracoid, ensuring it is in a central location from medial to lateral. Place the guide on the clavicle in the intended position in line with the coracoid process under fluoroscopic guidance.
- Advance the 2.4-mm guide pin through four cortices and until it can be seen exiting the inferior aspect of the coracoid process in the intended location. Use fluoroscopic imaging to confirm the location and remove the guide. Over-drill the superior cortex of the clavicle for flush seating of the Arthrex Knotless AC Joint TightRope "top hat."
- Remove the central sleeve of the drill guide and insert a nitinol wire into the drill guide and retrieve it out the low anterolateral cannula (Fig. 4.54A). Shuttle the suture limbs of the Arthrex Knotless AC joint Tightrope through the clavicle and coracoid process and retrieve it out the low anterolateral portal.
- Load a cortical button onto the suture limbs and, with the help of a KingFisher grasper, shuttle them through the low anterolateral cannula and seat them at the base of the coracoid process (Fig. 4.54B).
- Carefully tension the suture limbs and seat a "top hat" within the superior clavicle to allow complete reduction of the acromioclavicular joint. Confirm this fluoroscopically. Set aside the suture limbs for later knot tying.
- Create the tunnels for graft passage starting medially. Place a switching stick just medial to the TightRope location, starting at the posterior aspect of the clavicle and advancing inferiorly to exit on the medial aspect of the coracoid process. Advance an arthroscopic cannula dilator over the switching stick until it is visualized medial to the coracoid process. Remove the switching stick and place an Arthrex FiberStick into the dilator and retrieve it out the low anterolateral cannula. Repeat the process starting just lateral to the TightRope and anterior to the clavicle and advancing the switching stick lateral to the coracoid process (Fig. 4.54C). Retrieve the second FiberStick out the low anterolateral cannula.
- Whip stitch both ends of an anterior tibial tendon allograft with Arthrex FiberLoop suture. Shuttle the graft using the medial FiberStick suture, bringing the graft posterior to the clavicle and medial to the coracoid process; continue until all suture limbs are retrieved out anterolateral cannula (Fig. 4.54D).
- Use the lateral FiberStick suture to shuttle the graft around the coracoid process, exiting anterior to the clavicle

(Fig. 4.54E). The graft lies over the cortical button on the inferior surface of the coracoid process (Fig. 4.54F).
- Complete the tensioning of the TightRope and cut and tie the remaining sutures. Tie the graft over the clavicle and secure it to itself with two figure-of-eight No. 2 FiberWire sutures (Fig. 4.54G). Cut and discard excess graft. Obtain final fluoroscopic images.
- Close the clavipectoral fascia with No. 0 Vicryl suture, and the remainder of the wounds in standard fashion.

POSTOPERATIVE CARE Patients are kept in sling immobilization for 6 weeks to limit gravity forces placed on the operative construct. Hand, wrist, and elbow range of motion exercises, as well as pendulum exercises, are initiated immediately postoperatively. Physical therapy is begun at 4 weeks with gentle shoulder passive range of motion exercises, and at 6 weeks unrestricted active motion is begun. Strengthening exercises are initiated at 10 to 12 weeks (Fig. 4.54H).

CALCIFIC TENDINITIS OF THE ROTATOR CUFF

Although the exact cause of calcific tendinitis of the rotator cuff is unknown, many investigators believe that local tissue hypoxia and degeneration result in the calcium deposits. During the acute resorptive phase of calcific tendinitis, patients may have pain, inflammation, and limited range of motion of the shoulder, all of which mimic an acute infection. Conservative treatment of this painful condition consists of intermittent icing, antiinflammatory drugs, and occasionally a local injection of a long-acting anesthetic into the subacromial space. The use of corticosteroid injections is controversial and may prolong the painful resorptive phase of calcific tendinitis. Oral narcotics for pain often are necessary during the acute phase.

Anteroposterior radiographs with the shoulder in internal and external rotation and an axillary lateral view are helpful in identifying the area of calcification. The supraspinatus tendon and the subscapularis tendon are commonly involved. If surgical intervention is necessary, arthroscopic release of the calcification may be beneficial.

RELEASE OF CALCIFIC TENDINITIS

TECHNIQUE 4.29

- Standard arthroscopy portals are used for thorough intraarticular evaluation. The undersurface of the supraspinatus tendon when involved with calcific tendinitis may have an appearance of a strawberry lesion or hyperemic inflamed area, and the tendon in this area may be frayed. A fullness or slight bulge in the tendon also may be visible.
- If identified, lightly debride the area with a full-radius resector and mark this with a No. 1 PDS placed through a spinal needle and left in place when the needle is retracted. View the lesion through a subacromial portal and use an anterolateral accessory portal for instrumentation.

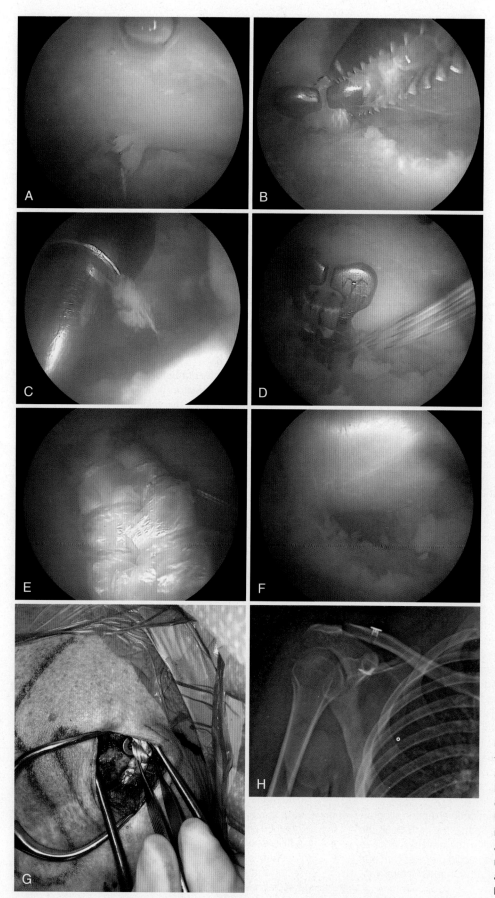

FIGURE 4.54 Acromioclavicular joint reconstruction. **A,** Drill guide is used to drill through four cortices of the clavicle and coracoid. Drill sleeve is removed and Nitinol wire or Arthrex FiberStick is retrieved out low anterolateral portal. **B,** Cortical button is guided into position on inferior portion of coracoid using a KingFisher grasper. **C,** Graft passage around clavicle is facilitated with help of dilation using switching stick and arthroscopic cannula dilator. **D,** Graft passage around clavicle is facilitated with the help of dilation using a switching stick and arthroscopic cannula dilator. **E,** Graft is being shuttled around lateral aspect of coracoid process. **F,** Graft overlies cortical button and is seated flush on inferior surface of coracoid process. **G,** Graft is secured to itself using multiple nonabsorbable sutures. Graft overlies "top hat" seated on the superior cortex of clavicle decreasing risk of implant irritation. **H,** Final postoperative radiograph showing completed arthroscopically assisted AC joint reconstruction. Note anatomic alignment of AC joint. **SEE TECHNIQUE 4.27.**

Release the calcification into the subacromial bursa with a spinal needle or arthroscopic knife.

- For larger lesions, use a small curet to open the area in line with its fibers to release the calcification. Place a small, full-radius resector over the lesion to suction the pasty material from the cuff and lightly debride this area to stimulate a healthy response. Repair of the small partial tear usually is unnecessary.
- If there is evidence of impingement with fraying of the undersurface of the acromion and its counterpart near the rotator cuff, perform arthroscopic acromioplasty.
- Approach calcification of the subscapularis tendon through an anterolateral portal to view the subscapularis bursa and subscapularis tendon. Use the standard anterior portal to place a full-radius resector down into the bursa into the site of the subscapularis tendon inflammation, and lightly debride and release the calcification.

POSTOPERATIVE CARE Active-assisted range-of-motion exercises are used to regain full motion as quickly as possible. As symptoms subside, progressive strengthening exercises for the cuff are performed, avoiding exercises in the impingement position.

OSTEOARTHRITIS

Weinstein et al. reported 25 patients with arthroscopic debridement for degenerative arthritis. Treatment consisted of lavage, removal of loose bodies, debridement of degenerative labral tears and chondral lesions, and debridement of partial rotator cuff tears. They reported 80% good results and 20% unsatisfactory results when evaluating pain relief, function, and range of motion. At an average follow-up of 34 months, 76% of patients maintained pain relief.

This technique (Fig. 4.55) may be beneficial in patients in whom conservative therapy has failed but who are not candidates for total joint arthroplasty. The best results may be expected in patients who have had a recent exacerbation of symptoms as opposed to patients who have had a gradual, long-term, progressive worsening of the condition. Few studies specific to microfracture of the glenoid and humeral head are available, but, as in other joints, best results can be expected for local unipolar defects in patients younger than 50 years of age. Small humeral head defects fare better than glenoid defects. For glenoid defects associated with a Bankart lesion, advancement of the labrum to cover or decrease the size of the defect can be used. Aggressive microfracture will cause a stress riser in the glenoid and should be avoided.

POSTERIOR OSSIFICATION OF THE SHOULDER (BENNETT LESION)

The Bennett lesion was originally believed to be calcification caused by a traction injury in the area of the triceps tendon insertion. Ferrari et al. described the arthroscopic findings in seven pitchers with Bennett lesions, all of whom had posterior intraarticular changes, including posterior labral injury and posterior undersurface rotator cuff damage. The extraarticular calcification seen on radiography was not visible arthroscopically and was not treated. The frayed labrum and rotator cuff were debrided, and a rehabilitation program was started. Six of the seven athletes were able to return to preinjury levels of competition. Warren suggested that in athletes with evidence of posterior labral injury some may have a partially detached posterior capsule. This injury may be in the spectrum of lesions described by Burkhart and Morgan as a peel-back lesion associated with extreme external rotation in sports requiring overhead motion. They suggested reattachment of this posterior capsule to a "freshened" glenoid. If capsular attachment is necessary, the glenoid can be freshened with a full-radius resector through a posterior portal with the arthroscope in the anterior portal. The capsule can be approximated to the glenoid with an arthroscopic absorbable suture anchor technique using accessory posterior portals for instrumentation and an anterior portal for viewing or a posterolateral portal 1 cm anterior and lateral to the posterolateral corner of the acromion.

SPINOGLENOID CYST

In the past, treatment of a spinoglenoid cyst with associated suprascapular nerve symptoms focused on excision of the cyst with repair of the labrum. Most of the cysts are secondary to flap tears. A series by Youm, Matthews, and El Attrache evaluated 10 patients treated with arthroscopic decompression of the cyst and labral repair. All patients were satisfied with their treatment, and eight of the 10 had MRI evidence of the cyst completely resolving. All six patients who had external rotation weakness regained normal function and had normal electromyographic studies. It seems that decompression should be done when it can be safely performed while decorticating the neck and making a small puncture into the cyst, decompressing it at the time of repair. Nevertheless, the main part of the treatment has been shown to be a labral repair, and results are excellent with repair of the SLAP lesion.

SHOULDER CONTRACTURES

Shoulder contractures may be caused by trauma, surgery, or inflammation. Many of these conditions are preventable or treatable by intensive, goal-oriented physical therapy. A

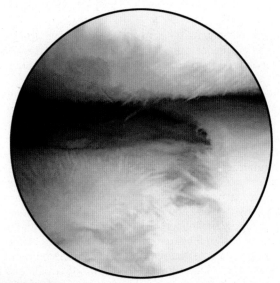

FIGURE 4.55 Arthroscopic debridement for osteoarthritis.

particularly troublesome form of contracture is that associated with diabetes mellitus. The presentation typically is one of gradual progression of idiopathic adhesive capsulitis owing to a marked thickening and loss of viscoelastic properties of the joint capsuloligamentous complex. Scarlat and Harryman noted that patients who had symptoms for more than 6 months were less likely to respond favorably to manipulation than were patients with posttraumatic or postsurgical stiffness. In our experience, patients with symptoms of more than 4 months' duration combined with rotation of less than 30 degrees and flexion of less than 100 degrees generally respond poorly to therapy. These patients and all patients with capsulitis should be monitored closely in therapy. If a patient is not gaining significant motion (10 to 15 degrees over 2 weeks) over a 4-week period, manipulation or surgical intervention should be contemplated early. Scarlat and Harryman recommended early prophylactic range-of-motion programs for patients with diabetes, particularly type 1, and early treatment with manipulation and complete arthroscopic release to prevent chronic painful symptoms. In their study, approximately 20% of the patients required early remanipulation, and these patients did best if the second procedure was done 3 to 4 years after the first. The guidelines listed in Box 4.3 can be used to approach the difficult problems associated with shoulder contractures.

BOX 4.3

Guidelines for Treatment of Shoulder Contractures

1. The patient must fully understand the potential surgical procedures, including open techniques, and the difficult postoperative course.
2. Initial portals are placed superiorly 1.5 cm below the acromion and 1.5 cm below the acromioclavicular joint. Sharp trocars may be necessary to penetrate the thickened contracted capsule carefully.
3. Selective arthroscopic releases may accomplish the following gains in motion (Bennett):
   Rotator interval: external rotation
   Inferior capsule: external rotation, flexion, internal rotation
   Posterosuperior capsule: internal rotation
4. Patients with diabetes require complete circumferential release if manipulation does not restore full motion.
5. Postsurgical contractures usually require a combined arthroscopic and open release. A subscapularis lengthening may be necessary to restore external rotation.
6. If arthroscopic visualization is poor, convert to an open procedure. If an arthroscopic release is to be performed in the 5-o'clock to 7-o'clock position at the inferior capsule, stay within 1 cm of the labrum and carefully separate capsule from muscle to protect the axillary nerve.
7. Postoperative pain control is obtained with interscalene block, passive range of motion, careful follow-up, and early 3- to 4-week reintervention with arthroscopic procedures when indicated.

CAPSULAR RELEASE

TECHNIQUE 4.30

(SCARLAT AND HARRYMAN)

- Begin by performing a bilateral range-of-motion examination with the patient under anesthesia and then attempt gentle manipulation.
- Make a posterosuperior portal after marking the surgical anatomy.
- Insert a tapered-tip trocar through the soft spot at the posterosuperior aspect of the glenohumeral joint. Use a sharp trocar to pierce the thickened posterior capsule if necessary, but immediately switch back to the blunt tapered tip before advancing into the joint.
- Advance the scope toward the rotator interval. In very stiff shoulders there is no room below the biceps tendon, but the scope can be advanced above the biceps tendon toward the rotator interval capsule.
- Use a Wissinger rod to create an anterosuperior portal from inside out. Alternatively, this portal can be made outside in by making a portal 1.5 cm anterior to the acromioclavicular joint and passing a sharp trocar through the rotator interval capsule under direct view. Insert a 30-degree arthroscope through the anterosuperior portal to view the posterosuperior capsule adjacent to the glenoid labrum.
- Retract the posterior cannula to release the contracted posterosuperior capsule using capsular release forceps. These forceps are specially designed to free the capsule from the subjacent rotator cuff musculature and to resect the thick capsule widely. The labrum should be left entirely intact. Some authors prefer electrocautery for the release.
- After the posterosuperior quadrant has been released, release the posterior capsule in an inferior direction as far as visibility allows.
- Exchange the arthroscope in position and excise the anterosuperior rotator interval capsule. To avoid additional bleeding, do not use a motorized shaver for debridement except for sucking out pieces of capsule. Next, resect the anterior capsule farther inferiorly, continuing with the middle glenohumeral ligament and extending toward the anteroinferior glenohumeral ligament. Alternatively, a 70-degree arthroscope can be used to assist in viewing the release in an inferior direction.
- Retract the arthroscope posteriorly to view the intact and contracted posteroinferior capsule.
- Use a spinal needle to locate a second posteroinferior portal for placement of a second posterior cannula.
- When portal access is established, insert the capsular release forceps and retract the cannula. Close the capsular release forceps and separate the rotator cuff musculature and neurovascular structures from the external surface of the contracted capsule before resecting the capsular tissue. Insert and retract the cannula alternately with the capsular release forceps. Use a suction shaver to extract tissue fragments effectively. Direct the cutting orifice of the motorized shaver toward the labrum to avoid nerve or vascular injury.

- Perform the inferior capsular release no more than 1 cm from the inferior labrum to avoid risk to the neurovascular structures. Use the maximal length of the angulated capsular release forceps to continue release of the capsule. As the release continues from posterior to anterior, the inferior border of the subscapularis is encountered. Continue the release into the anteroinferior quadrant. In this location, the inferior glenohumeral ligament is quite thick.
- Position the arthroscope to view the upper rolled border of the subscapularis tendon and place a second antero-inferior portal from outside to inside just above the subscapularis tendon. When the portal is established, use the anterosuperior portal for arthroscopic viewing and position the capsular release forceps through the anteroinferior portal to resect the inferior glenohumeral ligament from the deep surface of the subscapularis muscle.
- Completely release the thick capsuloligamentous structure until a direct connection is made between the anterior and posterior release. The humeral head does not drop inferiorly and does not fully rotate until the inferior glenohumeral ligament is completely divided.
- After the release has been connected circumferentially around the joint, finish with a synovectomy and wide resection of the capsular margins to prevent early scar formation and restricted capsular volume.
- When the intraarticular capsular release is complete, view the subacromial space. Usually, significant adhesion contractures of the humeroscapular motion interface are seen in patients with prior surgical intervention. These adhesions connect the deep surface of the deltoid to the rotator cuff, and because they prevent rotating or gliding motions, they limit the shoulder range.
- Through an axillary deltopectoral approach, perform a complete lysis of adhesions between the bursal surface around the proximal humerus and surfaces of the entire rotator cuff, coracoacromial arch, coracoid base, and conjoined tendon.

POSTOPERATIVE CARE A supraclavicular catheter is placed before surgery under ultrasound guidance. It is left in place for pain management for the first 48 to 72 hours after surgery. After surgery, the patient and family members are instructed on immediate active-assisted range-of-motion exercises to be repeated continuously throughout the day. Physical therapy for passive- and active-assisted range of motion is started within 24 hours.

We recommend reexamination within 3 weeks. The stretching exercises must be performed in all four quadrants, five times a day, with five repetitions of each stretching maneuver.

SUPRASCAPULAR NERVE ENTRAPMENT

Suprascapular nerve entrapment has drawn more attention in recent literature as a cause of persistent parascapular and posterior shoulder pain associated with massive cuff tears and traction placed on the nerve by the retracted cuff. Other causes of suprascapular nerve entrapment include ganglia in or around the suprascapular notch and altered anatomy of the notch involving transverse scapular ligament thickening and constricting bony anatomy of the notch. Lafosse et al. suggested that chronic pain and electrodiagnostic evidence of suprascapular nerve compression refractory to conservative management are indications for nerve release.

SUPRASCAPULAR NERVE RELEASE
TECHNIQUE 4.31

(LAFOSSE, TOMASI, AND CORBETT)
- Place the patient in a beach-chair position with the arm held in flexion and with 3 kg of longitudinal traction. Position the suprascapular nerve portal between the clavicle and the scapular spine, approximately 7 cm medial to the lateral border of the acromion. This portal is approximately 2 cm medial to the Neviaser portal. Warner et al. found that the suprascapular notch is approximately 4.5 cm from the posterolateral acromion. This portal is created under direct visualization through an outside-in technique.
- After inspection of the glenohumeral joint through the posterior portal, introduce the arthroscope into the subacromial space through the lateral portal. Use a shaver and radiofrequency device through the posterior portal to remove the anteromedial bursa and provide access to the suprascapular notch. Because swelling during the procedure adds significantly to the difficulty of gaining adequate exposure to the transverse scapular ligament, distal clavicular resection or subacromial decompression, if it is to be performed, should be done after the suprascapular nerve decompression.
- Once the anteromedial bursectomy has been completed, switch the arthroscope to the lateral portal. Create an anterolateral portal at the anterolateral corner of the acromion. This portal is optimal for completing the dissection of the transverse scapular notch with a shaver and radiofrequency devices.
- First, identify the coracoacromial ligament and follow its course to the base of the coracoid. Next, identify the coracoclavicular ligaments (conoid and trapezoid) by carrying the dissection posteriorly and medially. The medial border of these ligaments at the base of the coracoid defines the lateral insertion of the superior transverse scapular ligament. The transverse scapular ligament is identified as the medial continuity of the conoid ligament above the scapular notch (Fig. 4.56A).
- Once visualization of the transverse scapular ligament is adequate, use an 18-gauge spinal needle to guide the placement of the new suprascapular nerve portal through the trapezius at an angle orthogonal to the suprascapular fossa and slightly anteriorly toward the transverse scapular notch. The portal is located approximately 7 cm medial to the lateral border of the acromion and approximately 2 cm medial to the Neviaser portal. If the spinal needle is oriented correctly, the tip of the needle should be visualized immediately anterior to the anterior border of the supraspinatus muscle. Take care not to damage the spinal accessory nerve as it traverses near the medial border of the scapula; the portal should be more than 5 cm medial to the suprascapular nerve.

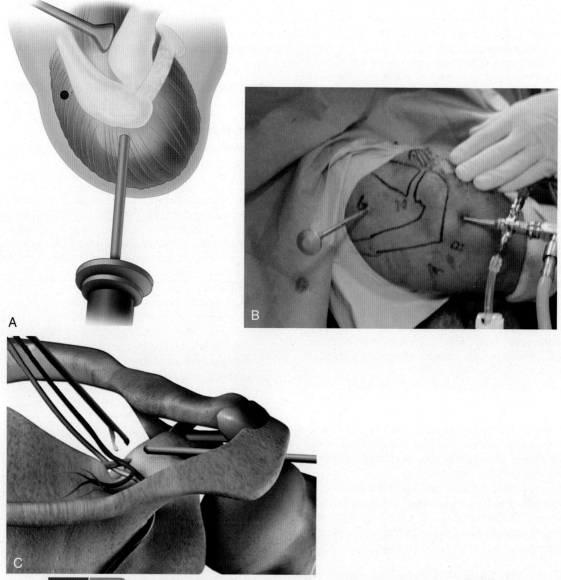

FIGURE 4.56   **A,** Superior view of portals for suprascapular nerve decompression (red dot, standard posterior portal). **B,** Portals on right shoulder. **C,** Portals and instrument positioning. Viewing through lateral portal, all other devices are passed through suprascapular nerve portal. (From Lafosse L, Tomasi A, Corbett S, et al: Arthroscopic release of suprascapular nerve entrapment at the suprascapular notch: technique and preliminary results, *Arthroscopy* 23:34, 2007.) **SEE TECHNIQUE 4.30.**

- Once the spinal needle has been appropriately positioned, use a knife to incise the skin and blunt dissection through the trapezius and surrounding soft tissues to the suprascapular nerve with a trocar. Use the blunt trocar to dissect the fatty tissues that surround the suprascapular nerve within the transverse scapular notch and to further clarify the borders of the transverse scapular ligament. The suprascapular artery is easily visualized superior to the ligament, and the suprascapular nerve is identified as it travels underneath the ligament (Fig. 4.56B). If necessary, use radiofrequency or shaver devices to enhance the dissection but be sure that the instruments remain superior

and lateral to the conoid ligament insertion at the base of the coracoid to avoid injury to the suprascapular artery.

- Once the ligament and nerve are identified, position the blunt tip of the trocar lateral to the suprascapular nerve within the transverse scapular notch to protect the suprascapular nerve during transection of the ligament. To perform the ligament release, make a second portal approximately 1.5 cm lateral to the suprascapular nerve portal to introduce the arthroscopic scissors. Release the transverse scapular ligament (Fig. 4.56C).

- After release of the transverse scapular ligament, assess the decompression with gentle manipulation of the suprascapular nerve within the scapular notch. If there is residual compression of the nerve, usually resulting from bony hypertrophy within the suprascapular notch, perform a notchplasty along the lateral border of the suprascapular notch with a burr.

- Close the portals with an absorbable subcutaneous suture.

POSTOPERATIVE CARE Patients are discharged on the day of surgery. They are instructed to wear a sling for the first 48 to 72 hours for comfort, although there is no structural reason to restrict activity. Pendulum exercises and active motion are encouraged on the first postoperative day, and patients are permitted to progress their activity without restrictions thereafter. Follow-up should be in 6 weeks and 6 months.

SCAPULOTHORACIC BURSECTOMY

Snapping scapula syndrome usually results from scapular dysfunction or dyskinesis, and 90% to 95% of patients have pain relief with conservative measures. Patients with persistent symptoms should be evaluated with MRI or CT for detection of any bony abnormalities. When secondary gain is ruled out and extensive conservative treatment fails, good results can be obtained with arthroscopic bursectomy and superior angle restoration by an expert arthroscopist.

TECHNIQUE 4.32

(MILLETT ET AL.)
- Place the patient prone and prepare and drape the operative extremity and posterior thorax in a sterile fashion.
- Place the dorsum of the operative hand posteriorly on the mid-lumbar spine, creating winging of the scapular and increasing the potential space between the scapula and chest wall for portal placement.
- Establish an initial viewing portal approximately 3 cm medial to the inferomedial angle of the scapula and insert a 30-degree arthroscope.
- Establish a second working portal using triangulation with the assistance of a spinal needle approximately 3 cm medial to the scapula, just caudal to the scapular spine.
- After diagnostic arthroscopy confirms bursal hypertrophy, use a shaver and radiofrequency ablator to clear inflamed bursal tissue and any fibrous bands in the area of the patient's symptoms as previously determined by preoperative anesthetic injections.
- Expose the superomedial angle of the scapula by careful partial removal of the underlying muscular attachments with a radiofrequency probe.
- Resect any bony prominence in this region with a shaver and high-speed arthroscopic burr.
- Place spinal needles outlining the border of the scapula to mark the extent of the planned resection. Use a high-speed burr to remove a triangular section of bone, typically 2 cm (anteroposterior) × 3 cm (mediolateral).

- Perform a dynamic examination of the scapula to ensure that no mechanical crepitation or other abnormalities remain.
- Close the portals and apply a sling to the affected extremity.

POSTOPERATIVE CARE Full range of motion is allowed, and early scapular protraction and retraction are encouraged. Return to activities usually can be permitted at 8 weeks after surgery.

COMPLICATIONS

Complications after diagnostic and operative shoulder arthroscopy are as uncommon as they are in other joints. The less frequent use of shoulder arthroscopy by the average orthopaedic surgeon may contribute to an increased incidence of complications, however. Portal placement for shoulder arthroscopy is more difficult than for the knee because there are fewer bony landmarks and more muscle mass to traverse. Maneuvering the arthroscope is more difficult in the shoulder than the knee because the joint is surrounded by thick layers of musculotendinous cuff and capsular tissue. New advanced procedures are being done by more surgeons, and in some procedures the learning curve may be quite steep. This in itself results in increased procedure failures and increased intraarticular damage.

Many potential arthroscopic complications can be eliminated before they occur by thoroughly examining the causes of recurrence. Treating bony lesions and hyperlaxity with standard arthroscopic techniques will certainly result in a high failure rate. In appropriately chosen patients in whom repair was obtained with good arthroscopic technique, the chance of recurrent instability is comparable with open techniques. Likewise, overconstrained joints usually can be avoided by carefully evaluating and choosing appropriate patients on whom to perform interval closures and plication procedures.

Neurologic injuries can occur from traction or pressure and are normally transient. Injury to the suprascapular nerve can occur because it resides less than 2 cm medial to the glenoid articular surface along the scapular neck, and the axillary nerve can also be injured because it is 3 cm or more from most portals. Care in marking landmarks and portal position is critical. Finally, the subclavian vein is within 1 cm of the 5-o'clock portal; thus, to preserve the vein and the integrity of the subscapular muscle, the portal is mainly a percutaneous portal for anchor placement. Although the neurovascular structures are at risk for injury with anterior portal placements that are too medial or inferior, neurologic complications seem to result more often from excessive traction on the shoulder and improper positioning. Paulos and Franklin reported an approximately 30% incidence of transient paresthesias in the upper extremity after shoulder arthroscopy using traction. Klein et al. reported a 10% incidence of transient paresthesias and palsies combined. They also used cadaver shoulders to study the strain on the brachial plexus that results from traction loads applied at various arm positions and to correlate this with visibility through the arthroscope. The most common arthroscopic shoulder position of 30 degrees of forward flexion and 70 degrees of abduction produced the highest average strain on the brachial plexus. They recommended placing the shoulder in either 45 degrees of forward flexion and 90 degrees of abduction or 45 degrees of forward flexion and 0 degrees of abduction to maximize visibility with minimal strain to the brachial plexus. We typically place the shoulder in 30 to 70 degrees of abduction with 10 to 13 lb of traction and have not had any significant neurologic sequelae.

Infection should be an infrequent complication because of the limited exposure, the rich vascularity around the joint, and the dilutional effect of the irrigating solution. Infection can occur, however, with violations of sterile technique. Careful preparation and draping minimize fluid leakage and contamination through the drapes to unsterile areas. *Propionibacterium acnes* is a low-virulence organism associated with shoulder procedures. Completely sealing the axilla with sterile gauze and sterile drapes helps decrease possible exposure.

Chondrolysis can be a severely debilitating complication. The risk factors are postarthroscopic infusion of local anesthetic, particularly in young patients when suture anchors are used.

Thromboembolic events have been reported in patients having shoulder arthroscopy. Kuremsky et al. reported a 0.31% prevalence in patients after shoulder arthroscopy. Deep vein thrombosis occurred in both the ipsilateral upper and lower extremities. Four of six patients had a pulmonary embolism and three of them had identifiable risk factors. Routine use of lower extremity serial compression devices may be beneficial, particularly if risk factors are evident.

Lo and Burkhart reported fluid retention and weight gain after arthroscopy as common, although transient, complications of shoulder arthroscopy. In a study of 53 patients, the average weight gain caused by arthroscopy fluid was 4.2 ± 3.8 lb (range: 0 to 14.5 lb). All of these fluid retention problems resolved rapidly postoperatively but could be a potential problem in a cardiac-compromised patient.

Currently, the most frequent complication of shoulder arthroscopy is failure of the procedure. Earlier stabilization techniques with transglenoid sutures had failure rates ranging from 4% to 40%. To prevent suture loosening and subsequent instability, appropriate tension should be placed on the sutures and meticulous intraarticular knot-tying techniques should be used. The surgeon should be skilled in the tying of two basic knot types—a nonsliding knot and a sliding knot. The nonsliding knot can be used for any application. The sliding variety is a good choice when the suture slides easily through the anchor and soft tissues. A variety of arthroscopic knots can be used, but the surgeon's or Revo knot is the standard, most secure knot with a tight suture loop and no slippage (Fig. 4.57). According to a study by Lo and Burkhart evaluating loop and knot security, locking-sliding knots such as the Duncan loop (Fig. 4.58), SMC (Fig. 4.59), and Roeder (Fig. 4.60) knots are secure when three reversing half-hitches are placed on alternating posts and are tied over the knot. The Roeder and SMC knots are locking-sliding knots.

When tying arthroscopic intraarticular knots, the initial knot should be either a slipknot with two half-hitches thrown in the same direction over the same post or a fisherman's knot (Duncan loop). The initial slip knot is secured by three reversing half-hitched throws over alternating posts. The post suture is held under tension while the knot pusher is used to tease the slip knot down securely; the hitch suture is pushed to the side and past the point of the knot to tie the throw securely. The post changes from one suture strand to the other

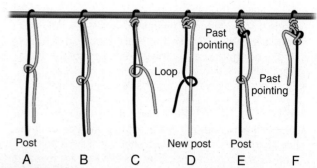

FIGURE 4.57 Revo nonsliding knot. Place knot pusher on post strand. **A,** Throw underhand loop (first half-hitch) around post, and advance loop into operative cavity, alternating tension on each strand until first half-hitch is tightened down on tissue to be opposed. **B,** Withdraw knot pusher while maintaining tension on post strand, and throw another underhand half-hitch around same post. Push it into joint until knot has seated. **C,** Maintain tension on post strand, and this time overhand throw around same post and push down into place. Tension knot by past-pointing, accomplished by passing knot pusher beyond knot sequence and applying tension on both strands while holding pusher in position beyond knot. Knot pusher is switched to second limb, which is designated as new post. **D,** Throw an underhand half-hitch around new post and tension. **E,** Switch knot pusher to original post, and throw an overhand hitch and tension. **F,** Alternatively, pull half-hitches into joint by placing knot pusher on loop strand ahead of loop and drag loop into position. Tighten knot by past-pointing on each loop. Cut tails of suture 3 to 4 mm from knot.

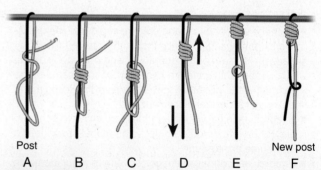

FIGURE 4.58 Duncan loop sliding knot. Verify that suture is free to slide and there is no evidence of twists or soft-tissue entanglements between suture and tissue to be apposed. Begin with two uneven parallel sutures, with post being half as long as loop as it protrudes from operative cannula. **A,** Grasp sutures between thumb and index finger, creating small loop by passing loop strand over post. **B,** Follow this by succession of four loops around post and loop strands. **C,** Pass tail of loop strand through original loop created, and pull on loop limb to tighten knot configuration. **D,** When it is tightened, gently advance knot by pulling on post. Maintain tension on post during locking sequence. Place series of half-hitches to lock this knot. **E,** Place first half-hitch on same post strand by passing it under post. **F,** Change post, and place opposite throw (overhand) over new post. Tension and advance into position. Continue sequence, alternating posts and direction of loop thrown to give total of three or four half-hitches on top of sliding knot to prevent slippage of this knot.

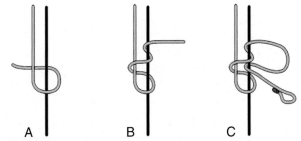

FIGURE 4.59 SMC knot. **A,** Underhand throw with loop strand under loop and post strands. **B,** Second underhand throw with loop strand under post strand. **C,** Underhand throw with loop strand under post strand behind second throw. (From Kim SH, Ha KI: The SMC knot—a new slip knot with locking mechanism, *Arthroscopy* 16:563, 2000.)

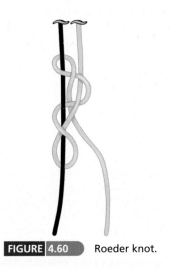

FIGURE 4.60 Roeder knot.

with each throw of the suture. This may also be achieved by alternating tension on the two suture ends; the suture tail under tension serves as the post suture. Recommendations of Loutzenheiser et al. are as follows: (1) always switch the post for every throw after securing the first half-hitch following a slipknot, (2) always reverse the half-hitch direction, over and then under the post, for each half-hitch throw, (3) use at least three half-hitches on alternating posts, and (4) reverse loops to secure slip knots. They also recommended practicing and examining pusher-tied knots for consistency before attempting them clinically.

Other important points for secure knot tying are as follows: (1) the suture must slide through the anchor eyelet, allowing for an initial slip knot; (2) the knot passer must pass all the way down the post suture without obstruction; and (3) no excessive tension should be placed on the soft tissue being sutured. Tension can be relieved by decreasing traction and internally rotating the shoulder and by placing a tension suture or grasper on the soft tissue while tying the suture. Absorbable monofilament PDS maintains 40% to 50% strength at 6 weeks but can elongate up to 30% when placed under tension. Although the PDS is easier for passing and tying knots, it also slips and elongates easier than nonabsorbable suture. We reserve its use for plication techniques and to assist in passing anchor sutures through the capsule.

As skill levels and understanding of the pathoanatomy have increased, the failure rates have come more in line with those of the open techniques.

ELBOW

Arthroscopic evaluation and treatment of the elbow have advanced in popularity and in sophistication. New portals and more advanced surgical techniques have been described, and a better understanding of the pathologic findings has been obtained.

INDICATIONS

Elbow arthroscopy has been found to be helpful in the following situations: (1) evaluation and removal of loose bodies; (2) evaluation and treatment of osteochondritis dissecans of the capitellum; (3) evaluation and treatment of chondral or osteochondral lesions of the radial head; (4) excision of osteophytes from the humerus and olecranon; (5) partial synovectomy, especially in rheumatoid disease; (6) debridement and lysis of adhesions around the elbow in posttraumatic or degenerative disease; (7) tennis elbow release; and (8) evaluation of a painful elbow when other diagnostic tests are inconclusive. Use of the arthroscope also has been described for debridement of inflamed olecranon bursae, stabilization procedures, and treatment of some intraarticular fractures.

Contraindications are few but include bony ankylosis or severe fibrous ankylosis that prevents safe introduction of the arthroscope. Previous surgery that alters normal elbow anatomy, such as anterior transposition of the ulnar nerve, also eliminates certain portals and may be a relative contraindication to arthroscopy. As with other joints, elbow arthroscopy should not be done in the presence of a periarticular infection.

PATIENT POSITIONING AND ANESTHESIA

Elbow arthroscopy can be done with the patient supine, prone, or in the lateral decubitus position on a standard operating room table. A tourniquet is used to control bleeding and is placed as high as possible on the arm to avoid crowding the operative field. Usually, general anesthesia is used because it affords complete muscle relaxation and eliminates intraoperative patient discomfort.

■ SUPINE POSITION

With the patient supine, the hand and forearm are placed in a sterile, waterproof stockinette suspension device connected to a rope and pulley system with 5 to 6 lb of weight for balanced suspension. The patient is positioned so that the arm hangs free off the side of the table, with the shoulder in neutral rotation and 90 degrees of abduction (Fig. 4.61). The elbow is flexed at 90 degrees. This position provides access to both sides of the elbow and relaxes the neurovascular structures in the antecubital fossa. The surgeon sits on a rolling stool with the elbow at chest level so that he or she can easily move to either side of the elbow (Fig. 4.61).

The monitor is placed on the opposite side of the patient, and 4-mm, 30-degree and 2.7-mm, 70-degree wide-angle arthroscopes are used. Maintaining established portals with interchangeable cannulas or cannulas with rubber diaphragms is essential to reduce the risk of damaging adjacent neurovascular structures with repeated passage of instruments and decreases fluid extravasation with its risk of neurovascular

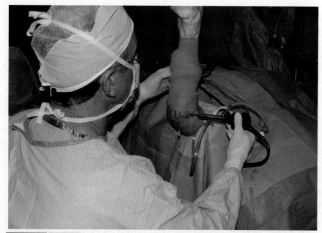

FIGURE 4.61 Setup for patient in supine position with elbow maintained in 90 degrees of flexion and shoulder in 90 degrees of abduction by overhead traction.

compression in the antecubital fossa. Use of a video-dedicated arthroscope also is recommended to decrease fogging. Inflow may be by gravity or by arthroscopic pump with low pressure at 40 to 50 mm. Throughout the procedure, the amount of fluid extravasation and the tension of the soft tissues, especially in the antecubital fossa, should be carefully monitored. If extravasation becomes excessive, the procedure should be aborted.

■ PRONE POSITION

Poehling et al. introduced the use of the prone position for elbow arthroscopy in 1989. They recommended this operative position on the basis of their impression that it improves arthroscopic mobility, makes joint manipulation easier, improves access to the posterior aspect of the joint, and provides more complete viewing of the intraarticular structures. The patient is placed prone on chest rolls, and a tourniquet is applied around the proximal arm. An arm board is placed parallel to the operating table at the level of the arm. The shoulder and proximal arm are elevated on a sandbag placed on the arm board. No traction is used, and the arm is positioned with the shoulder in neutral rotation and 90 degrees of abduction. The elbow is flexed 90 degrees with the hand pointing toward the floor. The surgeon stands with the operating table at chest level to prevent contamination of the dependent hand. The monitor and other equipment are placed across from the surgeon (Fig. 4.62).

After induction of anesthesia, the arm is prepared in the usual fashion and waterproof drapes are applied. After the arm is exsanguinated and the tourniquet is inflated, bony landmarks and portal sites are outlined with a marking pen: laterally, the lateral epicondyle and the radial head; medially, the medial epicondyle; and posteriorly, the olecranon tip. The most commonly used portals are the direct lateral, anterolateral, anteromedial, proximal medial, posterolateral, and straight posterior (Fig. 4.63).

■ LATERAL DECUBITUS POSITION

The lateral decubitus position for elbow arthroscopy was developed as a modification of the prone position. Placing the patient in the lateral decubitus position allows easy access

to the posterior compartment and maintains mobility of the patient for induction and maintenance of anesthesia during the procedure. The patient is kept in the lateral decubitus position with the help of a beanbag and kidney rest. The tourniquet is applied high around the arm, and the arm is placed over a bolster attachment to the bed. The bolster should be small enough to be out of the operative site and to allow the elbow to hang freely at 90 degrees of flexion with unobstructed access to anterior and posterior portals. Takahashi et al. advocated traction to assist in joint visualization. We have not used traction, but a small amount of manual distraction may improve exposure in some instances.

PORTAL PLACEMENT

The *direct lateral portal* is located in the lateral soft spot where elbow effusions are visible, palpable, and often aspirated. The portal is located in the center of the triangle formed by the lateral epicondyle, radial head, and tip of the olecranon. This spot can be precisely located by palpating the posterior articulation of the radiocapitellar joint. The portal is made just posterior and proximal to this joint. Instruments in this portal traverse skin, a small amount of subcutaneous tissue, the anconeus muscle, and the joint capsule. The elbow is distended initially through this portal.

The *anterolateral portal,* traditionally the standard diagnostic portal, usually is the first established after elbow distention. Anterolateral portals may include (1) the traditional distal anterolateral portal 2 to 3 cm distal and 1 cm anterior to the lateral epicondyle, (2) the midanterolateral portal just proximal and approximately 1 cm anterior to the palpable radiocapitellar joint, and (3) the proximal anterolateral portal 2 cm proximal and 1 cm anterior to the lateral epicondyle, as described by Field et al. These authors believe that this proximal portal is technically easier to establish and allows superior joint exposure compared with other anterolateral portals. The proximal anterolateral portal provides the safest distance from the radial nerve but can make instrumentation in the medial compartment more difficult than the midanterolateral portal. We no longer use the distal anterolateral portal because of its proximity to the radial nerve but prefer the midanterolateral portal (Fig. 4.64). The anterolateral portal traverses the extensor carpi radialis brevis muscle and passes beneath the radial nerve. Lynch et al. reported that instruments might pass within 4 mm of the radial nerve when the elbow is not adequately distended. If the elbow is flexed 90 degrees and maximally distended, however, the distance between the radial nerve and the cannula averaged 11 mm. Field et al. evaluated the distance from the cannula to the radial nerve with all three anterolateral portals. They found the distance to be greatest from the proximal anterolateral portal, averaging 13.7 mm with the elbow flexed; the nerve was an average of 7.2 mm from the distal anterolateral portal and 10.9 mm from the midanterolateral portion. All authors emphasize the importance of 90 degrees of elbow flexion and joint distention to move the radial nerve anteriorly out of the path of the trocar entering the joint. The skin incisions should be made carefully with a No. 11 blade, avoiding deep penetration to protect the lateral and posterior antebrachial cutaneous nerves. A small hemostat is used to spread down to the capsule before using a blunt trocar to enter the joint.

The *anteromedial portal* is located 2 cm distal and 2 cm anterior to the medial epicondyle. This portal approximates the medial extension of the flexor crease of the elbow

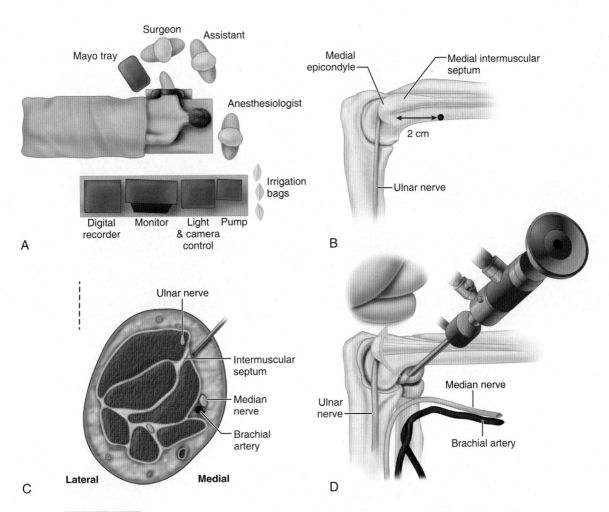

FIGURE 4.62 **A,** Operating room setup with patient prone on chest rolls. For added mobility, shoulder and proximal arm are elevated on sandbag. Tourniquet is placed on proximal arm. All equipment is mounted on portable rolling platform. **B,** Proximal medial portal is located 2 cm proximal to medial humeral epicondyle, just anterior to medial intermuscular septum. **C,** Cross-sectional view of proximal medial portal. Sheath and blunt trocar are inserted anterior to intermuscular septum and in contact with anterior humerus, directed toward radial head, avoiding injury to neurovascular structures. **D,** Proximal medial portal provides full view of anterior joint. Gravity protects median nerve and brachial artery.

(see Fig. 4.63A). It passes through the tendinous portions of the pronator teres and the radial aspect of the flexor digitorum sublimis before penetrating the medial capsule. Lynch et al. showed that cannulas pass a mean distance of 14 mm posterior to the median nerve and 17 mm posterior to the brachial artery when the elbow is flexed 90 degrees and the joint is maximally distended. The medial antebrachial cutaneous nerve and basilic vein are vulnerable with an incision deeper than the skin layer. These structures often can be transilluminated with the arthroscope in the lateral portal before establishing the medial portal.

The *proximal medial portal* (or supracondylar anteromedial portal) (see Fig. 4.63A), with the patient prone, has been recommended by Poehling et al. This portal is located 2 cm proximal and anterior to the medial epicondyle. It is imperative to palpate the position of the ulnar nerve before establishing this or any other medial portal. To avoid injury to the many cutaneous nerves, only the skin is incised longitudinally

with the tip of a No. 11 blade. The cannula is inserted anterior to the intermuscular septum to avoid injury to the ulnar nerve and should maintain contact with the anterior humerus to protect the median nerve and brachial artery. The cannula is directed toward the radial head during insertion. This portal allows better viewing of the entire elbow joint than the traditional anteromedial portal. If an anterior pathologic condition is identified, surgical instruments are introduced through an anterolateral portal.

To establish the two posterior portals with the patient supine, the elbow is flexed to 45 to 60 degrees to relax the triceps muscle and allow distention of the posterior aspect of the elbow joint. The *posterolateral portal* is located 2 to 3 cm proximal to the olecranon tip and just lateral to the border of the triceps tendon along the lateral supracondylar ridge (see Fig. 4.63A). If the posterior aspect of the radiocapitellar joint requires visualization and instrumentation, the portal for placement of the arthroscope should be made just proximal to

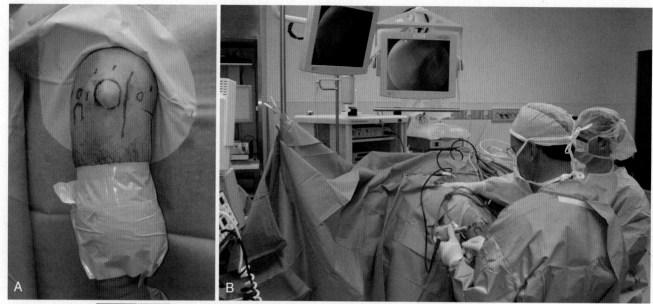

FIGURE 4.63 **A,** Portals are marked for arthroscopy with patient prone. Laterally, anterior midlateral and anterior proximal lateral portals are marked. Direct lateral portal also is indicated just posterior to outline of radiocapitellar joint. Medially, ulnar nerve and medial epicondyle are carefully marked. Flexor crease of elbow is noted. Proximal medial portal is made 2 cm proximal to epicondyle. Direct posterior and posterolateral portals are 2.5 to 3 cm proximal to tip of olecranon with elbow in 30 degrees of flexion and patient supine. **B,** Operating room setup for elbow arthroscopy with patient prone.

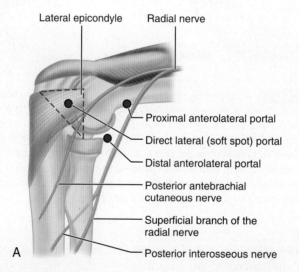

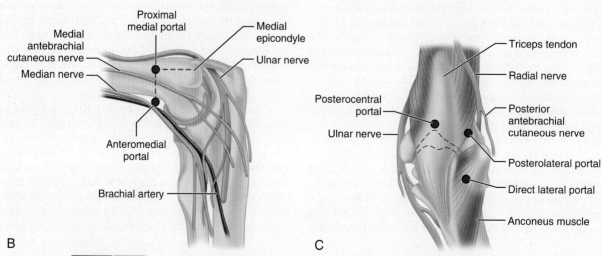

FIGURE 4.64 Portal sites on lateral **(A)**, medial **(B)**, and posterior **(C)** aspects of elbow.

the tip of the olecranon in line with the radial gutter, whereas instrumentation should be carried out through a direct lateral portal. The posterior antebrachial and the lateral brachial cutaneous nerves are at risk with deep incisions. The ulnar nerve is 2.5 cm medial to the center of the elbow joint and can be damaged if the cannula passes too far medially.

The *straight posterior portal* is placed 2 to 3 cm proximal to the olecranon tip and approximately 2 cm medial to the posterolateral portal, with the patient supine and the elbow at 45 degrees of flexion. With the patient prone and the elbow in 90 degrees of flexion, the portals are made 2 to 3 proximal to the olecranon tip centered in the triceps tendon (see Fig. 4.63A). It is used if a second operative portal is needed posteriorly. The ulnar nerve is at risk if the portal is placed too far medially. The portal is established under direct vision with the arthroscope in the direct lateral or posterolateral portal. Appropriate position of the portal can be confirmed by placement of a spinal needle. In severely arthrofibrotic elbows, sometimes the direct posterior portal can be established more easily than the posterolateral portal and use of a 2.7-mm arthroscope can make entrance to the posterior compartment easier. An accessory posterior "retractor" portal 2 cm more proximally can be made to place a Howarth elevator. Likewise, anteromedial or anterolateral retractor portals can be made 2 to 3 cm proximal to their respective arthroscopy portals.

EVALUATION OF THE ELBOW

ARTHROSCOPIC ELBOW EXAMINATION
TECHNIQUE 4.33

ANTERIOR PORTAL
- Begin by distending the elbow joint. Insert an 18-gauge spinal needle at the direct lateral portal, and aim it directly toward the center of the joint. The needle passes between the olecranon, radial head, and distal humerus. Avoid extending it too far anteriorly and entering the soft tissues in the antecubital fossa. Extraarticular swelling from infiltration of irrigant into these anterior soft tissues can collapse the anterior joint space. Using a 60-mL syringe and connective tubing, distend the elbow with fluid. Free backflow of fluid confirms proper intraarticular location of the needle. Maximally distend the joint with 20 mL of fluid to displace the neurovascular structures anteriorly in the antecubital fossa and to increase the space available in the anterior aspect of the joint.
- Leaving the first needle in place and maintaining distention, insert a second 18-gauge spinal needle through the midanterolateral portal. Aim this needle toward the center of the joint; free backflow of the solution confirms an intraarticular location.
- Remove the needle and incise the skin with the tip of a No. 11 blade by pulling the skin against the cutting edge. Use a mosquito hemostat to dissect bluntly down to the fascia to minimize the chance of injury to cutaneous or radial nerves (Fig. 4.65).

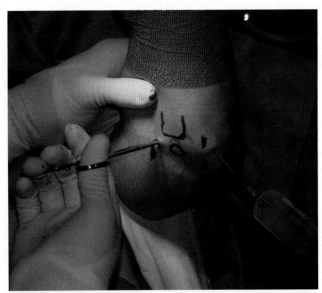

FIGURE 4.65 Hemostat being used for blunt dissection down to joint capsule with elbow distention through direct lateral portal. **SEE TECHNIQUE 4.32.**

- Pass the arthroscopy cannula with a blunt trocar along the same course as the needle, just proximal and anterior to the radiocapitellar articulation. Use the trocar to capture the joint capsule laterally; increase the angle of insertion to approximately 70 degrees to horizontal, moving toward the center of the joint. It is important to prevent the trocar from skiving more medially before penetrating the joint capsule. If this occurs, viewing and instrumentation from the anterolateral portal are compromised.
- Insert the arthroscope through this cannula with inflow through the arthroscope. This portal allows examination of the coronoid process of the ulna and the trochlear ridge (Fig. 4.66A).
- Examine the capsule medial to the articulation. Timmerman and Andrews showed that the anterior 10% to 15% of the anterior bundle of the ulnar collateral ligament can be seen in some elbows. Synovitis or capsular damage in this area may indicate medial instability. Confirm instability by releasing traction, supinating the forearm, and applying valgus stress to the elbow at varying degrees of flexion from 30 to 90 degrees. According to Andrews and Baumgarten, opening of the joint medially of more than 1 mm indicates medial laxity. Flexing and extending the elbow also allows viewing of the trochlea. Retracting the arthroscope brings the radial head into view, and the radioulnar articulation is viewed as the forearm is pronated and supinated.
- Turn the scope to observe the capsule and its insertion on the distal humerus. Observe the adequacy of the coronoid fossa. Embedded loose bodies, osteophytes, and adhesions may impinge the coronoid as the elbow is fully flexed.
- The anteromedial portal can be established with the Wissinger rod technique or under direct arthroscopic vision through the anterolateral portal. Some authors believe the anteromedial or the proximal medial portal should be

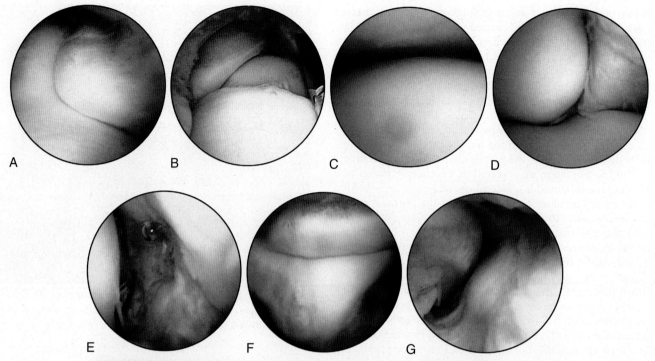

FIGURE 4.66   **A,** View of medial side of elbow with coronoid process on right and trochlea on left. **B,** Anterior aspect of elbow viewed from medial portal with coronoid and trochlea in foreground and radiocapitellar joint. Annular ligament is clearly seen. **C,** Radiocapitellar joint with varus stress applied to expose undersurface of radial head. **D,** With elbow flexed 90 degrees, patient supine, and 2.7-mm arthroscope in direct lateral portal, articulation of three bones is seen. Radial head is superior left, ulna is superior right, and capitellum is inferior. **E,** Bare area of olecranon is right inside with trochlea on left. Scope is in direct lateral portal. **F,** Posterior compartment viewed through posterolateral portal. Tip of olecranon is superior, trochlea is inferior, and olecranon fossa is in foreground. **G,** Medial gutter viewed through posterolateral portal with posterior aspect of ulnar collateral ligament on right and distal humerus on left. **SEE TECHNIQUE 4.32.**

established first in the manner described for the anterolateral portal.

■ With the Wissinger rod technique, push the arthroscope up to the medial capsule at the desired location for the medial portal, remove the arthroscope, and hold the cannula flush against the capsule. Insert the Wissinger rod and advance it until it tents the skin medially, incise the skin, and push the rod through the skin. Place a cannula sheath over the rod, and advance it into the joint. Remove the rod, and the portal is established.

■ Alternatively, an 18-gauge spinal needle can be inserted through the anticipated anteromedial portal site into the joint while confirming a satisfactory position arthroscopically. After the skin is incised and the fascia is reached with a hemostat, insert a blunt trocar following the same course as the needle, heading toward the center of the joint. Push the blunt trocar against the capsule where the exactness of the entry point can be confirmed proximal and anterior to the articulation, allowing maneuverability. Withdraw the arthroscope from harm's way before pushing the cannula while twisting back and forth to penetrate the joint capsule. This method prevents the cannula

from sliding anteriorly over the joint capsule and damaging neurovascular structures.

■ Leaving the cannula in the anterolateral portal, the arthroscope can be switched to the anteromedial portal to view the radioulnar and radiocapitellar articulations and the annular ligament (Fig. 4.66B). Extending the elbow reveals more of the capitellum, and pronating and supinating the forearm exposes more of the radial head. Chondromalacia of the radiocapitellar joint may develop as a result of repetitive trauma from throwing or racquet sports. Osteophytes and loose bodies likewise may form. By placing varus stress to the joint, the articular surface of the capitellum can be seen better as the elbow is extended (Fig. 4.66C). The annular ligament can be examined using the shaver tip or blunt cannula to lift the capsule anteriorly and distally over the radial head. The anterolateral capsule and gutter should be examined for synovitis. According to Andrews and Baumgarten, a synovial plica in the lateral gutter may be a normal finding. With repetitive trauma, this band may become thickened and fibrotic and may need to be excised. Slowly retracting the arthroscope and turning the lens toward the ulna reveals the coronoid process.

DIRECT LATERAL PORTAL

- This portal is made proximal and posterior to the radio-capitellar articulation, just posterior to the previously established anterolateral portal (see Fig. 4.63A). Use a blunt trocar to enter the joint carefully to avoid scuffing the articular cartilage. Become anatomically oriented by finding the two articulations and the posterior aspect of the radiocapitellar and the radioulnar articulations (Fig. 4.66D).
- Examine the concavity of the radial head articulating on the convex capitellum. Turn the lens to look anteriorly and gently move the elbow through flexion and extension to examine the surface of the capitellum. Examine for chondromalacia and any chondral defects producing instability and incongruence. Probe osteochondritis dissecans lesions through an accessory portal and evaluate the stability of the articular cartilage. Sweep the scope back posteriorly to the area of the two articulations.
- Examine the articulation between the olecranon and the trochlea. Small loose bodies may hide in this area. A normal bare area exists in the olecranon articulation at the site of the physeal scar (Fig. 4.66E). Follow the articulation proximally to view the posteromedial olecranon tip. Chondromalacia of the olecranon tip may progress to osteophyte formation, which is indicative of posteromedial elbow impingement. This spectrum of lesions is a continuum of a pathologic response related to medial elbow laxity from repetitive throwing.
- Sweep the arthroscope more proximally and turn the lens to observe the anticipated site of establishment of the posterolateral portal.

POSTE OLATERAL PORTAL

- The posterolateral portal can be established under arthroscopic guidance with the arthroscope in the direct lateral portal and the lens directed posteriorly. First insert an 18-gauge needle, aiming toward the olecranon fossa, and confirm a satisfactory position. If the direct lateral portal is to be a working portal as for treating an osteochondritis dissecans lesion, the posterolateral portal should be made at or just proximal to the olecranon tip in line with the radial gutter. A 70-degree arthroscope is inserted and directed toward the radiocapitellar joint for visualization. This allows separation of the scope and the working portal for easier triangulation.
- Incise the skin and use a small hemostat to spread down to the capsule. Use a blunt trocar to enter the joint. The arthroscopic view includes the olecranon fossa, olecranon tip, and posterior trochlea (Fig. 4.66F) and a portion of the posterior band on the ulnar collateral ligament (Fig. 4.66G). Loose bodies frequently gravitate to the posterior compartment, and osteophytes form on the posteromedial tip of the olecranon. Palpation along the ulnar nerve locates it immediately superficial to this posteromedial osteophyte, separated only by the joint capsule, and the proximity of this nerve should be considered when using motorized instruments or osteotomes posteriorly.
- If a second operative portal is needed, establish the straight posterior portal under arthroscopic guidance as described.

POSTOPERATIVE CARE Rehabilitation begins immediately. The patient is encouraged to move the elbow within the postoperative dressing as soon as pain and swelling permit. Flexibility and strengthening exercises are begun when pain and swelling are sufficiently diminished.

LOOSE BODIES

Removal of loose bodies probably is the most common indication for elbow arthroscopy. When symptoms of pain, catching, and limited range of motion persist, a thorough arthroscopic examination is indicated. According to Andrews and Carson, only approximately 38% of loose bodies are obvious on plain radiographs, and CT arthrography detects 72% (Fig. 4.67).

In addition to the location of the loose body, the site of origin should be identified. Osteocartilaginous loose bodies often result from osteochondritic lesions of the capitellum, osteochondral fractures as a result of lateral compression injuries, and synovial diseases such as synovial chondromatosis. Loose bodies may be embedded in the fibrous tissue in the coronoid, radial, or olecranon fossa and may be missed at arthroscopy if these areas are not thoroughly examined and probed. Release of the soft tissue with a shaver or arthroscopic scissors is necessary to free these loose bodies for removal. Small loose bodies may be found in the olecranon-trochlear articulation or in the radiocapitellar articulation. When large bodies are located in a difficult site for retrieval, they should be moved to a more easily accessible area. This can be accomplished through an accessory portal or by uncoupling the arthroscope from its sheath, rotating and pulling the scope back a few millimeters into the sheath, and using the arthroscope sheath to push the loose body to an accessible location. If turbulence is making loose body entrapment difficult, the inflow can be reduced or turned off. Occasionally, loose bodies are too large to be extracted through the arthroscopic portal; these can be broken using an arthroscopic burr and removed piecemeal, or they can be left in place until the rest of the arthroscopic procedure is completed and then removed through longitudinal extension of the capsular incision with a Kocher clamp (Fig. 4.68). This prevents extravasation of fluid into the anterior soft tissues during the remainder of the arthroscopic procedure and decreases the risk of neurovascular compromise.

PANNER DISEASE AND OSTEOCHONDRITIS DISSECANS

Panner disease is an idiopathic osteochondrosis with diffuse involvement of the capitellum usually occurring in patients 6 to 8 years old. With conservative treatment, this disease is self-limiting, and usually no residual joint problems occur. Osteochondritis dissecans develops in a more localized area in preadolescents or adolescents when the capitellum is closer to maturity and has less potential for healing and remodeling (Fig. 4.69). Osteochondritis dissecans has been related to activities involving repetitive compression and shear forces to the radiocapitellar joint, such as gymnastics, baseball pitching, racquet sports, and weight lifting.

Osteochondritis dissecans generally presents in the 10- to 17-year age group, with males being more frequently affected. Symptoms present as lateral-sided elbow pain, exacerbated

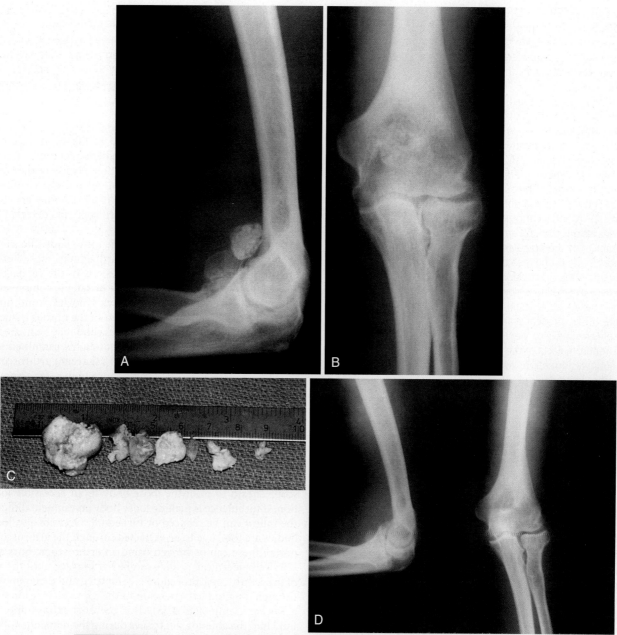

FIGURE 4.67 **A,** Lateral radiograph of elbow shows large anterior loose body and defect of radial head. **B,** Anteroposterior radiograph shows large loose body in coronoid fossa. **C** and **D,** After removal of loose bodies and resection of defect from radial head.

by repetitive loading activities, such as baseball pitching or gymnastics. Physical examination reveals tenderness over the capitellum with pain to active compression tests. Active compression testing is performed by resisted elbow extension while pronating and supinating with the fist clenched. O'Driscoll also described the radial shear test, with valgus stress applied during passive flexion and extension of the elbow, producing radial-sided pain or grinding. The presence of an effusion and loss of 20 degrees are poor prognostic signs according to Takahara et al. The examination is completed with a moving valgus stress test to evaluate ulnar collateral ligament stability.

Radiographic examination of the adolescent elbow should include anteroposterior views with the elbow in 45 degrees of flexion, extension, and a lateral view. Comparison views of

the opposite elbow also can be helpful for evaluating articular surfaces. MRI is the imaging modality of choice to determine the treatment course and to evaluate persistent elbow pain that cannot be diagnosed with plain radiographs. MRI findings of an unstable osteochondritis lesion of the capitellum are described by Kijowski and DeSmet as (1) a line of high-signal intensity deep to the fragment as seen on a T2-weighted image, (2) an articular fracture indicated by high-signal intensity passing through the subchondral bone plate, (3) a focal osteochondral defect, and (4) a 5-mm fluid-filled cyst deep to the lesion.

When determining conservative versus surgical intervention, lesions can be divided into stable and unstable as per Takahara et al. in his study of 106 patients with osteochondritis dissecans. Stable lesions that healed completely presented

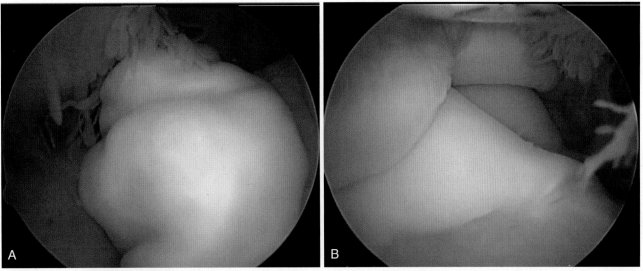

FIGURE 4.68   **A,** Large loose body in anterior elbow compartment. **B,** Anterior compartment after removal of loose body.

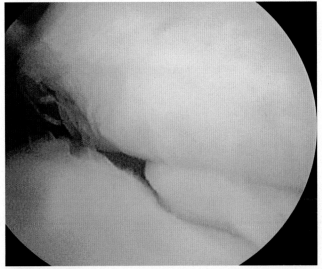

FIGURE 4.69   Partially detached osteochondritis dissecans of the capitellum.

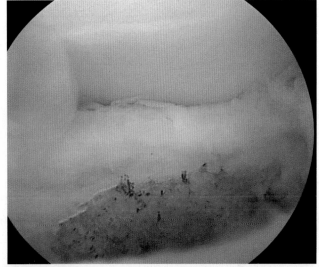

FIGURE 4.70   Microfracture of crater of osteochondritis dissecans lesion less than 1 cm in size with stable lateral rim.

initially with an open capitellar physis, localized flattening or radiolucency of the subchondral bone, and good elbow motion. Unstable lesions for which surgery provided better results had one of the following findings: a capitellum with a closed physis, fragmentation, restricted elbow motion of 20 degrees or more, or an effusion.

Our surgical guidelines for unstable lesions depend on arthroscopic evaluation, MRI findings, and Baumgarten, Andrews, and Satterwhite graded lesions as 1 to 5 arthroscopically: grade 1, articular softening; grade 2, fraying or fissuring but with the cartilage cap intact; and grades 3 to 5, degrees of disruption of the articular cartilage, with grade 5 being a displaced lesion. Likewise, the International Cartilage Research Society graded cartilage lesions of osteochondritis dissecans as 1 to 4, with grade 1 being intact cartilage, grade 2 being partially detached, grade 3 being detached but in the crater, and grade 4 being displaced from the crater. When arthroscopically evaluating the lesion, size, containment, and radial head

engagement of the lesion are important prognostic factors. Capitellar defects larger than 50% of the articular surface, loss of lateral buttress containment of more than 6 or 7 mm, or engagement of the radial head after debridement of the lesion are poor prognostic factors, according to Ahmad et al. They suggested that during evaluation of the engagement of the radial head the elbow should be placed in extension and pronated and supinated and then put through a full arc of motion to see if the radial head engages into the capitellar defect after debridement. With engagement, loss of lateral containment, or more than 50% involvement of the capitellum, either fragment fixation or, more commonly, osteochondral transfer is best to prevent further symptoms and the potential for further degenerative joint changes.

Follow-up studies of fragment fixation are variable. Most fragments tend to have chondral degenerative changes or minimal bone to provide secure fixation and thus most commonly are treated with either microfracture (Fig. 4.70) or

TABLE 4.9	
Treatment Protocol for Fragment Fixation	
Stable (Takahara; DeSmet—MRI)	Rest, controlled motion brace, follow healing at 6 weeks, MRI at 3 months, return to activity when healed and asymptomatic
Unstable—ICRS grading system	
Grade 1	Drill 0.062-inch Kirschner wire
Grades 2–4 Contained lesion, stable articulation	Microfracture
Grades 2–4 Unstable articulation, excellent quality cartilage and bone	Consider screw fixation; healing somewhat guarded
Grades 2–4 Unstable articulation, unipolar lesion	Osteochondral transfer
Grades 2–4 Unstable articulation, bipolar lesion	Debridement and microfracture, activity modification

osteochondral transfer, depending on the size and containment of the lesion. Our algorithm for a treatment protocol is shown in Table 4.9.

ARTHROSCOPIC TREATMENT OF OSTEOCHONDRITIS DISSECANS

TECHNIQUE 4.34

- Place the patient supine with the arm held in balanced suspension, with 5 to 6 lb of traction, the shoulder in 90 degrees of abduction, and the elbow in 90 degrees of flexion.
- Distend the elbow through a soft spot portal before making any other portals. Generally, five portals are necessary to fully visualize and treat the elbow in this condition.
- Make a midanterolateral portal using a spinal needle to enter the joint and a No. 11 blade to create the portal. A 4-mm arthroscope is used to view the anterior portion of the joint for loose bodies and to determine the extent of the osteochondritis dissecans lesion; it can be visualized if the elbow is placed near extension. An anteromedial portal can be used for probing the defect if necessary. Look for a pathologic plica above the lateral gutter that can cause popping across the edge of the capitellum; this should be resected with a shaver.
- Make a posterolateral portal just lateral to the tip of the olecranon and pass a small cannula with a blunt obturator so as to place it into the radiocapitellar area. Use a 70-degree scope to view the articulation.
- Using a spinal needle, identify the site for a direct lateral portal that should be placed at an angle that allows for

best manipulation and debridement or fixation of the osteochondritis dissecans lesion. Make an accessory lateral portal 1 cm ulnarward or 1 cm distal to the direct lateral portal if necessary.

- Resect the synovium and the fat pad in the area as well as any plica along the radiocapitellar articulation with a full radius resector. Fully visualize and probe the defect for continuity and to evaluate cartilage cap fragmentation. If the lesion is firm, stable, and just has some slight softening, arthroscopic drilling can be performed through one of the dual lateral portals.
- Use a 0.062-inch Kirschner wire to perforate the surface; a small drill guide should be used to protect the soft tissue while drilling. Perforations are spaced 3 mm apart to drill the entire defect.
- In the case of an unstable lesion, thoroughly evaluate the integrity of the articular cartilage, the amount of capitellum involved, whether the lesion is contained by a lateral buttress, and whether there is sufficient good-quality bone for screw fixation. In the rare instance that there is good-quality tissue of sufficient size to hold a screw, then a cannulated bioabsorbable screw can be inserted to secure the lesion.
- For grade II to IV defects with a contained lesion and a stable radiocapitellar articulation, debride the defect to a nice stable rim followed by microfracture. If there is a defect involving more than 50% of the capitellum with radial head engagement into the defect that results in catching and popping with pronation and supination of the arm and with the elbow in near extension or with flexion and extension, then perform an osteochondral transfer procedure as described in Technique 4.35. The osteochondral transfer procedure should be performed using an autograft from the intercondylar notch or from the lateral aspect of the lateral femoral condyle. This has been shown to be technically possible arthroscopically, but generally it should be done as an open procedure to get the precise smooth placement of the grafts in the capitellum.

POSTOPERATIVE CARE After drilling or microfracture of the elbow, early gentle range of motion of the elbow is started. The elbow is not loaded and neither are any strengthening exercises performed until full motion is obtained at least 6 weeks from the procedure. Return to activity from both of these procedures is in 3 to 4 months when symptoms have resolved and strength has been obtained. For osteochondral autograft transfer procedures, general range of motion is started early, with strengthening at 6 weeks and return to activity at 4 to 6 months when the graft has been incorporated.

OSTEOCHONDRAL AUTOGRAFT TRANSFER

Tsuda et al. described arthroscopic-assisted visualization and open osteochondral transfer in three nonathletes with osteochondritis dissecans of the elbow. Iwasaki et al. used a posterolateral column approach described by Mansat and

Morrey to perform mosaicplasty on eight patients who were baseball players. Seven of the eight had good-to-excellent results at 24-month follow-up. They used the Timmerman and Andrews scale, and their patients averaged improvement from 140 to 183 on a 200-point scale with 200 being normal. Yamamoto et al. reported 2-year follow-up in 18 teenage baseball players with osteochondritis dissecans who had an osteochondral transfer procedure. Nine had grade III lesions, and nine had grade IV lesions. Six of the nine patients with grade III lesions and eight of the nine with grade IV lesions were able to return to their previous levels of sports. They also noted that three of the grade IV lesions with wide defects had persistent evidence of articular irregularities on MRI at follow-up. At short-term follow-up, these lesions, which were associated with compression and shear forces from pitching, were satisfactorily treated with autogenous osteochondral transfers.

TECHNIQUE 4.35

(YAMAMOTO ET AL.)

- Perform arthroscopy of the elbow joint through the medial portal and inspect the joint cavity.
- Observe the osteochondritis dissecans lesions through a posterolateral approach or posterior approach.
- In the posterolateral approach, divide the anconeus muscle and extensor carpi ulnaris and preserve the lateral collateral ligament as much as possible. Separate the anterior joint capsule and expose the radiohumeral joint.
- In the posterior approach, fully flex the elbow and make a posterior longitudinal skin incision. Separate the anconeus muscle and joint capsule to view the osteochondritis dissecans lesion.
- The Osteochondral Autograft Transfer System (Arthrex, Inc., Naples, FL) is used for harvest and transfer of the osteochondral autografts.
- For grade IV or small grade III lesions, determine the sizes (using sizers) and numbers of the osteochondral grafts that would adequately cover the defect.
- Create the recipient sockets in the lesion with the recipient graft harvester. A cannulated drill can be used to create the recipient socket in a lesion with sclerotic changes by drilling to the base of the socket before insertion of the graft for bone marrow stimulation.
- Arthroscopically harvest osteochondral grafts of about 10 mm in length from the intercondylar notch of the lateral femoral condyle or lateral side of the patellofemoral joint.
- Measure the depth of the recipient socket with a calibrated alignment stick, match the length of the osteochondral graft, and transfer the graft. In grade IV lesions with a wide osteochondral defect, only part of the articular surface can be restored with this technique. For large grade III lesions, appropriate osteochondral grafts are transferred for the purpose of stabilizing the lesion.

POSTOPERATIVE CARE After surgery, a cast or soft splint is applied and worn for 2 weeks. Range-of-motion exercises are started at 3 weeks. Patients are allowed underhand tossing 2 months after surgery, and gentle overhand throwing is allowed after 3 months. Full throwing is allowed after 6 months.

THROWING INJURIES

Injuries to the elbow from throwing include compression and shear injuries to the radiocapitellar joint on the lateral side of the elbow, incompetence and disruption of the ulnar collateral ligament, and posteromedial impingement with osteophyte formation as described by Cain et al. and others. Loose bodies may be found anteriorly or posteriorly; small loose bodies may be found along the posterior radiocapitellar joint and the trochlear articulation. If elbow pain does not respond to rest and symptomatic treatment, MR arthrography is indicated. In young patients, radiographs of the elbow may show osteochondritis dissecans or physeal nonunion of the olecranon. In older patients, stress fractures of the olecranon may be found on radiographs or MRI. Arthroscopy is indicated when a pathologic process is found on MRI or when pain or inability to throw persists despite normal conservative measures.

EVALUATION OF ULNAR COLLATERAL LIGAMENT FUNCTION

The functional integrity of the anterior bundle of the ulnar collateral ligament can be evaluated by releasing traction on the extremity, supinating the forearm, and flexing the elbow to 70 degrees during arthroscopy. Valgus stress is applied to the joint as the ulnohumeral articulation is observed through the anterolateral portal. Normally, the ulnohumeral joint opens less than 1 mm with stress. Opening of more than 1 to 2 mm, according to Andrews and Baumgarten, indicates functional instability (Fig. 4.71). Incomplete undersurface tears of the ulnar collateral ligament, as described by Timmerman and Andrews, may not open to valgus stress. Ligamentous or capsular damage in the area of the ulnar collateral ligament may be present with these injuries. Treatment depends on the symptoms and the future goals of the athlete and is described in other chapter.

POSTERIOR ELBOW IMPINGEMENT

When a radiograph or MRI shows a posteromedial osteophyte, arthroscopic removal through a posterolateral and direct posterior portal is indicated. Careful, full evaluation

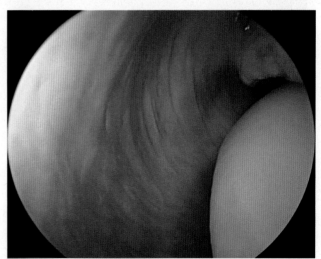

FIGURE 4.71   Arthroscopic examination showing medial instability to stress examination at 70 degrees of flexion. Note 2-mm opening between coronoid and trochlea.

of the elbow is indicated as previously noted. When resecting the olecranon osteophyte, studies by Kamineni et al. have shown that it is safe to remove the osteophyte and no more than 3 mm of bone at the tip of the olecranon. More aggressive removal of the tip of the olecranon results in increased stress to the ulnar collateral ligament and the potential for further problems.

REMOVAL OF OLECRANON TIP AND OSTEOPHYTES

TECHNIQUE 4.36

- Place the patient supine, prone, or lateral as desired.
- View the anterior compartments through proximal anterolateral and anteromedial portals. Posterior and posterolateral portals are used to perform the posterior procedure (see Technique 4.32).

- After fully examining the anterior compartment, turn attention to the posterior compartment. Observe the posteromedial and posterolateral gutters and radiocapitellar joint to ensure that there are no loose bodies.
- Remove any identified osteophyte of the tip of the olecranon with a small arthroscopic osteotome or small burr (Fig. 4.72). No more than 2 to 3 mm of bone should be removed.
- Smooth chondral lesions of the articular surface, and if exposed bone is encountered, use a microfracture technique.

POSTEROLATERAL SYNOVIAL PLICA SYNDROME

Posterolateral elbow pain, persistent pain, and popping with extension may be caused by osteochondritis dissecans, chondromalacia, or possibly synovial plica syndrome. Although rare, it is an entity that occurs in athletes from repetitive trauma to the outside part of the elbow, such as in throwing or golfing. Posterolateral pain and tenderness along the radiocapitellar joint and anconeus fossa area and pain on extension

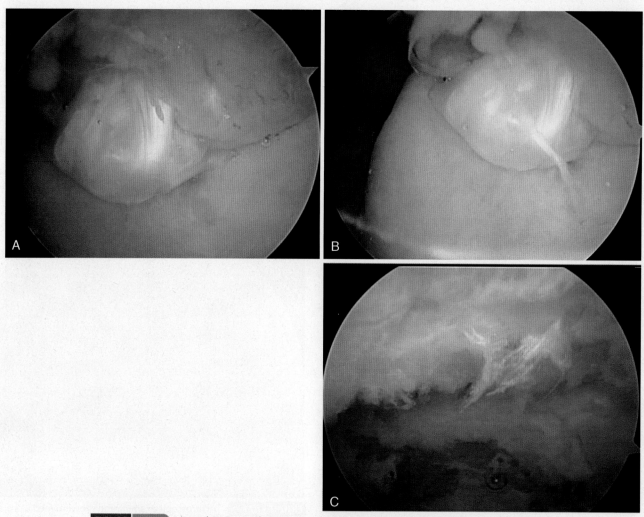

FIGURE 4.72 **A** and **B,** Osteophyte at tip of olecranon superiorly; trochlea is inferior in this supine patient. **C,** Tip of olecranon after osteophyte resection. **SEE TECHNIQUE 4.34.**

of the elbow with intermittent popping are best treated conservatively initially with antiinflammatory agents, relative rest, and a flexibility program. Intraarticular injection of cortisone in this area also can be helpful. Persistent pain despite conservative treatment may be an indication for arthroscopic examination of this area if an MRI shows evidence of thickening of the capsule of 3 mm on axial views indicating a pathologic plica of the posterolateral compartment. Posterolateral pain also may be caused by posttraumatic instability and should be thoroughly evaluated with preoperative and arthroscopic provocative tests for instability.

RESECTION OF THICKENED PATHOLOGIC SYNOVIAL PLICA

TECHNIQUE 4.37

- Examine the elbow anteriorly and posteriorly using multiple portals. The anterolateral aspect of the elbow is visualized through an anteromedial portal.
- If a pathologic catching or popping of plica is noted when the radiocapitellar joint is evaluated, debride the joint and shave the thickened plica through an anterolateral portal. Evaluate the posterior compartment of the radiocapitellar joint through a posterolateral portal with a 70-degree, 2.7-mm arthroscope. Resect the thickened pathologic tissue using a shaver or small basket through a direct lateral portal.

POSTOPERATIVE CARE Postoperatively, the patient is placed in a sling for 3 to 5 days to allow settling of the elbow, and early active range of motion is started, followed by a progressive strengthening program, starting at 3 weeks. Return to sports generally is allowed in 2 to 3 months.

RADIAL HEAD RESECTION

Radial head resection may be indicated for malunited head fractures or for painful arthritic changes. The radial head and a portion of the neck can be resected using an arthroscopic burr in the anterolateral portal and the arthroscope in the anteromedial portal. The radial head is removed in a piecemeal fashion past the level of the sigmoid notch of the ulna. A partial synovectomy may be necessary to adequately examine the radial head and the annular ligament, which should be left intact. After resection is completed, the forearm is pronated and supinated as the elbow is moved through a range of motion to ensure that no impingement occurs.

ARTHROFIBROSIS

Arthrofibrosis is a relatively common complication of elbow fractures and dislocations. For patients with mild symptoms, aggressive conservative treatment, including physical therapy and orthoses, may be sufficient; however, in patients with severe involvement, surgery generally is indicated. Good results can be obtained using arthroscopic treatment. In arthrofibrotic elbows, however, the ability to distend the joint capsule and to identify normal anatomic landmarks may be compromised. When performing procedures on arthrofibrotic elbows, a thorough familiarity with elbow arthroscopy and elbow anatomy is necessary. One should be prepared to perform an open procedure if adequate vision cannot be obtained. Delayed-onset ulnar neuritis may occur following release. Blonna et al. described delayed-onset ulnar neuritis in 11% of 235 patients with release of elbow contractures. A rapid-onset form of sensorimotor deficit and motion loss occurred in the first week in 60% of those with delayed-onset neuritis; these were treated with urgent nerve transfer. The rest of the patients had mild, nonprogressive or slowly progressive sensory changes. Risk factors were heterotopic ossification, preoperative neuropathy, and preoperative arc of motion of less than 100% flexion. Ulnar nerve release or transfer should be performed to prevent delayed-onset neuritis.

ARTHROSCOPY FOR ARTHROFIBROSIS

TECHNIQUE 4.38

(PHILLIPS AND STRASBURGER)

- After the usual portals have been established, distend the joint with sterile lactated Ringer solution through the soft spot (direct lateral) portal at the center of the triangle formed by the radial head, the lateral epicondyle, and the tip of the olecranon.
- Insert a spinal needle medially and posteriorly toward the center of the elbow joint to confirm the midanterolateral portal.
- Using a No. 11 blade, make a skin incision and use small hemostats to dissect the soft tissues down to the area of the joint capsule, avoiding injury to the antecubital cutaneous nerve.
- Enter the joint with a blunt trocar. Using the trocar, "capture" the capsule just anterior and proximal to the capitellum, with the cannula directed toward the center of the joint. Palpate the joint itself with the trocar to confirm entry into the joint. In an arthrofibrotic joint, the area of vision may be very limited initially, and the position of the portal and intraarticular placement of the trocar must be carefully evaluated.
- Make the medial portal under direct vision using a spinal needle. To increase visibility, place a 4.5-mm full-radius resector through the anteromedial portal and carefully resect the fibrotic tissue from the anterior part of the joint (Fig. 4.73A).
- Remove any loose bodies and fully debride the anterior fibrous tissue, using a combination of a full-radius resector and electrocautery through the anteromedial and anterolateral portals (Fig. 4.73B).
- Re-create the coronoid fossa using the resector, and, if necessary, resect bony hypertrophy from the area with a burr. Relieve impingement of the coronoid by partially resecting its tip (Fig. 4.73C). Ensure that the radioulnar joint is free of bony and soft-tissue impingement and that all loose bodies are removed.

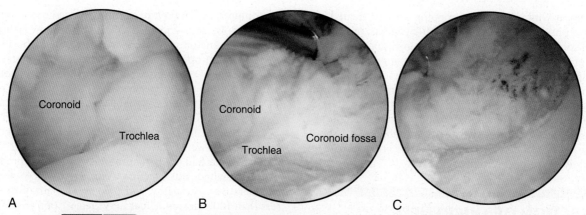

FIGURE 4.73   **A,** Arthrofibrotic joint with coronoid on left and trochlea on right and extensive fibrosis superiorly. **B,** After resection of fibrotic tissue and release of distal capsular insertion onto humerus. Coronoid fossa is filled by large osteophyte. **C,** Coronoid fossa after resection of osteophyte and recreation of fossa to allow elbow flexion. **SEE TECHNIQUE 4.36.**

- Use the resector to strip the capsule proximally off the distal humerus for approximately 2.5 cm proximal to the olecranon fossa until the posterior fibers of the brachialis muscles are identified proximally. Protect the muscle and the overlying median nerve. Complete the release using a small elevator and basket; to perform an adequate release, a 1-cm capsulotomy of the anterior capsule from medial to lateral is necessary. Do not stray distally where the radial nerve would come more into play.
- Debride the posterior compartment and remove loose bodies through a direct posterior portal and a posterolateral portal made under direct vision.
- After resecting the scar tissue from the olecranon fossa to improve visibility, change the scope to the posterolateral portal and place the resector or burr through the direct posterior portal to complete the procedure. Carefully release the contracture with a full-radius resector and use blunt mobilization to release the posterolateral and posteromedial gutters. Do not use the shaver in the area of the ulnar nerve, which is in close proximity medially.
- At this time, if you wish to expose the ulnar nerve through a small medial incision, use a posterior retractor portal made about 2 cm proximal to the direct posterior portal. A small retractor-elevator can be placed here and used to increase visualization and help prevent any injury to the ulnar nerve.
- Use an osteotome to resect any impingement of the olecranon tip in the fossa or osteophyte formation and complete the resection with an arthroscopic burr.
- To relieve bony hypertrophy creating impingement of the olecranon fossa, enlarge the fossa with a burr.
- When the procedure is complete, place a drain in the direct posterior portal and close the portals with nylon sutures.
- Manipulate the elbow to gain maximal motion and splint in maximal extension.

POSTOPERATIVE CARE The splint is left in place for 24 hours. Gentle active and passive range-of-motion exercise of the elbow is begun. A removable extension splint is worn between exercise periods. In patients with extensive posttraumatic arthrofibrosis and severe loss of flexion and extension, use of an elbow continuous passive motion machine may be helpful to maintain range of motion during the first 3 weeks after surgery. At 1 week after surgery a Joint Active System (Joint Active Systems, Effingham, IL) brace is used for 30 minutes three times a day for extension and flexion. Active and passive range-of-motion exercises are performed for 20 minutes four to five times a day at home, and supervised physical therapy is continued three times a week. An antiinflammatory drug is prescribed for the first 3 weeks to decrease inflammation and the risk of myositis.

OSTEOARTHRITIS

Arthroscopic debridement for osteoarthritis is as described for arthrofibrosis. Loose bodies and osteophytes are removed from anterior and posterior compartments, focusing on recreating the normal-shaped coronoid and olecranon tissue. Preoperative three-dimensional CT examination greatly improves the accuracy and reliability of bone resection and improves functional outcomes. Arthroscopic radial head resection can produce good pain relief and functional motion in patients with radiocapitellar arthritis and can safely be performed by an experienced arthroscopist.

SYNOVECTOMY

When indicated for rheumatoid arthritis or other inflammatory conditions of the elbow, arthroscopic synovectomy can be done using all the standard portals. The entire joint can be evaluated, and a subtotal synovectomy can be done with a full-radius resector (Fig. 4.74). Adequate vision should be maintained at all times using retractors when necessary. Care must be taken when working anteriorly to prevent damage to the neurovascular structures because often the capsule is thin. Posteromedially, a whisker shaver should be used if a motorized shaver is necessary. Lee and Morrey reported 93% good-to-excellent short-term results in 14 arthroscopic synovectomies in 11 patients. At 42 months, only 57% maintained these results, however. Four required total elbow replacement. These authors pointed out the importance of weighing the short-term gains against the potential serious complications from this procedure.

TENNIS ELBOW

Arthroscopic release for lateral epicondylitis has been shown to be safe in both anatomic and clinical studies (Fig. 4.75). Most patients are able to return to work within 2 to 3 weeks, and grip strength generally is nearly equal to that of the unoperated extremity. With appropriate therapy regimens, continued improvement can be expected for 3 to 6 months.

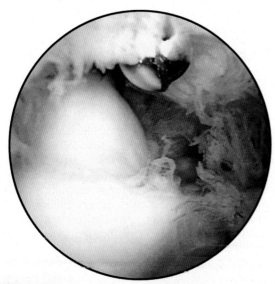

FIGURE 4.74 Extensive synovitis of anterior compartment in retired Major League pitcher with persistent pain, popping, and swelling of elbow. Partial synovectomy was done and loose bodies were removed.

ARTHROSCOPIC TENNIS ELBOW RELEASE

TECHNIQUE 4.39

(BAKER AND CUMMINGS)

- After intubation, place the patient prone on the operating table. Place two rolled towels longitudinally under the patient's thorax. Pad all bony prominences well. Position the affected extremity with the ipsilateral shoulder abducted to 90 degrees, and support the arm with a precut foam holder.
- After marking anatomic landmarks and portal sites, distend the joint with 20 to 30 mL of saline through an 18-gauge needle introduced through the direct lateral portal.
- Establish the proximal medial or superomedial portal, which is located approximately 2 cm proximal to the medial epicondyle and 1 cm anterior to the intermuscular septum. Introduce the trocar and sheath anterior to the intermuscular septum, maintaining contact with the anterior aspect of the humerus at all times as the trocar is directed toward the radial head. Insert a 2.7-mm, 30-degree arthroscope into the joint and perform the diagnostic portion of the procedure.
- After the pathologic tissue is identified, establish the superolateral portal with an 18-gauge needle through the lesion. Using a full-radius resector, excise the capsule to identify the undersurface of the extensor carpi radialis brevis tendon. View the origin of the extensor carpi radialis brevis.
- Using a curet and motorized shaver, debride the capsule and the pathologic tendinous attachment of the extensor carpi radialis brevis and decorticate the lateral epicondyle. Decortication of the lateral epicondyle and lateral epicondylar ridge can be done with an arthroscopic burr, handheld instruments, or electrocautery. Although a 30-degree arthroscope is adequate to view around the corner for most of the procedure, a 70-degree arthroscope may be required in rare instances.

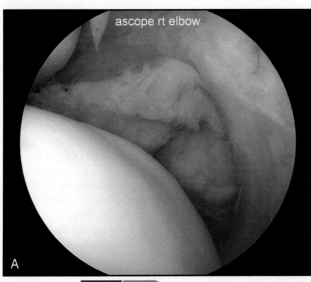
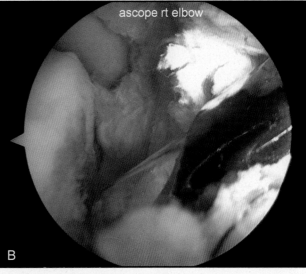

FIGURE 4.75 Tennis elbow release. **A,** Undersurface tear. **B,** Debridement and release.

- After release of the extensor carpi radialis brevis tendon and decortication of the lateral epicondyle, view the overlying muscle belly of the extensor musculature. Protect the lateral ulnar collateral ligament by limiting the amount of posterior resection.

POSTOPERATIVE CARE Postoperatively, the arm is placed in a sling with the elbow in 90 degrees of flexion. Gentle active and passive range-of-motion exercises are encouraged. The patient progresses to wrist extension-strengthening exercises and overall upper extremity rehabilitation exercises.

OLECRANON BURSITIS

Chronic recalcitrant olecranon bursitis generally can be treated effectively with a small open excision when necessary. Some surgeons have tried arthroscopic bursectomy in an attempt to circumvent healing problems. With the small number of studies and with complications similar to those reported for open techniques, the relative value of arthroscopic bursal resection remains to be determined.

ARTHROSCOPIC BURSECTOMY

TECHNIQUE 4.40

(BAKER AND CUMMINGS)
- After intubation, place the patient prone on the operating table. Make three arthroscopic portals: lateral, proximal central, and distal central. Use a standard No. 11 surgical blade and a hemostat to spread the soft tissue. Do not use medial portals because of the risk of injury to the ulnar nerve.
- Perform a total bursectomy, exchanging operative and viewing portals as necessary. Removal of the bursal tissue is complete when an increase in light can be seen through the skin and the triceps tendon and muscle can be seen. Excise only minimal subcutaneous fat. Remove spurs on the olecranon tip with an arthroscopic burr.
- Close the arthroscopic portals with 3-0 nylon sutures.
- Postoperative anesthetic injections rarely are used because of the need for an immediate neurologic evaluation. Apply a compression dressing.

POSTOPERATIVE CARE The compression dressing is removed at 7 to 10 days postoperatively. Mobilization of the extremity should be started immediately.

ARTHROSCOPIC-ASSISTED INTRAARTICULAR FRACTURE CARE

There are a few case reports of arthroscopic-assisted intraarticular fracture evaluation and treatment (see **Video 4.3**). Most commonly, arthroscopy has been shown to be beneficial in removal of small capitellar or radial head fragments. Radial head resection can be accomplished if a significant medial capsular injury has not occurred that might allow excessive fluid extravasation. Limited internal fixation can be accomplished with cannulated screws. In more extensive fractures involving significant soft-tissue injuries, the benefit of arthroscopy is outweighed by the associated risks. When contemplating arthroscopic fracture care, one should be fully prepared to abort the procedure when visualization is poor or fluid extravasation is significant.

PYARTHROSIS

Arthroscopic irrigation and debridement of periarticular matter can be used to treat early pyarthrosis. When extensive swelling and distention of landmarks have occurred, an open procedure is preferable. Cultures should be obtained at the time of debridement, and appropriate antibiotics should be instituted. A drain is placed in the anterior and posterior compartments. The drains are removed in 48 hours, and active range-of-motion exercise is begun if signs of infection are receding. If the infection has not improved, irrigation and debridement are repeated.

COMPLICATIONS

Complications of elbow arthroscopy are the same as for other arthroscopic procedures, including infection, instrument breakage, iatrogenic scuffing of articular surfaces, tourniquet problems, and neurovascular injuries. In a report from the Mayo Clinic, Kelly et al. noted a 1% incidence of true complications that adversely affected the outcome. They reported a 10% incidence of lesser problems that increased postoperative morbidity without causing long-term sequelae. Similarly low complication rates have been reported in children. Intravia and Mirzayan reported a 7.4% risk of nerve injury, the ulnar nerve being most commonly injured in children and adults. Arthrofibrosis and heterotopic ossification were other common complications.

Neurologic problems are the most commonly reported complications. Savoie and Field reported about a 3% prevalence of neurologic complications in a review of 465 arthroscopic procedures, most of which were transient injuries. Jones and Savoie reported one posterior interosseous nerve injury from an arthroscopic release. They recommended a more proximal lateral portal to increase the distance from the radial nerve. Horiuchi et al. reported arthroscopic synovectomies in 29 elbows. They noted that care must be taken when working anteriorly because of the thinness of the brachialis muscle; particular caution must also be exercised posteromedially. They did not try to perform a full synovectomy in this area, and they did not perform a capsular release. They started immediate range of motion in the postoperative period. As noted, the proximity of the nerves with the thinness of the capsule increases the risk for neurologic injury with this procedure, and it should be attempted only when proficiency in elbow arthroscopy has been obtained.

Various neurologic injuries have been reported, including transient low radial nerve and transient low median nerve palsies, neuroma of the medial antebrachial cutaneous nerve, and injuries to the ulnar, radial, and median nerves. Postoperative paresthesias and dysesthesias also have been reported, probably caused by the tourniquet, fluid extravasation, blunt trauma, or traction.

To prevent serious complications from elbow arthroscopy, surgeons should be familiar with the anatomy and perform procedures in accordance with their ability. Recommendations previously described in the text bear repeating. Recommendations for avoiding complications include carefully drawing anatomic landmarks, palpating the ulnar nerve location, obtaining adequate capsular distention, placing the elbow in 90 degrees of flexion, placing more proximal portals, not using pressurized infusion (low flow of 40 to 45 mL/min or gravity can be used safely), protecting the posterior interosseous nerve by pronation, using a retractor to lift the capsule away from debridement instruments, keeping instrument tips in view at all times, avoiding suction around nerves, and avoiding local anesthesia that can confuse postoperative evaluation.

WRIST

Indications and techniques for wrist arthroscopy are described in other chapter.

REFERENCES

SHOULDER

Abrams JS, Song FS: Arthroscopic repair techniques for massive rotator cuff tears, *Instr Course Lect* 61:121, 2012.

Abrams JS, Bradley JP, Angelo RL, et al.: Arthroscopic management of shoulder instabilities: anterior, posterior, and multidirectional, *Instr Course Lect* 59:141, 2010.

Accousti KJ, Flatow EL: Technical pearls on how to maximize healing of the rotator cuff, *Instr Course Lect* 56:3, 2007.

Acid S, Le Corroller T, Aswad R, et al.: Preoperative imaging of anterior shoulder instability: diagnostic effectiveness of MDCT arthrography and comparison with MR arthrography and arthroscopy, *AJR Am J Roentgenol* 198:661, 2012.

Adams CR, Schoolfield JD, Burkhart SS: Accuracy of preoperative magnetic resonance imaging in predicting a subscapularis tendon tear based on arthroscopy, *Arthroscopy* 26:1427, 2010.

Ahmad S, Haber M, Bokor DJ: The influence of intraoperative factors and postoperative rehabilitation compliance on the integrity of the rotator cuff after arthroscopic repair, *J Shoulder Elbow Surg* 24:229, 2015.

Ahmed I, Ashton F, Robinson CM: Arthroscopic Bankart repair and capsular shift for recurrent anterior shoulder instability: functional outcomes and identification of risk factors for recurrence, *J Bone Joint Surg Am* 94:1308, 2012.

Amirtharaj MJ, Wang D, McGraw MH, et al.: Trends in the surgical management of acromioclavicular joint arthritis among board-eligible US orthopaedic surgeons, *Arthroscopy* 34:1799, 2018.

Athwal GS, Sperling JW, Rispoli DM, Cofield RH: Deep infection after rotator cuff repair, *J Shoulder Elbow Surg* 16:306, 2011.

Bahk MS, Karzel RP, Snyder SJ: Arthroscopic posterior stabilization and anterior capsular plication for recurrent posterior glenohumeral instability, *Arthroscopy* 26:1172, 2010.

Barber FA, Field LD, Ryu RKN: Biceps tendon and superior labrum injuries: decision making. In Sperling JW, editor: *AAOS Instructional Course Lectures shoulder and elbow volume 2*, Rosemont, IL, 2010, American Academy of Orthopaedic Surgeons.

Barber FA, Herbert MA, Hap O, et al.: Biomechanical analysis of pullout strengths of rotator cuff and glenoid anchors: 2011 update, *Arthroscopy* 27:895, 2011.

Bedi A, Dines J, Dines DM, et al.: Use of the 70° arthroscope for improved visualization with common arthroscopic procedures, *Arthroscopy* 26:1684, 2010.

Beitzel K, Cote MP, Apostolakos J, et al.: Current concepts in the treatment of acromioclavicular joint dislocation, *Arthroscopy* 29:387, 2013.

Beitzel K, Sablan N, Chowaniec DM, et al.: Sequential resection of the distal clavicle and its effects on horizontal acromioclavicular joint translation, *Am J Sports Med* 40:681, 2012.

Bilsel K, Yildiz F, Kapicioglu M, et al.: Efficacy of bone marrow-stimulating technique in rotator cuff repair, *J Shoulder Elbow Surg* 26:1360, 2017.

Boileau P, Mercier N, Old J. Arthroscopic Bankart-Bristow-Latarjet (2B3) procedure: how to do it and tricks to make it easier and safe, Orthop Clin North Am 41:1381, 2010.

Boileau P, O'Shea K, Vargas P, et al.: Anatomical and functional results after arthroscopic Hill-Sachs remplissage, *J Bone Joint Surg Am* 94:618, 2012.

Boileau P, Parratte S, Chuinard C, et al.: Arthroscopic treatment of isolated type II SLAP lesions, *Am J Sports Med* 37:929, 2017.

Burkhart SS, Hartzler RU: Superior capsular reconstruction reverses profound pseudoparalysis in patients with irreparable rotator cuff tears and minimal or no glenohumeral arthritis, *Arthroscopy* 35:22, 2019.

Boykin RE, Friedman DJ, Higgins LD, Warner JJP: Suprascapular neuropathy, *J Bone Joint Surg* 92A:2348, 2010.

Carter CW, Moros C, Ahmad CS, Levine WN: Arthroscopic anterior shoulder instability repair: techniques, pearls, pitfalls, and complications. In Sperling JW, editor: *AAOS Instructional Course Lectures shoulder and elbow volume 2*, Rosemont, IL, 2010, American Academy of Orthopaedic Surgeons.

Chalmers PN, Erickson BJ, Verman NN, et al.: Incidence and return to play after biceps tenodesis in professional baseball players, *Arthroscopy* 34:747, 2018.

Ciccotti MG, Kuri JA, Leland JM, et al.: A cadaveric analysis of the arthroscopic fixation of anterior and posterior SLAP lesions through a novel lateral transmuscular portal, *Arthroscopy* 26:12, 2011.

Ciccotti MG, Neuman B, Boisvert CB, et al.: Paper #196: results of arthroscopic repair of type II slap repairs in overhead athletes: assessment of return to pre-injury playing level and satisfaction, *Arthroscopy* 27, 2011:e201.

Cohen SB, Valko C, Zoga A, Dodson CC: Posteromedial elbow impingement: magnetic resonance imaging findings in overhead throwing athletes and results of arthroscopic treatment, *Arthroscopy* 27:1364, 2011.

Cuff DJ, Pupello DR: Prospective evaluation of postoperative compliance and outcomes after rotator cuff repair in patients with and without workers' compensation claims, *J Shoulder Elbow Surg* 21:1728, 2012.

Davidson J, Burkhart SS: The geometric classification of rotator cuff tears: a system linking tear pattern to treatment and prognosis, *Arthroscopy* 26:417, 2010.

Dein EJ, Huri G, Gordon JC, et al.: A humerus fracture in a baseball pitcher after biceps tenodesis, *Am J Sports Med* 42:877, 2014.

DeLong JM, Jiang K, Bradley JP: Posterior instability of the shoulder: a systematic review and meta-analysis of clinical outcomes, *Am J Sports Med* 43:1805, 2015.

Denard PJ, Brady PC, Adams CR, et al.: Preliminary results of arthroscopic superior capsule reconstruction with dermal allograft, *Arthroscopy* 34:93, 2018.

Denard PJ, Burkhart SS: Arthroscopic revision rotator cuff repair, *J Am Acad Orthop Surg* 19:657, 2011.

Denard PJ, Lädermann A, Burkhart SS: Prevention and management of stiffness after arthroscopic rotator cuff repair: systematic review and implications for rotator cuff healing, *Arthroscopy* 27:842, 2011.

Diaz M, Shi B, Belkoff S, et al.: Open sub-pectoral biceps tenodesis: a biomechanics comparison of interference screw and various fixation techniques, *Orthop J Sports Med* 5(7 Suppl 6), 2017.

Dickens JF, Kilcoyne KG, Tintle SM, et al.: Subpectoral biceps tenodesis, *Am J Sports Med* 40:2337, 2012.

Dickens JF, Owens BD, Cameron KL, et al.: Return to play and recurrent instability after in-season anterior shoulder instability: a prospective multicenter study, *Am J Sports Med* 42:2842, 2014.

Di Giacomo G, Itoi E, Burkhart SS: Evolving concept of bipolar bone loss and the Hill-Sachs lesion: from "engaging/non-engaging" lesion to "on-track/off-track" lesion, *Arthroscopy* 30:90, 2014.

Dines DM, Moynihan DP, Dines JS, McCann P: Irreparable rotator cuff tears: what to do and when to do it: the surgeon's dilemma. In Sperling JW, editor: *AAOS Instructional Course Lectures shoulder and elbow volume 2*, Rosemont, IL, 2010, American Academy of Orthopaedic Surgeons.

Driscoll MD, Burns JP, Snyder SJ: Arthroscopic transosseous bony Bankart repair, *Arthrosc Tech* 4:e47, 2015.

Duerr RA, Nye D, Paci JM, et al: Clinical evaluation o f an arthroscopic knotless suprapectoral biceps tenodesis technique: loop and tack tenodesis, *Orthop J Sports Med* 6:2325967118779786, 2018.

Dumont GD, Fogerty S, Rosso C, et al.: The arthroscopic Latarjet procedure for anterior shoulder instability:5-year minimum follow-up, *Am J Sports Med* 42:2560, 2014.

Dunne KF, Knesek MJ, Tjong VK, et al.: Arthroscopic treatment of type II superior labral anterior to posterior (SLAP) lesions in a younger population: traditional repair versus biceps tenodesis with accelerated rehabilitation, *Orthop J Sports Med* 5(7 suppl 6):2325967117S00394, 2017.

Duquin TR, Buyea C, Bisson LJ: Which method of rotator cuff repair leads to the highest rate of structural healing? A systematic review, *Am J Sports Med* 38:835, 2010.

Duralde XA, McClelland WB: The clinical results of arthroscopic transtendinous repair of grade III partial articular-sided supraspinatus tendon tears, *Arthroscopy* 28:160, 2012.

Dzugan SS, Savoie FH, Field LD, O'Brien MJ: Arthroscopic treatment of combined lateral epicondylitis and posterolateral rotatory instability of the elbow (SS-51), *Arthroscopy* 27:e57, 2011.

Euler SA, Smith SD, Williams BT, et al.: Biomechanical analysis of subpectoral biceps tenodesis, *Am J Sports Med* 43:69, 2014.

Farmer KW, Uribe JW, Moser MW, et al.: Glenoid fracture after arthroscopic Bankart repair: case series and biomechanical analysis, *J Surg Orthop Adv* 23:155, 2014.

Faruqui S, Wijdicks C, Foad A: Sensitivity of physical examination versus arthroscopy in diagnosing subscapularis tendon injury, *Orthopedics* 37:e29, 2014.

Foad A, Wijdicks CA: The accuracy of magnetic resonance imaging and magnetic resonance arthrogram versus arthroscopy in the diagnosis of subscapularis tendon injury, *Arthroscopy* 28:636, 2012.

Forsythe B, Guss D, Anthony SG, Martin SD: Concomitant arthroscopic SLAP and rotator cuff repair, *J Bone Joint Surg* 92A:1362, 2010.

Forsythe B, Scott D, Martin MD: Concomitant arthroscopic SLAP and rotator cuff repair: surgical technique, *J Bone Joint Surg* 93A:1, 2011.

Forsythe B, Zuke W, Go B, et al.: Randomized prospective analysis of arthroscopic suprapectoral and open subpectoral biceps tenodesis: 1 year follow-up, *Orthop J Sports Med* 5(7 suppl 6):2325967117S00211, 2017.

Franceshi F, Papalia R, Rizzello G, et al.: Remplissage repair—new frontiers in the prevention of recurrent shoulder instability: a 2-year follow-up comparative study, *Am J Sports Med* 40:2462, 2012.

Friedman JL, FitzPatrick JL, Rylander LS, et al.: Biceps tenotomy versus tenodesis in active patients younger than 55 years: is there a difference in strength and outcomes?, *Orthop J Sports Med* 3:2325967115570848, 2015.

Gamradt SC: Short-term positive effects of platelet-rich plasma in arthroscopic rotator cuff repair, *J Bone Joint Surg* 93A:1, 2011.

Gerber C, Catanzaro S, Betz M, et al.: Arthroscopic correction of the critical shoulder angle through lateral acromioplasty: a safe adjunct to rotator cuff repair, *Arthroscopy* 34:771, 2018.

Gerber C, Snedeker JG, Baumgartner D, Viehöfer AF: Supraspinatus tendon load during abduction is dependent on the size of the critical shoulder angle: a biomechanical analysis, *J Orthop Res* 32:952, 2014.

Ghodadra N, Gupta A, Romeo AA, et al.: Normalization of glenohumeral articular contact pressures after Latarjet or iliac crest bone-grafting, *J Bone Joint Surg* 92A:1478, 2010.

Giles JW, Puskas GJ, Welsh MF, et al.: Suture anchor fixation of bony Bankart fractures: comparison of single-point with double-point "suture bridge" technique, *Am J Sports Med* 41:2624, 2013.

Gombera MM, Kahlenberg CA, Nair R, et al.: All-arthroscopic suprapectoral versus open subpectoral tenodesis of the long head of the biceps brachii, *Orthop J Sports Med* 3(Suppl 3):2325967115S00011, 2015.

Gottschalk MB, Karas SB, Ghattas TN, et al.: Subpectoral biceps tenodesis for the treatment of type II and IV superior labral anterior and posterior lesions, *Am J Sports Med* 42:2128, 2014.

Gowd AK, Liu JN, Cabarcas BC, et al.: Current concepts in the operative management of acromioclavicular dislocations: a systematic review and meta-analysis of operative techniques, *Am J Sports Med* 363546518795147, 2018, [Epub ahead of print].

Griesser MJ, Harris JD, McCoy BW, et al.: Complications and re-operations after Bristow-Latarjet shoulder stabilization: a systematic review, *J Shoulder Elbow Surg* 22:286, 2013.

Griffin JW, Cvetanovich GL, Riboh JC, et al.: Biceps tenodesis is a viable option for management of proximal biceps injuries in patients less than 25 years of age, *Orthop J Sports Med* 5(3 suppl 6):2325967117S0011, 2017.

Grumet RC, Bach BR, Provencher MT: Arthroscopic stabilization for first-time versus recurrent shoulder instability, *Arthroscopy* 26:239, 2010.

Hein J, Reilly JM, Chae J, et al.: Retear rates after arthroscopic single-row, double-row, and suture bridge rotator cuff repair at a minimum of 1 year of imaging follow-uup: a systematic review, *Arthroscopy* 31:2274, 2015.

Hirahara AM, Andersen WJ, Panero AJ: Superior capsular reconstruction: clinical outcomes after minimum 2-year follow-up, *Am J Orthop (Belle Mead NJ)* 46:266, 2017.

Hovelius L, Sandström B, Olofsson A: The effect of capsular repair, bone block healing, and position on the results of the Bristow-Latarjet procedures (study III): long-term results in 319 shoulder, *J Shoulder Elbow Surg* 21:647, 2012.

Huang AL, Thavorn K, van Katwyk S, et al.: Double-row arthroscopic rotator cuff repair is more cost-effective than single-row repair, *J Bone Joint Surg Am* 99:1730, 2017.

Jackson TJ, Hammarstedt JE, Vemula SP, Domb BG: Acetabular labral base repair versus circumferential suture repair: a matched-paired comparison of clinical outcomes, *Arthroscopy* 31(9):1716, 2015.

Jensen G, Millett PJ, Tahal DS, et al.: Concomitant glenohumeral pathologies associated with acute and chronic grade III and grade V acromioclavicular joint injuries, *Int Orthop* 41:1633, 2017.

Jiang CY, Zhu YM, Liu X, et al.: Do reduction and healing of the bony fragment really matter in arthroscopic bony Bankart reconstruction? A prospective study with clinical and computed tomography evaluations, *Am J Sports Med* 41:2617, 2013.

Kang HJ, Park MJ, Ahn JH, Lee SH: Arthroscopic synovectomy for the rheumatoid elbow, *Arthroscopy* 26:1195, 2010.

Kaplan K, El Attrache NS, Vazquez O, Chen YJ: Knotless rotator cuff repair in an external rotation model: the importance of medial-row horizontal mattress sutures, *Arthroscopy* 27:471, 2011.

Katthagen JC, Bucci G, Moatshe G, et al.: Improved outcomes with arthroscopic repair of partial-thickness rotator cuff tears: a systematic review, *Knee Surg Sports Traumatol Arthrosc* 26:113, 2018.

Keener JD, Wei AS, Kim HM, et al.: Revision arthroscopic rotator cuff repair: repair integrity and clinical outcome, *J Bone Joint Surg* 92A:590, 2010.

Khazzam M, Jordanov MI, Cox CL, et al.: SARL: Shoulder acronyms: a review of the literature, *Arthroscopy* 27:542, 2011.

Kim SJ, Jung M, Lee JH, et al.: Arthroscopic repair of anterosuperior rotator cuff tears: in-continuity technique vs. disruption of subscapularis-supraspinatus tear margin: comparison of clinical outcomes and structural integrity between the two techniques, *J Bone Joint Surg Am* 96:2056, 2014.

Koh KH, Kang KC, Kim TK, et al.: Prospective randomized clinical trial of single versus double-row suture anchor repair in 2- to 4-cm rotator cuff tears: clinical and magnetic resonance imaging results, *Arthroscopy* 27:453, 2011.

Kowalsky MS, Keener JD: Revision arthroscopic rotator cuff repair: repair integrity and clinical outcome: surgical technique, *J Bone Joint Surg* 93A:62, 2011.

Kuremsky MA, Cain EL, Fleischl JE: Thromboembolic phenomena after arthroscopic shoulder surgery, *Arthroscopy* 27:1614, 2011.

Lädermann A, Denard PJ, Burkhart SS: Mid-term outcome of arthroscopic revision repair of massive and nonmassive rotator cuff, *Arthroscopy* 27:1620, 2011.

Lafosse L, Boyle S: Arthroscopic Latarjet procedure, *J Shoulder Elbow Surg* 19:2, 2010.

Lafosse L, Boyle S, Gutierrez-Aramberri M, et al.: Arthroscopic Latarjet procedure, *Orthop Clin North Am* 41:393, 2010.

Lafosse L, Lanz U, Saintmard B, Campens C: Arthroscopic repair of subscapularis tear: surgical technique and results, *Orthop Traumatol Surg Res* 96S:S99, 2010.

LaFrance R, Madsen W, Yaseen Z, et al.: Relevant anatomic landmarks and measurements for biceps tenodesis, *Am J Sports Med* 41:1395, 2013.

Lee SJ, Min YK: Can inadequate acromiohumeral distance improvement and poor posterior remnant tissue be the predictive factors of re-tear?

Preliminary outcomes of arthroscopic superior capsular reconstruction, *Knee Surg Sports Traumatol Arthrosc* 26:2205, 2018.

Leroux T, Chahal J, Wasserstein D, et al.: A systematic review and meta-analysis comparing clinical outcomes after concurrent rotator cuff repair and long head biceps tenodesis or tenotomy, *Sports Health* 7:303, 2014.

Lim S, AlRamadhan H, Kwak JM, et al.: Graft tears after arthroscopic capsule reconstruction (ASCR): pattern of failure and its correlation with clinical outcome, *Arch Orthop Trauma Surg* 139:231, 2019.

Lopez-Vidriero E, Costic RS, Fu FH, et al.: Biomechanical evaluation of 2 arthroscopic biceps tenodeses, *Am J Sports Med* 38:146, 2017.

Lorbach O, Kieb M, Raber F, Busch LC: Comparable biomechanical results for a modified single-row rotator cuff reconstruction using triple-loaded suture anchors versus a suture-bridging double-row repair, *Arthroscopy* 28:178, 2012.

MacDonald PB, Altamimi S: Principles of arthroscopic repair of large and massive rotator cuff tears. In Sperling JW, editor: *AAOS Instructional Course Lectures shoulder and elbow volume 2*, Rosemont, IL, 2010, American Academy of Orthopaedic Surgeons.

MacDonald P, McRae S, Leiter J, et al.: Arthroscopic rotator cuff repair with and without acromioplasty in the treatment of full-thickness rotator cuff tears, *J Bone Joint Surg* 93A:2011, 1953.

Mall NA, Kim M, Keener JD, et al.: Symptomatic progression of asymptomatic rotator cuff tears, *J Bone Joint Surg* 92A:2623, 2010.

Marecek GS, Weatherford BM, Fuller EB, Saltzman MD: The effect of axillary hair on surgical antisepsis around the shoulder, *J Shoulder Elbow Surg* 24:804, 2015.

Mazzocca AD, Bollier M, Fehsenfeld D, et al.: Biomechanical evaluation of margin convergence, *Arthroscopy* 27:330, 2011.

Mazzocca AD, Cote MP, Arciero CL, et al.: Clinical outcomes after subpectoral biceps tenodesis with an interference screw, *Am J Sports Med* 46:1922, 2017.

McCromick F, Nwachukwu BU, Solomon D, et al.: The efficacy of biceps tenodesis in the treatment of failed superior labral anterior posterior repairs, A, *J Sports Med* 42:820, 2014.

McCormick F, Nwachukwu BU, Solomon D, et al.: The efficacy of biceps tenodesis in the treatment of failed superior labral anterior posterior repairs, *Am J Sports Med* 42:820, 2014.

McCrum CL, Alluri RK, Mirzayan R: Nerve injury with long head of the biceps tenodesis, *Orthop J Sports Med* 5(7 suppl 6):2325967117S00397, 2017.

McElvany MD, McGoldrick E, Gee AO, et al.: Rotator cuff repair: published evidence on factors associated with repair integrity and clinical outcome, *Am J Sports Med* 43:491, 2015.

McFarland EG, Selhi HS, Keyurapan E: Clinical evaluation of impingement: what to do and what works. In Sperling JW, editor: *AAOS Instructional Course Lectures shoulder and elbow volume 2*, Rosemont, IL, 2010, American Academy of Orthopaedic Surgeons.

Menge T, Horan MPM, Mitchell J, et al.: Two-year outcomes following arthroscopic treatment for snapping scapula syndrome, *Orthop J Sports Med* 4:7, 2016.

Menge TJ, Horan MP, RTahal DS, et al.: Arthroscopic treatment of snapping scapular syndrome: outcomes at minimum of 2 years, *Arthroscopy* 33:726, 2017.

Meyer DC, Farshad M, Amacker NA, et al.: Quantitative analysis of muscle and tendon retraction in chronic rotator cuff tears, *Am J Sports Med* 40:606, 2012.

Meyer DC, Wieser K, Farshad M, Gerber C: Retraction of supraspinatus muscle and tendon as predictors of success of rotator cuff repair, *Am J Sports Med* 40:2242, 2012.

Mihata T, Lee TQ, Hasegawa A, et al.: Arthroscopic superior capsule reconstruction eliminates pseudoparalysis in patients with irreparable rotator cuff tears, *Orthop J Sports ed* 5(3 Suppl 3):2325967117S00119, 2017.

Mihata T, Lee TQ, Itami Y, et al.: Arthroscopic superior capsule reconstruction for irreparable rotator cuff tears. A prospective clinical study in 100 consecutive patients with 1 to 8 years of follow-up, *Orthop J Sports Med* 4(3 Suppl 3):2325967116S00076, 2016.

Mihata T, Lee TQ, Watanabe C, et al.: Clinical results of arthroscopic superior capsule reconstruction for irreparable rotator cuff tears, *Arthroscopy* 29:459, 2013.

Mihata T, McGarry MH, Pirolo JM, et al.: Superior capsule reconstruction to restore superior stability in irreparable rotator cuff tears: a biomechanical cadaveric study, *Am J Sports Med* 40:2248, 2012.

Millett PJ, Gaskill TR, Horan MP, et al.: Technique and outcomes of arthroscopic scapulothoracic bursectomy and partial scapulectomy, *Arthroscopy* 28:1776, 2012.

Mohtadi NG, Chan DS, Hollinshead RM, et al.: A randomized clinical trial comparing open and arthroscopic stabilization for recurrent traumatic anterior shoulder instability: two-year follow-up with disease-specific quality-of-life outcomes, *J Bone Joint Surg* 96:353, 2014.

Moor BK, Bouicha S, Rothenfluh DA, et al.: Is there an association between the individual anatomy of the scapula and the development of rotator cuff tears or osteoarthritis of the glenohumeral joint? A radiological study of the critical shoulder angle, *Bone Joint J* 95B:935, 2013.

Moravek JE, Budge MD, Wiater JM: Current concepts in subacromial impingement and the role of acromioplasty, *Shoulder Elbow* 4:244, 2017.

Neyton L, Barath J, Nourissat G, et al.: Arthroscopic Latarjet tecniques: graft and fixation positioning assessed with 2-dimensional computed tomography is not equivalent with standard open technique, *Arthroscopy* 34:2032, 2018.

Nho SJ, Delos D, Yadav H, et al.: Biomechanical and biologic augmentation for the treatment of massive rotator cuff tears, *Am J Sports Med* 38:619, 2010.

Oh JH, Kim JY, Choi JH, et al.: Is arthroscopic distal clavicle resection necessary for patients with radiological acromioclavicular joint arthritis and rotator cuff tears? A prospective randomized comparative study, *Am J Sports Med* 42:2567, 2014.

Oh JH, Kim SH, Shin SH, et al.: Outcome of rotator cuff repair in large-to-massive tear with pseudoparalysis: a comparative study with propensity score matching, *Am J Sports Med* 39:1413, 2011.

Owens BD, Campbell SE, Cameron KL: Risk factors for anterior glenohumeral instability, *Am J Sports Med* 42:2591, 2014.

Park HB, Gwark JY, Im JH, et al.: Factors associated with atraumatic posterosuperior rotator cuff tears, *J Bone Joint Surg Am* 100:1397, 2018.

Park JS, Kim SH, Jung HJ, et al.: A prospective randomized study comparing the interference screw and suture anchor techniques for biceps tenodesis, *Am J Sports Med* 45:440, 2016.

Park MJ, Tjoumakaris FP, Garcia G, et al.: Arthroscopic remplissage with Bankart repair for the treatment of glenohumeral instability with Hill-Sachs defects, *Arthroscopy* 27:1187, 2011.

Pauly S, Kraus N, Greiner S, et al.: Prevalence and pattern of glenohumeral injuries among acute high-grade acromioclavicular joint instabilities, *J Shoulder Elbow Surg* 22:760, 2013.

Pennington WT, Gibbons DJ, Bartz BA, Dodd M: Comparative analysis of single-row versus double-row repair of rotator cuff tears, *Arthroscopy* 26:1419, 2010.

Peters KS, Lam PH, Murrell GAC: Repair of partial-thickness rotator cuff tears: a biomechanical analysis of footprint contact pressure and strength in an ovine model, *Arthroscopy* 26:877, 2010.

Petersen SA, Murphy TP: The timing of rotator cuff repair for the restoration of function, *J Shoulder Elbow Surg* 20:62, 2011.

Piasecki DP, Verma NN, Nho ST, et al.: Outcomes after arthroscopic revision rotator cuff repair, *Am J Sports Med* 38:40, 2010.

Plath JE, Feucht MJ, Bangoj R, et al.: Arthroscopic suture anchor fixation of bony Bankart lesions: clinical outcome, magnetic resonance imaging results, and return to sports, *Arthroscopy* 31:1472, 2015.

Ponce BA, Hosemann CD, Raghava P, et al.: Biomechanical evaluation of 3 arthroscopic self-cinching stitches for shoulder arthroscopy, *Am J Sports Med* 39:188, 2011.

Provencher MT, Arciero RA, Burkhart SS, et al.: Key factors in primary and revision surgery for shoulder instability. In Sperling JW, editor: *AAOS Instructional Course Lectures shoulder and elbow volume 2*, Rosemont, IL, 2010, American Academy of Orthopaedic Surgeons.

Provencher MT, McCormick F, Dewing C, et al.: A prospective analysis of 179 type 2 superior labrum anterior and posterior repairs, *Am J Sports Med* 41:880, 2013.

Rains DD, Rook GA, Wahl CJ: Pathomechanisms and complications related to patient positioning and anesthesia during shoulder arthroscopy, *Arthroscopy* 27:532, 2011.

Randelli P, Ragone V, Carminati S, et al.: Risk factors for recurrence after Bankart repair: a systematic review, *Knee Surg Sports Traumatol Arthrosc* 20:2129, 2012.

Rhee PC, Spinner RJ, Bishop AT, et al.: Iatrogenic brachial plexus injuries associated with open subpectoral biceps tenodesis, *Am J Sports Med* 41:2048, 2013.

Robertson WJ, Griffith MH, Carroll K, et al.: Arthroscopic versus open distal clavicle excision: a comparative assessment at intermediate-term follow-up, *Am J Sports Med* 39:2415, 2011.

Robinson CM, Seah M, Akhtar MA: The epidemiology, risk of recurrence, and functional outcome after an acute traumatic posterior dislocation of the shoulder, *J Bone Joint Surg Am* 93:1605, 2011.

Robinson CM, Shur N, Sharpe T, et al.: Injuries associated with traumatic anterior glenohumeral dislocations, *J Bone Joint Surg Am* 94:18, 2012.

Sahajpal DT, Blonna D, O'Driscoll SW: Anteromedial elbow arthroscopy portals in patients with prior ulnar nerve transposition or subluxation, *Arthroscopy* 26:1045, 2010.

Saridakis P, Jones G: Outcomes of single-row and double-row arthroscopic rotator cuff repair: a systematic review, *J Bone Joint Surg* 92A:732, 2010.

Schroeder AJ, Bedeir YH, Schumaier AP, et al.: Arthroscopic management of SLAP lesions with concomitant spinoglenoid notch ganglion cyst: a systematic review comparing repair alone to repair with decompression, *Arthroscopy* 34:2247, 2018.

Sears BW, Lazarus MD: Arthroscopically assisted percutaneous fixation and bone grafting of a glenoid fossa fracture nonunion, *Orthopedics* 35, 2012:e1279.

Seroyer ST, Nho SJ, Provencher MT, Romeo AA: Four-quadrant approach to capsulolabral repair: an arthroscopic road map to the glenoid, *Arthroscopy* 26:555, 2010.

Shaha JS, Cook JB, Song DJ, et al.: Redefining "critical" bone loss in shoulder instability: functional outcomes worsen with "subcritical" bone loss, *Am J Sports Med* 43:1719, 2015.

Shi LL, Mullen MG, Freehill MT, et al.: Accuracy of long head of the biceps subluxation as a predictor for subscapularis tears, *Arthroscopy* 31:615, 2015.

Shin SJ: A comparison of 2 repair techniques for partial-thickness articular-sided rotator cuff tears, *Arthroscopy* 28:25, 2012.

Shin SJ, Kim NKL: Complications after arthroscopic coracoclavicular reconstruction using a single adjustable-loop length suspensory fixation device in acute acromioclavicular joint dislocation, *Arthroscopy* 31:816, 2015.

Shin SJ, Kook SH, Rao N, Seo MJ: Clinical outcomes of modified Mason-Allen single-row repair for bursal-sided partial-thickness rotator cuff tears: comparison with the double-row suture-bridge technique, *Am J Sports Med* 43:1976, 2015.

Shon MS, Koh KH, Lim TK, et al.: Arthroscopic partial repair of irreparable rotator cuff tears: preoperative factors associated with outcome deterioration over 2 years, *Am J Sports Med* 43:1965, 2015.

Silberberg JM, Moya-Angeler J, Martin E, et al.: Vertical versus horizontal suture configuration for the repair of isolated type II SLAP lesion through a single anterior portal: a randomized controlled trial, *Arthroscopy* 27:1605, 2011.

Slabaugh MA, Nho SJ, Grumet RC, Wilson JB: Does the literature confirm superior clinical results in radiographically healed rotator cuffs after rotator cuff repair? *Arthroscopy* 26:393, 2010.

Smith CD, Dugas JR, Emblom BA, et al.: Biceps tenodesis in pitchers, *Orthop J Sports Med* 5(7 Suppl 6):2325967117S00212.

Sonnabend DH, Howlett CR, Young AA: Histological evaluation of repair of the rotator cuff in a primate model, *J Bone Joint Surg* 92B:586, 2010.

Spiegl UJ, Smith SD, Todd JN, et al.: Biomechanical comparison of arthroscopic single- and double-row repair techniques for acute bony Bankart lesions, *Am J Sports Med* 42:1939, 2014.

Strauss EJ, Salata MJ, Kercher J: The arthroscopic management of partial-thickness rotator cuff tears: a systematic review of the literature, *Arthroscopy* 27:568, 2011.

Su F, Kowalczuk M, Ikpe S, et al.: Risk factors for failure of arthroscopic revision anterior shoulder stabilization, *J Bone Joint Surg Am* 100:1319, 2018.

Tao MA, Garrigues GE: Arthroscopic-assisted fixation of Ideberg type III glenoid fractures, *Arthrosc Tech* 4:e119, 2015.

Tashjian RZ, Granger EK, Barney JK, et al.: Functional outcomes after arthroscopic scapulothoracic bursectomy and partial superomedial angle scapulectomy, *Orthop J Sports Med* 1:2325967113505739, 2013.

Tasaki A, Morita W, Yamakawa A, et al Combined arthroscopic Bankart repair and coracoid process transfer to anterior glenoid for shoulder dislocation in rugby players: evaluation based on ability to perform sport-specific movements effectively, *Arthroscopy* 31:1693, 2015.

Thomazeau H, Courage O, Barth J, et al.: Can we improve the indication for Bankart arthroscopic repair? A preliminary clinical study using the ISIS score, *Orthop Traumatol Surg Res* 96:S77, 2010.

Tierney JJ, Curtis AS, Scheller AD: *The insertional anatomy of the rotator cuff: an anatomic study*, Boston, 2000, Paper presented at the Boston Shoulder Symposium.

Tischer T, Vogt S, Kreuz PC, Imhoff AB: Arthroscopic anatomy, variants, and pathologic findings in shoulder instability, *Arthroscopy* 27:1434, 2011.

Tokish JM, Tolan SJ, Lee J, et al.: Treatment of biceps lesions in the setting of rotator cuff repair: when is tenodesis superior to tenotomy?, *Orthop J Sports Med* 5(7 suppl 6):2325967117S00399, 2017.

Tompane T, Carney J, Wu WW, et al.: Glenoid bone reaction to all-soft suture anchors used for shoulder labral repairs, *J Bone Joint Surg Am* 100:1223, 2018.

Toussaint B, Schnaser E, Bosley J, et al.: Early structural and functional outcomes for arthroscopic double-row transosseous-equivalent rotator cuff repair, *Am J Sports Med* 39:1217, 2011.

van den Ende KIM, McIntosh AL, Adams JE, Steinmann SP: Osteochondritis dissecans of the capitellum: a review of the literature and a distal ulnar portal, *Arthroscopy* 27:122, 2011.

van der Veen HC, Collins JP, Rijk PC: Value of magnetic resonance arthrography in post-traumatic anterior shoulder instability prior to arthroscopy: a prospective evaluation of MRA versus arthroscopy, *Arch Orthop Trauma Surg* 132:371, 2012.

van Grinsven S, Hagenmaier F, van Loon CJ, et al.: Does the experience level of the radiologist, assessment in consensus, or the addition of the abuction and external rotation view improve the diagnostic reproducibility and accuracy of MRA of the shoulder? *Clin Radiol* 69:1157, 2014.

van Nielen D, Wilson M, Hammond J, et al.: Biceps tenodesis vs repair for type II SLAP tears in patients under 30 years-old, *Orthop J Sports Med* 5(7 Suppl 6):2325967117S00395,

van Oostveen DPH, Timmerman OPP, Burger BJ, et al.: Glenoid fractures: a review of pathology, classification, treatment, and results, *Acta Orthop Belg* 80:88, 2014.

Vavken P, Sadoghi P, Palmer M, et al.: Platelet-rich plasma reduces retear rates after arthroscopic repair of small- and medium-sized rotator cuff tears but is not cost effective, *Am J Sports Med* 43:3071, 2015.

Verma NN, Bhatia S, Baker CL, et al.: Outcomes of arthroscopic rotator cuff repair in patients aged 70 years or older, *Arthroscopy* 26:1273, 2010.

Voos JE, Livermore RW, Feeley BT, et al.: Prospective evaluation of arthroscopic Bankart repairs for anterior instability, *Am J Sports Med* 38:302, 2010.

Wang J, Ma JX, Zhu SW, et al.: Does distal clavicle resection decrease pain or improve shoulder function in patients with acromioclavicular joint arthritis and rotator cuff tears? A meta-analysis, *Clin Orthop Relat Res* 476:2402, 2018.

Warth RJ, Spiegl UJ, Millett PJ: Scapulothoracic bursitis and snapping scapula syndrome, *Am J Sports Med* 43:236, 2014.

Weber SC, Payvandi S, Martin DF, Harrast JJ: SLAP lesions of the shoulder: incidence rates, complications, and outcomes as reported by ABOS part II candidates (SS-19), *Arthroscopy* 26:e9, 2010.

Werner BC, Brockmeier SF, Gwathmey FW: Trends in long head biceps tenodesis, *Am J Sports Med* 43:570, 2014.

Werner BC, Evans CL, Holzgrefe RE, Tuman JM, et al.: Arthroscopic suprapectoral and open subpectoral biceps tenodesis: a comparison of minimum 2-year clinical outcomes, *Am J Sports Med* 42:2583, 2014.

Werner BC, Miller MD, Lyons ML, et al.: Biceps tenodesis. How low do you go? A comparison of location between arthroscopic suprapectoral and open subpectural techniques, *Orthop J Sports Med* 1(Suppl 4): 2325967113S00087, 2013.

Wiater BP, Neradilek MB, Polissar NL, Matsen FA: Risk factors for chondrolysis of the glenohumeral joint: a study of three hundred and seventy-five shoulder arthroscopic procedures in the practice of an individual community surgeon, *J Bone Joint Surg* 93A:615, 2011.

Wolf EM, Siparsky PN: Glenoid avulsion of the glenohumeral ligaments as a cause of recurrent anterior shoulder instability, *Arthroscopy* 26:1263, 2010.

Yamakado K, Hayashi S, Katsuo SI: Histopathology of the residual tendon in high-grade articular-sided partial-thickness rotator cuff tears (PASTA lesions), *Arthroscopy* 27:e34, 2011.

Yamamoto N, Mineta M, Kawakami J, et al.: Risk factors for tear progression in symptomatic rotator cuff tears: a prospective study of 174 shoulders, *Am J Sports Med* 45:2524, 2017.

Yoon JP, Chung SW, Kim JY, et al.: Outcomes of combined bone marrow stimulation and patch augmentation for massive rotator cuff tears, *Am J Sports Med* 44:963, 2016.

ELBOW

Adams JE, King GJ, Steinmann SP, et al.: Elbow arthroscopy: indications, techniques, outcomes, and complications, *J Am Acad Orthop Surg* 22:810, 2014.

Ahmad CS, Conway JE: Elbow arthroscopy: valgus extension overload, *Instr Course Lect* 60:191, 2011.

Ahmad CS, Vitale MA: Elbow arthroscopy: setup, portal placement, and simple procedures, *Instr Course Lect* 60:171, 2011.

Ahmad CS, Vitale MA, El Attrache NS: Elbow arthroscopy: capitellar osteochondritis dissecans and radiocapitellar plica, *Instr Course Lect* 60:181, 2011.

Alvi HM, Kalainov DM, Biswas D, et al.: Surgical management of symptomatic olecranon traction spurs, *Orthop J Sports Med* 2:2325967114542775, 2014.

Andelman SM, Meier KM, Walsh AL, et al.: Pediatric elbow arthroscopy: indications and safety, *J Shoulder Elbow Surg* 26:1862, 2017.

Baker CL, Romeo AA, Baker CL: Osteochondritis dissecans of the capitellum, *Am J Sports Med* 38:1917, 2010.

Bexkens R, van den Bekerom MPJ, Eygendaal D, et al.: Topographic analysis of 2 alternative donor sites of the ipsilateral elbow in the treatment of capitellar osteochondritis dissecans, *Arthroscopy* 34:2098, 2018.

Blackwell JR, Hay BA, Bolt AM, et al.: Olecranon bursitis: a systematic review, *Shoulder Elbow* 6:182, 2014.

Blonna D, Huffman GR, O'Driscoll SW: Delayed-onset ulnar neuritis after release of elbow contractures: clinical presentation, pathological findings, and treatment, *Am J Sports Med* 42:2113, 2014.

Blonna D, Wolf JM, Fitzsimmons JS, O'Driscoll SW: Prevention of nerve injury during arthroscopic capsulectomy of the elbow utilizing a safety-driven strategy, *J Bone Joint Surg Am* 95A:1373, 2013.

Dugas JR, Looze CA, Jones CM, et al.: Ulnar collateral ligament repair with internal brace augmentation in amateur overhead throwing athletes, *Orthop J Sports Med* 6(7 Suppl 4):2325967118S00084, 2018.

Dugas JR, Walters BL, Beason DP, et al.: Biomechanical comparison of ulnar collateral ligament repair with internal bracing versus modified Jobe reconstruction, *Am J Sports Med* 44:735, 2015.

Erickson BJ, Chalmers PN, Bush-Joseph CA, et al.: Ulnar collateral ligament reconstruction of the elbow. A systematic review of the literature, *Ortho J Sports Med* 3:2325967115618914, 2015.

Gancarczyk SM, Makhni EC, Lombardi JM, et al.: Arthroscopic articular reconstruction of capitellar osteochondral defects, *Am J Sports Med* 43:2452, 2015.

Hasham AA, Kalainov DM, Biswas D, et al.: Surgical management of symptomatic olecranon traction spurs, *Ortho J Sports Med* 2(7):2325967114542775, 2014.

Intravia J, Mirzayan: Elbow arthroscopy complications in pediatrics and adults, *Orthop J Sports Med* 5(7 Suppl 6):2325967117S00402, 2017.

Iwasaki N, Kato H, Ishikawa J, et al.: Autologous osteochondral mosaicplasty for osteochondritis dissecans of the elbow in teenage athletes: surgical technique, *J Bone Joint Surg* 92A:208, 2010.

Intravia J, Mirzayan R: Elbow arthroscopy complications in pediatrics and adults, *Orthop J Sports Med* 5(7 Suppl 6):2325967117S00402, 2017.

Jinnah AH, Luo TD, Wiesler ER, et al.: Peripheral nerve injury after elbow arthroscopy: an analysis of risk factors, *Arthroscopy* 34:1447, 2018.

Koehler SM, Walsh A, Lovy AJ, et al.: Outcomes of arthroscopic treatment of osteochondritis dissecans of the capitellum and description of the technique, *J Shoulder Elbow Surg* 24:1607, 2015.

Leong NL, Cohen JR, Lord E, et al.: Demographic trends and complication rates in arthroscopic elbow surgery, *Arthroscopy* 31:1928, 2015.

Miyake J, Shimada K, Oka K, et al.: Arthroscopic debridement in the treatment of patients with osteoarthritis of the elbow, based on computer simulation, *Bone Joint J* 96-B:237, 2014.

Mommma D, Iwasaki N, Oizumi N, et al.: Long-term stress distribution patterns across the elbow joint in baseball players assessed by computed tomography osteoabsorptiometry, *Am J Sports Med* 39:336, 2011.

Moon JG, Biraris S, Jeong WK, Kim JH: Clinical results after arthroscopic treatment for septic arthritis of the elbow joint, *Arthroscopy* 30:673, 2014.

Murthi AM, Keener JD, Armstrong AD, Getz CL: The recurrent unstable elbow: diagnosis and treatment, *Instr Course Lect* 60:215, 2011.

Noonburg GE, Baker CL: Elbow arthroscopy. In Sperling JW, editor: *AAOS Instructional Course Lectures shoulder and elbow volume 2*, Rosemont, IL, 2010, American Academy of Orthopaedic Surgeons.

O'Brien MJ, Lee Murphy R, Savoie 3rd FH: A preliminary report of acute and subacute arthroscopic repair of the radial ulnohumeral ligament after elbow dislocation in the high-demand patient, *Arthroscopy* 30:679, 2014.

O'Holleran JD, Altchek DW: Elbow arthroscopy: treatment of the thrower's elbow. In Sperling JW, editor: *AAOS Instructional Course Lectures shoulder and elbow volume 2*, Rosemont, IL, 2010, American Academy of Orthopaedic Surgeons.

Oki G, Iba K, Sasaki K, et al.: Time to functional recovery after arthroscopic surgery for tennis elbow, *J Shoulder Elbow Surg* 23:1527, 2014.

Osbahr DC, Dines JS, Breazeale NM, et al.: Ulnohumeral chondral and ligamentous overload: biomechanical correlation for posteromedial chondromalacia of the elbow in throwing athletes, *Am J Sports Med* 38:2535, 2010.

Pierce TP, Issa K, Gilbert BT, et al.: A systematic review of tennis elbow surgery: open versus arthroscopic versus percutaneous release of the common extensor origin, *Arthroscopy* 33:1260, 2017.

Raphael BS, Weiland AJ, Altchek DW, Gay DM: Revision arthroscopic contracture release in the elbow resulting in ulnar nerve transection: how to avoid complications: surgical technique, *J Bone Joint Surg* 93A:100, 2011.

Ruchelsman DE, Hall MP, Youm T: Osteochondritis dissecans of the capitellum: current concepts, *J Am Acad Orthop Surg* 18:557, 2010.

Sardelli M, Tashjian RZ, MacWilliams BA: Functional elbow range of motion for contemporary tasks, *J Bone Joint Surg* 93A:471, 2011.

Steinmann SP, King GJW, Savoie FH: Arthroscopic treatment of arthritic elbow. In Sperling JW, editor: *AAOS Instructional Course Lectures shoulder and elbow volume 2*, Rosemont, IL, 2010, American Academy of Orthopaedic Surgeons.

Uchilda S, Utsunomiya H, Taketa T, et al.: Arthroscopic fragment fixation using hydroxyapatite/poly-L-lactate acid thread pins for treating elbow osteochondritis dissecans, *Am J Sports Med* 43:1057, 2015.

Vavken P, Müller AM, Camathias C: First 50 pediatric and adolescent elbow arthroscopies: analysis of indications and complications, *J Pediatr Orthop* 36(4):400, 2016.

Walters BL, Cain EL, Emblom BA, et al.: Ulnar collateral ligament repair with internal brace augmentation, *Orthop J Sports Med* 4(3 Suppl 3):2325967116S00071, 2016.

Wang J, Qi W, Shen X, et al.: Results of arthroscopoic ficaction of Mason type II radial head fractures using Kirschner wires, *Medicine (Baltimore)* 97, 2018:e0201.

Yoon JP, Chung SW, Yi JH, et al.: Prognostic factors of arthroscopic extensor carpi radialis brevis release for lateral epicondylitis, *Arthroscopy* 31:1232, 2015.

The complete list of references is available online at Expert Consult.com.

MICROSURGERY

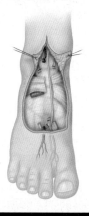

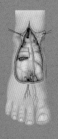

Microsurgery techniques are being applied to an expanding range of orthopaedic problems. Now the term *supermicrosurgery*, coined by Koshima et al., is used to apply to the anastomosis of submillimeter vessels that is necessary in distal replants and perforator flaps. The discussion presented in this chapter includes microsurgical procedures appropriate for surgery of the hand, including the repair of small vessels and nerves; the transfer of composite tissue grafts using microvascular techniques in the upper and lower extremities; and our approach to the replantation of amputated parts.

Microsurgery includes surgical procedures for structures so small that magnification by an operating microscope is required for their performance. Although many procedures can be performed using magnifying loupes of 5×,

magnification of 16× to 40× is provided by the microscope and is essential when working with structures less than 2 mm in diameter. For dissection and exposure of the small nerves and vessels, magnification of 6× and 10× is used most often, and for microsurgical repair of vessels and nerves, magnification of 16× and 25× is used. For surgical procedures requiring an assistant who also must see the microsurgical field, a double binocular microscope (diploscope) is essential. A triploscope also is available for use with a second assistant or an observer. Additional ports are available for television, movies, and photography. Electrical foot controls help to adjust focus and magnification.

Regardless of their proficiency with the techniques of hand surgery, surgeons should not expect to master microsurgery immediately. The acquisition of microsurgical

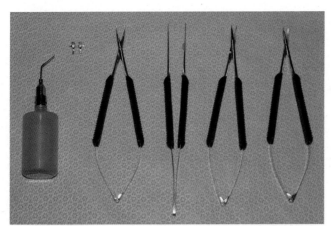

FIGURE 5.1 Instruments for microsurgery including vessel and nerve repair: small ophthalmic irrigator, vascular clamp, microneedle holder, jeweler's forceps, and microscissors.

techniques requires many hours of practice in the animal laboratory before sufficient skill is mastered to apply the techniques to a patient. Approximately 6 to 8 hours of daily practice in the laboratory for 2 to 3 weeks are required. Thereafter, regular clinical or laboratory practice is essential to maintain proficiency. Some surgeons require longer training, and some are unable to master the technique even after long hours of practice. Because many hours are frequently required for microsurgical procedures, the efficiency of the surgeon and the team is of prime consideration in keeping operating time to a minimum.

Factors that fatigue and lower the efficiency of the surgeon must be eliminated. Bracing the elbows on a stable platform, maintaining a posture that is comfortable, and minimizing tremor by obtaining adequate rest and by avoiding caffeine just before surgery all are helpful. Extraneous movements are amplified when viewed through the microscope and should be avoided. Surgeons must discipline themselves to maintain constant visual contact with the operating field through the microscope and depend on a practiced awareness of the location of their unseen hands and their relationship to the field and the microscope.

A simplified approach to instrumentation is preferred. Two or three straight and curved jeweler's forceps and microscissors are sufficient basic instruments for most microsurgical procedures (Fig. 5.1). Modified jeweler's forceps also are used as bipolar coagulation forceps for precise coagulation of small vessels.

Microvascular clamps of several designs are available. Clamps with a closing pressure of less than 30 g/mm² are preferable for small vessels. This pressure generally allows control of bleeding without damaging the vascular intima. Microirrigating cannulas and dilating probes are additional useful instruments.

Fine suture material is available with diameters of 18 to 35 μm swagged onto atraumatic needles with diameters of 50 to 139 μm. Nylon sutures designated as 9-0, 10-0, 11-0, and 12-0 are commercially available.

Detailed discussions of microsurgical history, microscopes, microsurgical instruments, needles, sutures, training methods, and techniques are found in many of the references at the end of this chapter.

MICROVASCULAR TECHNIQUES

MICROVASCULAR ANASTOMOSIS (END-TO-END)

TECHNIQUE 5.1

- Expose the selected vessel by careful dissection under magnification, using the operating microscope for dissection of vessels less than 2 mm in diameter.
- Using jeweler's forceps and microscissors, carefully remove the loose connective tissue surrounding the vessel.
- Mobilize each end of the vessel proximally and distally to obtain adequate length for anastomosis.
- Cauterize tethering side branches with bipolar electrocautery and continue mobilization until the vessel ends can be easily approximated with minimal or no tension.
- Place a contrasting colored rubber or plastic sheet behind the vessel to help make it easier to see.
- Frequently irrigate the operative field with heparinized lactated Ringer solution.
- Remove sufficient adventitia from the vessel ends to expose all layers of the vessel wall. Adventitia can be removed by careful circumferential trimming or by applying traction to the adventitia and transecting it in a manner similar to circumcision (Fig. 5.2A and B). Magnification of 6× to 10× usually is sufficient for this dissection.
- After the adventitia has been trimmed, continue to irrigate the field intermittently with heparinized lactated Ringer solution.
- Inspect the vascular intima using magnification of 25× and 40× and resect the vessel wall until the cut ends appear normal. Appose the vessel ends with a clamp approximator.
- Use interrupted sutures to prevent vascular constriction and place each suture through the full thickness of the vessel wall (Fig. 5.2C to F). Chen et al. showed in a rabbit model that a continuous suture technique significantly reduced anastomosis time and obtained similar patency rates as an interrupted suture technique in arteries larger than 0.7 mm and veins larger than 1 mm; however, we have not incorporated this technique into our practice.
- Place the first two sutures approximately 120 degrees apart on the vessel's circumference. Leave the ends of these sutures long for use as traction sutures.
- Rotate the clamp approximators to expose the posterior vessel wall and place a stitch 120 degrees from the initial two stitches.
- Place additional stitches in the remaining spaces to complete the anastomosis (Fig. 5.2G and H). Arteries 1 mm in diameter usually require 5 to 8 stitches, and veins usually require 7 to 10 stitches.
- Vessels can be dilated gently by inserting the tips of jeweler's forceps or specially designed dilators. The walls of the vessels can be grasped gently, but avoid rough ma-

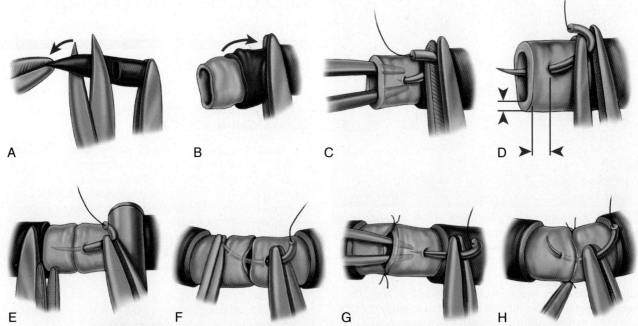

FIGURE 5.2 Microvascular anastomosis, basic steps. **A,** Adventitial excision. Traction is applied to adventitia, and it is excised sufficiently to avoid intrusion into vascular lumen. **B,** Appearance of vessel end after adventitial excision. **C,** Placement of initial suture. Forceps can be used as counterpressor agents without internal damage. **D,** Needle is passed through full thickness of vessel wall some distance from cut edge that is slightly greater than thickness of vessel wall. **E,** Passage of needle through opposite end of vessel is accomplished at similar distance from cut edge. **F,** Forceps, used as counterpressor agents, assist in passage of needle through opposite end of vessel. **G** and **H,** After completion of initial sutures, vessel is stabilized, allowing completion of even anastomosis. **SEE TECHNIQUE 5.1.**

nipulation of the intima. To overcome vascular spasm, apply topical lidocaine or papaverine.

- After the completion of the vascular anastomosis, remove the clamp downstream from the anastomosis first, then remove the clamp that is upstream.
- Minimal bleeding between stitches is of no concern, but excessive bleeding should be rapidly controlled by reapplication of clamps or inflation of a pneumatic tourniquet. Place additional stitches in the areas of leakage, remove the clamps again, and deflate the tourniquet.
- After bleeding from the suture line has stopped, assess the patency of the anastomosis by occluding a segment of vessel with forceps distal to the anastomosis. Gently strip blood from the segment from proximal to distal. Release the proximal clamp. Rapid filling of the emptied segment indicates a patent anastomosis.
- The suture line should be even, and there should be no anastomotic stenosis, dilation proximally, or stenosis distally. Small platelet clots around the anastomosis are to be expected, but avoid occlusion of the anastomosis by irrigating with heparinized solution or by gentle milking of the vessel.
- After the anastomosis, close the soft tissue over the vessels as soon as possible to avoid drying of the vessel wall.

MICROVASCULAR END-TO-SIDE ANASTOMOSIS

TECHNIQUE 5.2

- After dissecting and mobilizing the vessels as described in Technique 5.1, carefully excise a small longitudinal elliptical portion of the recipient vessel wall using microscissors (Fig. 5.3).
- Cut the end of the vessel that is to be attached to the recipient vessel at an angle of about 45 degrees.
- Begin the anastomosis by placing sutures at the proximal and distal ends of the ellipse. Leave the suture ends long for traction and complete the anastomosis by placing sutures evenly along the opening between the traction sutures.
- Release the occluding clamps or release the tourniquet and assess the patency and flow.

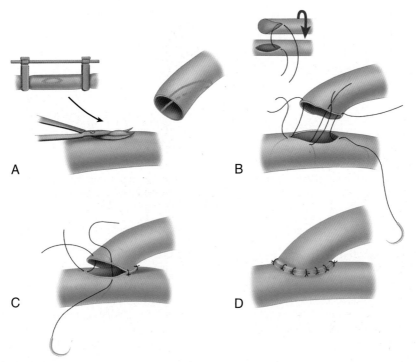

FIGURE 5.3 Microvascular end-to-side anastomosis. **A,** With microvascular scissors, small ellipse of vessel wall is excised between microvascular clips *(upper left).* Suitable fit of recipient vessel is achieved with oblique cut to match elliptical defect in vessel wall *(upper right).* Vessel also can be trimmed transversely to provide 90-degree anastomosis. **B,** Suture line begins with sutures placed at each end of openings. Suture ends are left long temporarily for traction. **C,** Suture line continues, placing interrupted stitches around anastomosis. **D,** Completed end-to-side microvascular anastomosis. **SEE TECHNIQUE 5.2.**

MICROVASCULAR VEIN GRAFTING

TECHNIQUE 5.3

- When end-to-end vessel anastomosis cannot be performed without tension, bone shortening and vein grafting may be necessary (Fig. 5.4). Many sizes of veins are available on the dorsum of the hand, on the dorsal and volar aspects of the forearm, and on the dorsum of the foot, so the vein graft can roughly approximate the diameter of the recipient vessel. This helps avoid thrombosis as a result of turbulence.
- When vein grafts are harvested, cauterize small side branches with bipolar forceps well away from the main vein wall.
- After the grafts have been removed, reverse them end to end for use as interposition grafts for arterial reconstruction; reversal is unnecessary when they are used for venous reconstruction. Reversal avoids obstruction of blood flow by the valves in these small veins.
- The technique for suture anastomosis of a vein graft is similar to that described for end-to-end repair.
- Gently perfuse the vein graft with heparinized Ringer solution and perform the proximal anastomosis.
- Release the occluding vascular clamps to confirm the flow through the graft.

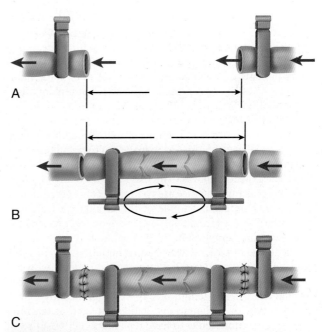

FIGURE 5.4 Microvascular vein graft. **A,** Vessel ends excised, leaving gap. *Arrows* show direction of flow in vessel. **B,** Vein graft harvested and reversed to allow flow through valves. Microvascular clips help stabilize and control vessels and graft. **C,** Microvascular clips in place; anastomoses have been completed. Valves in vein graft allow for proper direction of blood flow. **SEE TECHNIQUE 5.3.**

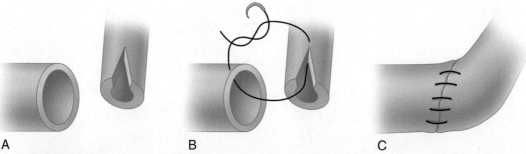

FIGURE 5.5   Ridha, Morritt, and Wood spatulated end-to-end microvascular anastomosis. **A,** Longitudinal incision in smaller diameter vessel to increase luminal circumference to match that of opposing vessel. **B,** First suture being placed at apex of incision on smaller vessel. **C,** Completed anastomosis.

- Reapply the clamps and perform the distal anastomosis.
- Release the clamps again to show flow across both anastomoses.
- Accommodate discrepancies in diameter by cutting the vessel ends obliquely or in a fish-mouth configuration.
- As an alternative, the spatulated technique can also be used. Create a longitudinal incision in the smaller vessel, place the first suture in the apex of the slit, and complete the anastomosis (Fig. 5.5).

REPLANTATION

Since the first pioneering efforts in 1962, digits, hands, feet, and limbs have been successfully replanted by surgeons around the world, including Kleinert, Bunke, Urbaniak, Meyer, and Millesi. Atroshi and Rosberg reviewed epidemiologic data from different countries and found that 85% to 95% of replantations occur in young men with a mean age of 25 to 30 years. In the studies that included children, 3% to 10% of patients were younger than 10 years of age. The main mechanisms of injury reported in the series of replantations were guillotine (14% to 53%), crush (11% to 62%), and avulsion (16% to 29%). The overall rate of attempted replantation has had a downward trend despite the 2013 mandate by the American College of Surgeons to make microvascular service available at all times at Level 1 trauma centers in the United States. The expectation was to increase the rate of digit replantation by concentrating the case volume. A cohort study using the National Inpatient Sample of the Healthcare Cost and Utilization Project found 9407 patients who were treated for upper extremity amputation, 1361 of whom had replantation. The mean age of patients who had replantation was 36 years (range, 0 to 86 years), and the mean age of patients who did not have replantation was 44 years (range, 0 to 104 years). Hospital charges and length of stay were significantly higher for patients with replantations. Patients treated at teaching facilities were more likely to have replantation (19%, 1088 of 5795 patients) than those at a nonteaching facility (7%, 252 of 3386 patients). Large hospitals and urban hospitals were more likely to perform replantation. Payer status affected replantation rates, with fewer replants being performed in self-pay, Medicare, and Medicaid patients compared with other payer status.

RESULTS

Overall survival rates reported by U.S. and foreign surgeons vary from slightly better than 50% to 92% for replanted and revascularized parts. The success rate of digital replantations at two U.S. academic Level 1 trauma centers recently was reported as 57% (69 of 135 digits).

Major limb replantations have a reported survival rate of nearly 40% to 80% and better. Results of replantation of above-elbow amputations are mixed compared with those of below-elbow replantations. There is some variation in reported results, with limb survival ranging from 61% to 88% in above-elbow replantations and 36% to 90% for below-elbow replantations.

Success of digital and limb replantations cannot be measured by survival alone. In the final analysis, success is measured better by the extent of return of useful function. Although it is of some value to compare the replanted part with the normal uninjured part, it is more meaningful to compare the replanted part with amputation or prosthetic function at the level in question. Insofar as function was concerned in one study, good or excellent outcomes were achieved in 36% to 50% of replanted limbs compared with prosthetic limbs in which no good results were obtained. Others have suggested that similar functional results between the two can be expected. Most authors use different grading systems based on factors such as ability to return to work, return of muscle function, range of motion, sensibility, ability to perform activities of daily living, and patient satisfaction. Chen et al. developed criteria for the evaluation of function that are ideal for assessing multisystem injury and are general enough to allow comparison of results within complex injury groups (Table 5.1). Several studies have reported successful return of function after replantation in 62% to 78% of patients. Jones, Schenck, and Chesney used a scoring system to evaluate patients who had undergone replantation compared with a group of patients who had amputations at similar levels. In their small group of patients, they found grip strength to be better in patients who had replanted thumbs or replanted multiple digits than in patients with amputations. Grip strength in patients with single-digit replantation was not significantly different, however, from patients with amputations. Patients with replanted multiple digits had a small functional advantage over patients with amputations. Their study also reinforced the concept that amputated thumbs should be replanted if possible, although the type of

TABLE 5.1	
Chen Criteria for Evaluation of Function after Extremity Replantation	
GRADE	**FUNCTION**
I	Able to resume original work; ROM > 60% of normal; complete or nearly complete recovery of sensibility; muscle power grade 4–5
II	Able to resume some suitable work; ROM > 40% of normal; nearly complete sensibility; muscle power grade 3–4
III	Able to carry out activities of daily living; ROM >30% of normal; partial recovery of sensibility; muscle power grade 3
IV	Almost no usable function of survived limb

ROM, Range of motion.
From Chen CW, Qian YQ, Yu ZJ: Extremity replantation, *World J Surg* 2:513, 1978.

amputation is a significant factor in the survival of replanted digits. Only 12% of replanted digits survived in crushing or avulsion amputations in one study, and the survival rate was significantly better if the injury occurred proximal to the metacarpophalangeal joint. In minimally damaged amputations, only the time between injury and surgery was significantly related to survival. Most patients who have had parts replanted are satisfied with the reattached part and would undergo replantation again; however, some were dissatisfied because of emotional stress, financial loss, and number of subsequent surgeries required.

Although most workers are able to return to some form of work, our experience suggests that the more proximal the injury, the less likely it is that the patient will be able to return to former employment in a reasonable time.

Cold intolerance is experienced by almost all replantation patients; however, it usually is not incapacitating. It may take 2 years or more to improve if at all, and patients may perceive moderate improvements because of change in habits. Most patients regain protective sensibility, but two-point discrimination, especially in more proximal injuries, is rarely less than 10 mm. Fine tactile discrimination rarely returns. Most patients have some residual limitation of movement, especially if a joint has been injured and if the flexor tendon injury in the hand lies between the metacarpophalangeal and proximal interphalangeal joints.

Functional results after major limb replantations vary with the age of the patient, the level of the injury, and the mechanism of injury. Generally, the more distal the injury, the sharper the injuring mechanism, and the younger the patient, the better the outlook (96% excellent results in children). This seems to be largely the result of the dependence on nerve regeneration for return of sensibility and motor function. The results of replantations are poorer if the amputation is above the elbow, if the elbow joint is involved, or if the injury is through the muscular portion of the proximal forearm. Transmetacarpal amputations carry a poor prognosis for replantation because of injury to the intrinsics. Functional outcomes at a mean of 4 years (range, 1 to 7 years) after replantations of radiocarpal amputations in six patients were reported by Patel et al. Total active motion of the hand was

38% (range, 26% to 59%) and grip strength was 9% (range, 0% to 18%) as compared with the contralateral extremity. Tip and key pinch were not achieved. Mean two-point discrimination was 10.6 mm (range, 8 to 12 mm). All outcome scores, including the Disabilities of Arm, Shoulder, and Hand score, showed moderate disability (mean, 76; range, 45 to 82).

Despite the guarded outlook regarding more proximal amputations, some patients achieve useful function that is significantly better than that obtained with a prosthesis.

REPLANTATION TEAM
Replantation of amputated upper extremity parts should be done by surgeons who are trained in surgery of the hand and upper extremity. In addition, digital replantation requiring the use of the operating microscope should be done by surgeons who have exhibited the ability to perform reliable microvascular anastomoses with a predictable patency rate of 90% or better.

Although replantation can be done by one surgeon with highly trained and motivated assistants, it is more desirable to use rotating teams of surgeons. During the microvascular portions of the procedure, at least one of the scrubbed surgeons should be proficient at microvascular and microneural repairs. The replantation surgeons should be available on a rotating basis 24 hours a day except in unavoidable circumstances. Assistants who are familiar with the sequence of events, instruments, and other equipment required for replantation procedures should be available. Finally, it is important that the hospital be able to support such an undertaking with surgical suites and an intensive care unit available around the clock and with nursing and anesthesia personnel to provide the essential care before, during, and after the procedure.

GENERAL CONSIDERATIONS
The function anticipated after replantation must be better than that with a prosthesis or an amputation, and the difference must be worth the risk, time, and expense. The potential for the replanted part to regain useful motion and sensibility must be assessed carefully before committing the patient to a long and difficult course of rehabilitation. The following factors generally are evaluated for replantation of an amputated part:

- Age of patient
- Severity of injury
- Level of amputation
- Part amputated
- Interval between amputation and time of replantation (especially warm ischemia time)
- Multiple or bilateral amputations
- Segmental injuries to the amputated part
- Patient's general condition, including other major injuries or diseases
- Rehabilitation potential of patient (occupation and intelligence)
- Economic factors

These considerations are expanded on in the discussions of indications and contraindications that follow.

INDICATIONS AND CONTRAINDICATIONS
Because the final decision regarding replantation rests with the patient and the surgeon, there are no absolute indications for replantation of an amputated part. The following

discussion reflects our present practice combined with the published recommendations of the previously noted authors. The factors discussed should be taken as relative guides based on current knowledge and experience.

AGE

Replantations have been reported in patients a few weeks old and in patients older than 70 years. The young patient poses particular problems, especially regarding digital replantations, because of the increased technical difficulty in microvascular anastomoses of their smaller digital vessels. Postoperative anxiety may contribute to vasospasm, and rehabilitation of children may be less predictable than rehabilitation of adults. Nevertheless, satisfactory functional results have been reported, and most authors consider replantation over amputation of almost any part, including lower extremity parts, in children. The success rate of distal fingertip replantations in children has been reported to be higher than in adults and may be undertaken by a skilled replant surgeon. Vessel size in children may be 0.5 mm, making it difficult to place a clamp on the distal segment, and either a volar venous anastomosis or controlled bleeding is necessary for venous outflow.

The upper age limit beyond which replantation should not be considered has not been clearly established. Poor nerve regeneration and joint stiffness limit the functional outcome. Replantation above the elbow, through the elbow, or through the proximal forearm results in little promise for hand function in the elderly; however, the elbow may be preserved in anticipation of a subsequent below-elbow amputation to allow more satisfactory prosthetic fitting. Because the potential for return of sensibility and motion is better after replantation at and beyond the tendinous portion of the forearm, older patients may be considered as serious replantation candidates if their injuries are more distal. Data from the Nationwide Inpatient Sample over a 10-year period from 1998 to 2007 revealed no difference in perioperative complications or mortality between patients younger than 65 years of age and those older than 65 years of age after replantation of fingers or thumbs. Age is not an absolute contraindication to very distal replantation. The patient's physiologic status, the presence of other diseases, and general level of activity also should weigh heavily in the evaluation.

SEVERITY OF INJURY

The types of injuries that have the best outlook regarding survival and return of function after replantation include (1) clean, sharp "guillotine" amputations, (2) minimal local crush amputations, and (3) avulsion amputations with minimal proximal and distal vascular injury. Ideally, significant additional injury to the limb should not be present, especially of the vessels, proximally and distally. Crushed and avulsed vessels require debridement and the use of interpositional vein grafts as needed. Ring avulsion-degloving injuries may be revascularized and salvaged; however, if the skin has been completely degloved, or if the digit has been amputated, vein grafts may be required, and the outlook for useful function is extremely uncertain. Ring avulsion amputations through the joint usually are best treated by closure of the amputation. Injuries contaminated extensively with soil, especially from a barnyard, carry a high risk of significant infection and should be evaluated carefully before replantation.

LEVEL OF INJURY AND PART AMPUTATED

Replantation near the shoulder generally carries a poor prognosis regarding hand function because of unpredictable nerve regeneration, muscle atrophy, and joint stiffness. Amputations through the humerus, elbow, and proximal forearm have the potential for successful replantation and useful function, especially in a young, healthy patient, and especially if the injury is clean and sharp. The patient should be young enough and motivated enough to be able to await nerve regeneration sufficient for return of function. Replantation more distally, whether through the distal forearm, wrist, metacarpals, or digits, also should be seriously considered because generally the potential for sensory and motor return is good (Fig. 5.6). Replantation just above the elbow, through the elbow joint, or in the proximal forearm has a guarded prognosis in older patients because of questionable nerve regeneration, limitation of elbow motion, and persistence of intrinsic muscle atrophy. Replantation for salvage of the elbow for later below-elbow prosthetic fitting may be feasible in selected patients.

Thumb amputations at almost any level should be considered for replantation despite nerve and tendon avulsion and joint involvement (Fig. 5.7). If the thumb can be revascularized, sensibility can be restored with nerve grafts or a neurovascular island pedicle transfer if needed, and motion can be achieved with tendon grafts or transfers. Replantation may not be successful after amputations caused by roping injuries with crush and avulsion components. Replantation of single and multiple digits distal to the flexor digitorum sublimis insertion should be expected to achieve satisfactory function (Fig. 5.8), but amputations at a more proximal level, especially through the proximal interphalangeal joint, usually result in poor function. They are usually stiff and tend to impair the overall function of the remaining digits by getting in the way. The amputated thumb is the exception to this generalization. Although many patients do well without replantation of single-digit amputations, such a replantation may be worthwhile for some musicians, individuals with other special occupations, some children, and for other aesthetic or social reasons. Replantation of a single digit also may be helpful if the remaining attached digits are severely damaged, especially with tendon and nerve injury over the proximal phalanx. If multiple digits have been amputated, replantation of at least two digits in the long and ring positions provides a good combination of digits to use with the thumb for pinch and for power grip. Occasionally, amputations through the distal phalanx may best be treated by replantation, and success with fingertip replantation has been reported. Hattori et al. believe that amputation proximal to the lunula is a relative indication for replantation. Except in some centers, these distal replantations are not performed because of the degree of difficulty in identifying and anastomosing suitable vessels, longer surgery time, longer time off from work, and higher costs. Indications for fingertip replantation remain controversial.

In bilateral amputations, replantation on each side should provide better function than bilateral prostheses. If replantation is not suitable or possible because of extensive injuries on one side, the best side should be selected, and at times parts from one side may be attached to the opposite, more suitable stump. Although amputations through the joints impair the movement of those joints, a satisfactory limb can result through arthrodesis, excisional or fascial arthroplasty, or, in ideal circumstances, silicone implant arthroplasty.

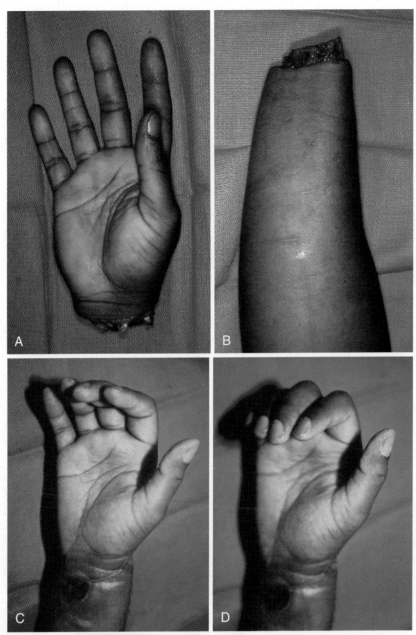

FIGURE 5.6 **A-D,** Hand replantation (see text).

■ WARM ISCHEMIA (ANOXIC) TIME

Because irreversible necrotic changes begin in muscle after 6 hours of ischemia without cooling (at 20°C to 25°C), it is preferable to begin the replantation of parts amputated proximal to the palm within this time. With cooling (to 4°C), this time may be extended to 12 hours. For parts with no muscle (digits), the allowable warm ischemia time may be 8 hours or more. With cooling, this has been extended to longer than 30 hours. Although replantation of parts containing small amounts of muscle, such as the hand, probably is less risky, larger parts such as the forearm and arm above the elbow probably should not be replanted if they cannot be revascularized 6 to 8 hours after amputation. The risk of renal damage resulting from myoglobinuria, acidosis, and hyperkalemia is increased after the replantation of a part with significant amounts of necrotic muscle. The risk of infection also is greater, and the long-term outlook for a functional limb is poor.

■ PREEXISTING DEFORMITY OR DISABILITY

If the amputated part was already deformed or disabled because of some congenital or acquired disorder, satisfactory function is unlikely to be achieved by replantation. Conditions that would fit this situation include, but are not limited to, scar deformity and contracture caused by previous burns or mangling injury, significant residual deficits from spinal cord or peripheral nerve injuries, and deformities as a result of stroke.

■ CONDITIONS THAT MIGHT PRECLUDE REPLANTATION

In the same accident that causes the amputation of a part, patients at times sustain significant intracranial, thoracic, cardiovascular, or major intraabdominal visceral injuries requiring lengthy lifesaving operations. In such circumstances, a

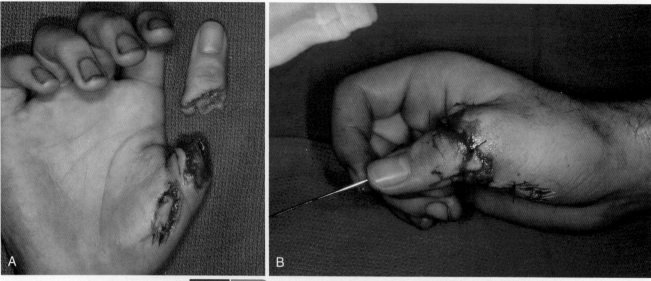

FIGURE 5.7   **A** and **B,** Thumb replantation (see text).

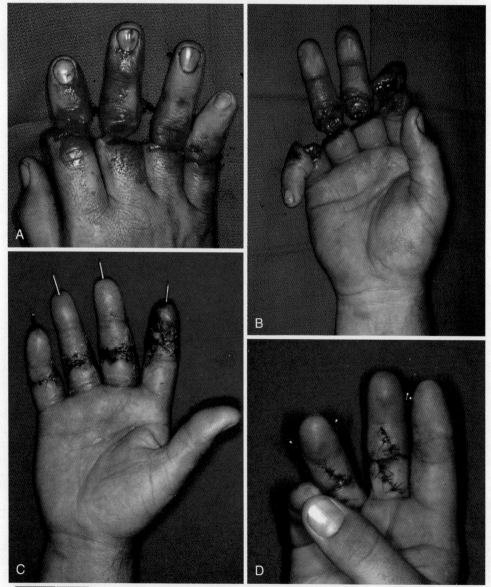

FIGURE 5.8   Multiple-digit replantation in 20-year-old man with saw injury. **A** and **B,** Multiple digits amputated distal to flexor sublimis insertion. **C,** Finger flexion and extension 7 months after replantation. **D,** Sensory return allows for useful finger function.

major limb replantation may be impossible because of excessive ischemia time. Digits may be cooled to 4°C in a refrigerator and saved for replantation later if technically feasible and if the patient's condition permits.

Patients with preexisting diseases that typically affect peripheral blood vessels are probably poor replantation candidates, especially if their vessels have an unsatisfactory appearance when inspected under the operating microscope. Patients with diabetes mellitus, rheumatoid arthritis, lupus erythematosus, other collagen vascular diseases, and significant atherosclerosis fit into this category. Severe chronic or uncompensated medical illnesses, such as coronary artery disease, myocardial infarction, peptic ulcer disease, malignant neoplasms, and chronic renal or pulmonary disease, may increase the anesthetic risk enough to preclude replantation.

Considerable judgment is required when assessing patients with psychiatric illnesses who have amputated parts. If the amputation event is an act of self-inflicted mutilation or attempted suicide during a psychiatric episode that can be treated and stabilized, replantation carries considerable risk of failure. If the amputated part is a focus in the patient's mental illness, it is likely that the part, if replanted, will be reinjured. If the amputation occurs as a true inadvertent accident, especially in a patient whose mental illness is compensated, the outlook for replantation might be better. Valid psychiatric evaluation of patients with amputated parts in an emergency department is extremely difficult. The inability of patients with profound psychiatric illness to understand their delicate postoperative condition and to cooperate with the difficult rehabilitation process further complicates their care as replant patients.

MANAGEMENT AND TRANSPORTATION OF PATIENT AND PART

At the scene of the injury and in the outlying hospital, the patient's condition is of utmost importance. Major injuries other than the amputated part should take precedence, and the patient's condition should be stabilized. Major stump bleeding should be controlled with pressure. No attempt should be made to clamp or ligate vessels. A pressure dressing should be applied for transporting the patient to an institution with replantation capabilities. If bleeding is persistent, the temporary use of a pneumatic tourniquet or blood pressure cuff is helpful. Elastic tourniquets should not be applied; they may be covered later with bandages and forgotten.

As noted, cooling of the amputated part to about 4°C is important to prolong the viability of the part. After the part has been found, it can be rinsed gently with sterile saline, lactated Ringer, or other physiologic solutions so that excess contamination is removed. The part should be treated in one of two ways: (1) it can be wrapped with sterile gauze or other clean material, soaked in sterile lactated Ringer or saline, and placed in a plastic bag, which is then sealed, or (2) it can be immersed in a plastic bag containing a physiologic solution such as lactated Ringer or saline. The bag is placed on ice in an insulated container so that the part is not touching the ice to avoid freezing of the part. Dry ice should not be used; neither should the part be warmed. Nonphysiologic solutions such as alcohol and formaldehyde should not be used on the amputated part.

No attempt should be made to clamp, dissect, ligate, or cannulate vessels on the amputated part because this further damages vessels that may be essential to revascularization of the part. If the part has been incompletely severed, it should be handled gently. Care should be taken to correct any kinking of the soft tissues or rotation that might compromise marginal arterial or venous flow. Sterile bandages moistened with a physiologic solution should be applied to the limb and the injured part and an ice pack applied to the latter. The limb should be supported with padded splints and a nonconstricting wrapping for the trip to the hospital.

When the patient is stable with an intravenous infusion in place, the patient along with the part can be transported. Although air transportation may be preferable for patients traveling great distances, especially in limb amputations, ground transportation is suitable if the patient can reach the replantation team in 2 to 3 hours and if the amputated parts are digits that have been appropriately cooled. The receiving institution and replantation team should be contacted and alerted that the patient is being sent.

Finally, it is preferable for the patient and family to understand that the patient is being referred to another hospital and other surgeons who have the capability to reattach parts and who will evaluate the particular situation and make appropriate recommendations regarding treatment. This understanding helps to minimize unrealistic expectations of patients, family, and friends, who usually are quite distraught. In a 2010 report from one tertiary replant center, 65% of patients transported by air for possible replantation did not have replantation, with injury characteristic being the main contraindication. Delaying digital replantation overnight so that a suitable operating room and rested replantation team are available is an acceptable practice and may be beneficial as long as the amputated part is properly preserved.

PREOPERATIVE PREPARATION

Some aspects of preoperative, intraoperative, and postoperative management vary slightly among institutions; however, general agreement has been reached on many of the basic principles regarding replantation. Having two teams to deal with replantation candidates from the time of their arrival in the emergency department is most helpful. While one team evaluates and prepares the patient, the other team assesses the amputated part.

Patient assessment and preparation should include (1) a history of the injury and medical history, including serious illnesses or previous injuries to the amputated part; (2) physical examination, especially to exclude injuries to other major organ systems; and (3) stabilization and resuscitation of the patient with the institution of an intravenous infusion, appropriate antibiotics, and tetanus prophylaxis. Blood typing and crossmatching are done, and transfusions are given if needed. An indwelling urinary catheter may be inserted in the emergency department or in the surgical suite. Radiographs of the amputated part, the amputation stump, the chest, and other areas as indicated should be obtained in the emergency department. The patient and family are advised of the nature of the injury, the uncertainties regarding survival of the part and return of function, the possible duration of the replantation operation, the possibility of repeated operations, and the likelihood that the replanted part will never be normal.

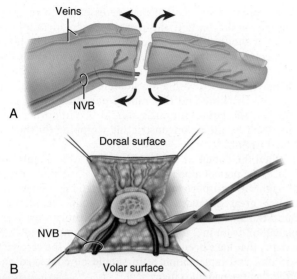

A, Veins, NVB

B, Dorsal surface, NVB, Volar surface

FIGURE 5.9 Dissection of amputated digit. **A,** Incisions on radial and ulnar midline allow reflection of dorsal and palmar flaps. **B,** Structures to be repaired are carefully and gently dissected using microsurgical instruments and meticulous technique. *NVB,* Neurovascular bundle. **SEE TECHNIQUE 5.4.**

PREPARATION FOR REPLANTATION

TECHNIQUE 5.4

- While the patient is being assessed and prepared, another surgeon on the replantation team takes the amputated part to the surgical suite to clean it and to evaluate the extent of injury.
- Clean the part and keep it cool by placing ice in a pan, covering the ice with a sterile plastic drape, and placing a sterile drape sheet over the plastic and ice. Place the part on the drape sheet for dissection under loupe or microscope magnification.
- Dissect the amputated part to allow exposure of the arteries, veins, nerves, tendons, joint capsule, periosteum, and other salvageable soft tissues. In digits, exposure usually is best achieved using midlateral incisions in the radial and ulnar aspects allowing reflection of dorsal and palmar flaps (Fig. 5.9). Although digital arteries and nerves are usually found with ease, locating satisfactory veins is more difficult. Careful, gentle, and meticulous dissection is required to locate these.
- Carefully preserve the small structures and use sutures of 8-0 or 9-0 nylon to mark them so that they can be located easily for nerve repair and vascular anastomoses.
- Although multiple vein grafts can be used to provide tension-free anastomoses, it is our practice to shorten bone, usually in the part of the digit having the most bone to spare. In digits, this shortening rarely exceeds 1 cm.
- Place internal fixation in the digit. We usually insert a longitudinal Kirschner wire combined with an obliquely crossing Kirschner wire. Occasionally, interosseous wires are used near joints. Plates and screws usually are not needed.

- If the amputation has occurred through a joint, or if the extensor mechanism is irreparable, prepare for arthrodesis.
- If the amputation is clean and sharp, perfusing the digital arteries before anastomosis usually is unnecessary.
- If the part has been crushed or avulsed, evidence of distal injury may be seen in the form of ecchymoses along the vessels or abrasions and lacerations. In these situations, gently perfuse the digital artery and vascular tree using a small Silastic catheter and heparinized Ringer solution or saline. If there is no return of the perfusate, or if it extravasates from distally injured vessels, blood flow is unlikely to be maintained after anastomosis. Perfusion for brief periods may be helpful in rinsing blood and metabolites from the vascular tree of amputated hands, forearms, and arms.
- The approach to the structures of the amputated hand and more proximally amputated parts usually is made through generally accepted incisions that allow extensive exposure of the structures to be identified and repaired.
- While the amputated part is being dissected, the patient usually is given an axillary brachial plexus block with the long-acting local anesthetic bupivacaine. This provides satisfactory anesthesia for digital or hand replantation in most adults and older children. For proximal amputations, younger children, anxious patients, and prolonged surgery as in multiple digital or bilateral amputations, general anesthesia frequently is preferable.
- Pad the operating table well and apply a warming blanket to prevent body cooling during prolonged surgery.
- Use a pneumatic tourniquet to provide a bloodless field for initial dissection of the stump and to control any subsequent significant bleeding.
- When the patient is comfortable, thoroughly cleanse the stump with an antiseptic solution, usually a povidone-iodine solution, and irrigate with normal saline.
- The stump is dissected by a hand surgeon who has microsurgery training and experience.
- Using gentle and meticulous technique, identify the arteries, veins, and nerves with magnifying loupes or the operating microscope and tag them with sutures of 8-0 or 9-0 nylon.
- Dissect tendons and hold them with 4-0 nylon sutures for later repair.
- Before initiating reattachment, free clots from the proximal arterial stumps and open the stumps to allow free arterial flow. If no satisfactory flow can be achieved, additional dissection, vessel resection, and possibly vein grafting may be needed.

ORDER OF REPAIR

After all structures have been thoroughly cleansed, debrided, and identified, repair is begun. As indicated in the discussion that follows, certain conditions or circumstances dictate a variation in the order of repair. The following is our usual order of repair of damaged structures. Discussions of digit, hand, and arm replantations are included.

1. Shorten and internally fix bone.
2. Repair extensor tendons.
3. Repair flexor tendons (2 and 3 may be reversed, or flexor tendon repair may be delayed).

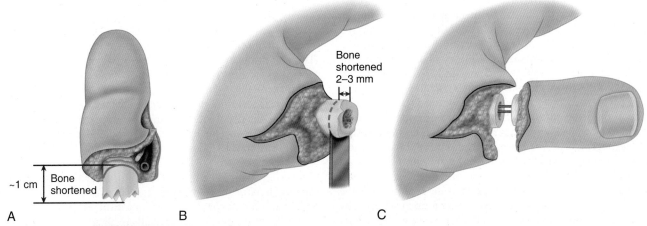

FIGURE 5.10   Bone management. **A,** In digits, shortening of 1 cm usually allows tension-free vessel anastomosis without excessively impairing hand function. **B,** Shortening of thumb proximal phalanx with oscillating saw in 2- to 3-mm increments until satisfactory shortening is achieved. **C,** Bone fixation with longitudinal Kirschner wires usually is sufficient.

4. Repair arteries.
5. Repair nerves.
6. Repair veins.
7. Close or cover wound.

If time permits, we often repair the veins immediately after extensor tendon repair. This minimizes repositioning of the hand and allows for venous anastomosis in a bloodless field. It also may minimize venous congestion. Also, if time permits, it is easier to repair the nerve just before repairing the artery.

In distal thumb amputations, it may be easier to anastomose interpositional vein grafts to the terminal branch of the ulnar digital artery and largest vein before performing osteosynthesis. The proximal anastomoses can be performed dorsally and proximal to the area of injury.

MANAGEMENT OF BONES AND JOINTS

The periosteum is stripped minimally. Bone is shortened to permit tension-free vascular anastomoses and nerve repairs (Fig. 5.10A). Initial bone shortening reduces the size of the soft-tissue defect, allows maximal soft-tissue debridement, and changes crush injuries to guillotine injuries. If vein grafts are used, the need for bone shortening is minimized, but survival depends on the patency of the two anastomoses of the graft, rather than one. Additional time is required to harvest the vein and to perform the anastomoses. Vein grafting may be necessary, however, if the amputation has occurred near an undamaged joint.

Shortening of an amputated thumb should be kept to a minimum (Fig. 5.10B). We have found that shortening of a digit much more than 1 to 1.5 cm at times impairs the function of the digit. Amputations damaging digital joints usually are treated by primary arthrodesis (Fig. 5.11C), but joint motion can be preserved by the insertion of a Silastic implant. This method probably is best reserved as a primary procedure for amputations that are sharp and clean and when occupational requirements are best satisfied by having mobile joints.

Bone fixation in digits and metacarpals usually is achieved by using two parallel medullary axial Kirschner wires or a single axial Kirschner wire supplemented by an

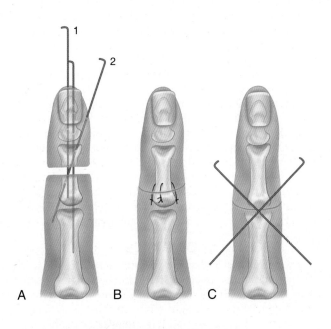

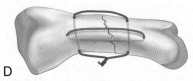

FIGURE 5.11   Bone fixation. **A,** Fixation usually is achieved with two parallel Kirschner wires (1) or single Kirschner wire supplemented with oblique wire (2). **B,** Wire loop fixation suitable for amputation near undamaged joint. **C,** Primary arthrodesis with crossed wires for amputation through irreparably damaged joint. **D,** Intraosseous wires.

oblique Kirschner wire to control rotation (Fig. 5.11A; see Fig. 5.10C). Wires should be placed to allow joint motion, if possible. Occasionally, when the amputation is near an undamaged joint, wire loops through drill holes are used (Fig. 5.11B). Care must be taken to maintain axial alignment and rotational control, especially when dealing with multiple digital amputations. We have not found it necessary to use plates and screws for digital or metacarpal fixation during replantation. This is an acceptable but often time-consuming technique. Periosteal suture with 4-0 or 5-0 absorbable suture may be done after bone fixation. Whitney et al. evaluated clinical results after use of single and crossed Kirschner wires and intraosseous wires with and without Kirschner wire support (Fig. 5.11D). Although initial results showed similar early angulation deformities in all groups, intraosseous wires were found to have the lowest nonunion and complication rates.

Management of the skeleton in more proximal amputations is more varied and requires more skill in the handling of medullary fixation devices, bone plates, and screws than in distal amputations. If the amputation level is through the carpus, shortening may be achieved and motion preserved by excision of carpal bones and temporary fixation with transarticular Steinmann pins. Amputations through the forearm and arm usually are shortened 2 to 5 cm to allow tension-free vessel anastomoses and nerve repairs.

For amputations through the forearm, generally accepted principles of internal fixation are applied; however, time constraints frequently dictate modifications. Distal radial metaphyseal amputations usually are fixed with Steinmann pins; plates and screws are used less often. We have also used intraosseous wiring occasionally with success. Amputations more proximally are fixed with plates and screws on both bones, intramedullary fixation with Rush rods or Steinmann pins in both bones, or combinations, such as a plate and screws for the radius and intramedullary fixation for the ulna. Medullary screws combined with wire loops are used for olecranon amputations. If the elbow joint is comminuted, an attempt is made to salvage sufficient bone to allow subsequent elbow arthroplasty. Amputations through the humerus are usually fixed with plates and screws; however, fracture configuration and time considerations may require interfragmentary Steinmann pins or intramedullary rods.

TRANSPOSITION OF DIGITS

Because of extensive damage to amputated parts or to the amputation stump, anatomic restoration of digits is sometimes impossible. In these situations, a functioning part may be restored by moving digits from their original anatomic position to a more suitable position. In bilateral digital amputations, parts from one hand may be better replanted to the opposite hand. Priority should be given to restoration of the thumb position with provision for a digit in the index or long position for pinch. Consideration also should be given to providing long, ring, and little digits for cup restoration. When digital transposition is considered in bilateral amputations, the dominant hand is given priority if possible.

TENDON REPAIR

During replantation, damaged structures are usually repaired in a serial fashion from the skeletal plane to more superficial planes. This may delay repair of vessels in the sequence so that deeper structures can be repaired without jeopardizing vascular anastomoses.

■ FLEXOR TENDONS

If the amputating injury involves crushing or avulsion of the part, and if the amputation is through the digits proximal to the flexor digitorum sublimis insertion or if tendon substance has been lost, flexor tendons usually are not repaired primarily. Delayed tendon grafting is planned in these circumstances. At times, silicone rods may be inserted at the time of replantation in anticipation of two-stage tendon grafting. The condition of the wound, extent of contamination, and potential for infection should be considered before silicone rod placement.

A flexor tendon injured distal to the flexor sublimis insertion near the distal interphalangeal joint is reattached with a pull-out wire. In injuries over the middle phalanx, the distal tendon stump is tenodesed to bone or tendon sheath.

If the flexor tendons have been sharply severed, both tendons are usually repaired primarily in injuries at the proximal phalanx or more proximally. Waikakul et al. found that repair of the proximal flexor digitorum profundus to the distal flexor digitorum superficialis resulted in a better overall arc of motion than did repair of both tendons in zone 2 amputation and expedited this portion of the replantation. Our usual tenorrhaphy involves a modified Kessler technique with 4-0 polyester fiber (Mersilene) sutures. The technique of first placing separate sutures in each end of the tendon allows nerve and vessel repair and subsequent tying of the sutures as advocated by Urbaniak. This helps prevent obstruction of the repair of vessels and nerves by the flexed finger. Similar configurations or mattress double right-angle sutures are used more proximally at the wrist and in the distal forearm. When technically feasible, the digital flexor sheath is repaired with 5-0 or 6-0 nonabsorbable sutures, usually nylon. If the flexor tendons have been injured at the myotendinous junction, the tendon is reattached in a fish-mouth configuration with mattress sutures to the muscle belly.

■ EXTENSOR TENDONS

Extensor tendons are repaired using nonabsorbable 4-0 sutures. Injuries to the extensor tendons between the metacarpophalangeal joint and the wrist extensor retinaculum are usually repaired with mattress sutures. Extensor tendons injured at the extensor retinaculum usually require excision of a portion of the retinaculum to aid in repair and subsequent tendon gliding. A mattress stitch usually suffices at this level and more proximally at the myotendinous junction. This injury at the myotendinous level is repaired with insertion of the tendon into the muscle belly in a fish-mouth configuration, reinforced with mattress sutures.

VESSEL REPAIR

Identifying the volar digital arteries is usually easier than finding suitable veins for anastomosis. The arteries lie just dorsal to the volar digital nerves. Although both digital arteries can usually be identified with ease, hypoplastic vessels on the radial side of the index finger and the radial side of the thumb have been common in our experience. In the thumb, the princeps pollicis artery can provide sufficient blood flow from the dorsum if no palmar arteries are suitable for repair.

■ ORDER OF VESSEL REPAIR

Surgeons' preferences differ regarding the order in which the vessels should be repaired. The approach may vary depending on the location of the amputation. In the digits, our practice is to repair the arteries first. This allows assessment of adequacy of flow across the anastomosis and through the digit before proceeding with the replantation. If veins are repaired first, one has to await arterial anastomosis to determine whether or not blood will flow through the digit and across the venous anastomosis. Performing arterial repair first also allows the dorsal veins to fill, aiding in the identification of hard-to-find veins. In fingertip amputations, identification of a central artery arising from the distal transverse palmar arch formed by the radial and ulnar digital arteries may be required. It is located in the midline of the pulp just volar to the distal phalanx and is about 0.85 mm. The dorsal terminal vein can be identified in the midline distal to the distal interphalangeal joint and is formed by a confluence of veins from the nail wall. It is approximately 1 mm in diameter at the level of the distal interphalangeal joint. Koshima et al. reported a useful technique of delayed venous repair for distal replantations. They allowed venous engorgement to occur after arterial repair and returned the patient to the operating room the following day for venous anastomosis of dilated veins.

If the amputation has occurred through the palm, wrist, forearm, or more proximally, and if the limb can be safely revascularized, sometimes blood loss can be minimized if two or three large veins can be repaired before the arterial repair. This rarely should be done if the ischemia time is 6 hours or more. If considerable time has passed after amputation, repairing the artery first shortens the ischemia period and minimizes the risk from revascularization of a part containing dying muscle. Carotid endarterectomy shunts and ventriculoperitoneal shunts can be used to make arterial connections if the ischemia time is 6 hours or more. Release of excessive amounts of potassium, lactic acid, and myoglobin should be avoided. If the artery is repaired first in such circumstances, venous repair should follow as soon as possible to avoid excessive blood loss. In such a situation, the use of a pneumatic tourniquet helps to control bleeding.

Large and small parts may benefit from perfusion of the artery, using a small, soft Silastic catheter and heparinized lactated Ringer solution. Crushed small parts and large, muscle-containing parts may have a better chance for survival if they are perfused gently with a heparinized solution. Gentle dilation and irrigation of the cut ends of the vessels help to clear the field of thrombogenic material.

VESSEL REPAIR IN REPLANTATION

TECHNIQUE 5.5

- After the arteries have been identified and marked with a small suture, dissect the veins from the dorsal skin flap. Three or four suitable veins usually are found on the dorsum of the digit between the metacarpophalangeal joint and the midportion of the middle phalanx. Distal to this point, only one or two suitable veins may be present. Although volar veins can be seen, they are frequently less than 1 mm in diameter and may not be suitable for anastomosis. Mark the veins with small sutures and proceed to prepare the vessels for anastomosis.
- Dissection of the vessels in the palm, on the dorsum of the hand, and in the forearm is less tedious than in the digits because of the larger vessel size. This dissection frequently requires a midpalmar incision paralleling the skin creases and curved or zigzag incisions on the dorsum of the hand and forearm.
- After all the arteries and veins have been identified and marked with sutures, mobilize them by dissecting them free from the surrounding tissues using gentle and meticulous technique. Transect small side branches and tributaries using ligatures, metal clips, or bipolar electrocautery, depending on the size of the branch being sacrificed. This mobilization aids in a tension-free anastomosis.
- When the vessels have been mobilized, the size of the gap between the vessel ends determines whether the anastomoses can be accomplished without additional bone shortening or the use of an interpositional vein graft.
- Free the vessel of any adventitia that may be causing constriction and excise the adventitia from the cut ends of the vessels.
- Irrigate the vessel with heparinized saline, 100 U/mL.
- Use magnification, including the operating microscope, to determine the extent of vessel wall injury. If evidence of thrombosis in the wall is found or if the intima has been damaged, excise the damaged segment. If an avulsion seems to have caused the intima to be pulled out of the vessel ("telescoped"), excise that portion of the vessel as well. Extensive avulsing or crushing injuries may cause vessel wall injury sufficient to preclude a successful anastomosis.
- After the vessel preparation has been completed, anastomose the vessels in the order noted previously. Attempt to repair both digital arteries and as many veins as possible, preferably two veins per artery. Use the small vessel-approximating clips on the digital vessels. Similar clips are available for the larger vessels. Keep in mind the length of time these clips are in place, especially on small (1 mm) vessels; time elapsed should be kept to a minimum, preferably less than 30 minutes.
- After the vascular clips are released, bathe the vessel in lidocaine or bupivacaine to minimize spasm.
- For digital vessels, use 10-0 or 11-0 monofilament sutures. In the hand, wrist, and distal forearm, 7-0 to 9-0 sutures are suitable, whereas vascular injuries near the elbow and more proximally require larger sutures, in the 6-0 and 7-0 range. Most digital arteries require 6 to 8 sutures; digital veins require 8 to 10 and sometimes more. Expect a small amount of blood leakage; this usually stops in a few minutes.
- If spasm is encountered, apply warm saline, topical lidocaine, papaverine, reserpine, and magnesium sulfate to relieve the spasm. Although intraoperative and postoperative systemic heparinization has been widely used, we have used low-molecular-weight dextran and aspirin for anticoagulation.
- At times, the arteries and veins are so damaged that no satisfactory proximal vessel is available to suture to the distal vessel or vessel debridement would leave a gap too large to correct by simple end-to-end repair. Techniques such as interpositional grafting with arterial segments and reversed segments of vein, vein harvesting and shifting in the injured digit, and transposition of arterial and venous pedicles from adjacent, uninjured digits may help to salvage an otherwise nonviable digit (Fig. 5.12). Vein grafts usually are harvested from unsalvageable amputated

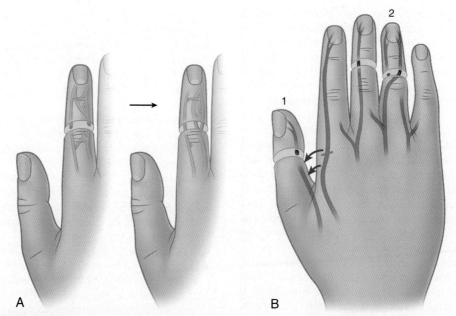

FIGURE 5.12 Vessel shifting. **A,** Dorsal veins mobilized to provide additional distal veins for proximal anastomosis. **B,** Arteries mobilized to allow shifting of artery from intact digit to vascularize thumb (1) and within same digit to vascularize distal amputated part (2). **SEE TECHNIQUE 5.5.**

parts, the dorsum of the hand or forearm, and the foot. In some situations, a single vein graft anastomosed to a single digital artery proximally may be attached to two digital arteries distally, using side-to-end anastomoses or a Y configuration of the graft. When vein grafts are used, care should be taken to maintain the proper (reversed) flow direction so that flow is not obstructed by venous valves. The harvested vein grafts should have approximately the same diameter as the recipient vessel.

NERVE REPAIR FOR REPLANTATION

TECHNIQUE 5.6

- With the dorsal and palmar skin flaps retracted, locate the digital nerves in the palmar flap, superficial to the digital arteries. Usually the nerves can be repaired easily after the arterial anastomoses.
- Gently dissect the nerves free of the surrounding connective tissue and mobilize them so that they can be repaired without excessive tension. Occasionally, it may be necessary to transect small side branches for sufficient mobilization of a nerve.
- When the proximal and distal ends of the nerve have been mobilized, inspect them using the operating microscope or magnifying loupes and trim 3 to 5 mm of nerve from each end.
- If the injury has been sharp, the nerves usually are repaired primarily. Use two to four epineurial stitches of 9-0 or 10-0 monofilament suture material to align carefully and approximate the fascicles.

- For more proximal injuries, dissect the respective nerve trunks using standard palmar incisions, paralleling the skin creases in the palm and extending proximally up the forearm. In a nerve trunk in the palm, at the wrist, and more proximally, use a "group fascicular" or peripheral fascicular stitch.
- If the amputated part has been avulsed, or if significant crushing makes the extent of intraneural injury unclear, several techniques may be useful.
- Trim the nerve ends proximally and distally so that normal-appearing nerve can be identified. Insert a nerve graft and secure it with microsuture techniques. Nerve grafts can be harvested from unreplantable amputated parts, the lateral antebrachial cutaneous nerve, and the sural nerve. Because of the additional operating time required for nerve grafting and the uncertainty regarding the extent of intraneural injury, we generally do not include primary nerve grafting in the replantation procedure. Instead, suture the ends of the avulsed or crushed nerve together with an 8-0 mattress suture, anticipating later nerve exploration, debridement, repair, or grafting.
- As an alternative, if the nerve ends cannot be brought together, secure them to the adjacent soft tissues so that they can be easily identified and mobilized later for nerve grafting.
- After all structures have been repaired, close the skin primarily if the procedure has been completed promptly, if no excessive swelling is present, and if the skin edges can be approximated without tension.
- In the digits and more proximal sites, some areas can be left open to heal by secondary intention or to be covered with skin grafts. Nerves, vessels, bone, joints, and tendons should not be exposed if the wounds are left open.
- Satisfactory alternatives include closure with Z-plasties; local rotation of skin; remote, two-stage pedicle flaps;

single-stage transfer of composite tissue (free flaps); and split-thickness skin grafts. In our experience, primary remote pedicle flaps and free flaps have not been needed. A combination of skin flap rotation, split-thickness skin graft, and leaving the wound partially open has been satisfactory.

- Apply medicated petrolatum gauze to the skin wounds and use a bulky dressing to cover the dorsal and palmar surfaces. Fluffed cotton or synthetic material provides a soft and gently conforming dressing. Moisten the padding with physiologic saline or lactated Ringer solution to allow blood to be absorbed into the bandage more readily and to permit the bandage to conform more easily to the contours of the part. Avoid localized pressure at all times.

POSTOPERATIVE CARE The part is adequately padded, and a plaster splint is applied to the palmar surface to support the fingers, hand, and wrist. Excessive tightness or constriction is avoided when securing the bandage. The fingertips and small areas of skin are left exposed for evaluation of the circulation. During the first week, the bandage is moistened with physiologic solutions every 8 hours to prevent dried blood from forming circumferential crusts that might have a constricting effect. Although early and frequent dressing changes may be necessary for the assessment of the circulation or to determine the source and extent of any bleeding, our policy has been to delay the initial dressing change for at least 1 week in uncomplicated replantations. This decreases the risk of disturbing the fragile vascular anastomoses and lessens the chance of stimulating vascular spasm.

The replanted part usually is positioned with the hand at heart level as long as the appearance of the part is satisfactory. If the replanted part appears congested and cyanotic because of venous obstruction, elevation on several pillows may be helpful. If the part becomes pale because of arterial insufficiency, depression of the part below the level of the heart may be required to enhance arterial flow. Depending on the extent of the injury, the patient usually is kept at bed rest for the first 3 to 7 days.

Maintaining a warm room, prohibiting smoking by the patient and visitors, and advising abstinence from caffeine-containing beverages are measures that help to prevent vasospasm in the early postoperative period. Vasospasm related to pain and emotional distress may be prevented or minimized through the use of appropriate narcotic analgesics and sedative medications such as chlorpromazine (25 mg four times daily).

Nerve blocks are beneficial in the postoperative period for the prevention of vasospasm. If small Silastic catheters are left adjacent to the median and ulnar nerves, 4 to 5 mL of bupivacaine 0.25% injected every 6 to 8 hours may be sufficient. Stellate ganglion sympathetic blocks or axillary brachial plexus blocks with bupivacaine are carried out once or twice daily in situations in which it is necessary to control vasospasm.

Various anticoagulants alone or in combination have been administered by different surgeons. Heparin, low-molecular-weight dextran, aspirin, dipyridamole, and sodium warfarin (Coumadin) have been most popular. Heparin has been advocated in injuries thought to be at high risk for thrombosis, especially in replantations with extensive crushing or avulsing injuries, replantations showing poor flow from the cut ends of vessels before anastomosis, replantations with poor or equivocal flow across completed anastomoses, and replantations done in small children. It has been our practice to use dextran, 500 mL every 24 hours (10 mL/kg/day in children) for 3 days, combined with aspirin, 300 mg twice daily for 5 to 7 days. Antibiotics are administered routinely for 1 week after surgery. The use of vacuum-assisted closure (VAC) in complex open injuries has been shown to be safe and beneficial in promoting granulation tissue. Low intermittent pressure (75 mm Hg) settings, avoidance of circumferential dressings, and delay of application until the first dressing change should be considered.

MANAGEMENT OF CIRCULATORY COMPROMISE AFTER REPLANTATION

If the replanted part shows signs of inadequate circulation, prompt evaluation and management of the problem might allow salvage of a part that otherwise would be lost. Mechanical monitors of skin temperature, oxygen tension, hydrogen and fluorescein dilution, and other factors (see Monitoring Techniques after Microvascular Surgery later in this chapter) in many instances are sufficiently sensitive to detect significant changes in blood flow before clinically apparent ischemic changes develop. If the part is cool and has developed the pallor and loss of turgor consistent with arterial insufficiency, or if it is cyanotic, congested, and turgid consistent with venous obstruction, several measures can be helpful in relieving the problem before the patient is taken to the operating room for exploration.

The room should be comfortably warm, and the patient should have sufficient analgesic medication and be sufficiently sedated to minimize emotional distress. As noted previously, the part should be elevated well above the level of the heart to enhance venous drainage. Medical-grade leeches (Hirudo medicinalis) are effective in relieving venous congestion; however, they may be a source of infection and should not be used in the presence of nonviable tissue. If arterial insufficiency is suspected, placing the part in a dependent position may be beneficial. Splints and dressings are loosened or removed to ensure that nothing is causing direct pressure on the vessels and that nothing is constricting the limb. Using gentle digital pressure, the arteries are lightly "milked" from proximal to distal and the veins are "milked" from distal to proximal.

In distal injuries, if Silastic catheters have been left adjacent to the median or ulnar nerves, 4 to 5 mL of 0.25% bupivacaine is injected. Stellate ganglion sympathetic blocks and brachial plexus blocks also have been useful, especially in patients with troublesome vessel spasm. Although it is not part of our usual routine, many surgeons with extensive experience find it useful to administer heparin intravenously as a bolus of 3000 to 5000 U when attempting to salvage a failing replanted part.

If the replanted part does not respond to these measures, the surgeon must decide, based on knowledge of the injury and experience, whether returning to the operating room to explore the vessels is worthwhile. This decision should be made promptly when definite signs of impaired circulation are evident. Reoperation is more likely to be successful if done within 4 to 6 hours of the development of signs of ischemia.

REOPERATION

TECHNIQUE 5.7

- Although the clinical signs may indicate whether the problem is arterial or venous, when the decision to reoperate is made, all anastomoses are evaluated.
- Inspect the arterial anastomoses to determine patency.
- If one or more arterial anastomoses are not patent, excise the anastomoses, ensure that there is adequate "spurting" flow proximally, and repair the vessels.
- If proximal flow is inadequate, or the proximal artery appears excessively damaged, dissect more proximally, find good arteries, and interpose a reversed segment of vein graft.
- Similar problems may be encountered in the distal arteries. If good arterial trunks cannot be found, search for other arteries to substitute. Repair any vein graft as needed. Assess the arterial flow and perfusion distally and the appearance of the part.
- Inspect all venous anastomoses to assess patency. If flow cannot be restored despite all efforts, consider reamputation.
- If on initial inspection all arterial anastomoses are patent and none seem to have spasm, torsion, pressure, or thrombosis proximally or distally, attention should be directed to the veins.
- If all venous anastomoses are patent, the veins proximal and distal to the anastomoses should be inspected to exclude compression, torsion, and thrombosis. If areas of thrombosis are found, excise those segments and repair the vessel end-to-end or interpose vein grafts. If the venous anastomoses are found to be obstructed by thrombi, excise and repair them end to end or with vein grafts.
- Evaluate arterial and venous flow and the appearance of the part. If all available and suitable veins have been located, repaired, or grafted, and satisfactory flow cannot be restored, consider reamputation.
- For digital injuries, techniques such as pulp incisions and wedge excision of the nail to allow venous oozing may allow sufficient flow to persist long enough for a digit to survive. In such patients, the hemoglobin and hematocrit should be monitored closely so that blood volume loss can be corrected promptly.

COMPLICATIONS

Although circulatory compromise related to the vessel repairs is the most pressing complication after replantation, other complications that occur in the early postreplantation period include bleeding, skin necrosis, ischemia caused by muscle compartment swelling, and infection. Excessive bleeding may be from vessels that have not been cauterized, or it may be caused by anticoagulant therapy. Significant skin necrosis usually occurs after closure of skin that initially appears viable but later undergoes necrotic changes resulting from the magnitude of the injury sustained at the initial traumatic amputation. Additional debridement and secondary closure with local flaps or skin grafts may be required. Significant sepsis is rare after replantation and usually is managed satisfactorily with appropriate systemic antibiotics, wound debridement, and drainage

as needed. Although ischemia may be caused by excessive muscle compartment pressure, this usually occurs in major limb replantations and can be treated with appropriate fasciotomies in the arm, forearm, and hand. These early complications may require wound inspection and dressing changes with the patient under anesthesia in the first week after replantation.

Later complications, such as nonunion and malunion of bones, tendon adherence, joint stiffness, and delay in return of nerve function, usually can be managed with the usual techniques appropriate to these problems. In nonunion and malunion, bone grafts and internal fixation may be required. Tendon adhesions with loss of excursion may require tenolysis and, in some situations, tendon grafting as one-stage or two-stage procedures. Stiff joints may require capsulotomy, or if sufficient damage has occurred, interposition arthroplasty may salvage motion in selected patients. If a primary neurorrhaphy fails to show return of function in a reasonable length of time, or if the nerves are not repaired as part of the original replantation, reexploration and repair or interpositional nerve grafting may be necessary. The nature and timing of specific reconstructive procedures depend on the individual patient's problems and needs and the judgment and experience of the surgeon.

REHABILITATION

The specific rehabilitation program for each patient depends on many factors, especially the patient's needs and motivation and the extent of injury to the part. Generally, no attempt is made to begin significant movement of bone, joint, or tendon for the first 3 weeks after replantation. Then, depending on the extent of injury, most replantation patients are treated in a manner similar to most patients with combined tendon, bone, and nerve injuries. After the first 3 weeks, most patients are encouraged to participate in a graduated program of active, active-assisted, and protected passive stretching and range-of-motion exercises supplemented by appropriate dynamic and static bracing and splinting.

MONITORING TECHNIQUES AFTER MICROVASCULAR SURGERY

After microvascular procedures such as replantation and free composite tissue transfer, a reliable monitoring system should be established for the replanted or transferred tissue. Although the clinical determination of the color, capillary refill, temperature, and turgor is easily made, there is room for error because of the subjective nature of these factors, especially color and temperature. This, combined with the possibility that considerable ischemic injury may occur before clear clinical signs are present, has led to the development and use of a variety of mechanical monitoring devices and techniques, including ultrasonic and laser Doppler probes, plethysmography, skin temperature probes, transcutaneous oxygen tension measurements, hydrogen washout techniques, and skin fluorescence measurements.

The Doppler probe and plethysmographic techniques are reasonably accurate indicators of arterial flow; however, they are not as accurate when venous flow is to be assessed. Although the transcutaneous oxygen tension determination, the hydrogen washout method, and the skin fluorescence measurement all have been found to be useful and sensitive assays of changes in the microcirculation, the use of skin temperature monitoring probes is presently a simple and reliable adjunct to the clinical evaluations. With separate temperature probes attached to the revascularized tissue, adjacent normal tissue, and the dressing, relative and absolute changes in the temperature can be monitored constantly. A decrease in the temperature of the replanted digit to less than 30°C or a decrease of more than 2°C or 3°C less than the normal digit is considered a sign of circulatory compromise.

Transcutaneous oxygen measurements show changes in oxygen tension several hours before the onset of clinical signs of ischemia and before temperature changes occur. This and other techniques hold promise for the development of monitoring techniques with increasing sensitivity.

REVASCULARIZATION

Partial amputation or devitalization of tissues from serious vascular interruption can occur without complete detachment of the part. Some of these parts with impaired circulation ultimately may survive, but there may be persistent ischemia that later causes disabling cold intolerance and atrophy or contracture of the intrinsic muscles of the hand. Digits with impaired circulation show extremely slow return of the normal pink color after blanching by pressure. The management of these hand injuries is essentially the same as for replantation; however, a longer interval from the time of the accident to the anastomosis of the vessels may be tolerated, and the procedure can be done by one team. The same postoperative routine is carried out as described previously. When radial and ulnar arteries are severed at the wrist, usually at least one should be repaired. If viability of the hand is questionable, both the radial and the ulnar arteries should be repaired.

SPECIAL TECHNIQUES

For distal fingertip amputations in which microvascular anastomosis is impossible, Brent described the "pocket technique." This technique involves debriding and deepithelializing the amputated part, reattaching it as a composite graft, and burying it in a contralateral chest wall subcutaneous pocket for 3 weeks. It is then removed, and the viable tip skin is grafted. Lee et al. used this technique with an abdominal pocket. Muneuchi et al. reported poor results with this technique in seven fingers and did not recommend it for injuries at or proximal to the lunula. To avoid shoulder and elbow stiffness, Arata et al. modified this procedure by using the ipsilateral palm as the pocket site. In their 16 patients, complete survival was seen in 13, with the remaining three showing partial necrosis.

POCKET TECHNIQUE FOR MICROVASCULAR ANASTOMOSIS

TECHNIQUE 5.8

(ARATA ET AL.)

FIRST OPERATION

- With the use of wrist or upper arm block anesthesia and a pneumatic tourniquet applied to the upper arm, wash the amputated part and the amputation stump with normal saline and remove the nail.
- Reduce fractured bone segments and stabilize them with Kirschner wires, cutting the wire as short as possible.
- Reattach the amputated part to the amputation stump without vascular anastomosis.
- After reattaching the amputated part to the digit, use a scalpel to deepithelialize the amputated part to the mid-dermal layer.
- Make a 2-cm transverse incision in the ipsilateral palm and bluntly undermine the subcutaneous layer to form a pocket.
- Insert the reattached part into the pocket and suture the finger to the palmar skin 2 mm proximal to the reattached level to prevent the inserted digit from pulling out of the pocket.
- Apply a light compressive gauze dressing without splinting.

SECOND OPERATION

- Sixteen to 20 days after the first operation, carefully remove the replanted part from the palmar pocket and suture the palmar skin.
- Change the dressing to a wet dressing and encourage active exercise of the injured finger.
- At approximately 2 weeks after the second operation, epithelialization should be complete and the replanted part gradually gains stability.

Another technique described for replanting distal fingertip amputations involves anastomosing a volar radial vein to the proximal digital artery to create an arteriovenous anastomosis. Venous drainage is accomplished by a transverse tip incision. Yabe et al. reported four fingertip replantations; three survived, and one developed partial necrosis.

SINGLE-STAGE TISSUE TRANSFER (FREE FLAPS)

Before the development of microvascular techniques, remote pedicle flaps were used to cover major soft-tissue defects. In 1946, Shaw and Payne reported their extensive experience with tubed pedicle flaps based on the superficial epigastric and superficial circumflex arterial circulations. Based on that report, their analysis of the deltopectoral flap of Bakamjian, and their own experience with the groin pedicle flap, McGregor and Morgan explained the differences between random pattern and axial pattern flaps. The random pattern flap relies on no specific established pattern of circulation. A length-to-width ratio of greater than 2:1 increases the risk of failure of a random flap. An axial pattern flap relies on a definite and usually consistent arterial supply centered on one or more arteries. There are no rigid length-to-width ratio requirements for axial pattern flaps. These flaps generally are considered to be cutaneous or myocutaneous, depending on the pattern of their arterial circulation. Cutaneous flaps rely on a constant circulation from a single artery passing through the underlying subcutaneous tissue, supplying the overlying skin through the dermal-subdermal vessels. The myocutaneous flap receives its cutaneous arterial supply from deep vessels that perforate the muscle and fascia to reach the skin (Fig. 5.13). Perforator flaps, first described by Koshima and Soeda, are skin or subcutaneous tissue flaps that are based on

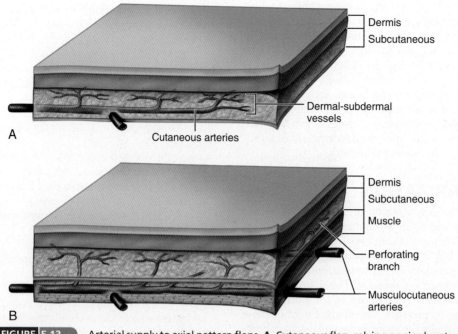

FIGURE 5.13 Arterial supply to axial pattern flaps. **A,** Cutaneous flap, relying on single artery supplying dermal and subdermal vessels. **B,** Myocutaneous flap, relying on deep musculocutaneous arteries perforating muscle and fascia to overlying skin.

a single vascular tributary and its cutaneous perforator vessels. The intervening fascia or muscle is not elevated with the flap, thus allowing for less donor-site morbidity and better recipient-site contouring without a longer and more tedious dissection. Common perforator flaps include the deep inferior epigastric artery perforator flap, anterolateral thigh flap, thoracodorsal artery perforator flaps, and superior-inferior gluteal artery perforator flaps.

Although various workers have described many free flaps from a variety of donor sites and with many different uses, this section discusses the flaps with proven application to reconstructive surgery in the extremities.

INDICATIONS AND ADVANTAGES

The traditional indications for pedicle flaps are similar to the indications for free flaps, and pedicle flaps may be preferred in young children, electrical burn patients, fingertip amputations, and preparation for toe-to-hand microvascular transfers.

Each case must be considered individually. Current indications for free flaps include, but are not limited to, the following:

1. Secondary and, in some situations, primary coverage of extensive skin and soft-tissue loss with exposure of essential structures (e.g., blood vessel, nerve, tendon, bone, and joint)
2. Coverage of a soft-tissue bed unsatisfactory for later reconstructive procedures (e.g., scar, chronic draining ulcers, and chronic osteomyelitis that prevent tendon grafts, tendon transfers, nerve repairs or nerve grafts, bone stabilization, and bone grafting)
3. Replacement of unstable area scars after burns, irradiation, radical surgery for cancer, and scar contracture
4. Coverage situations for which a suitable random or axial pattern flap is unavailable

5. Coverage situations in which immobilization of the extremities for prolonged periods in awkward positions is undesirable or impossible
6. Restoration of specific tissue to satisfy a functional need (e.g., sensation in the hand or the plantar surface of the foot, digital reconstruction in the hand, replacement of major skeletal muscle loss in the forearm, replacement for bone loss in the upper and lower extremities, replacement of lost or destroyed joints in the fingers, replacement of functioning epiphyses in the hand and forearm, and correction of congenital and developmental deformities including radial club-hand and congenital pseudarthrosis of the tibia)

The advantages free flaps seem to have over more traditional techniques include the following:

1. They usually are done as single-stage procedures.
2. The choice of a donor site usually is not as restrictive.
3. There usually is more versatility regarding the matching of the color, texture, thickness, and hair distribution of the donor area with the recipient area.
4. In many situations, the donor site can be closed primarily, without resorting to skin grafts.
5. Most donor sites are left with an acceptable appearance.
6. Well-vascularized tissue with a permanent blood supply can replace ischemic or avascular tissue.
7. When indicated, a vascularized bone graft, functioning joints, epiphyses, and skeletal muscle can be electively included in the composite graft used to reconstruct a limb.
8. Prolonged immobilization in awkward positions is not required, allowing the patient more freedom in daily activities.
9. Joints adjacent to the recipient area are mobilized earlier than after conventional techniques, preventing joint stiffness and contractures.
10. Hospital stays usually are shortened.

CONTRAINDICATIONS AND DISADVANTAGES

Although absolute contraindications to the use of free flaps are few, the surgeon should have reservations regarding their use in the following situations:

1. The surgeon has neither microsurgical training nor microsurgical experience.
2. Institutional support for a reconstructive microsurgical program is insufficient.
3. No suitable recipient vessels are available in the area requiring coverage or tissue reconstruction.
4. Previous trauma or irradiation to the recipient area may have damaged the vessels sufficiently to preclude their use.
5. If only one major artery to the foot or the hand is present, the use of it as the recipient vessel for a free flap may jeopardize the viability of the foot or hand, even though an end-to-side anastomosis is used.
6. Age alone may not constitute a contraindication; however, if major systemic illnesses create a major anesthetic risk for the patient, an alternative method of treatment should be considered.
7. If systemic illnesses, such as atherosclerosis, vasculitis, or other lesions, have caused damage to the vascular system, microvascular procedures, although not certain to fail, are more likely to fail than are those done when the vessels are not diseased.
8. If previous operative procedures have been done in the donor area, the donor vessels may have been damaged, precluding the use of that specific donor site.
9. Obesity makes dissection of vascular pedicles difficult or impossible. Bulky, obese flaps are awkward to manipulate and difficult to place without causing tension, torsion, or disruption of anastomoses. The fat at times causes obstruction of a clear view of the vascular pedicles, preventing the performance of satisfactory anastomoses.

The disadvantages of free tissue transfer include the following:

1. The initial operation usually is longer than are operations for conventional flaps. Free flap procedures take 4 to 10 hours, depending largely on the flap selected and the experience of the surgical team.
2. The operations may be difficult and tedious.
3. Two teams of surgeons usually are required.
4. If vascular thrombosis occurs, the risk of complete loss of the free flap is considerable.
5. Reportedly, the overall risk of free flap failure compared with conventional techniques is greater. A 10% to 30% failure rate for free flaps is cited by Sharzer et al. In addition, the reoperation rate after free flap transfers may be 25%.
6. Postoperative vascular complications, which usually occur in the first 24 hours, may be seen 10 days after the procedure.

SELECTION OF FREE FLAPS

Numerous free flaps have been described. The selection of one specific flap over another is influenced by many factors. Specific tissue requirements at the recipient site are important: Is full-thickness coverage needed? Would a skin graft or conventional flap suffice? Is a free flap really needed? Is the need only for simple coverage? How thick and how large should the coverage be? Is skin sensibility, bone, joint, nerve, or functioning muscle needed? In general, free skin flaps are selected rather than free muscle flaps when dead space is minimal and skin and subcutaneous tissue must be matched to restore cutaneous sensibility.

The condition and availability of donor and recipient vessels are important considerations in the determination of which flap would be best in a given situation. Generally, the simplest procedure should be chosen that would fulfill the tissue requirements of a specific recipient area. The flap should be designed so that if it fails, a satisfactory salvage procedure is possible. In most situations, a major factor in flap selection is likely to be the experience of the individual surgeon using specific flaps.

Single-stage transfers of composite tissue grafts (free flaps) are discussed here as they apply to repair and reconstruction of traumatic, infectious, neoplastic, congenital, and developmental problems in the upper and lower limbs. The simplest procedures, including local and remote pedicle flaps, should be considered first. In circumstances precluding more traditional techniques, microsurgical procedures should be considered, and in some situations, priority should be given to the use of free flaps.

■ UPPER EXTREMITY

In the upper extremity, free tissue transfer has proved to be useful in the simple coverage of soft-tissue defects, the restoration of sensibility, the reconstruction of bony defects, the replacement of nonfunctioning skeletal muscle units, and thumb and digital reconstruction by toe transfers. The transfers of vascularized toe joints to finger joints and toe and fibular physes to digital and forearm physes show promise in the management of additional difficult reconstructive problems in the upper extremity.

Currently, free flaps used most often in the upper extremity include the lateral arm flap, the anterolateral thigh flap, and the dorsalis pedis cutaneous flap for soft-tissue coverage. The dorsalis pedis flap has an added advantage of having nerve supply through the deep and superficial peroneal nerves that can be used in restoring sensibility to the hand. For large defects with considerable dead space, especially around the elbow, free muscle transfers, including the latissimus dorsi, serratus anterior, and rectus abdominis, are helpful. The gracilis, latissimus dorsi, and pectoralis major muscles have been used to restore skeletal muscle function to the forearm. All or portions of the great, second, and third toes have been used successfully for thumb and finger reconstruction. Vascularized bone grafts using rib, iliac crest, and fibula have been used for bone reconstruction in the upper limb and hand.

Most soft-tissue defects in the upper extremity can be treated with direct closure, skin grafts, local flaps, or distant pedicled flaps, and these remain the procedures of choice if they are technically possible. Immediate free flap coverage can be performed in the upper extremity. Radical initial debridement of all nonviable and potentially nonviable tissue and an experienced and well-staffed microvascular team are necessary for this approach.

■ LOWER EXTREMITY

In the lower extremity, requirements for soft-tissue coverage in the management of osteomyelitis have been satisfied by using the latissimus dorsi muscle, the serratus anterior muscle, the rectus abdominis muscle, the gracilis muscle, the tensor fasciae latae muscle, the free groin cutaneous flap, and the scapular cutaneous flap. The dorsalis pedis cutaneous flap also has been used as a neurovascular cutaneous flap to provide sensibility to the plantar surface of the foot. Although the rib and iliac crest have been used to reconstruct bony defects in the lower extremity, the curvature and relative weakness of these bones limit their usefulness. The vascularized fibula has been applied successfully to a variety of bony problems in the lower extremity, including defects caused by tumor surgery, trauma, and congenital anomalies, such as congenital pseudarthrosis of the tibia. Although the vascularized fibula has been used in the treatment of osteonecrosis of the femoral head, the results are inconclusive to date because long-term results in significant numbers of patients have not been accumulated.

Several authors have discussed the use of free flaps in the management of posttraumatic chronic osteomyelitis. Myocutaneous flaps seem to be more resistant to infection than random pattern flaps. Some preliminary reports using microvascular skin and myocutaneous flaps in the treatment of osteomyelitis were optimistic, although others were not. Major complications, flap failure, and recurrent infections have been reported. Gordon and Chiu in a study of 14 infected tibial nonunions concluded that free muscle transfer alone was effective in managing infected nonunions without segmental bone loss. For small defects (<3 cm), they recommended a posterolateral bone graft after successful free flap coverage. Segmental defects of the fibula and tibia were best treated with a subsequent free fibular transfer.

For large soft-tissue defects (>15 cm), the latissimus dorsi is the preferred muscle flap. For smaller distal lower extremity defects after procedures such as sequestrectomy for osteomyelitis, muscle flaps such as the gracilis, serratus anterior, or rectus abdominis may be preferable.

PREOPERATIVE REQUIREMENTS

Proficiency in microvascular techniques and familiarity with the vascular anatomy of the various free flaps acquired through cadaver dissection are necessary.

The candidate for a free flap must be evaluated before surgery. The patient should be healthy enough to tolerate a potentially lengthy procedure. Surgical debridement of all unhealthy tissue should be completed before free flap coverage, and the patient should have demonstrably normal donor and recipient vasculature out of the zone of injury. The adequacy of vessels can be estimated by clinical palpation of peripheral pulses, the Allen test in the hand, and the use of the ultrasonic Doppler probe. These methods are considered inadequate by some surgeons who favor preoperative angiography, especially in a traumatized extremity, to help assess the condition of the recipient vessels. However, preoperative angiography may cause damage to the recipient vasculature, and at times surgical exposure is the only way to assess the vessels. Venography may help determine the adequacy of the deep venous system if the superficial system is incompetent. Although it may be difficult to assess the vasculature with angiography, if there are any questions regarding the donor site, angiography may be helpful.

Before the operation, the patient is informed of the risks, hazards, and potential problems involved in such procedures. In addition, laboratory studies, including assessment of bleeding and clotting factors, and adequate blood replacement arrangements should be made.

GENERAL PLAN OF PROCEDURE

Excessively cold temperatures are avoided in the operating room. The patient is placed on a heating and cooling blanket. Body temperature is monitored with rectal or esophageal probes. If the planned procedure is expected to last several hours, an indwelling urinary catheter is inserted. After the induction of the anesthetic, the patient is positioned appropriately to permit access to the recipient and the donor sites. Bony prominences and neurovascular structures are padded to avoid excessive pressure. The recipient defect is mapped by measuring it and drawing it out on the patient, and the mapped defect is superimposed on the donor area so that the donor area can be determined to fit when transferred. The general courses of the donor and recipient vessels are identified by palpation and with a Doppler probe, and the courses are marked with a skin marker. In the extremities, a pneumatic tourniquet is used to maintain a bloodless field during most of the dissection. After major structures have been identified, the tourniquet is intermittently inflated and deflated as needed.

Two teams usually are preferred for free tissue transfers, especially for larger transfers. One team prepares the recipient area by debriding scar and all necrotic tissue, including bone. All recipient vessels are exposed to determine that arterial and venous pedicles of appropriate lengths are available. If venous grafts seem to be needed, they should be harvested before the delivery of the donor tissue to minimize the ischemia time of the tissue. Care is taken in this dissection to avoid stripping the vessel clean because this may cause refractory vessel spasm, precluding the planned tissue transfer. In the extremities, if the circulation to the limb depends on a single artery, the decision must be made regarding the use of the artery through an end to-end or an end-to-side anastomosis, or whether the artery should be used at all. If nerve or tendon repairs are planned, those structures are identified as well.

While one team is working on the recipient area, a second team dissects the donor area, usually using the identified course of the donor artery as the axis for the outlined flap of tissue. The approach to the free flap usually begins at the vascular pedicle. If suitable arteries and veins are identified, the dissection of the flap proceeds. If no satisfactory vessels are found on the first side of the body to be dissected, the opposite side may be explored if patient positioning and preoperative planning permit.

After the flap has been elevated, it is left attached to its vascular pedicle until the recipient site has been completely prepared and it is certain that the recipient vessels are capable of supplying sufficient circulation to the donor tissue through the pedicle to maintain its viability. When it is certain that preparation of the recipient area and the recipient vessels has been completed, and that the donor vascular pedicle is long enough, the pedicle is transected. The artery usually is clamped and transected first to allow time for venous drainage to occur. The veins are clamped next and transected. The flap is now ready for attachment to the recipient site. The donor team delivers the flap to the recipient team. While the flap is being attached to the recipient area, the donor team closes the donor-site wound. Although this usually can be done by direct approximation of the wound edges, at times split-thickness skin grafts may be required.

The recipient team loosely attaches the flap to the recipient site with sutures placed at widely spaced intervals around its periphery, sufficient to hold the flap in place to prevent shear on the vessels and disruption of anastomoses. The flap is positioned so that the vessel anastomoses can be done conveniently. Perfusion of the flap with various solutions usually is not required.

The sterilely draped operating microscope is brought into the surgical field, and attention is turned to dissecting the perivascular adventitia and soft tissue away from the vessels. This dissection is done gently to avoid undue trauma to the vessel walls. Microvascular anastomoses are carried out first on the artery and next on the veins. It sometimes is helpful to keep the microvascular clips on the artery until at least one venous anastomosis is completed so that the flap does not become congested by the arterial inflow while the veins are being sutured. Because of potential injury to the vessel wall, the clip should not be left attached too long.

Anastomoses should be done on as many vessels as are available and suitable. Two-vein anastomosis is preferred to one-vein anastomosis, but is not essential for flap survival.

At the time of the anastomoses, anticoagulation therapy may be started; heparin or low-molecular-weight dextran can be used. Patency is assessed by removing the vascular clips from the artery and the vein. If the flap is being perfused through the anastomoses, the patency test of the artery shows flow across the repair, and the emptying veins rapidly fill. A pink, warm flap, with rapid capillary refill and no demonstrable venous congestion is a good indicator of satisfactory perfusion in most situations. Other indicators of satisfactory flow include bleeding from the skin edges of the flap and rapid, bright red bleeding from small stab wounds made in the margins of the flap.

If flow into the flap is questionable, a Doppler probe can be used to detect flow, although this may not be reliable. Similarly, patients may be given intravenous fluorescein, and the flap can be assessed for fluorescent perfusion using an ultraviolet light. If arterial spasm occurs, it can be relieved at times by using topical papaverine or lidocaine. Stellate sympathetic ganglion blocks may be helpful if problems caused by vessel spasm continue in the upper extremity.

When satisfactory arterial and venous flow has been established, attention can be turned to additional reconstructive procedures, such as bone, tendon, or nerve grafts and tendon transfers, if circumstances permit. If the situation does not permit these more extensive procedures, they should be delayed until another time. The margins of the flap are next sutured in place. Ideally, the vessels should be covered by the skin of the transplanted flap or the local skin in the recipient area. Split-thickness skin grafts may be required to cover exposed areas not completely covered by the free flap. To allow easier inspection of the flap after surgery, we do not routinely cover free muscle transfers with a split-thickness skin graft during the initial procedure. Care is taken to avoid excessive tension so that the vessels are not occluded by the pressure of overlying skin or muscle. If needed, a small suction drain may be left beneath the flap well away from the vascular anastomoses to avoid their disruption on removal of the drain.

When the dressing is applied, whether in the upper or lower limb, care should be taken to avoid excessive pressure on the flap or constriction of the limb proximal to the flap. Our practice is to apply a wide-mesh petrolatum gauze to the wound edges and over skin grafts. This is covered with a loose bandage of gauze. Next, cotton cast padding is evenly applied to allow the application of a plaster splint to support the hand and wrist, or the foot and ankle, depending on the specific situation. Although the manner in which a patient awakens from the anesthetic is difficult to control predictably, every effort should be made to avoid violent straining, shivering, and flailing about, which sometimes accompany this stage of the procedure.

GENERAL POSTOPERATIVE CARE

Placing the patient in an intensive care unit should ensure regular monitoring of vital signs and the vascularity of the flap. If the patient has medical illnesses that require special monitoring techniques, the intensive care setting is probably the safest place. After an uncomplicated operation, if the nurses and house staff are familiar with administering this type of postoperative care, the patient may be cared for safely in a hospital room. The room is kept warm; excessive cooling is avoided to prevent cold-induced vasospasm. The room is kept quiet, and visitors are kept to a minimum to prevent emotional upsets that might lead to vasospasm. Cigarette smoking by the patient and visitors is prohibited to avoid nicotine-induced vasospasm. Cold drinks and those containing caffeine also are avoided.

Medications usually include antibiotics, sedatives, analgesics, and different combinations of anticoagulant medications. Anticoagulation routines vary, depending on the preference of the individual surgeon. In some patients, no significant anticoagulant medication is given. Some experienced surgeons use heparin routinely. Others use low-molecular-weight dextran, and our current practice is to give dextran, 500 mL, every 24 hours for at least 3 days. In addition, aspirin usually is added in doses of 300 mg twice daily.

The involved part usually is kept at the level of the heart or slightly elevated to avoid venous congestion. If the flap seems to be ischemic, the part can be lowered to improve arterial flow. If the flap becomes congested, the part is elevated well above the level of the heart to improve drainage. If the flap appears to be in jeopardy, a great deal of time should not be spent in carrying out these maneuvers because reexploration is likely to be required, and valuable time may be lost awaiting improvement.

The circulation of the flap can be monitored satisfactorily using a variety of techniques. Regardless of the techniques used, regular clinical evaluations by the surgical and nursing staff are essential.

MONITORING

Currently available monitoring techniques include ultrasound and laser Doppler scanning, digital plethysmography, radioisotope clearance assays, fluorescein perfusion monitoring, transcutaneous oxygen tension monitoring, and photoplethysmography. Continuous temperature monitoring is widely used and currently seems to be the simplest method for assessing temperature of replanted digits and vascularized free flaps. The use of three temperature probes is required. One is placed on the replanted digit or hand, a second is placed on an adjacent or an opposite digit, and a third is placed on the bandage for monitoring the ambient temperature. The normal digital temperature ranges from 30°C to 35°C. Replanted digits should have temperatures within 2°C to 3°C of the control digit. If the temperature of the replanted digit decreases to less than 30°C, thrombosis on the arterial or venous side is likely, and reexploration of the replanted part or free flap should be considered.

If sufficient clinical signs of ischemia accompany the indications of ischemia by any mechanical monitoring device, the patient should be returned to the surgical suite for exploration of the anastomoses. If the flap is pale without capillary refill or is cyanotic and congested, if bright red bleeding is absent when the flap is punctured with a No. 11 blade, or if a deep purple ooze occurs, the flap is in jeopardy, and reexploration is indicated.

If arterial thrombosis is identified, the arterial anastomosis and at least one venous anastomosis should be excised. This excision allows assessment of perfusion of the flap after the arterial anastomosis is repeated. If venous thrombosis is the problem, excising the venous anastomosis is helpful to allow free bleeding from the flap for several minutes to determine satisfactory flap perfusion and adequate back bleeding from the flap before repeating the venous repair. If vessel torsion or tension is found to have caused thrombosis over a segment of the vessel, interpositional vein grafting may be required to salvage the flap. The wounds are bandaged as noted previously, and the postoperative routine is resumed.

Mobilization of the part is resumed, commensurate with the part receiving the tissue transfer. If a simple soft-tissue cover has been provided, the parts can be mobilized as soon as wound healing and edema permit. If vascularized bone or functioning muscle has been transferred, mobilization depends on the requirements of these procedures. If a free muscle transfer has been performed, the patient routinely is returned to the operating room at 2 to 3 days for any necessary further debridement and split-thickness skin grafting of the flap. The specific routines used are discussed in the following sections covering the specific free tissue transfer procedures.

FREE GROIN FLAP

The iliofemoral (groin) pedicle flap, popularized by McGregor and Jackson, has been applied extensively for repair and reconstruction in the upper extremity. Since the report in 1973 by Daniel and Taylor describing its successful use as a free flap, many surgeons have found it useful for coverage problems encountered in reconstruction of the head, neck, and trunk and in the upper and lower extremities. The free groin flap also has been beneficial for coverage of the exposed tibia and for problems in the foot, especially over the heel. In some situations requiring a bone graft, the underlying iliac crest may be included with the groin flap, using the superficial circumflex iliac artery or the deep circumflex iliac artery.

Advantages ascribed to the free groin flap include its potentially large size, its location in an area with sparse hair distribution, minimal donor-site morbidity, its multiple arterial and venous systems, the potential for incorporating bone with the overlying skin, and its proven applications as a traditional pedicle flap before the development of microvascular surgical techniques. Disadvantages include its potential excessive thickness in obese patients, problems with color matching, its usually short vascular pedicle, difficulty in dissection of the vessels, its lack of satisfactory innervation, and the likelihood that previous surgical procedures in the inguinal region might have damaged the essential vessels. Primarily because of its short and unpredictable vascular

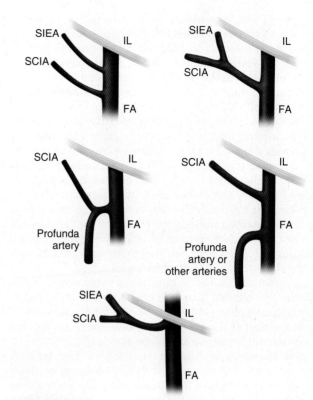

FIGURE **5.14**   Vascular anatomy of groin flap. Variations identified in arterial pedicle supplying ilioinguinal region. *FA*, Femoral artery; *IL*, ilioinguinal ligament; *SCIA*, superficial circumflex iliac artery; *SIEA*, superficial inferior epigastric artery.

pedicle, the groin flap has lost some of its initial popularity as a free tissue transfer.

■ VASCULAR ANATOMY

The iliofemoral flap, as usually described, receives its principal arterial supply from the superficial circumflex iliac artery, branching from the femoral artery. Anatomic studies reveal variations in the arterial supply, with the superficial inferior epigastric artery contributing significantly at times (Fig. 5.14). Taylor and Daniel found the origin of the superficial circumflex iliac and the superficial inferior epigastric arteries to have one of three patterns (Fig. 5.15). In 48% of their specimens, there was a common origin of the superficial circumflex iliac and the superficial inferior epigastric arteries. In 35% there was a large superficial circumflex iliac artery and absent superficial inferior epigastric artery. Separate origins were found for both arteries in 17%. The arteries arose from vessels other than the femoral artery at times, and the relationships were symmetric in about one third of the specimens. The diameters of the vessels were 1.1 to 1.4 mm.

The superficial circumflex iliac artery passes from its origin superficial to the femoral nerve, remaining subfascial until it reaches the lateral border of the sartorius, where it passes through the deep fascia into the subcutaneous tissue, supplying the dermal-subdermal plexus lateral to the anterior superior iliac spine. The flap is drained through the relatively constant superficial inferior epigastric and the variable superficial circumflex iliac veins. These veins may enter the femoral vein separately, usually on its anterior surface. They also may be found to join at the saphenous bulb. The vascular axis of

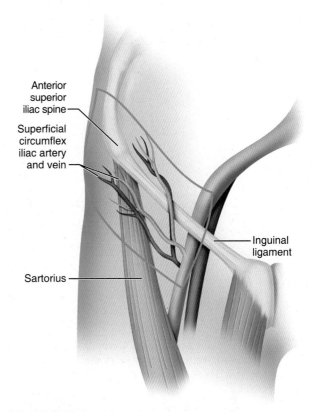

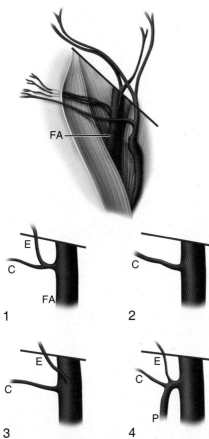

FIGURE 5.15 Interrelated origins of superficial circumflex iliac *(C)* and superficial inferior epigastric *(E)* arteries from femoral artery *(FA)* or another parent artery *(P). 1,* Common origin; *2,* compensatory superficial circumflex iliac with absent superficial inferior epigastric; *3,* separate origins; *4,* origin from parent vessel other than femoral artery.

FIGURE 5.16 Anatomy of groin flap. Flap outline is centered on axis of superficial circumflex iliac vessels perforating sartorius fascia near lateral border of sartorius muscle. **SEE TECHNIQUE 5.9.**

the superficial circumflex iliac artery begins about 5 cm inferior to the inguinal ligament and generally is oriented parallel to the inguinal ligament toward the anterior superior iliac spine and the inferior angle of the scapula.

When a groin flap is being designed, this general alignment should be kept in mind. If the iliac crest is to be included in the flap, it may be supplied sufficiently by the overlying skin and superficial circulation; however, Taylor, Townsend, and Corlett have shown the importance of the osseous circulation from the deep circumflex iliac vessels. The dissection of these vessels is accomplished through the inguinal region.

DISSECTION FOR FREE GROIN FLAP

TECHNIQUE 5.9

- Position the patient supine with a generous rolled towel or sandbag beneath the ipsilateral buttock.
- Prepare and drape the skin to allow surgical access to the inferior costal margin superiorly, the pubic tubercle

medially, the circumferential thigh and knee distally, and the flank posteriorly. Having the thigh within the surgical field allows easy abduction and external rotation during pedicle exposure and flexion for donor-site closure.
- Before beginning the dissection of the vessels, use the Doppler probe to identify and outline the course of the superficial circumflex iliac artery. Using paper, plastic sheeting, or other suitable material, outline the recipient defect and place the pattern in the inguinal region, generally paralleling the inguinal ligament and lying along the course of the superficial circumflex iliac artery (Fig. 5.16). Groin flaps 30 cm × 20 cm can be harvested; however, the portion of the flap that is lateral to the anterior superior iliac spine is a random pattern flap, and its length-to-base width ratio must be 1.5 to 1 or less.
- Begin the approach to the vessels from the medial or the lateral end of the flap. Daniel and Taylor and Harii and Ohmori favored beginning the dissection at the lateral end of the flap, fearing damage to the artery, failure to identify the vessels, and interference with use of the flap as a pedicle flap should microvascular transfer be impossible. O'Brien et al. recommended beginning the dissection at the medial end so that the suitability of the arterial trunk can be determined. Jackson also pointed out that four situations might make the vascular trunk unsuitable for microvascular transfer: (1) the presence of multiple small veins unsuitable for anastomosis; (2) a single small

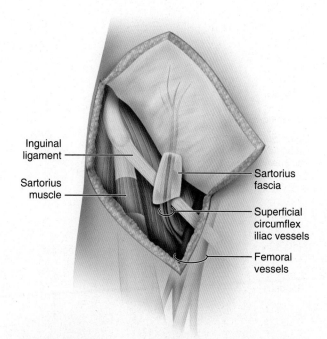

Inguinal ligament

Sartorius muscle

Sartorius fascia

Superficial circumflex iliac vessels

Femoral vessels

FIGURE 5.17 Groin flap dissection. Sartorius fascia has been dissected up with cutaneous flap protecting superficial circumflex iliac artery and vein. **SEE TECHNIQUE 5.9.**

vein; (3) several arteries, none large enough for anastomosis; and (4) one extremely narrow artery.

- Generally, we favor starting on the medial end of the flap to assess the vessels. If care is taken and the vessels are unsuitable for anastomosis, a pedicle flap still can be fashioned if the area to be covered is in the upper extremity. Both approaches are described here because some situations may make the use of one technique better than the other. In either case, the landmarks to keep in mind are the pubic tubercle, the anterior superior iliac spine, the inguinal ligament, and the pulsation of the femoral artery.
- When beginning the dissection medially, make a longitudinal incision over the femoral artery, centered about 5 cm inferior to the inguinal ligament. Use gentle sharp and blunt dissection and stay to the medial side of the femoral artery, watching carefully for the superficial circumflex iliac artery to arise from the medial or anterior aspect of the femoral artery (Fig. 5.17).
- Identify the veins and dissect them gently as well.
- Follow the superficial circumflex iliac artery as it passes laterally. Include the fascia overlying the sartorius until the artery can be seen to pass through the fascia into the subcutaneous fat near the lateral border of the sartorius. Before reaching that point, incise the outline of the flap on the skin as needed to permit identification of the vessels and the muscular landmarks.
- After the vascular pedicle has been dissected and suitable arteries and veins have been identified, the entire skin flap can be incised and elevated. The vessels are not transected until preparation of the recipient area is completed and suitable recipient vessels have been identified. If the vessels are unsatisfactory for a microvascular transfer and

if the recipient area is on the upper extremity, a pedicle flap still can be fashioned with the dissected flap.
- When the dissection is begun from the lateral end of the flap, a pattern matching the recipient area also is outlined over the inguinal region. As noted, the axis of the flap is centered about 5 cm inferior to the inguinal ligament. The margins of the flap, as outlined, are incised, leaving a medial skin bridge intact.
- Dissect from lateral to medial, carrying the deep fascia with the flap as the lateral border of the sartorius is crossed.
- After the vessels are reached and identified, follow the superficial circumflex iliac artery across the femoral triangle superficial to the iliacus and the femoral nerve to the femoral artery.
- Locate the superficial inferior epigastric vein on the anterior aspect of the femoral vein in the same area.
- Evaluate the size of the vessels. If spasm is apparent, apply topical papaverine or lidocaine to relieve it.
- If the vessels are satisfactory, the medial skin bridge can be transected; however, the vessels should not be sectioned until the recipient area is prepared for the skin transfer. If the vessels are unsuitable for microvascular anastomosis, the flap can be used as a pedicle flap if the defect is in the upper extremity.
- If the defect to be covered is in the lower extremity and the vessels are unsuitable for anastomosis, another donor site must be selected or the procedure must be abandoned, regardless of which approach is used for the vessels.
- After the groin flap has been isolated on its vessels and the recipient site has been prepared, transect the artery first to allow additional venous drainage, and then transect the veins.
- Apply suture tags to the vessels to avoid losing them if they retract into the subcutaneous tissue.
- Place the free flap into the recipient defect, oriented so that the flap vessels match the recipient vessels.
- Place several anchoring sutures in the margins of the flap to avoid its being dislodged while the anastomoses are being performed.
- Suture the artery and the veins as promptly as possible to avoid venous congestion in the flap.
- While one team is working on the vessels, the other team closes the groin donor defect. This usually can be done by side-to-side direct closure of the wound. Tension on the wound is minimized by undermining the skin margins and by flexing the hip to allow closure of the wound.

POSTOPERATIVE CARE The general care of the patient is essentially the same as that already outlined. The circulation to the flap is monitored, and the hip is maintained in a flexed posture for 5 to 7 days, at which time gradual extension is begun and continued for another 7 to 10 days.

ANTEROLATERAL THIGH FLAP

This fasciocutaneous flap was first described by Song et al. for reconstruction of burn contractures affecting the head and neck, and it has been described in hand reconstruction. The flap has been found to be reliable, with no failures in seven patients. Advantages of this flap include its potential size (≤800 cm²), its long vascular pedicle (≤15 cm), and its use as a possible flow-through flap to revascularize a digit. It also is potentially sensate through the lateral femoral cutaneous nerve, as reported by Maamoon in his description of its use to cover weight-bearing areas of the foot. The flap tends to be thick, although using it as a fascial flap with skin grafting obviates this problem. Dissection may be difficult if the perforators pass through the vastus lateralis. Kimata et al. found in 74 patients that perforators were absent in 4 (5.4%), and musculocutaneous perforators were present in 81.9%. This flap is considered unsuitable for use in obese patients, particularly women, and in men with extremely hairy thighs. Comparing the anterolateral thigh (ALT) flap to the latissimus dorsi flap for lower extremity coverage, Philandrianos et al. found no difference in bone healing, infectious bone complications, or flap healing; however, the ALT flap provided a better cosmetic result.

■ VASCULAR ANATOMY

The free ATL flap is based off the descending branch of the lateral circumflex femoral artery. The descending branch passes between the rectus femoris and the vastus lateralis and has an internal diameter of greater than 3 mm. After supplying the major branch to the rectus femoris, it provides perforators to the skin that pass through the intermuscular septum or through the anterior 4 cm of the vastus lateralis. The largest perforator reaches the deep fascia at a point 2 cm lateral and 2 cm distal to the midpoint of a line drawn between the anterior superior iliac spine and the superolateral border of the patella. Venous drainage is through one or two venae comitantes accompanying the descending branch of the lateral circumflex femoral artery. The descending branch of the lateral circumflex femoral artery is accompanied by motor nerve branches to the vastus lateralis, which should be preserved during the dissection.

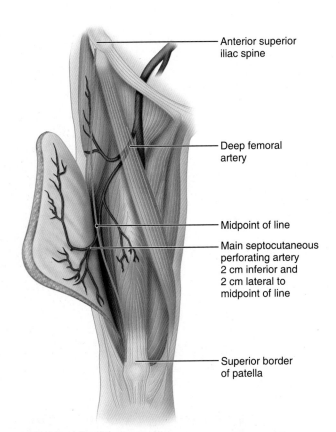

FIGURE 5.18 Skin marking of anterolateral thigh flap. Flap elevation is accomplished with use of Esmarch tourniquet secured to Steinmann pin in anterior superior iliac spine. **SEE TECHNIQUE 5.10.**

Labels in figure:
- Anterior superior iliac spine
- Deep femoral artery
- Midpoint of line
- Main septocutaneous perforating artery 2 cm inferior and 2 cm lateral to midpoint of line
- Superior border of patella

DISSECTION FOR ANTEROLATERAL THIGH FLAP

TECHNIQUE 5.10

(JAVAID AND CORMACK)

FLAP PLANNING

- Before surgery, detect the location of the perforators with a Doppler probe using an 8-MHz transducer and mark them on the skin.
- At surgery, determine the defect and expose the potential recipient site artery and vein.
- Join the site for the anastomoses to the defect with a suitable incision. Avoid tunneling under intact skin bridges where the vascular pedicles may be compressed when the skin tightens secondary to postoperative swelling.
- Create a paper pattern that covers the defect and the anastomosis site to determine if the flap and its vascular pedicle is going to be of a "tadpole" or "mushroom" configuration.

- Place the paper pattern on the thigh in the appropriate position relative to the principal perforator and the pedicle to achieve the right configuration.

FLAP ELEVATION

- With the patient supine, apply a sterile Esmarch tourniquet secured to a Steinmann pin in the anterior superior iliac spine (Fig. 5.18). Begin flap elevation at its medial edge where skin and deep fascia are incised.
- The lateral cutaneous nerve of the thigh is encountered in its downward course from the anterior superior iliac spine and can be dissected free of the anterior margin of the flap or included if a neurosensory flap is planned.
- Continue the elevation to expose the intermuscular septum between the rectus femoris and vastus lateralis, which is explored for the descending branch.
- Continue exploration until the septocutaneous perforators or the muscle-perforating vessels from the descending branch of the lateral circumflex femoral vessels can be seen. Ligate and divide any branches to muscle that are not passing through to supply the skin.
- If accessory septocutaneous perforators are found arising above and below the main perforator, two or more can be preserved to increase the vascular connecting points between the flap and its pedicle in larger flaps.

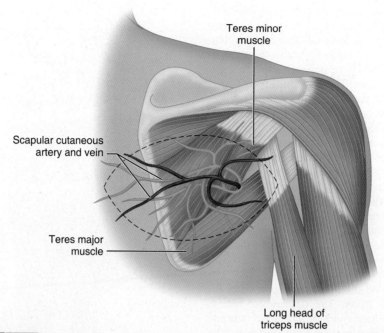

Teres minor
muscle

Scapular cutaneous
artery and vein

Teres major
muscle

Long head of
triceps muscle

FIGURE 5.19   Cutaneous scapular artery and two accompanying veins exit through triangular space and supply skin superficial to inferior two thirds of scapula. Scapular flap is designated by *dashed circle*. **SEE TECHNIQUE 5.11.**

- If no septocutaneous perforators are present, carefully dissect out perforators from the anterior part of the vastus lateralis as they pass through on their way to the skin.
- When the vascular supply to the flap is ensured, incise the posterior and distal parts of the flap.
- Remove the Esmarch tourniquet and develop the pedicle farther proximally with a skin incision if a "tadpole" flap configuration is required. Do not carry the dissection of the pedicle above the point where the arterial branch to the rectus femoris arises and its venous drainage joins because this is the sole supply to the rectus femoris and must not be compromised. At about this level, the venae comitantes of the descending branch may unite to form a single vein before joining with veins from the rectus femoris.
- Usually the skin defect on the thigh cannot be closed directly, partly because the harvest of some of the deep fascia allows the muscle to bulge and hinder closure. Advance the skin edges and suture them to the muscle to reduce the overall size of the defect and cover the remaining area with a meshed split-thickness skin graft taken from the medial aspect of the same thigh.

SCAPULAR AND PARASCAPULAR FLAP

Cutaneous flaps based on the circumflex scapular arterial system include the cutaneous scapular flap and the cutaneous parascapular flap. The scapular flap is considered a versatile cutaneous flap that can cover a defect measuring 10 × 16 cm. Functional donor-site morbidity is not appreciable. The skin is thin and hairless, although the hilum may be fairly bulky. The pedicle is long and constant, with a length of 4 to 9 cm.

The scapular flap can be elevated and dissected quickly and is suitable for small areas of skin loss. Its disadvantages include its lack of a cutaneous nerve as an innervated flap and

the tendency for the donor-site scar to spread, limiting its usefulness in women.

■ VASCULAR ANATOMY

The cutaneous scapular flap receives its circulation through the transverse cutaneous branch of the circumflex scapular artery and accompanying veins. The circumflex scapular artery is a major branch of the subscapular artery, and the branches of the circumflex scapular artery have several terminal branches (Fig. 5.19). The more superior branches supply portions of the supraspinatus and infraspinatus muscles. An inferior or infrascapular branch supplies the muscles and skin to the inferior angle of the scapula. A descending branch divides into the cutaneous parascapular artery, which continues inferiorly along the border of the latissimus dorsi muscle and a transverse branch, the cutaneous scapular artery.

The cutaneous scapular artery passes through the triangular space formed by the teres minor superiorly, the teres major inferiorly, and the long head of the triceps laterally. Two veins accompany the circumflex scapular artery.

DISSECTION FOR SCAPULAR AND PARASCAPULAR FLAP

TECHNIQUE 5.11

(GILBERT; URBANIAK ET AL.)
- Place the patient prone or in the lateral decubitus position on an axillary pad, allowing mobility of the chest so that the patient can be turned prone if needed. If the flap is to be used for upper extremity coverage, the contralateral

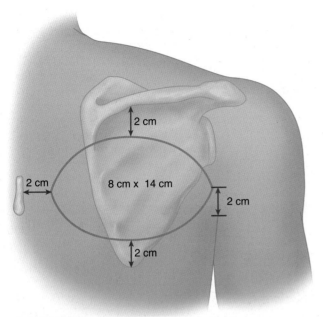

FIGURE 5.20 "Rule of twos" is helpful in outlining scapular flap. Medial border may extend 2 cm lateral to the spinous processes and lateral border 2 cm superior to posterior axillary crease. Inferior border may extend 2 cm superior to inferior edge of scapula and superior border 2 cm inferior to spine of scapula. **SEE TECHNIQUE 5.11.**

shoulder serves as the donor. In situations in which the posterior tibial artery is the recipient vessel, the contralateral shoulder should serve as the donor site. If the anterior tibial-dorsalis pedis system is to be used, the donor site is the ipsilateral scapular area.

- Drape the arm free so that it can be moved through a full range of motion, especially adduction and abduction, to allow dissection of the vascular pedicle.
- Place the patient's arm at his or her side and make an outline of the flap in a transversely oriented direction centered over the scapula. Urbaniak et al. pointed out the usefulness of the "rule of twos" in outlining the scapular flap (Fig. 5.20). The medial border extends to within 2 cm of the vertebral spinous processes. The lateral border extends to within 2 cm superior to the posterior axillary crease. The inferior border extends to within 2 cm superior to the inferior angle of the scapula, and the superior border extends to within 2 cm inferior to the spine of the scapula.
- Make a skin incision and elevate the flap, beginning on the medial border approximately 2 cm lateral to the vertebral spinous processes.
- Incise the lateral, superior, and inferior borders of the flap. Use loupe magnification to aid in the dissection.
- Retract the deltoid muscle superiorly and identify the teres minor, the long head of the triceps, and the teres major forming the triangular space.
- Retract the long head of the triceps laterally, the teres minor superiorly, and the teres major inferiorly.
- Expose the circumflex scapular artery and its venae comitantes by dissecting along the inferior border of the teres minor in the interval superficial to the fascia of the teres minor (see Fig. 5.19).

- After the flap has been completely excised and mobilized so that it is attached only to its vascular pedicle, determine that the recipient site is prepared, dissect the pedicle proximally, and section the vessels, cauterizing and ligating or applying a hemoclip to the central stump and microvascular clips to the flap pedicle.
- Close the donor site by mobilizing the skin edges and inserting drains as needed.
- Nassif et al. described a parascapular flap, receiving its vascular supply through the cutaneous parascapular artery, a branch of the circumflex scapular artery. The orientation of this flap is more vertical, and it parallels the anterior margin of the latissimus dorsi muscle. The reader is referred to the references for the details of this flap.

LATERAL ARM FLAP

The lateral arm flap is a fascial or fasciocutaneous flap based on the posterior radial collateral artery, which is a direct continuation of the profunda brachii. Its maximal dimension is limited (10 cm × 15 cm); however, it has the advantage of supplying a relatively thin flap that can be reinnervated through the posterior cutaneous nerve of the arm. Also, it can be harvested from the same side as the injured forearm or hand, eliminating multiple surgical sites. If harvested as a fascial flap, it may provide thin pliable coverage for hand and finger defects. The chief disadvantages are the relatively short (2 to 6 cm) pedicle and variable vessel diameter (1 to 3 mm). Flap bulkiness may be an issue; however, this is outweighed by the versatility of the lateral arm flap. In reviewing the outcome of 123 lateral arm free flaps, Graham et al. thought that this flap is best limited to male patients in whom primary closure of the donor site is possible.

■ VASCULAR ANATOMY

The profunda brachii artery courses along the spiral groove of the humerus and passes through the lateral intermuscular septum just distal to the deltoid insertion. At this point, it branches into a smaller anterior radial collateral artery and a larger posterior radial collateral artery (Fig. 5.21). The anterior radial collateral artery accompanies the radial nerve and courses anterior to the brachioradialis. The posterior radial collateral artery courses posterior to the brachioradialis along the lateral intermuscular septum, giving off small cutaneous branches that supply the lateral arm flap. It eventually anastomoses with the interosseous recurrent artery around the lateral epicondyle. The posterior radial collateral artery is accompanied by the posterior cutaneous nerve of the arm, which innervates the distal skin of the flap, and the posterior cutaneous nerve of the forearm and two large venae comitantes, each approximately 2 mm in diameter.

DISSECTION FOR LATERAL ARM FLAP

TECHNIQUE 5.12

- Prepare and drape free the entire upper extremity up to the axilla with the patient in the supine position. Apply a sterile tourniquet if available to provide a bloodless field.

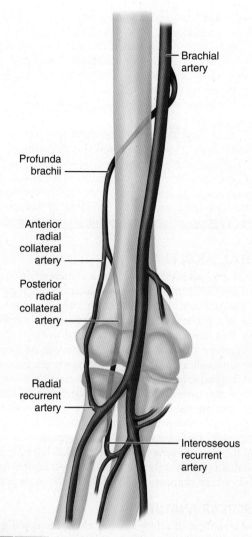

FIGURE **5.21** Vascular anatomy of lateral arm flap.

It is easier to carry out the dissection with the arm resting on the chest with the elbow in flexion.
- Center the flap over the lateral intermuscular septum, which courses from the deltoid insertion to the lateral epicondyle (Fig. 5.22A).
- Incise the posterior margin of the flap through the fascia overlying the triceps muscle.
- Carry the dissection anteriorly between the triceps and its fascia until the lateral intermuscular fascia is encountered. Identify the cutaneous branches of the posterior radial collateral artery within the septum (Fig. 5.22B).
- Bluntly separate the septum from the triceps to its full depth and note the course of the posterior radial collateral artery within the septum.
- Continue the dissection proximally along the vascular pedicle between the triceps and deltoid (Fig. 5.22C).
- Identify and protect the radial nerve. Identify the posterior cutaneous nerve of the arm, which enters the skin flap proximally and superficial to the triceps fascia. This may be divided proximally and used for sensory reinnervation.

- Incise the anterior margin of the flap and elevate it with the underlying fascia off the brachialis and brachioradialis posteriorly to the lateral intermuscular septum.
- Ligate and divide the posterior radial collateral artery and venae comitantes, which extend distal to the flap margins (Fig. 5.22D).
- Proximally, divide the anterior radial collateral artery, and when adequate pedicle length has been gained, divide the profunda brachii and its venae comitantes. The posterior cutaneous nerve to the forearm usually is included within the flap, although it can be preserved.
- Close the wound primarily over suction drains if the flap width is less than 6 cm, or skin graft it if necessary.

MUSCLE AND MUSCULOCUTANEOUS FREE FLAPS

Muscle and musculocutaneous free flaps are useful in two ways. They have been widely applied for coverage of soft-tissue defects in the upper and lower extremities and in the reconstruction of contour in soft-tissue defects in the head, neck, and trunk. Their second major area of usefulness is in the transfer of functioning neuromuscular units to replace paralyzed muscular units in the face and extremities. Muscle flaps tend to atrophy with time, diminishing in bulk, and donor site functional deficits usually are insignificant. Unless restoration of local sensibility is required, a muscle flap usually is preferable to a cutaneous flap for free tissue transfer.

LATISSIMUS DORSI TRANSFER

Building on the 1896 reports of Tansini, who used the latissimus dorsi muscle pedicle flap for breast reconstruction, and on the extensive use of the latissimus dorsi as a muscle pedicle flap for trunk and head and neck reconstruction, Baudet et al., Harii et al., and Maxwell et al. showed the successful transfer of the latissimus dorsi muscle as a free flap. This myocutaneous free flap has been used extensively for soft-tissue coverage problems because of its large size and long, reliable pedicle of adequate vessel diameter.

■ VASCULAR ANATOMY

Arising from the thoracolumbar fascia, the iliac crest, and the lower three ribs, the latissimus dorsi muscle covers most of the lower portion of the posterior trunk and passes laterally to insert on the inferior portion of the bicipital groove of the humerus. The principal vascular supply to the latissimus dorsi is through the thoracodorsal branch of the subscapular artery with its venae comitantes. The thoracodorsal artery courses just deep to the anterior margin of the latissimus dorsi and enters the muscle on its deep surface 8 to 12 cm from the insertion (Fig. 5.23).

If the thoracodorsal artery is taken below the circumflex scapular branch, it has a diameter of 1.5 to 3 mm. Secondary vascular pedicles enter the muscle medially from the perforating branches of the lumbar and posterior intercostal arteries. The thoracodorsal nerve follows the artery and has two to three fascicles with a diameter of about 2 mm. All of the

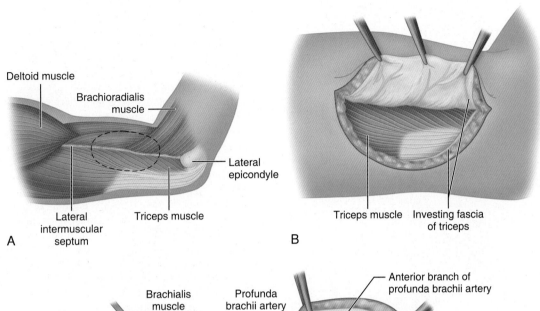

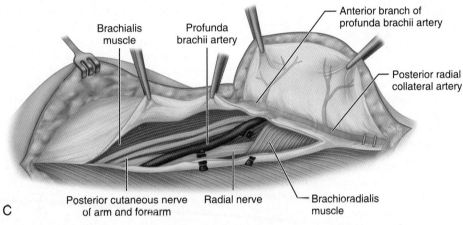

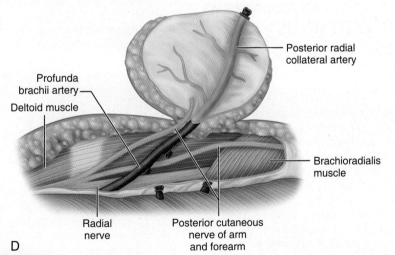

FIGURE 5.22   **A,** Outline of lateral arm flap centered over lateral intermuscular septum (dashed circle). **B,** Initial posterior incision and elevation of flap deep to triceps fascia showing cutaneous branches of posterior radial collateral artery within lateral intermuscular septum. **C,** Exposure of vascular pedicle. **D,** Flap elevated on its pedicle with posterior cutaneous nerves to arm and forearm. **SEE TECHNIQUE 5.12.**

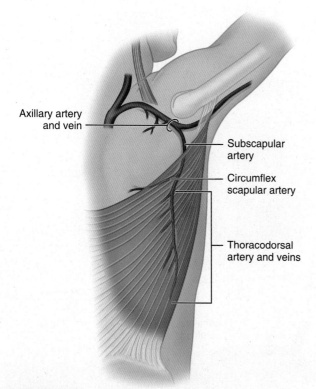

Axillary artery and vein

Subscapular artery

Circumflex scapular artery

Thoracodorsal artery and veins

FIGURE 5.23 Latissimus dorsi vascular supply. Thoracodorsal branch of subscapular artery with venae comitantes enters muscle on its deep surface 8 to 12 cm from humeral insertion. Thoracodorsal nerve (not shown) accompanies artery.

muscle with most of its overlying skin can be transferred with the thoracodorsal neurovascular bundle. Skin flaps of varying sizes may be oriented over the muscle as needed.

DISSECTION FOR LATISSIMUS DORSI TRANSFER

TECHNIQUE 5.13

- Place the patient in the lateral decubitus position, maintaining this position with sandbags and kidney rests.
- Prepare and drape the patient, leaving the entire shoulder and thorax exposed anteriorly and posteriorly. Drape the entire upper extremity free so that it can be easily moved about.
- Draw a line along the anterior margin of the latissimus dorsi muscle from the anterior margin of the posterior axillary fold to the midportion of the iliac crest.
- Although most of the skin overlying the latissimus dorsi muscle can be transplanted, it usually is not required for upper extremity reconstruction. If an island of skin is to be taken for upper extremity coverage, it may be best designed over the anteroinferior aspect of the muscle (Fig. 5.24A). This allows direct closure of the donor site. If the flap is to be removed for coverage of larger defects (as in the lower extremity), larger skin islands may be outlined

(10 to 12 cm wide) or the muscle may be removed without its overlying skin and split-thickness skin grafts may be applied to the muscle belly after the flap has been attached to the recipient site.

- Make a curved incision, extending from the axilla, following the anterior margin, and include the outline of the skin flap.
- Identify the dorsal surface of the latissimus dorsi to avoid dissection of skin from the muscle.
- If only a muscle flap is to be harvested, make the incision along a line 3 cm posterior to the anterior margin of the latissimus dorsi (Fig. 5.24B).
- Separate the latissimus dorsi anteriorly from the serratus anterior muscle. Separate the anterior margin of the muscle from the posterior iliac crest distal to the skin island.
- Retract the muscle posteriorly and dissect deep to the muscle medially toward the spine. Ligate or cauterize perforating vessels entering the muscle medially. With the anterior margin and the distal attachments mobilized, the muscle can be manipulated freely to allow dissection of the neurovascular pedicle. Palpate the vascular pedicle proximally near the insertion and 1 to 2 cm from the anterior margin. Dissect carefully when mobilizing the pedicle.
- Using the bipolar cautery, cauterize branches perforating the chest wall musculature from the latissimus dorsi.
- Identify and preserve the long thoracic nerve to the serratus anterior deep and anterior to the thoracodorsal pedicle. Identify the nerve to the latissimus dorsi, accompanying the thoracodorsal pedicle.
- Dissect the pedicle proximal to the branch to the serratus anterior muscle to obtain a pedicle length of 8 to 12 cm (Fig. 5.24C). Unless the serratus is to be included in the muscle transfer, clamp and divide the anterior branch to the serratus anterior.
- If maximal pedicle length is required, dissect proximally, ligating and dividing the circumflex scapular branch, to include the entire subscapular artery as it arises off the axillary artery (Fig. 5.24D).
- After dissecting the neurovascular pedicle, proceed with the dissection medially and superiorly, releasing the proximal attachments of the muscle to the chest wall.
- Determine the amount of muscle required at the recipient site (arm or leg) and excise the medial margin of the skin flap down to the muscle.
- Suture the margins of the skin flap dermis to the fascia to avoid shear.
- Release the tendon at its insertion and section the neurovascular pedicle only when the recipient site has been completely prepared.
- If a functioning muscle is required, determine the maximal functional length, as noted in the discussion of transfer of functioning muscle to forearm (see later section on Functioning Neuromuscular Transfers).
- Transfer the muscle to the recipient site and close the donor site. A split-thickness skin graft may be required at the donor site, depending on the size of skin flap removed. Suction drainage is useful to avoid the development of a seroma or hematoma in the donor site.
- Shoulder mobilization can be begun on the day after surgery.

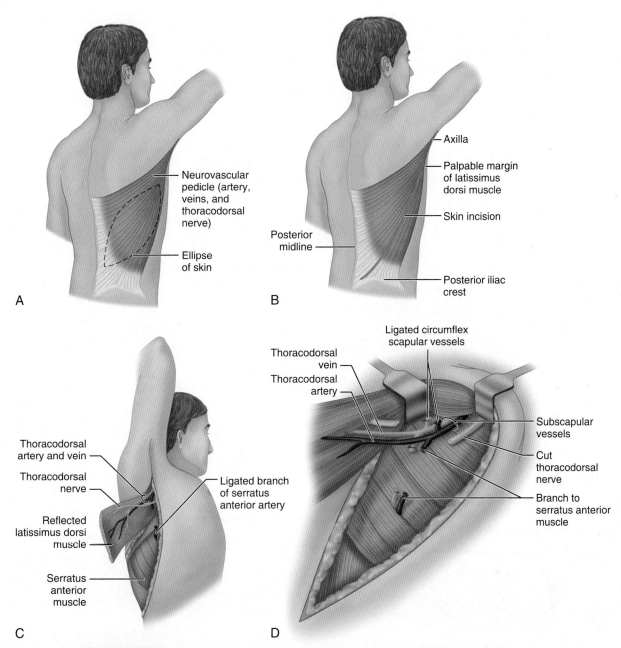

FIGURE 5.24 **A,** Latissimus dorsi musculocutaneous flap design *(dashed oval)*. Note skin flap along anterior inferior portion of muscle. **B,** Latissimus dorsi muscle flap incision is parallel and 3 cm posterior to anterior edge of muscle. **C,** Latissimus dorsi flap isolation. Distal and posteromedial portions have been released to allow for cephalad dissection of vascular pedicle. Anterior arterial branch to underlying serratus anterior is divided. **D,** Division of circumflex scapular artery allows dissection up to subscapular artery origin of axillary artery. **SEE TECHNIQUE 5.13.**

SERRATUS ANTERIOR FLAP

The first published report of the serratus anterior free flap was by Takayanagi and Tsukie in 1982. A musculocutaneous flap using the lower three muscular digitations, based on the thoracodorsal artery, was used to cover two lower extremity defects. Three major advantages of this flap noted by Brody et al. were (1) low donor-site morbidity, (2) easy divisibility of the three separate slips for contouring, and (3) durability and adhesion that provide a stable resurfacing for grasp. This is a relatively thin muscle with a long vascular pedicle, and it can be harvested through a relatively short

midaxillary incision. Removal of the lower three to four digitations has not been found to cause winging of the scapula, provided that the proximal portion of the long thoracic nerve is not injured.

■ VASCULAR ANATOMY

The serratus anterior originates from the first nine ribs to insert on the medial border of the scapula. The lower three to four digitations are primarily vascularized by a consistently present anterior branch of the thoracodorsal artery (Fig. 5.25). The upper six digitations receive their blood supply primarily from the lateral thoracic artery. The long thoracic nerve, which courses superficially along the serratus anterior and just anterior to the vascular pedicle, provides innervation to all digitations. A 15-cm vascular pedicle can be achieved by preserving the subscapular artery (2 to 3 mm in diameter) within the pedicle.

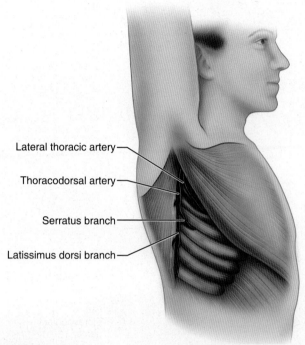

Lateral thoracic artery

Thoracodorsal artery

Serratus branch

Latissimus dorsi branch

FIGURE 5.25   Vascular anatomy of serratus anterior muscle.

DISSECTION FOR SERRATUS ANTERIOR FLAP

TECHNIQUE 5.14

- Position the patient in the lateral decubitus position.
- Prepare and drape the entire upper extremity along with the hemithorax.
- Make a linear incision along the midaxillary line centered over the sixth through tenth ribs (Fig. 5.26A). Deepen the incision anterior to the leading edge of the latissimus dorsi until the loose areolar tissue covering the serratus is encountered.
- Widely abduct the arm and, using careful blunt dissection, identify the thoracodorsal artery just beneath the latissimus dorsi muscle and its anterior branch to the serratus anterior (Fig. 5.26B). Just distal to the takeoff of this anterior branch, ligate and divide the thoracodorsal artery.
- Identify the thoracodorsal nerve by direct exposure or by using a nerve stimulator and carefully preserve it as the dissection is carried proximal along the thoracodorsal artery and vein.
- Trace the anterior branch distally to the point at which it enters the lower three to four digitations of the serratus anterior.
- Identify and protect the long thoracic nerve proximal to this point.
- Elevate the lower three to four digitations off the underlying ribs and intercostal muscles. Section the scapular insertion of this portion of muscle.

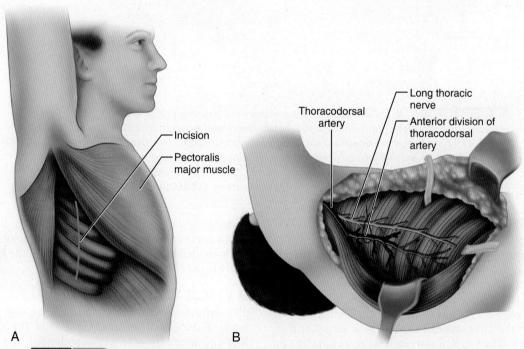

Incision

Pectoralis major muscle

Thoracodorsal artery

Long thoracic nerve

Anterior division of thoracodorsal artery

A   B

FIGURE 5.26   **A,** Skin incision for serratus anterior free flap. **B,** Dissection and isolation of serratus anterior free flap. **SEE TECHNIQUE 5.14.**

- Verify that the muscle is well perfused by its vascular pedicle and divide the pedicle.
- Take care to achieve meticulous hemostasis and close the wound over suction drainage.

TENSOR FASCIAE LATAE MUSCLE FLAP

Although its fascial surface may not adhere to a recipient site, the tensor fasciae latae muscle can be used for coverage of soft-tissue defects in the upper or lower extremity, as a sensory innervated flap, as a functioning neuromuscular unit, and as an osteomusculocutaneous flap incorporating a portion of the bone of the iliac crest. Its function as an innervated flexor substitute is limited because of its limited excursion; however, it has potential as an extensor replacement. A 10- × 30-cm skin flap centered over the midaxis of the muscle may be harvested with the underlying muscle.

■ VASCULAR ANATOMY

The tensor fasciae latae originates from the anterior portion of the iliac crest and inserts into the fascia lata of the thigh. It has a single major arterial supply, the transverse branch of the lateral femoral circumflex artery from the profunda femoris artery. The vascular pedicle enters at the midpoint of the muscle approximately 10 cm inferior to the iliac crest. The arterial supply lies deep to the rectus femoris muscle and gives branches to the rectus femoris, the vastus lateralis, and gluteus minimus muscles (see Fig. 5.27B). The venous drainage is through the two venae comitantes that accompany the arterial pedicle. A vascular pedicle 6 to 8 cm long can be dissected. The vessels have diameters of 2 to 2.5 mm.

The tensor fasciae latae receives its motor innervation through a branch of the superior gluteal nerve, which enters the muscle proximal to the vascular pedicle. The skin area of the muscle is located on the lateral thigh between lines extending from the anterior superior iliac spine and the lateral femoral condyle anteriorly and the greater trochanter posteriorly; it extends from the iliac crest to the knee. This skin receives its sensory innervation through the cutaneous branch of the T12 nerve and the lateral femoral cutaneous nerve. The branch of the T12 nerve enters the region in the subcutaneous tissue near the posterosuperior aspect of the flap, and the lateral femoral cutaneous nerve enters the medial portion of the flap in the subcutaneous tissue 8 to 10 cm distal to the anterior superior iliac spine.

DISSECTION FOR TENSOR FASCIAE LATAE MUSCLE FLAP

TECHNIQUE 5.15

- Outline on the proximal lateral thigh the area of skin required by the recipient area. The midaxis of the muscle flap and a musculocutaneous flap is along a line drawn from a point 3 cm posterior to the anterior superior iliac spine to the head of the fibula (Fig. 5.27A).

- Mark the location of the anticipated entrance of the vascular pedicle approximately 10 cm inferior to the anterior superior iliac spine. This point usually is located along a line drawn transversely and laterally from the pubic tubercle.
- If the transfer is to be a neurosensory, osteomusculocutaneous, or functional free flap, identify the areas of the lateral femoral cutaneous nerve anteromedially, the sensory branch of the T12 nerve posterolaterally, the anticipated location of the motor branch, and any required bone before making the skin incision.
- Plan the flap so that the required neurovascular repairs and bone placement if used can be located appropriately in the recipient site.
- Incise the anterior margin of the flap through the subcutaneous tissue and the underlying fascia lata (Fig. 5.27B).
- If sensory nerves are to be incorporated in the transfer, dissect and identify them at this point. The lateral femoral cutaneous nerve enters the flap 5 to 10 cm inferior to the anterior superior iliac spine. Identify the nerve in the subcutaneous tissue, dissect it proximally, and divide it, providing sufficient nerve for nerve repair before identification of the vascular pedicle.
- Continue the dissection anteriorly and medially deep to the fascia until the interval between the tensor and rectus femoris is encountered (Fig. 5.27C). This interval is usually obvious.
- Use blunt dissection to locate the transverse branches of the lateral femoral circumflex vessels deep to the rectus femoris.
- Identify the descending branch that courses distally into the vastus lateralis and ligate it.
- Trace the lateral femoral circumflex artery with its two venae comitantes medially beneath the rectus femoris to its origin off the profunda femoris. Take care not to injure the femoral nerve during this portion of the dissection.
- After the vascular pedicle has been clearly delineated, incise the posterior margin of the skin flap.
- Suture the margins of the skin flap to the muscle superiorly and to the fascia lata distally to avoid shear on the flap.
- Deepen the dissection through the interval between the gluteus maximus and the tensor and continue medially until the vascular pedicle is encountered (Fig. 5.27D). Protect the vascular pedicle with a retractor during this portion of the dissection.
- Section the tensor fasciae latae distally and develop the flap in a cephalad direction (Fig. 5.27E).
- Elevate proximally the superior margin of the flap and incise and divide the proximal muscle superior to the entrance of the vascular pedicle.
- If bone is to be included, carry the dissection more proximally after incision and elevation of the superior skin to the level of the iliac crest.
- Using an osteotome, include the tensor fasciae latae with the underlying iliac crest.
- Leave the vascular pedicle intact until the recipient site is completely prepared and then section the vessels for transfer.
- Close the wound over large suction drains.
- Hip and knee motion and weight-bearing ambulation can be started on the first postoperative day as allowed by the recipient site.

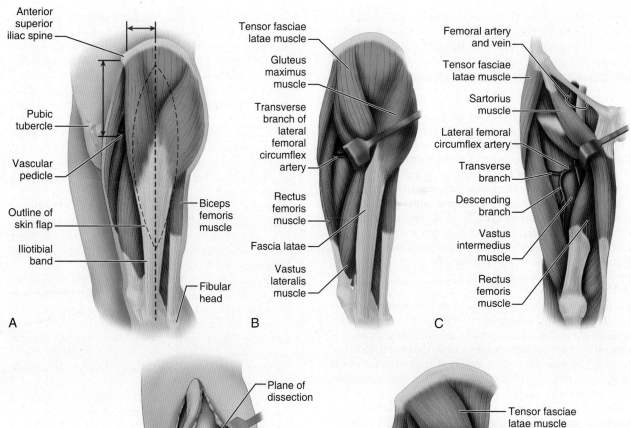

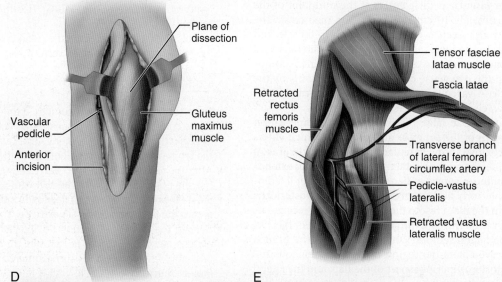

FIGURE 5.27 **A,** Landmarks and skin incision for tensor fasciae latae muscle or musculocutaneous flap. Note vascular pedicle at level of pubic tubercle. **B,** Dissection initially is carried out anteriorly and medially to identify transverse branch of lateral femoral circumflex artery deep to rectus femoris muscle. **C,** Isolation of vascular pedicle. **D,** Posterior dissection between tensor and gluteus maximus. **E,** Elevation of tensor flap from distal to proximal. **SEE TECHNIQUE 5.15.**

GRACILIS MUSCLE TRANSFER

The gracilis can be used as a free muscle or a musculocutaneous flap. Because it is fairly small with a long, narrow contour, it has only limited use for soft-tissue coverage, but is suitable for a free innervated functioning muscle transfer. Its vascular pedicle is short and based on a terminal branch of the medial femoral circumflex artery, which has a diameter of 1 to 2 mm. It is conveniently harvested with the patient in the supine position and has minimal donor-site morbidity.

▮ VASCULAR ANATOMY

Arising from the anterior body and the inferior ramus of the pubis and the ischium, the gracilis muscle passes distally in the medial thigh posterior to the adductor longus and sartorius muscles, inserting on the medial aspect of the proximal tibia posterior and deep to the sartorius tendon and anterior to the semitendinosus muscle insertion. Its innervation comes from a branch of the anterior division of the obturator nerve, which has two to four fascicles entering the muscle 6 to 10 cm from the origin.

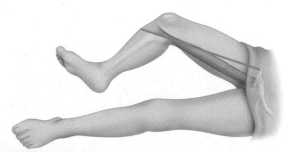

FIGURE 5.29   Gracilis muscle dissection. Gracilis muscle lies posterior to line drawn between adductor origin and tibial tuberosity. **SEE TECHNIQUE 5.16.**

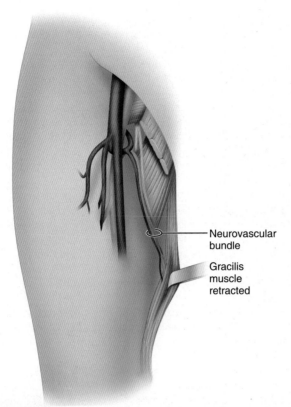

Neurovascular bundle

Gracilis muscle retracted

FIGURE 5.28   Gracilis muscle neurovascular pedicle. Major vascular pedicle to gracilis muscle enters in proximal third of muscle and includes a branch of medial femoral circumflex artery and tributary of femoral vein and anterior branch of obturator nerve.

The obturator nerve accompanies the dominant vascular pedicle, the medial femoral circumflex artery, and its venae comitantes arising from the profunda femoris artery and vein, 8 to 12 cm from the muscle origin (Fig. 5.28). A vascular pedicle can be obtained 4 to 6 cm long with a vessel diameter of 1 to 2 mm. Two minor vascular pedicles, branches of the superficial femoral artery, are located distally and may be sacrificed. No significant functional loss can be seen after removal of the gracilis muscle.

DISSECTION FOR GRACILIS MUSCLE TRANSFER

TECHNIQUE 5.16

- Prepare and drape the entire lower extremity, exposing the groin, thigh, and knee so that the limb can be easily moved about. Abduct and externally rotate the hip and flex the knee to allow access to the medial side of the thigh from the groin to the knee.
- Draw a straight line between the origin of the adductor longus and the tibial tuberosity. The gracilis muscle should lie posterior to such a line (Fig. 5.29).
- To remove a cutaneous flap with the muscle, center the outlined flap over the proximal muscle because skin flaps

in the distal portion have been found by Manktelow to be unreliable.
- After outlining the skin flap, make the skin incision along the line marked.
- Incise down to the gracilis muscle and suture the dermis at the margins to the underlying muscle.
- Dissect anterior to the gracilis muscle, separating the adductor longus muscle from the gracilis and retracting the adductor longus anteriorly. The neurovascular structures now can be seen entering the deep surface of the gracilis muscle.
- Ligate or cauterize the vascular side branches to allow the development of a long pedicle.
- Dissect the gracilis muscle free posteriorly and mobilize it proximally and distally by blunt digital dissection.
- Ligate or cauterize the lesser vascular pedicles as they are encountered distally on the deep surface of the muscle.
- If the muscle is to be transferred as a functioning muscular unit, determine its physiologic length by placing marking sutures as indicated in the transfer of functioning muscle to forearm (see later section on Functioning Neuromuscular Transfers).
- Make a short incision in the distal thigh, identify the gracilis tendon by blunt dissection, and section the tendon distally after determining the needed length.
- To avoid displacement of the muscle, suture it loosely in situ, leaving it attached to the remaining pedicle and origin until the forearm is prepared.
- Section the origin and the neurovascular pedicle and deliver the muscle unit to the recipient site.

RECTUS ABDOMINIS TRANSFER

The free rectus abdominis muscle flap was first described by Pennington, Lai, and Pelly in 1980 and since that time has gained increasing popularity primarily because of its large and consistent vascular pedicle based on the deep inferior epigastric artery and ease of dissection. It is easily dissected with the patient supine, and herniation is not a problem if the posterior rectus sheath is left intact and the anterior rectus sheath is repaired. There are few or no functional deficits caused by its use. Prior herniorrhaphy and transverse abdominal scars preclude its use. It also can be harvested as a musculocutaneous flap using as much overlying skin as would allow primary closure.

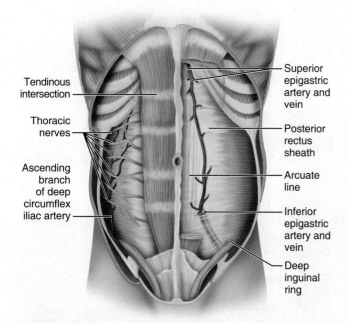

Tendinous intersection

Thoracic nerves

Ascending branch of deep circumflex iliac artery

Superior epigastric artery and vein

Posterior rectus sheath

Arcuate line

Inferior epigastric artery and vein

Deep inguinal ring

FIGURE 5.30 Anatomy of rectus abdominis muscle and its sheath.

■ VASCULAR ANATOMY

Each rectus abdominis muscle takes its origin along the pubic crest and inserts into the costal cartilages of the fifth, sixth, and seventh ribs (Fig. 5.30). The costal cartilages are fairly close together in this region, and the muscle insertion is practically horizontal. The muscle is fairly rectangular, measuring 7 to 10 cm wide × 30 cm long. It is enclosed within the rectus sheath. The anterior wall of the rectus sheath is complete throughout its length; however, the posterior wall is complete distally only as far as the arcuate line located halfway between the umbilicus and the pubis, at which point it is composed of transversalis and subserous fascia only. The muscle is divided into four or five transverse sections by tendinous intersections. One occurs at the level of the umbilicus and another at the inferior end of the xiphoid process; a third occurs at a point equidistant between these two, and another can occur between the umbilicus and the pubis. The deep inferior epigastric artery arises from the external iliac artery. It is 3 to 4 mm in diameter at its origin and is accompanied by two venae comitantes. It arises just deep to the inguinal canal, pierces the transversalis fascia, and enters the rectus sheath lateral and inferior to the arcuate line. It enters the rectus abdominis muscle along its deep surface, courses superiorly, and ramifies with branches from the superior epigastric artery. The muscle receives segmental innervation from the seventh through twelfth intercostal nerves.

DISSECTION FOR RECTUS ABDOMINIS TRANSFER

TECHNIQUE 5.17

- Position the patient supine and prepare and drape the entire abdomen from the costal margins above to the pubic tubercle below.

- Make a longitudinal paramedian incision from just below the costal margin to 3 to 4 cm proximal to the pubic tubercle (Fig. 5.31A).
- Deepen the incision through the anterior portion of the rectus sheath. Dissect the underlying rectus muscle from the rectus sheath primarily with blunt dissection.
- In the areas of the anterior transverse inscriptions, use sharp dissection to divide the inscriptions off the overlying anterior rectus sheath, being careful not to incise into the muscle itself.
- Clamp and cauterize the multiple perforating fasciocutaneous vessels as encountered.
- Retract the muscle medially and using blunt scissor dissection to identify the vascular pedicle located lateral and deep to the rectus in the inferior portion of the sheath (Fig. 5.31B). The pedicle enters the rectus muscle approximately at the junction of its middle and distal thirds.
- Trace the inferior epigastric artery and its venae comitantes laterally and inferiorly to their origin on the external iliac vessels.
- Section the muscle proximally and distally, protecting the vascular pedicle. Observe that the muscle is being adequately perfused throughout its length by the inferior epigastric vessels only.
- When the recipient bed is ready, ligate and divide the pedicle near its origin.
- Carefully inspect the posterior rectus sheath, and if it has been violated, repair it with a strong nonabsorbable suture to prevent herniation.
- Close the anterior rectus sheath with 3-0 nonabsorbable sutures over suction drainage.
- Complete the subcutaneous and skin closure in layers.

FUNCTIONING NEUROMUSCULAR TRANSFERS

Tamai et al., in 1970, first showed in a canine model that a functioning neuromuscular unit could be transplanted using microvascular anastomoses and nerve repairs at the recipient site. Functioning free muscle transfers can be used for replacement of the flexor and extensor compartments of the forearm, the muscles of facial expression, and the muscles in the extensor compartment of the leg.

Muscles that have been found useful for this procedure include the pectoralis major, latissimus dorsi, gracilis, rectus femoris, extensor digitorum brevis of the toes, and serratus anterior. The semitendinosus, tensor fasciae latae, and brachioradialis also can be used for functioning muscle transfers. The selection of a given muscle depends on the strength and excursion of the donor muscle, the skin coverage requirements, the motor nerve availability, and the location of the ends of the flexor tendons. The advantage of this procedure is the restoration of a functional deficit by transferring a viable muscle under voluntary control with little functional loss after transfer. The disadvantages include (1) the loss of a functioning muscle, (2) the long reinnervation time, (3) the requirement for microvascular skill, and (4) the length of the procedure.

If a simpler procedure, such as a tendon transfer, suffices to restore the desired function, it should be used in preference

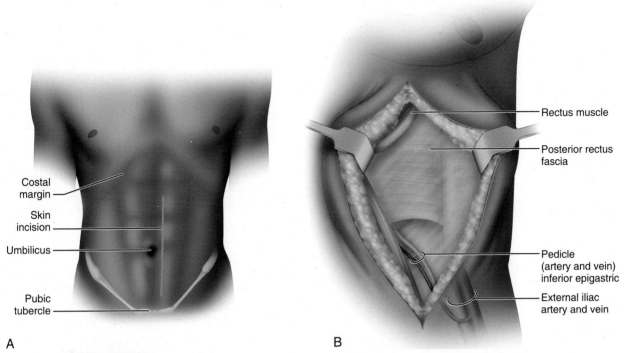

Costal margin

Skin incision

Umbilicus

Pubic tubercle

Rectus muscle

Posterior rectus fascia

Pedicle (artery and vein) inferior epigastric

External iliac artery and vein

A

B

FIGURE 5.31 **A,** Paramedian incision for harvesting rectus abdominis muscle. **B,** Rectus abdominis muscle flap isolation. Muscle is retracted medially, and inferior epigastric artery is seen entering posterior aspect of muscle within inferior lateral portion of sheath. **SEE TECHNIQUE 5.17.**

to a free muscle transfer. A high level of patient motivation is essential for these procedures to succeed.

The following should be considered in preoperative evaluation and planning. The needs and the neurovascular anatomy of the recipient site should be assessed carefully. A single, undamaged motor nerve should be available in the recipient area to supply the muscle transplant. In the forearm, median nerve branches to the flexor digitorum sublimis or the anterior interosseous nerves have been used most often. The status of recipient nerves should be evaluated carefully by history and physical examination, electromyography, and an exploratory surgical procedure if needed. Arteriography is indicated to assess recipient vessels and in some situations the donor vessels. The muscle to be transferred should be similar in size, strength, and excursion to the muscle to be replaced.

If a large muscle is required, the latissimus dorsi or pectoralis major muscle is preferred. If a small muscle is needed, the gracilis, serratus anterior, or extensor digitorum brevis may suffice. The muscle and the neurovascular pedicle should be easily accessible. The joints in the recipient extremity should be supple with a functional range of motion available in the elbow, wrist, and fingers. Stable proximal joints with balanced muscles should be present. Good skin covering the recipient site is required. If necessary, a skin island can be carried with the transferred muscle in most situations.

TRANSFER OF FUNCTIONING MUSCLE

The reader is referred to previous sections for details of harvesting a particular donor muscle. Before this procedure is begun, preparations should be made for appropriate

monitoring of vital signs and body temperature, appropriate padding of bony prominences, a heating blanket, and an indwelling urinary catheter. Two surgical teams permit a more efficient and prompt completion of the procedure and usually are essential.

TECHNIQUE 5.18

FOREARM PREPARATION

- Determine the general location of the recipient arteries and nerves, based on previous surgical procedures on the forearm, preoperative clinical examination, electromyography, and angiography.
- Fashion a paper template to assist in locating the neurovascular pedicle (Fig. 5.32). This also helps to determine the area of needed skin coverage.
- Use a pneumatic tourniquet to allow rapid initial dissection. Inflate and deflate the tourniquet as needed after the initial dissection.
- Usually an extensive curved or a zigzag incision is required for adequate exposure.
- Plan to use the radial or ulnar artery or a suitable large branch as a recipient vessel.
- On the flexor aspect, plan to expose the ulnar, median, and anterior interosseous nerves as needed. On the extensor surface, plan to use branches of the radial nerve.
- If extensive scarring is present, carefully dissect from normal, uninjured areas into the scarred areas to avoid injury to the recipient vessels and nerves.
- Exposure of the anterior interosseous nerve and artery may require section of the pronator teres in a Z configuration, allowing for later repair.

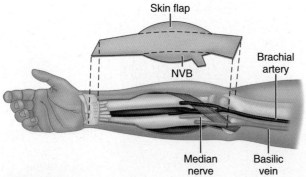

FIGURE 5.32 Free transfer, functioning muscle. Paper template assists in preoperative planning of skin coverage requirements, musculotendinous attachments, and neurovascular repairs. *NVB*, Neurovascular bundle. **SEE TECHNIQUE 5.18.**

- For venous drainage, use the venae comitantes of the arteries selected or superficial veins in the area.
- Expose the tendons of the flexor digitorum profundus, and mobilize them by dissecting them free from surrounding scar to ensure satisfactory gliding.
- Identify the flexor tendons distally for flap attachment and plan to expose the medial epicondyle and surrounding fascia for flexor replacement attachment.
- Expose the lateral epicondyle and the extensor origin for extensor replacement attachment.
- Plan to cover the distal flexor tendon repair with a local skin flap or with skin on the transplanted muscle.
- Cover the proximal belly of the transplanted muscle with a skin graft if needed.
- Before anastomosis, determine that the recipient artery shows free pulsatile flow.

TRANSFER OF FUNCTIONING MUSCLE TO FOREARM (MANKTELOW)

- After dissecting the donor muscle, leave it attached to its major vascular pedicle and at the origin and insertion until the recipient area in the forearm has been completely prepared. Determine that the recipient vessels are suitable for anastomosis and that all is ready for transfer to minimize the muscle ischemia time.
- The following method, as suggested by Manktelow, is helpful in determining the proper tension for attachment of the transferred muscle, especially if the extensor musculature is not intact. Position the extremity so that the muscle is fitted to its maximal physiologic length. For the latissimus dorsi and the pectoralis major, this would be maximal humeral abduction. For the gracilis, this would be with the knee fully extended (Fig. 5.33).
- With the arm in the appropriate position, place suture markers on the surface of the muscle at 5-cm intervals. After transfer and revascularization, this length can be restored by stretching the muscle from its new origin to its new insertion, reestablishing the 5-cm interval between the suture markers.
- When the length determinations have been made, detach the muscle from its origin and insertion, and carefully section the arteries, veins, and nerves.

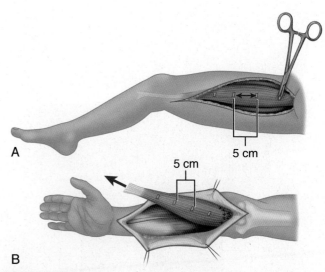

FIGURE 5.33 Free transfer, functioning muscle. **A,** Gracilis transfer. Pretransfer muscle length is determined by placing metal clips 5 cm apart in muscle. **B,** Transferred muscle attached proximally. Pretransfer length is restored with traction on muscle sufficient to restore 5-cm interval between metal clips. **SEE TECHNIQUE 5.18.**

- Immediately transfer the muscle to the arm in the best position for ease of neurovascular repair and attachment proximally and distally. This may require reversing the ends of the muscle so that the origin becomes the insertion.
- On the flexor surface, attach the origin to the medial epicondyle and surrounding fascia.
- On the extensor surface, attach the origin to the lateral epicondyle, fascia, and periosteum.
- Loosely suture the muscle in place to prevent its displacement during the neurovascular repairs.
- While the muscle is being attached by one team, the other team closes the donor site.
- Position the transferred muscle so that the arterial and venous anastomoses can be carried out easily (Fig. 5.34). Position the vascular repairs so that the nerve repairs are as close to the muscle as possible. This should shorten the period of muscle denervation. Manktelow reported a distance of 2 to 3 cm in most of his patients.
- Blood loss can be decreased by repairing one or more large veins before repairing the arteries; however, as long as the ischemia time is minimized, the order of repair is not critical. After completing the vascular repairs, connect the nerves with careful fascicular repair (see Primary Neurorrhaphy, earlier) using 10-0 or 11-0 nylon suture.
- Restore the predetermined 5-cm intervals on the muscle belly by pulling the transferred muscle out to length, and mark on the recipient tendons the appropriate locations for repair.
- Weave the flexor digitorum profundus tendons into the transplanted tendons as marked.
- Before attaching the recipient tendons to the donor flap, secure the recipient tendons to each other with a side-to-side suture. If the transferred muscle has no tendon, attach the recipient tendons by sewing them into the muscle and securing them with mattress sutures.

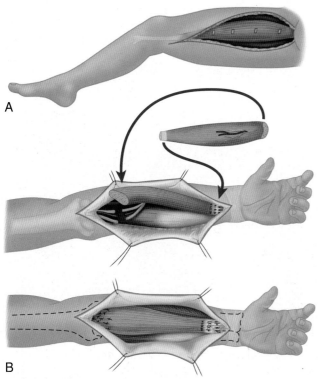

A

B

FIGURE 5.34 Free transfer, functioning muscle. **A,** Scheme of transfer of functioning gracilis muscle from right thigh, reversed to match for neurovascular repairs in left forearm. If ipsilateral gracilis muscle is used, reversal is unnecessary. **B,** Transfer is completed; muscle is attached to fascia and periosteum proximally and interwoven with flexor tendons distally. **SEE TECHNIQUE 5.18.**

- Cover the distal musculotendinous repair with a local skin flap or skin carried with the transferred muscle. Split-thickness skin grafts can be used to cover the muscles proximally.
- Close the wounds loosely to avoid constriction of vessels and apply plaster splints with the wrist and fingers moderately flexed to relieve tension on the muscle and tendon repairs.

POSTOPERATIVE CARE Maintain the systemic circulation with good peripheral perfusion, ensuring adequate hydration. A postoperative anticoagulation routine may be followed, depending on the training, experience, and preference of the surgeon.

Gentle passive stretching exercises are begun 3 weeks after the operation and are continued until a full range of motion is achieved. As reinnervation occurs, usually at 2 to 4 months, active finger flexion is begun. Usually by 6 to 12 months, daily exercises include active resistive exercises. Various physical therapy techniques to increase the strength and range of motion are used throughout the course. Muscle strength stabilizes 2 to 3 years after the transplantation.

FREE VASCULARIZED BONE TRANSPLANT

Ostrup and Fredrickson and Doi et al. were the first to report their experimental success using microvascular techniques to transfer ribs as bone grafts to the mandible of dogs. Their work showed that vascularized bone grafts remained viable, based on their medullary and periosteal circulation, and healed without undergoing "creeping substitution."

Taylor, Miller, and Ham, in 1975, were the first to report a clinical case of a free vascularized bone graft to reconstruct a large defect in a tibia in which conventional bone grafting techniques had failed. This technique is applicable to a variety of orthopaedic problems, including long bone defects after trauma, irradiation, and excision for tumor, congenital pseudarthrosis of the tibia, and congenital and acquired bony defects of the upper extremity. It also has been used as a concomitant vascular bone graft in a spine fusion for scoliosis. More recently, free vascularized grafts from the medial femoral condyle (MFC) harvested as either thin periosteal or corticoperiosteal grafts have proven useful in treatment of nonunions of the ulna, metacarpals, clavicle, tibia, humerus, mandible, and scaphoid.

As outlined by Taylor, the free vascularized bone graft (fibula) has the following advantages:
1. It is accomplished in a one-stage procedure.
2. The graft can be "doweled" into the tibia proximally and distally for stability during anastomoses.
3. Tubular bone is stronger than an onlay cortical bone graft.
4. Bleeding bone with endosteal and periosteal circulation is transferred to the recipient site.
5. If the anastomoses fail, the fibula can function as a traditional cortical bone graft.

The disadvantages cited include the following:
1. A long operation is required, limiting its application primarily to younger patients.
2. The procedure should be done electively.
3. Morbidity is created at the donor site, which may cause problems at the knee and ankle.
4. The patency of the anastomosis cannot be easily assessed.
5. A major vessel is sacrificed in the donor and the recipient limb.

The iliac crest, rib, and fibula currently are considered the best sources for vascularized bone grafts (Fig. 5.35). For most orthopaedic reconstructive procedures, the fibula is the preferred donor bone if its circulation has not been injured. The fibula has the following qualities:
1. It is a straight cortical bone.
2. A graft about 26 cm long can be harvested from an adult.
3. Muscle, an articular surface proximally, and, in a child, a proximal physis are available.
4. The vascular pedicle consists of the peroneal artery (1.5 to 2.5 mm in diameter) and its two venae comitantes (2 to 3 mm in diameter) and may be 1 to 5 cm in length.
5. The dissection is superficial and straightforward.
6. Complications are minimal, especially if the peroneal nerve and tibial vessels are protected.
7. Usually, overlying skin and nerve are unavailable.
8. It is useful for long bone defects.

The characteristics of the iliac crest graft include the following:
1. It is a curved and corticocancellous bone.
2. A length of 8 to 10 cm can be used.
3. Its vascular pedicle consists of the superficial circumflex iliac artery (0.5 to 3 mm in diameter) or the deep

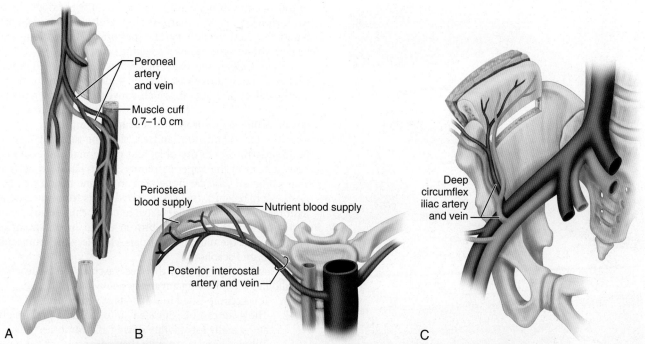

FIGURE 5.35 Vascularized bone grafts. Three sites considered best sources of vascularized bone, with blood supply shown. **A,** Fibula with peroneal vessels is preferred for long bone defects. **B,** Rib site with intercostal vessels. **C,** Iliac crest with deep circumflex iliac vessels shown. Sites depicted in **B** and **C** are preferred for shorter bone defects and mandibular reconstruction.

circumflex iliac artery and the superficial inferior epigastric veins (1.5 to 3 mm in diameter), and it is 1 to 5 cm in length.

4. If the superficial vessels are used, the dissection is superficial. If the deep vessels are chosen, the dissection is deep and tedious.
5. Overlying skin and cutaneous nerves are available.
6. Muscle, articular surface, and physes are unavailable.
7. Complications include abdominal wall hernia and neuromas in the cutaneous nerve stump.
8. It can be used as a composite bone and skin graft in the extremities and for mandibular reconstruction.

The rib as a free vascularized graft has the following characteristics:

1. It is a curved, membranous, flexible bone.
2. A length of 30 cm can be obtained.
3. Its vascular pedicle includes the posterior intercostal artery (1.5 to 2 mm in diameter) and single intercostal vein (1.2 to 2.5 mm in diameter) and may be 3 to 5 cm in length.
4. The dissection is deep and difficult, and tube thoracotomy may be required.
5. Complications may include pneumothorax.
6. The nerve, overlying skin, muscle, and an articular surface are available.
7. A physis is unavailable.
8. It is most applicable to mandibular reconstruction and to extremity injuries requiring composite skin and bone.

INDICATIONS

The transfer of a vascularized bone graft is indicated when traditional bone grafting techniques cannot be done, especially if soft-tissue coverage is inadequate. It also may be useful when traditional bone grafting techniques have failed. Its use for treatment of congenital pseudarthrosis of the tibia also has been reported, and it also is used for bony reconstruction after excision for tumors or conditions such as fibrous dysplasia.

PREOPERATIVE PLANNING

A bone graft donor site should be selected based on the needs of the recipient site. For a segmental defect or bone gap of 6 cm or less, traditional bone grafting techniques may suffice. For a defect 6 to 10 cm, the iliac crest or fibula may be appropriate. For a defect greater than 10 cm, a fibula is preferable as a vascularized bone graft.

Angiography of the donor and recipient limbs should be performed to permit planning and to obtain information regarding anomalous vascularity or vascular injury. The technique recommended by Taylor is to superimpose the image of the fibula with its vascular pedicle from the donor leg angiogram on the recipient leg radiograph. This permits planning for the placement of the anastomoses and an estimation of vessel size and bone needs. The procedure can be rehearsed in the anatomy dissecting room to enhance operative skills.

FREE VASCULARIZED FIBULAR TRANSFER

The fibula is the most common bone used for free vascularized osseous transfers. Its length and linear contour make it the preferred donor for long bone reconstruction. The fact that it is a strong cortical bone allows it to be rigidly fixed with plates and screws. It can be dissected rapidly under tourniquet control and is considered a fairly expendable bone. Its pedicle, consisting of the peroneal artery (1.5 to 3 mm) and its venae comitantes, is 6 to 8 cm long. The nutrient artery enters the bone in the middle third. About 26 cm of bone can be harvested. It can be elevated as a bone-muscle complex by incorporating the flexor hallucis longus or the soleus or as a bone-skin complex by incorporating the overlying skin. Two techniques for harvesting the fibula are described, one a posterior approach and the other a lateral. We prefer the lateral approach because it is much quicker and easier.

POSTERIOR APPROACH FOR HARVESTING FIBULAR GRAFT

TECHNIQUE 5.19

(TAYLOR)
- After administration of epidural or general anesthesia, place the patient prone and following the usual preparations, including insertion of an indwelling urinary catheter, abduct the legs onto separate tables. Two surgical teams operate simultaneously. Use pneumatic tourniquets to maintain a bloodless field.
- Start the incision in the popliteal fossa of the donor leg and extend it obliquely laterally toward the fibula and distally along the course of this bone.
- Make an incision between the soleus and peroneal muscles and extend this deep dissection medially into the popliteal fossa.
- Reflect skin flaps to expose the underlying muscle.
- Identify the lateral popliteal nerve and preserve its tibial and peroneal branches.
- Preserve the proximal peroneal and extensor muscle attachments to the tibia and the head of the fibula.
- Identify the anterior tibial vessels.
- Preserve a 5- to 10-mm sleeve of muscle on the lateral and anterior aspects of the fibula.
- Begin the posteromedial dissection posteriorly, detaching the lateral head of the gastrocnemius and the plantaris muscle from the femur and retracting the popliteal vessels and medial popliteal nerve medially.
- Divide the soleus muscle 1 to 2 cm parallel to the fibula and the posterior tibial vessels and follow the popliteal and posterior tibial vessels to the origin of the peroneal vessels.
- Trace the peroneal vessels to the origin of the flexor hallucis longus muscle distally and ligate the several large muscle branches to the soleus during this dissection.
- Using sharp dissection, carefully divide the flexor hallucis longus muscle along the course of the peroneal artery, leaving a 1-cm sleeve of muscle on the fibula.
- Divide the fibula proximally and distally at levels determined by the length required for the recipient bone.
- Preserve the proximal peroneal muscle attachment and the tibial collateral ligament for knee stability. Preserve the distal 25% of the fibula to retain ankle stability. In children, secure the distal fibula to the tibia with a transverse screw, taking care to avoid tilting the fibula.
- Beginning distally, divide the interosseous membrane and the posterior tibial muscle parallel to the fibula to isolate the fibula entirely on its vascular pedicle.

- Remove the periosteum from the proximal and distal 1 to 3 cm of the fibula to allow insertion of the fibula into the recipient bone.
- Release the tourniquet to permit hemostasis and to determine that the circulation to the fibula is adequate.
- Transect the vascular pedicle carefully and deliver the bone graft to the recipient site when it is completely prepared.
- Resection techniques are discussed subsequently.
- Close the donor defect over suction drainage tubes as needed.

POSTOPERATIVE CARE The postoperative care is the same as that described for the lateral approach described next.

LATERAL APPROACH FOR HARVESTING FIBULAR GRAFT

TECHNIQUE 5.20

(GILBERT; TAMAI ET AL.; WEILAND)
- Place the patient supine with the donor extremity flexed at the hip and the knee and the foot internally rotated slightly. Place a large sandbag under the ipsilateral buttock. During the initial portion of the dissection, use a pneumatic tourniquet to maintain a bloodless field.
- Make an incision centered on the fibula along the lateral aspect of the leg, extending from the neck of the fibula distally toward the ankle (Fig. 5.36A).
- Incise the skin and subcutaneous tissue to the superficial fascia over the interval between the peroneus longus and the soleus muscles.
- Incise the aponeurosis and dissect longitudinally posterior to the peroneus longus muscle and anterior to the soleus muscle (Fig. 5.36B).
- Identify the peroneus longus tendon in the distal part of the incision for orientation (Fig. 5.36C).
- Incise the fascia along the interval between the soleus muscle posteriorly and the peroneus longus muscle laterally.
- Elevate the soleus muscle in the distal portion of the wound with blunt dissection and proceed proximally until the origin of the soleus muscle on the proximal fibula is encountered.
- At this point, identify the peroneal vessels lying just deep to the soleus and nearly in contact with the fibula.
- When the pedicle has been identified, sharply incise the fibular origin of the soleus (Fig. 5.36D) to allow adequate posterior retraction of the soleus for later pedicle dissection.
- Identify the interval between the peroneal muscles and the flexor hallucis longus in the distal portion of the leg by observing the thin line of adipose tissue just posterior to the peroneals. The flexor hallucis longus is posterior to the peroneals, deep to the soleus covering the posterolateral surface of the fibula. The peroneal vessels course within the flexor hallucis muscle and are protected.

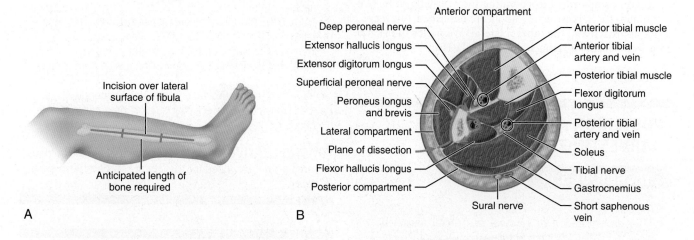

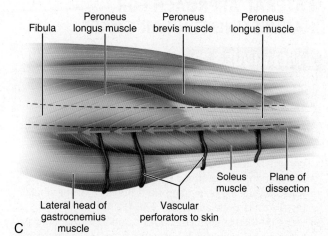

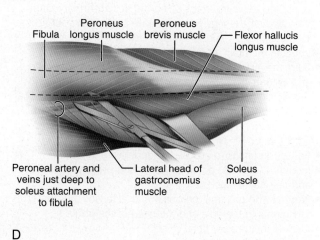

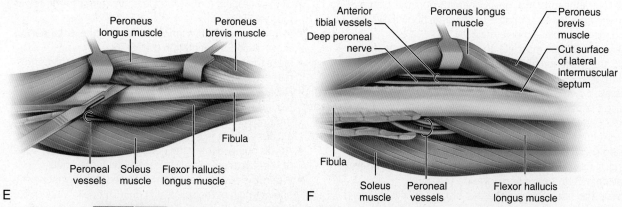

FIGURE 5.36 **A,** Vascularized free fibular transfer. Skin incision. **B,** Cross-sectional view of leg with planned course of dissection around fibula. **C,** Interval between soleus and peroneal muscles defined and developed. **D,** Peroneal vessels identified just distal and deep to fibular origin of soleus muscle in proximal part of dissection. Soleus origin released with scissor dissection. **E,** Anterior fibular dissection, releasing peroneal muscles in extraperiosteal fashion, protecting peroneal nerve proximally. **F,** Anterior dissection continues through anterior intermuscular septum, releasing anterior muscles off fibula and protecting deep peroneal nerve and anterior tibial vessels.

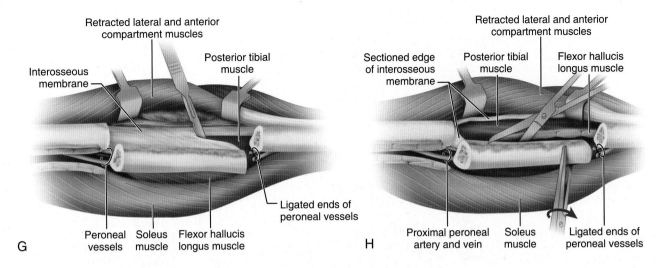

Retracted lateral and anterior compartment muscles

Interosseous membrane

Posterior tibial muscle

Peroneal vessels Soleus muscle Flexor hallucis longus muscle

Ligated ends of peroneal vessels

G

Retracted lateral and anterior compartment muscles

Sectioned edge of interosseous membrane

Posterior tibial muscle

Flexor hallucis longus muscle

Proximal peroneal artery and vein Soleus muscle Ligated ends of peroneal vessels

H

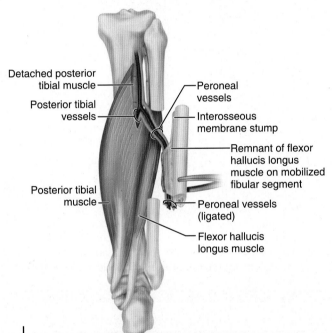

Detached posterior tibial muscle

Posterior tibial vessels

Posterior tibial muscle

Peroneal vessels

Interosseous membrane stump

Remnant of flexor hallucis longus muscle on mobilized fibular segment

Peroneal vessels (ligated)

Flexor hallucis longus muscle

I

FIGURE 5.36, Cont'd **G,** Distal and proximal osteotomies have been completed using Gigli saw. Peroneal vessels are seen ligated distally. Fibula is externally rotated for incision of intermuscular septum close to fibula. **H,** Posterior tibial muscle is released from fibula. **I,** Completed dissection after release of flexor hallucis longus, leaving thin layer of muscle to protect peroneal vessels. **SEE TECHNIQUE 5.20.**

- Retract the peroneal muscles anteriorly and sharply dissect them off the fibula in an extraperiosteal fashion (Fig. 5.36E). During this portion of the dissection, carefully identify and protect the superficial peroneal nerve in the proximal part of the wound where it is closely applied to the fibula and can be seen coursing distally within the peroneal muscles. The peroneal vessels are well protected posteriorly by the flexor hallucis longus.
- Continue the dissection anteriorly along the fibula and, as the anterior intermuscular septum is encountered, incise it close to the fibula.
- Elevate the anterior compartment in a similar extraperiosteal fashion as far as it can be exposed, protecting

the anterior tibial artery and deep peroneal nerve (Fig. 5.36F).
- Place a Gigli saw around the fibula where the proximal osteotomy is to be made. This should be within the proximal third of the fibula to be certain that the nutrient artery is included within the harvested segment. In placing the Gigli saw, retract the peroneal vessels posteriorly and the superficial and deep peroneal nerves with the anterior tibial vessels anteriorly.
- Bluntly develop an extraperiosteal plane closely around the fibula where the distal osteotomy is to be made.
- Osteotomize the fibula using a Gigli saw, protecting the surrounding soft tissues. Sharply elevate the flexor

hallucis longus off the fibula for a distance of 1 cm proximal and distal to the distal osteotomy site. Retract the fibula anteriorly and the flexor hallucis longus posteriorly to identify the peroneal vessels coursing close to the fibula. In the distal part of the leg, the peroneal vessels may have perforated the interosseous membrane to continue anteriorly. After identifying the peroneal vessels, ligate and divide them.

- Grasp the fibula with a bone clamp and externally rotate it to allow exposure and sharp release of any remaining anterior compartment muscles from it.
- Apply gentle lateral traction to the fibula and incise the interosseous membrane close to it from distal to proximal (Fig. 5.36G). Take care not to avulse the fibula from the peroneal vessel during this portion of the dissection.
- From anteriorly, release the posterior tibial muscle from the fibula while directly observing the peroneal vessels (Fig. 5.36H). Small muscular branches from the peroneal artery to the posterior tibial muscle should be clipped or cauterized with the bipolar cautery.
- Release the flexor hallucis longus from the fibula, leaving a thin layer of muscle adjacent to the peroneal vessels (Fig. 5.36I).
- At this point, the fibular graft is completely isolated on its vascular pedicle and should exhibit some bleeding on tourniquet release. We routinely allow the bone to be perfused at this point to minimize ischemic time. The peroneal artery and venae comitantes may be divided at their origin from the posterior tibial vessels.
- Obtain hemostasis. Loosely suture the flexor hallucis longus to the interosseous membrane and close the subcutaneous tissue and skin in layers over a suction drain. Do not attempt to close the fascia for risk of postoperative compartment syndrome.
- When harvested, fix the graft rigidly to the recipient bone, preferably by doweling each end of it into the medullary canal of the recipient bone and applying supplemental plates and screws. The method of fixation depends on recipient site factors. Give careful consideration to pedicle length and positioning in relation to the donor artery and vein before fixation. After fixation is complete, proceed with arterial and venous anastomoses.

POSTOPERATIVE CARE Immobilization should be applied according to the level of the bone graft. If the graft has been placed below the knee, a long leg cast with the knee flexed to prevent weight bearing should be worn for 3 to 5 months. A bone scan usually is obtained within the first week to evaluate perfusion of the graft. Union of the graft to the recipient bone should be determined by radiographic and clinical evaluation, and full weight bearing may be permitted when the graft begins to show signs of hypertrophy, which may require 15 months or more. Supplemental conventional bone grafting may be required. If the graft has been applied for knee fusion or to the femur, or the patient is a small child, a long leg cast with a pelvic band or a spica cast may be required to immobilize the part sufficiently to permit healing. When healing is progressing and the

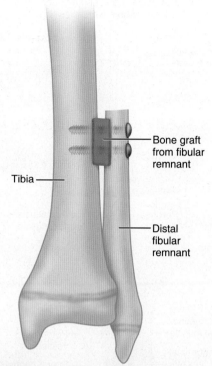

FIGURE 5.37 Fibular donor-site management in children should include distal tibiofibular fusion to prevent progressive valgus deformity. **SEE TECHNIQUE 5.21.**

bone is hypertrophying, an orthosis may be fitted and is worn until the limb is strong enough to support weight bearing.

Because of the risk of a valgus deformity of the ankle after removal of the fibular shaft in children with significant remaining growth, a distal tibiofibular fusion is recommended in this age group.

DISTAL TIBIOFIBULAR FUSION TO PREVENT PROGRESSIVE VALGUS DEFORMITY

TECHNIQUE 5.21

- After harvest of the fibular graft as just described, decorticate a 2- to 3-cm area of the adjacent surfaces of the tibia and fibula above the distal metaphysis.
- Place a 3-cm segment of the harvested fibula or of the remaining fibula between the tibia and fibula and insert two cortical screws across the fibula and the graft and into the tibia using AO lag techniques (Fig. 5.37).

POSTOPERATIVE CARE A long leg, bent-knee, non–weight-bearing cast is worn for 6 weeks, followed by a patellar tendon-bearing cast for an additional 6 weeks.

The bone of the iliac crest receives its blood supply through the cutaneous distribution of the superficial circumflex iliac artery, the muscular attachments of the tensor fasciae latae muscle, and, as shown by Taylor, Townsend, and Corlett, the deep circumflex iliac system that provides an optimal blood supply (see Fig. 5.35C).

FREE ILIAC CREST BONE GRAFT

TECHNIQUE 5.22

(TAYLOR, TOWNSEND, AND CORLETT; DANIEL; WEILAND ET AL.)

- With two surgical teams working, place the patient supine and administer a general anesthetic.
- Identify by palpation the femoral vessels and, using a Doppler probe, outline the course of the superficial circumflex iliac artery paralleling the inguinal ligament toward the iliac crest. If the superficial circumflex iliac system with overlying skin as an osteocutaneous flap is to be used, outline the skin flap and the course of the vessels.
- Make a vertical incision over the vessels medially and dissect and identify the superficial circumflex iliac artery and the inferior epigastric vein.
- Carry the dissection laterally from inferior to superior, incising the fascia at the point of vessel penetration near the lateral border of the sartorius muscle.
- Continue to elevate the skin flap superficial to the fascia as the dissection proceeds laterally and maintain the attachments of the skin and soft tissue to the iliac crest while this dissection is proceeding.
- When the flap has been elevated and the vessels have been identified and protected, osteotomize the iliac crest, obtaining sufficient bone for the planned reconstruction.
- Transfer the bone graft to the recipient site after the vessels have been transected.
- To use the deep circumflex iliac artery and vein, the dissection proceeds in a similar fashion. Identify the superficial circumflex iliac artery and vein and the inferior epigastric vein and proceed superior to the inguinal ligament, continuing the skin incision to allow exposure paralleling the inguinal ligament.
- Identify the deep circumflex iliac artery and vein as they arise from the external iliac artery and vein.
- Incise transversely the external oblique, internal oblique, and transversus abdominis muscles.
- Use blunt dissection to expose the preperitoneal fascia and expose the posterior aspect of the inner table of the iliac crest with its attached iliacus muscle.
- The deep circumflex iliac artery courses approximately 2.5 cm inferior to the iliac crest on its internal margin in a tunnel along the transversus abdominis and iliacus fasciae. Avoid injury to the spermatic cord, the vascular structures, and the genitofemoral branch of the femoral nerve.
- Outline the flap based on the deep circumflex artery and perform the osteotomy beginning on the lateral surface of the iliac crest and using an oscillating saw or an osteotome. Preserve the overlying skin or subcutaneous tissue and its attachment to the iliac crest to avoid injury to the nutrient vessels supplying the skin.

- The curvature of the ilium prevents the harvesting of grafts much longer than 10 to 12 cm. Osteotomy of the graft helps to straighten the curve.
- On the inner table of the iliac crest, retain the covering of the iliacus muscle to preserve the nutrient blood supply of the bone.
- The donor site can be closed primarily by flexing the hip.
- Place the bone graft in the recipient site. Fixation of the iliac crest graft into the recipient site may be more difficult than fixation of the fibula. Because the iliac graft is short, fixation by insetting or doweling may compromise length. Fixation also can be achieved using an external fixation device or a combination of fixation devices with screws. Difficulty may be encountered in attaching a plate to an iliac crest graft.

POSTOPERATIVE CARE Postoperative care is similar to that described for the fibular graft (see Technique 5.20).

FREE VASCULARIZED MEDIAL FEMORAL CONDYLE FLAP

The use of free vascularized periosteal and corticoperiosteal bone from the MFC was first described by Sakai in 1991 and has grown in popularity because of its reliable vascular pedicle and its use as an osteocartilaginous graft. Fuchs et al. described its use extensively in treatment of nonunions of the clavicle and scaphoid. Higgens and Burger described their technique and experience with its use as an osteocartilaginous flap for proximal scaphoid arthroplasty. Fifteen of 16 patients achieved osseous union with acceptable pain relief and motion. Donor-site complaints were transient and did not preclude a return to athletics.

The flap is based off the descending genicular artery (DGA), the superior medial genicular artery, or both. The DGA branches off the superficial femoral artery about 13 cm above the knee, just proximal to the adductor hiatus, and divides into two or three of the following branches: the osteoarticular branch, the muscular branch, and the saphenous branch. The DGA is present in about 90% of specimens. The osteoarticular branch arises about 11 cm above the knee lying just deep or lateral to the adductor magnus tendon along the posterior aspect of the medial intermuscular septum. The superior genicular artery is consistently present arising from the popliteal artery 5 cm above the knee to anastomose with the osteoarticular branch of the DGA and is dominant in 11% of specimens (Fig. 5.38).

HARVESTING OF MEDIAL FEMORAL CONDYLE CORTICOPERIOSTEAL FREE FLAP

TECHNIQUE 5.23   *Figure 5.39*

- Make a longitudinal incision in the distal medial thigh overlying the adductor magnus and sartorius muscles. Retract the adductor magnus anteriorly and the sartorius

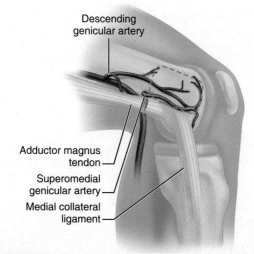

Descending
genicular artery

Adductor magnus
tendon

Superomedial
genicular artery

Medial collateral
ligament

FIGURE 5.38 Arterial anatomy medial femoral condyle.

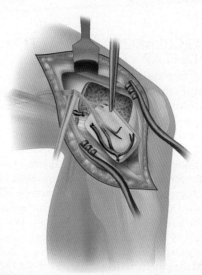

FIGURE 5.39 Flap elevated from medial femoral condyle. **SEE TECHNIQUE 5.23.**

posteriorly to expose the descending genicular vessels and the superior genicular vessels. Note the arcade of vessels formed by these two vessels over the MFC.

- Outline the proposed corticoperiosteal flap to include this network of vessels, taking care to preserve the medial collateral ligament. Limit the graft proximally at the metaphyseal diaphyseal junction.
- Elevate the periosteum with the underlying corticocancellous bone to the extent needed by the recipient site. A 5 × 7-cm graft is the maximal size.
- Dissect the descending genicular vascular pedicle proximally, ligating and dividing the saphenous and muscular branches, to its origin off the superficial femoral vessels in Hunter's canal. A 1- to 2-mm diameter vascular pedicle measuring approximately 7 cm in length may be obtained.
- Ligate and divide the superior genicular vessels unless they are to be used as a vascular pedicle as well.

MEDIAL FEMORAL CONDYLE CORTICOPERIOSTEAL FREE FLAP FOR SCAPHOID ARTHROPLASTY

TECHNIQUE 5.24

(HIGGINS AND BURGER)

The same surgical approach is used for harvesting the medial femoral condyle (MFC) flap and medial femoral trochlea (MFT) flap through the soft tissue. Iorio et al. described this surgical approach, including the potential use of a skin segment of the flap in the harvesting technique. The flap can be harvested with a skin segment overlying the medial aspect of the knee, based on a cutaneous branch from the descending genicular artery (DGA) pedicle. This allows surface monitoring of flap viability and makes closure of the skin over the anastomosis easier. Alternatively, the anastomosis can be monitored with an implantable Doppler monitor. Skin closure can be achieved with mobilization of local skin flaps or skin grafts if needed.

- Trace the DGA distally along the medial column of the femur to a broad filigree of blood vessels intimately adherent into the periosteum of the medial distal femur (Fig. 5.40A). The longitudinal branch supplies the region commonly used for harvest of the MFC osteoperiosteal flap. The perpendicular transverse branch typically traverses the metaphyseal region and densely supplies the periosteum surrounding the MFT on both its medial and proximal aspects. This is the vessel that is used.
- Before harvesting the flap, prepare the wrist dissection. The reconstruction can be done through a volar or dorsal approach, according to the surgeon's preference. The dorsal approach provides greater visualization of the scaphoid fossa and nearby snuffbox for microvascular anastomosis. The volar approach can be made through a less extensive exposure and permits screw placement from distal to proximal. In this approach arterial anastomosis can be done with an end-to-side anastomosis into the radial artery or end-to-end into the palmar branch of the radial artery.
- With either approach, confirm the absence of arthritis in the scaphoid fossa. If the scaphoid fossa is deemed adequate to proceed with reconstruction, carefully resect the proximal pole nonunion segment (Fig. 5.40B). Preserve the thin cartilaginous surface that effaces the midcarpal joint. The MFT flap provides a cancellous surface facing distally and will require the native scaphoid cartilage to maintain smooth articulation with the capitate.
- Preserve the most distal aspects of the dorsal and volar scapholunate ligaments in continuity with the distal rim of cartilage. This is done to provide a benefit of stability between the scaphoid and lunate and inhibit rotary instability of the scaphoid.
- Debride the proximal pole segment so that it extends well beyond the nonunion plane and includes a significant amount of the distal segment. The MFT flap provides a larger osteocartilaginous segment that permits creation of a defect large enough to permit ease of inset. Creating a larger defect and larger flap provides greater ease of fixation

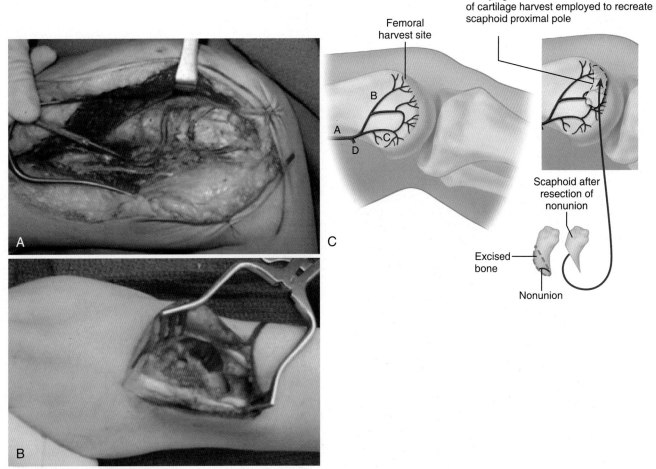

Shadow image of scaphoid is drawn overlying MFT to demonstrate orientation of cartilage harvest employed to recreate scaphoid proximal pole

Femoral harvest site

Scaphoid after resection of nonunion

Excised bone

Nonunion

FIGURE 5.40 **A,** Medial view of femur after elevation of vastus medialis. This exposure is much more extensive than that required for scaphoid reconstruction but is provided to demonstrate the vascular anatomy of the descending genicular artery (DGA) system. **B,** Dorsal approach to scaphoid nonunion after resection of proximal pole and nonunion site in preparation for reconstruction. Fingers are to left and forearm to right. Note generous resection and preservation of midcarpal articulating cartilage. **C,** Medial femoral trochlea (MFT) and planned portion of reconstructed proximal scaphoid. Portion of MFT and planned portion of reconstructed proximal scaphoid. Portion of MFT harvested to provide vascularized osteocartilaginous reconstruction of proximal scaphoid. *A,* descending geniculate artery; *B,* transverse branch; *C,* longitudinal branch; *D,* superomedial geniculate artery. (**C** from Bürger HK, Windhofer C, Gaggl AJ, et al: Vascularized medial femoral trochlea osteocartilaginous flap reconstruction of proximal pole nonunions, *J Hand Surg Am* 38:690, 2013.)

and the ability to provide an uninterrupted smooth cartilage surface for articulation with the scaphoid fossa. Preparation of the defect thus converts the difficult proximal pole fracture into a more manageable scaphoid waist osteosynthesis.

- With attention turned to the knee and the soft-tissue dissection completed, identify the DGA and suture-ligate it proximally from its origin off the superficial femoral artery within the adductor canal. This yields a lengthy pedicle beyond the requirements of the reconstruction. This length of pedicle is desirable because it provides the greatest caliber point of the DGA for microvascular anastomosis.
- After the DGA is ligated from the superficial femoral artery, reflect it distally. Ligate smaller branches as the dissection approaches the distal femur. As the DGA be-

comes intimately embedded in the periosteum, the two larger branches will become apparent. The longitudinal branch to the condyle can be suture-ligated.

- Continue harvest of the vessel using the transverse branch, which can be traced toward the medial trochlea. As the vessels become progressively smaller, perform dissection subperiosteally so as not to injure the small artery or veins. Leave the periosteal vessels adherent to the territory of bone and cartilage desired for harvest.
- Use a sagittal saw and osteotomes to harvest the most proximal portion of the cartilage-bearing segment of the MFT. The dimensions correspond as follows:
  - Measure the proximal-to-distal harvest to equal the radial-to-ulnar dimensions of the defect in the wrist.

- Measure the anterior-to-posterior harvest to equal the proximal-to-distal dimension of the defect in the wrist.
- Measure the medial-to-lateral harvest in the knee to equal the volar-to-dorsal dimensions of the wrist.
- Carefully harvest the segment to be in close approximation to the measured defect in the wrist. After the flap is elevated, close the capsule of the knee, followed by layered closure of the donor-site defect over a drain placed via counterincision.
- Fashion the osteocartilaginous segment to fit as precisely as possible into the defect created from resection of the proximal scaphoid (Fig. 5.40C). The convex surface of the flap apposes the concave scaphoid fossa of the radius, leaving a cancellous portion apposing the adjacent lunate as well as the preserved distal cartilaginous shell of the lesser curvature of the native scaphoid. A bone segment is usually affixed with a single cannulated screw driven from the dorsal or volar approach (surgeon's preference).
- Use intraoperative fluoroscopy to confirm satisfactory reconstruction of the scaphoid and implant placement.

MICROVASCULAR ANASTOMOSIS

- When the approach is made dorsally, the anastomosis usually is done in the end-to-side fashion to the radial artery in the snuffbox and associated veins. When the approach is made volarly, the arterial anastomosis usually is done in an end-to-end fashion into the palmar branch of the radial artery, with venous anastomosis into either deeper superficial vein in that region.
- If the skin can be closed without excessive tension, perform primary closure. If excessive tension of closure demonstrates compression of the vessels, a small skin graft can be used. Harvest of the flap with a small skin flap component will permit tension-free closure as well as a means of monitoring the flap postoperatively.

POSTOPERATIVE CARE Postoperatively, the patient's immobilization and radiographic monitoring are similar to those after other conventional means of scaphoid nonunion surgery. The patient is permitted to ambulate immediately after surgery. It is common for the patient to have some discomfort with ambulation, which resolves within 2 to 4 months. No knee brace or other immobilization of the knee is required.

COMPOSITE FREE TISSUE TRANSFERS FROM THE FOOT

The neurovascular supply to the structures of the foot makes it an unusually versatile donor site for many problems, especially in the foot and hand (Fig. 5.41). This section includes a discussion of the neurovascular anatomy of the foot as it pertains to the specific structures that are used most often as free tissue transfers. Also included are the advantages, disadvantages, various applications, and discussions of the various foot flaps, including dorsalis pedis, first web, pulp, "wraparound," bone and joint, epiphyseal, great toe, and second and third toe transfers.

NEUROVASCULAR ANATOMY

Standard anatomic textbooks describe the dorsalis pedis artery as a continuation of the anterior tibial artery that passes deep to the inferior extensor retinaculum. As the dorsalis pedis artery passes anterior to the ankle joint, it lies between the tendons of the extensor hallucis longus medially and the extensor digitorum longus laterally. Single accompanying veins lie on either side of the artery. The deep peroneal nerve lies immediately lateral to the artery. Passing over the tarsal bones, the dorsalis pedis artery gives off the medial and lateral tarsal arteries, and in the region of the bases of the metatarsals arises the arcuate artery, which passes laterally. The second, third, and fourth dorsal metatarsal arteries arise from the arcuate artery and descend to the dorsal surfaces of the respective dorsal interosseous muscles (Fig. 5.42).

The first dorsal metatarsal artery is the continuation of the dorsalis pedis artery. It runs distally, usually on the dorsal surface of the first dorsal interosseous muscle, and supplies branches to the dorsal skin, the first and second metatarsals, and the interosseous muscles. Near the first web space between the first and second toes, the first dorsal metatarsal artery divides into at least two branches, one passing deep to the tendon of the extensor hallucis longus, supplying the medial side of the great toe, and the other dividing to supply the adjacent sides of the great and second toes.

The deep plantar, or communicating, artery leaves the dorsalis pedis artery at the base of the first metatarsal and passes toward the plantar surface of the foot between the heads of the first dorsal interosseous muscle. It communicates with the lateral plantar artery and completes the plantar arterial arch. The deep plantar artery also supplies a branch to the medial side of the great toe. The first plantar metatarsal artery is the continuation of the deep plantar artery, which passes distally in the first interosseous space, divides, and supplies the adjacent sides of the great and second toes from the plantar side.

Important anatomic variations have been noted, however. The first dorsal metatarsal artery may lie superficial to or just within the substance of the first dorsal interosseous muscle in 78% to 88% of feet or may lie plantar to the first metatarsal (12% to 22%; Fig. 5.43). Variations include first metatarsal arteries lying plantar to the first metatarsal, absent first dorsal metatarsal arteries, and absent first dorsal and plantar metatarsal arteries (Fig. 5.44). Although the diameter of the dorsalis pedis artery may range from 1.8 to 3 mm, the artery also may be hypoplastic and narrow.

The venous drainage from the dorsum of the toes and foot flows into the dorsal venous arches, feeding the greater and lesser saphenous systems (Fig. 5.45). Additional venous drainage occurs through the veins accompanying the dorsalis pedis artery.

The dorsal surfaces of the toes and foot receive sensory innervation through the superficial peroneal nerve branches; the first web is innervated by the deep peroneal nerve, and the plantar surface is innervated by the digital branches of the medial plantar nerve (Fig. 5.46). All these nerves can be used to supply innervated flaps.

DORSALIS PEDIS FLAP

The advantages of the dorsalis pedis free tissue transfer are that it has a large-caliber arteriovenous pedicle, a long

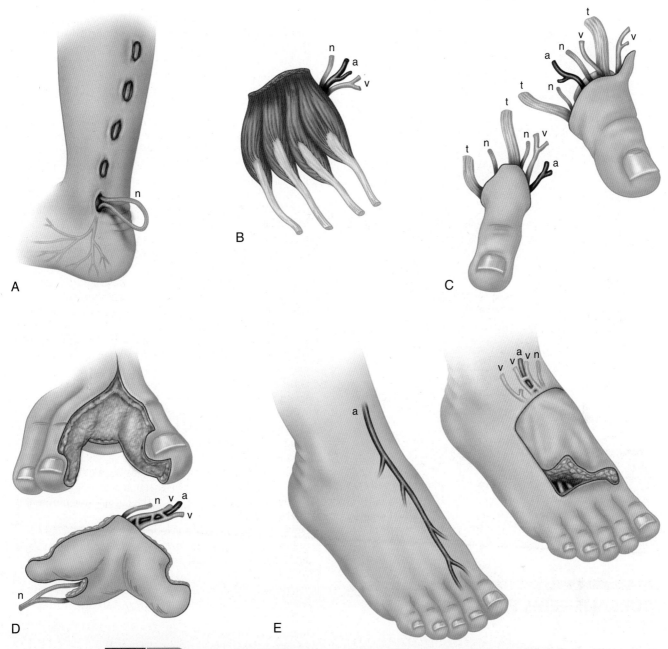

FIGURE **5.41** Foot as versatile donor source for free tissue transfers. **A,** Sural nerve graft. **B,** Extensor digitorum brevis muscle flap. **C,** First and second toe free tissue transfer. **D,** First web space free neurovascular flap. **E,** Dorsalis pedis cutaneous or cutaneous neurovascular free tissue flap. All these procedures require microsurgical techniques. *a,* Artery; *n,* nerve; *t,* tendon; *v,* vein.

pedicle can be obtained, it can be innervated, it is a thin flap, bone may be included, the donor site may be relatively inconspicuous after adequate healing, and in some patients a large (10 × 10 cm) flap can be obtained. Disadvantages include a technically difficult and tedious dissection, the possibility of a painful and hypertrophic donor-site scar, the frequently restricted size (7 × 7 cm or smaller), the inability to use the flap if the posterior tibial artery is absent or is not patent, and the inability to use the flap if the dorsalis pedis artery is not present or is not patent. The dorsalis pedis free flap is useful for coverage problems in the palm, the thumb web space, and the foot, especially in areas requiring protective sensation.

Because of the potential for variation in the vascularity of the foot, it is helpful to assess the dorsalis pedis artery with a Doppler probe and with arteriography of the donor foot obtained in two planes to show any variation that might preclude doing the procedure. If the flap is to be transferred to an area of a foot or hand that has been badly damaged, arteriography of the recipient area also is indicated to allow evaluation of those vessels. Separate teams of surgeons are needed to dissect the donor and recipient sites.

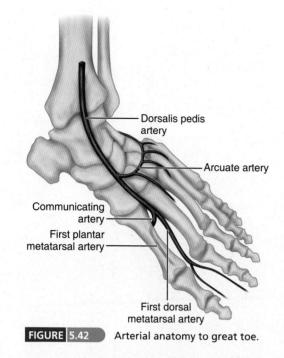

FIGURE 5.42 Arterial anatomy to great toe.

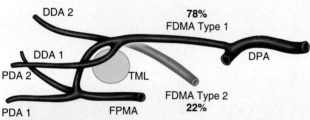

FIGURE 5.43 One scheme reported of variations in vascular supply to great toe. *DDA,* Dorsal digital artery; *DPA,* dorsalis pedis artery; *FDMA,* first dorsal metatarsal artery; *FPMA,* first plantar metatarsal artery; *PDA,* plantar digital artery; *TML,* transverse metatarsal ligament.

DORSALIS PEDIS FREE TISSUE TRANSFER

TECHNIQUE 5.25

- When the course of the dorsalis pedis artery has been determined, outline it with a skin-marking pencil. Determine the pattern of the dorsal veins by holding the foot in a dependent position to allow the veins to fill. Also outline the veins with a skin marker.
- Mark the margins of the flap based on the requirements of the recipient area (Fig. 5.47). Generally, the flap should neither extend more proximally than the extensor retinaculum nor extend more distally than about 2 cm distal to the palpable dorsalis pedis pulse or about the level of the metatarsophalangeal joints. Limiting the medial border to the extensor hallucis longus tendon and the lateral border to the fifth toe extensor digitorum longus tendon creates small flaps but usually prevents problems with the donor-site scar caused by denuding the medial side of the foot.

- Exsanguinate the limb by wrapping, inflate the pneumatic tourniquet, and begin the dissection on the medial side of the outlined flap. The dissection must be kept superficial to the extensor paratenon so that a satisfactory bed will be left for a split-thickness skin graft.
- Continue to dissect to the extensor hallucis longus tendon and divide the deep fascia over it.
- Dissect down to the periosteum overlying the first metatarsal and identify the dorsalis pedis artery with its veins and the deep peroneal nerve. If the flap is to be innervated, the branches of the superficial peroneal nerve are identified, transected proximally, and kept superficial to the plane of dissection while the flap is elevated.
- Continue the dissection laterally and distally to identify the beginning of the first dorsal metatarsal artery, the deep plantar (communicating) artery, and the arcuate artery. When the deep plantar artery has been identified, ligate and transect it.
- If bone is to be taken, at this point remove a portion or all of the second metatarsal and keep it with the flap.
- Continue to dissect distally, staying superficial to the paratenon without exposing tendon.
- Elevate and transect the extensor hallucis brevis tendon. Although the extensor hallucis brevis tendon is carried with the flap by some surgeons, it is sometimes useful to leave this muscle on the foot to assist in coverage of the tendon and bone.
- As the dissection is continued distally, keep the first dorsal metatarsal artery superficial to the plane of dissection and incise the margins of the flap to allow the flap to be elevated.
- When the distal limit of the flap has been developed, ligate and divide the distal arterial branches to the toes.
- Divide the distal skin margins of the flap and the proximal margins near the extensor retinaculum.
- If a long vascular pedicle is required, divide the extensor retinaculum in a Z-shaped fashion and dissect the dorsalis pedis and anterior tibial arteries, dividing the small side branches.
- Temporarily place a small vessel clip on the dorsalis pedis artery to ensure that the tibial artery is sufficient to vascularize the foot.
- Repair the extensor retinaculum.
- Determine that the dissection of the recipient site has been completed by the recipient site team; ligate and divide the dorsalis pedis artery, deliver the flap to the recipient site, and begin closure of the donor defect with a split-thickness skin graft.
- Place the flap in the recipient area, suture the distal margins so that the flap is not displaced while the vessels and nerves are being sutured, and complete the vascular anastomoses, usually repairing the arteries first, followed by the veins.
- Apply topical 2% lidocaine or papaverine to minimize vascular spasm.
- Suture nerves as needed and close the wounds.

POSTOPERATIVE CARE Appropriate bandages and splints are applied to the recipient area so that constriction is avoided and to allow examination of a portion of the flap. The general postoperative routine outlined previ-

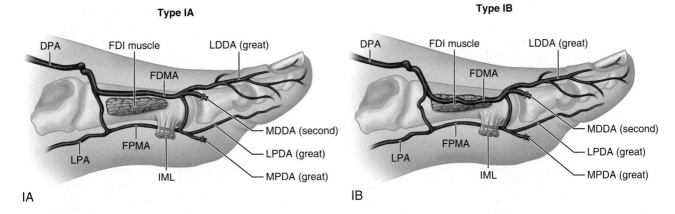

Type IA

Type IB

Type IIA

Type IIB

Type III

IA

IB

IIA

IIB

III

FIGURE 5.44 Anatomic variances of first metatarsal artery. *A,* Artery; *DPA,* dorsalis pedis artery; *FDI muscle,* first dorsal interosseous muscle; *FDMA,* first dorsal metatarsal artery; *FPMA,* first plantar metatarsal artery; *IML,* intermetatarsal ligament; *LDDA (great),* lateral dorsal digital artery to great toe; *LPA,* lateral plantar artery; *LPDA (great),* lateral plantar digital artery to great toe; *MDDA (second),* medial dorsal digital artery to second toe; *MPDA (second),* medial plantar digital artery to second toe.

ously usually is followed. A compression bandage is left on the donor foot, and the foot is kept elevated for 7 to 10 days to allow sufficient healing of the skin graft. An elastic wrap or elastic stocking is worn for 3 to 6 months to minimize donor-site scar hypertrophy and instability.

Activity is determined by the part that has received the reconstruction. In the hand, when the skin has healed and when sensation is returning, progressive rehabilitation of the hand can begin. In the foot or lower extremity, when healing has occurred and edema is resolving, a gradually progressive program of walking is followed, beginning with no weight bearing and prolonged elevation and progressing to full weight bearing to tolerance. If an innervated flap has been transferred to the foot, maximal participation in activities must await the return of sensation, and the foot should be protected with cushioned shoe inserts.

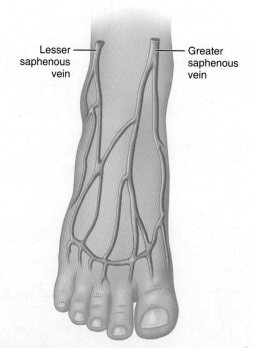

FIGURE 5.45 Venous drainage of foot. Tributaries to greater and lesser saphenous venous system used to drain dorsalis pedis and toe free flaps.

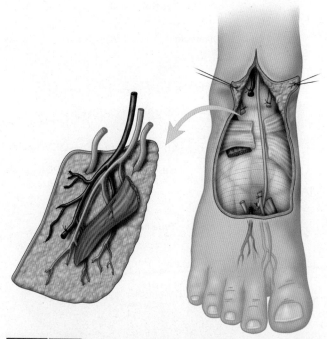

FIGURE 5.47 Dorsalis pedis flap dissection. Donor site usually requires skin grafting. **SEE TECHNIQUE 5.25.**

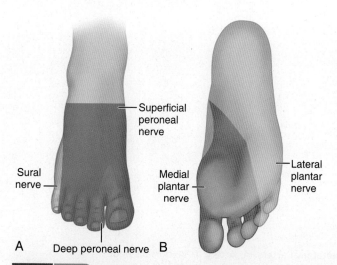

FIGURE 5.46 Cutaneous innervation of foot. **A,** Dorsal sensory supply of foot and toes. **B,** Plantar sensory supply of foot and toes.

FIRST WEB SPACE, PULP, AND HEMIPULP NEUROVASCULAR FREE FLAPS

The neurovascular supply to the web space between the great and second toes makes that area of the foot suitable for transfer to areas of the hand requiring restoration of sensibility, particularly the thumb. Based on their detailed anatomic studies of this region, Gilbert et al., in 1975, reported the first successful first web free tissue transfer. The advantages of using the first web and pulp donor area include the following:

1. The first web has a good potential for restoration of functional sensibility; the two-point discrimination on the toe pulps ranges from 10 to 18 mm.

2. The pulp skin is glabrous, closely approximating the digital skin.
3. The first web has a reliable blood supply.
4. The relatively large area available permits resurfacing the thumb, especially with the wraparound flap.
5. Larger areas may be covered by incorporating a dorsalis pedis flap with the first web space.
6. When successfully covered with a split-thickness skin graft, there is minimal donor-site morbidity.

The disadvantages are few and primarily involve the need to have a two-team approach to the procedures and the risks of vascular thromboses with loss of the entire flap. Delayed healing or failure of the skin graft to take in the donor site also can be troublesome. Limited usefulness from pain and hypersensitivity and cold intolerance have been reported.

May et al. found that the distal communicating artery, the terminal continuation of the first dorsal metatarsal artery, has three patterns of communication with the plantar digital arterial system (Fig. 5.48): (1) a distal communicating artery joining at the bifurcation of the first plantar metatarsal artery, (2) a distal communicating artery joining with the second plantar digital artery, and (3) a distal communicating artery joining with the second plantar digital artery. The dorsal portion of the first web also is supplied by the first and second dorsal digital arterial branches of the first dorsal metatarsal artery. These relationships and the possibility of other variations should be kept in mind when the dissections are done for these flaps.

As noted, the innervation of the adjacent sides of the great and second toes is supplied by three nerves. The most important innervation to the lateral side of the great toe pulp and the medial side of the second toe pulp is through the plantar digital branches of the common digital nerve to the first web space. The proper digital branches usually

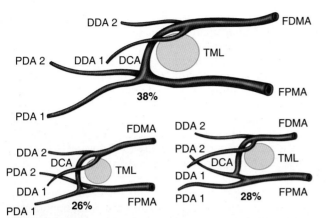

FIGURE 5.48 Variations in circulation to first web space. Three patterns of communication between distal communicating artery (DCA) and plantar digital arterial system have been identified. *DDA*, Dorsal digital artery; *FDMA*, first dorsal metatarsal artery; *FPMA*, first plantar metatarsal artery; *PDA*, plantar digital artery; *TML*, transverse metatarsal ligament.

are about 1 to 1.5 mm in diameter and can be dissected separately into the common digital nerve to give sufficient length to allow repair of the proper digital nerves of the thumb or finger in question. Two branches of the deep peroneal nerve enter the web space dorsally and supply the dorsal surfaces of the adjacent sides of the great and second toes. These branches also can be used to innervate a free web space flap. The superficial peroneal nerve terminal branches are extremely small and terminate too far to the dorsum to innervate the first web or pulp flaps.

NEUROVASCULAR FREE FLAP TRANSFER FIRST WEB SPACE

TECHNIQUE 5.26

- As with the dorsalis pedis flap, the arterial supply to the foot is assessed preoperatively with a Doppler probe and arteriography in two planes. If the first dorsal metatarsal artery is hypoplastic or absent, it may be necessary to use the first plantar metatarsal artery as the major arterial supply to the flap.
- On the skin, mark the course of the artery as determined by palpation of the pulse and the use of a Doppler probe. Identify the venous pattern by allowing the foot to hang over the edge of the operating table so that the veins fill; mark the course of the veins.
- Determine the amount of skin required by measuring the recipient area on the thumb or finger. Flaps measuring 6 × 10 cm to 8 × 12 cm can be obtained from the first web. If large amounts of skin are required, the dorsalis pedis skin flap may be included with the first web skin; this should be considered when planning the dissection.
- Outline the flap in the first web with a skin marker.

- Exsanguinate the limb by wrapping and inflate the pneumatic tourniquet.
- Begin the dissection over the artery with a curved or zig-zag incision on the dorsum of the foot between the first and second metatarsals.
- With careful and meticulous dissection, identify the dorsalis pedis artery, follow it to the deep plantar branch, ligate and divide the deep plantar branch, and follow the first dorsal metatarsal artery distally.
- Elevate and divide the extensor hallucis brevis tendon to allow exposure of the artery. Include the deep peroneal nerve with the arterial pedicle.
- As the dissection proceeds distally, elevate the skin flaps medially and laterally to identify the venous drainage. Usually, large veins can be found in the dorsum of the first web space, communicating with the large tributaries to the greater saphenous system on the medial side of the dorsum of the foot.
- If the first dorsal metatarsal artery is absent or hypoplastic, make a longitudinal plantar incision between the first and second metatarsals, communicating with the outline of the skin flap.
- Identify the plantar digital arteries, which can be found dorsal to their respective proper digital nerves. The plantar digital arteries and nerves can be dissected proximally so that the first plantar metatarsal artery and the common plantar digital nerve can be identified. Usually if the first dorsal metatarsal artery is hypoplastic, the first plantar metatarsal artery has a diameter large enough to allow anastomosis. Dorsal and plantar dissections should expose arteries, veins, and nerves for long enough to avoid the need for interpositional grafting.
- After developing the neurovascular pedicles, elevate the first web skin, maintaining a plane of dissection deep to the plane of the vessels and nerves so that they are carried with the skin without devascularizing it.
- While the donor site is being dissected, the hand recipient site is dissected and a split-thickness skin graft for the web space closure is obtained by the recipient site team.
- To harvest a pulp or hemipulp flap from the great or second toe (Fig. 5.49), outline the small amount of skin required for the recipient digit.
- The vascular dissection is identical to the web dissection until it approaches the web. At the first web, if the great toe is to be the donor, dissect the digital arterial and venous branches so that those to the lateral side of the great toe are carried with the flap.
- Handle the digital nerve branches in a similar manner by dissecting the plantar digital nerves proximally and separating the nerve to the lateral side of the great toe from the common digital nerve.
- If the second toe is to be the donor, dissect the nerves and vessels so that they are carried with the skin and pulp on the medial side of the second toe.
- If the recipient site is to be the thumb, carefully dissect and preserve the palmar digital nerves, the branches of the superficial radial nerve, the princeps pollicis artery, and dorsal digital and hand veins. If a finger is to receive the web or pulp flap, identify and mobilize the proper digital arteries, digital nerves, and dorsal veins for anastomosis.

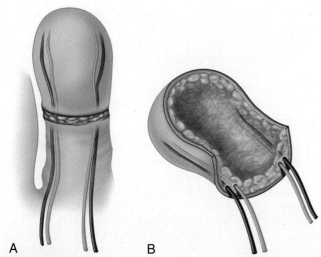

FIGURE 5.49 Scheme for pulp free flap. **A,** Flap outlined and toe dissection begun for skin flap. **B,** Flap separated from toe with digital arteries, venae comitantes, and nerves. **SEE TECHNIQUE 5.26.**

- While one team closes the donor defect with a skin graft, the other team loosely sutures the web, pulp, or hemipulp flap into the recipient defect. In the thumb, suture of the first dorsal metatarsal or plantar metatarsal arteries is done at the princeps pollicis or radial artery at the wrist by end-to-end or end-to-side anastomoses.
- Perform the venous repairs on the dorsum of the hand, anastomosing the saphenous system branches to the cephalic venous system.
- Suture plantar digital nerves to the palmar digital nerves on the palm side and the deep peroneal and superficial radial branches on the dorsum. In the fingers, suture the first dorsal metatarsal and the common or proper digital arteries.
- Suture the dorsal digital veins and the saphenous tributaries and the proper digital nerves to the plantar digital nerves.

POSTOPERATIVE CARE Postoperative care after first web, pulp, and hemipulp flaps is essentially the same as that for dorsalis pedis flaps (see Technique 5.26). The part is bandaged, splinted, immobilized, and monitored for the first 5 to 7 days. The routine is as described in the section on postoperative care. Because these flaps are transferred for restoration of sensibility as much as for coverage, it is essential that the patient protect the part from cutting, burning, and blistering until sensory return has begun.

GREAT TOE WRAPAROUND FLAP

In 1980, Morrison et al. described their experiences with a free vascularized composite tissue transfer from the great toe to wrap around a traditional, nonvascularized autogenous iliac crest bone graft for thumb reconstruction. This flap, which includes the toenail and the dorsal, lateral, and plantar skin of the great toe, is considered to be a good reconstructive procedure for the thumb amputated at or distal to the metacarpophalangeal joint. The advantages attributed to this flap include (1) restoration of length, overall size, sensibility, movement, and thumb cosmesis, (2) reliable neurovascular supply, (3) the need for only a single-stage procedure, (4) preservation of foot skeleton, (5) minimal to no gait disturbance, and (6) minimal donor-site morbidity. Disadvantages include (1) need for a two-team approach, (2) potential loss of entire flap because of thrombosis, (3) potential for bone graft resorption, (4) loss of interphalangeal motion, (5) potential for significant donor-site morbidity should the skin graft fail or if dissection is carried too far proximally, and (6) inability of use in young children because of the impossibility of estimating appropriate length. Although usually this option is reserved for reconstruction of thumbs with amputations distal to the metacarpophalangeal joint, amputation of the thumb proximal to the metacarpophalangeal joint is not an absolute contraindication for the wraparound free flap reconstruction.

As with most microvascular operations on the foot, the adequacy of the first dorsal metatarsal artery should be assessed by arteriography in two planes, Doppler probe and clinical palpation. In feet without a first dorsal metatarsal artery, plantar dissection may be required to gain access to the first plantar metatarsal artery. If the recipient hand has been extensively damaged, arteriography of the hand also may be needed. Preoperative measurements are made of the length and circumference of the normal thumb. The toe on the same side as the injured thumb is used to allow suture of the lateral plantar nerve to the ulnar digital nerve. Two surgical teams are used to hasten the procedure. One team dissects the foot, while the other dissects the hand and obtains the iliac crest bone graft.

GREAT TOE WRAPAROUND FLAP TRANSFER

TECHNIQUE 5.27

(MORRISON ET AL.; URBANIAK ET AL.; STEICHEN)

FOOT DISSECTION

- Outline the skin flap so that the entire great toe is degloved with the exception of a strip on the medial side and distal end of the toe (Fig. 5.50). The distal end of this strip should extend nearly to the lateral corner of the tip of the toenail. The width of this strip is determined by the amount of skin required to match the size of the normal thumb. A strip about 1 cm wide usually is left.
- The flap should not extend much proximal to the base of the great toe. Leave sufficient skin in the web space to aid in closure.
- Mark the course of the first dorsal metatarsal artery. By lowering the foot and using a venous tourniquet, outline the engorged dorsal veins on the foot.
- Make a longitudinal incision between the first and second metatarsals.
- Identify the dorsalis pedis artery.
- Dissect distally to the first dorsal metatarsal artery.

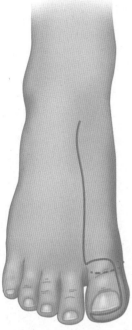

FIGURE 5.50 Wraparound flap. Skin flap is outlined to deglove entire great toe except thin strip extending to lateral corner of toenail. Width of strip (usually 1 cm) is determined by amount of skin needed for thumb. **SEE TECHNIQUE 5.27.**

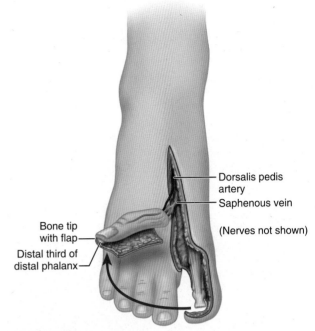

FIGURE 5.51 Wraparound flap. Dissection is complete with vascular pedicle intact. Nerves are not shown. Note tip of distal phalanx with flap. **SEE TECHNIQUE 5.27.**

- If the first dorsal metatarsal artery is volar, or if the plantar digital artery is dominant to the great toe, make a plantar incision into the first web space. Locate the lateral plantar artery in the first web and dissect proximally through a longitudinal incision.
- Ligate vascular branches to the second toe but preserve all branches to the flap.
- Follow the deep peroneal nerve lateral to the artery into the toe flap and divide the nerve proximally, securing a length appropriate to the requirements of the recipient site.
- Dissect the dorsal veins to the toe flap.
- Cauterize the side branches to obtain as much length as possible for the arterial and venous pedicles.
- If the plantar metatarsal artery is used, a vein graft may be required because of insufficient length.
- When the neurovascular pedicle has been dissected, make a transverse incision at the base of the toe but avoid damaging the veins draining the flap.
- Elevate the toe flap, open it, and identify the lateral plantar neurovascular bundle.
- Mobilize the neurovascular bundle and keep it intact with the flap.
- Dissect and identify the medial neurovascular bundle and keep it intact with the medial strip of skin.
- Separate the toe flap beneath the nail by gentle, sharp subperiosteal elevation beneath the nail plate. Avoid injury to the germinative layer of the nail.
- Remove with the flap about 1 cm of the distal tuft of the distal phalanx beneath the nail.
- Save the paratenon over the extensor hallucis longus to receive the split-thickness skin graft.

- Elevate the plantar surface of the flap, leaving the subcutaneous fat over the plantar surface of the toe. Avoid injury to the circulation to the medial skin strip.
- Dissect the lateral plantar digital nerve from the common digital nerve at an appropriate level.
- Unless the lateral plantar digital artery is to be the donor artery, coagulate and divide it.
- At this point, the flap should be free except for the vascular pedicle consisting of the dorsal digital branches of the first dorsal metatarsal artery and the venous tributaries to the saphenous system (Fig. 5.51).
- Release the tourniquet and confirm that the flap will be vascularized by the arteriovenous pedicle. It may take 30 to 60 minutes for the flap to turn pink. Bathing the vessels in warm saline and lidocaine may help relieve vascular spasm.
- When the flap turns pink, ensure that the hand preparation is complete, apply microvascular clips to the vessels, and ligate or apply a small hemoclip to the vessels before sectioning them (Fig. 5.52).
- Carefully apply a split-thickness skin graft to the great toe while the flap is being applied to the hand. Removal of 1 cm of the distal phalanx allows the rotation of the medial skin flap over the tip of the toe. Apply the split-thickness skin graft to the plantar, dorsal, and lateral surfaces of the great toe. Stent the graft as needed. Although advocated by Morrison et al., a cross toe flap usually is not needed to complete the great toe closure.

HAND DISSECTION

- The team responsible for the preparation of the hand also must obtain a corticocancellous iliac crest bone graft and sculpt it to the approximate length and thickness of the

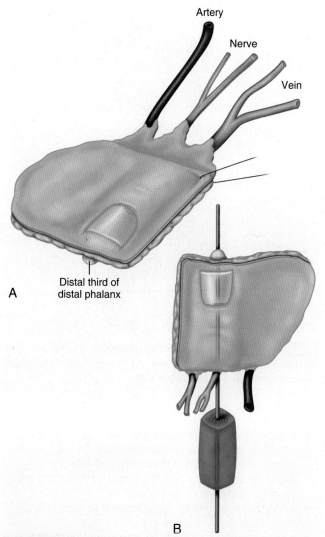

Artery

Nerve

Vein

Distal third of
distal phalanx

A

B

FIGURE 5.52 Wraparound flap. **A,** Dissection complete after section of nerve and vessels. Distal portion of distal phalanx remains with flap. **B,** Diagram of scheme for "skewering" distal end of distal phalanx, then iliac bone graft with Kirschner wire, allowing soft tissue to be "wrapped around" bone graft. **SEE TECHNIQUE 5.27.**

normal contralateral thumb. The tip of the normal thumb when adducted comes to within about 1 cm of the index proximal interphalangeal joint.
- On the hand, two areas require preparation (Fig. 5.53): the dorsoradial aspect just distal to the anatomic snuffbox and the amputation stump itself.
- With the pneumatic tourniquet inflated, make a longitudinal incision in the web space between the first and second metacarpals.
- Dissect and mobilize two or more dorsal hand veins.
- Between the first dorsal interosseous and the adductor pollicis muscles, identify and mobilize the princeps pollicis (first palmar metacarpal) artery.
- Identify the superficial radial nerve.
- Mobilize the arterial pedicle by dissecting it proximally to the level of the proposed anastomosis near the base of the thumb at the carpometacarpal or metacarpophalangeal joints.

- Dissect the thumb stump through a straight incision across its tip extending from midradial to midulnar, allowing the elevation of dorsal and volar subperiosteal flaps for about 1 cm.
- Expose and dissect the ulnar digital neuroma, and when the flap is ready for attachment, excise the neuroma.
- Excise any scar in the bone end and freshen the end to receive the iliac crest bone graft.
- Create a recess in the base of the proximal phalanx or the thumb metacarpal so that the bone graft may be placed into the recess and fixed there with Kirschner wires, screws, or small fragment plates and screws (Fig. 5.54).
- Ensure that the flap is perfused by its arterial pedicle.
- Transect the arteriovenous pedicle and mark the artery, veins, and nerves with sutures.
- Wrap the flap around the bone graft so that the lateral side of the flap is applied to the ulnar side of the bone graft. If the bone graft is too large, it should be trimmed as needed.
- Loosely suture the flap in place to align the nail in a dorsal orientation with the neurovascular pedicle in the first web of the hand.
- Using magnification, suture the ulnar digital nerve of the thumb to the lateral plantar digital nerve of the flap with 9-0 or 10-0 nylon.
- Suture the princeps pollicis (first palmar metacarpal) artery to the first dorsal metatarsal artery of the flap.
- Establish arterial flow and suture the dorsal veins.
- Suture the deep peroneal nerve to the branch of the superficial radial nerve.
- Place drains beneath the flap as needed, taking care to avoid placing a drain near the arteriovenous or nerve repairs. Apply a nonconstricting bandage to the hand and thumb, leaving sufficient surface exposed to allow for monitoring clinically and with devices.

POSTOPERATIVE CARE Aspirin (300 mg/day) and dextran (500 mL/day) are continued for the first 5 to 7 days. Some surgeons also give dipyridamole (Persantine, 50 mg twice daily). Heparin generally is not used. The donor foot and the hand are kept elevated for the first week. The skin color, turgor, and capillary refill are monitored. Skin temperature monitoring is an added measure. The patient's room temperature is kept at greater than 24°C (74°F). Appropriate hydration is maintained, and smoking by the patient and anyone entering the room is prohibited. The bandages and splints are changed after 7 to 10 days unless needed sooner. Active motion of the thumb is begun with protection after 3 weeks. When the foot wound has healed, progressive protected weight bearing is started, and the patient is allowed to increase activities gradually to tolerance. Shoe inserts to protect the great toe usually are not required.

THUMB AND FINGER RECONSTRUCTION

SINGLE-STAGE TRANSFER OF THE GREAT TOE

In 1967, Cobbett reported the first single-stage toe-to-hand transfer in a human, and at 30-year follow-up this patient was

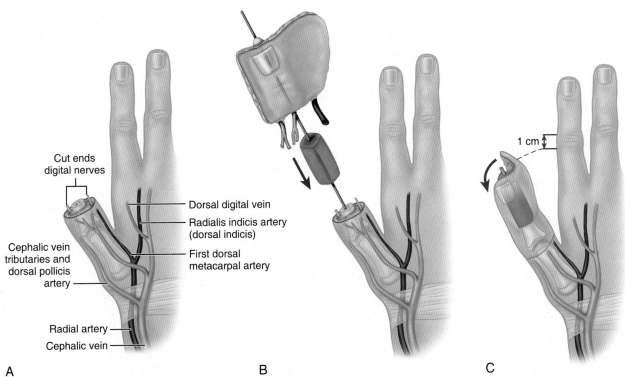

FIGURE 5.53 Wraparound flap hand dissection. **A,** Thumb stump exposed and dissected with midlateral incisions. Dorsum of first web space is dissected to locate cephalic vein and radial artery and branches. **B,** Scheme for attaching iliac bone graft to bone and soft tissue with Kirschner wire to allow nerve and vessel repairs. **C,** Iliac bone graft with soft tissue in place for "wraparound." Length of reconstructed thumb allows tip to come within about 1 cm of proximal interphalangeal joint of index finger. **SEE TECHNIQUE 5.27.**

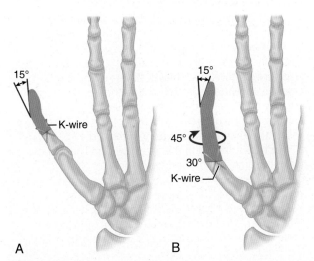

FIGURE 5.54 Fixation of iliac bone block. **A,** For amputation distal to metacarpophalangeal joint, iliac bone block is fixed parallel to long axis of proximal phalanx. **B,** For amputation at or proximal to metacarpophalangeal joint, iliac bone block is fixed in 30 degrees of flexion and 45 degrees of internal rotation. These positions allow opposition of reconstructed thumb to other fingers. *K-wire,* Kirschner wire. **SEE TECHNIQUE 5.27.**

gainfully employed as a timber checker, suggesting that favorable long-term results can be achieved.

Further advancements and refinements of the transfer of the great toe to the hand and the use of the second and third toes for thumb and finger reconstruction have been made, and the clinical usefulness of great toe transfer for thumb reconstruction and second toe or second-third toe combinations for finger and thumb reconstruction has been confirmed. Protective sensibility is regained, and pinch strength has been reported to be 40% to 80% of that on the opposite side. Almost all patients are pleased with the appearance of the reconstructed digit.

Biomechanical evaluations suggest that no significant limitation of ambulatory activities results from loss of the great toe. Significant donor-site morbidity in the form of delayed healing of skin grafted areas and residual hypertrophic scarring on the dorsum of the foot has been reported, however. These problems can be minimized by careful attention to the details of dissection, closure of the donor defect, and the postoperative routine.

■ INDICATIONS

Transfer of the great toe to the hand may be indicated to reconstruct the thumb after amputations from the level of the metacarpal base to the interphalangeal joint. This procedure may be indicated most often in hands with multiple injuries and multiple amputations because it provides an opposable thumb for the remaining digits. Toe-to-hand transfer is recommended for reconstruction of a thumb lost at or near the metacarpophalangeal joint when no adjacent digits are available for pollicization. Others believe that posttraumatic thumb loss, including loss of the entire first metacarpal, is better treated by pollicization or second toe transfer, because of impairment in ambulation caused by loss of the first metatarsal.

Before such a major reconstructive effort is begun, consideration should be given to the patient's age, motivation, occupation, and preferences regarding the donor site. The great toe is usually preferred as a donor for thumb reconstruction because the remaining toes usually are thinner and shorter than the thumb.

■ PREOPERATIVE PLANNING

As with other foot flaps, preoperative evaluation should include a thorough evaluation of the circulation to the foot, including clinical evaluation of the pulses, the use of the Doppler probe, and arteriography of the foot in two planes. In addition, arteriography of the hand should be done if there is any doubt regarding the status of potential recipient vessels. These procedures also help to document the adequacy of the posterior tibial arterial supply.

Although the ipsilateral great toe usually is used, if the medial skin of the foot will be needed for coverage on the reconstructed thumb, the contralateral great toe should be considered at times. Buncke found that clay models of the toe placed in the thumb position are helpful in making decisions regarding toe selection and the amount of skin required. If the great toe has an unacceptable size discrepancy, then the trimmed toe transfer as described by Wei et al. can be used. This technique has the advantage of the wraparound technique in matching thumb size while also allowing interphalangeal joint motion.

The soft-tissue requirements of the recipient area may be satisfied by traditional coverage techniques such as skin grafts or pedicle flaps before the thumb reconstruction or at the time of thumb reconstruction by incorporating a dorsal foot flap with the great toe transfer. Generally, it is preferable to allow for split-thickness skin grafting to be done on the recipient hand, rather than the donor foot because of the unpredictable results, especially on the dorsum of the foot.

SINGLE-STAGE GREAT TOE TRANSFER

TECHNIQUE 5.28

(BUNCKE, MODIFIED)
- Position the patient so that the donor foot and the recipient hand are easily accessible.
- Provide a padded operating table with a heating and cooling blanket and esophageal or rectal temperature probes.
- Monitor urinary output with an indwelling urinary catheter.
- Two surgical teams are required: one for the hand, the other for the foot.

- Using skin-marking pencils, outline incisions on the hand and foot, providing adequate soft-tissue coverage for both areas.

FOOT DISSECTION
- Based on the Doppler findings, outline the course of the dorsalis pedis artery. Allow the veins to fill by holding the foot in a dependent position over the edge of the operating table. The large superficial veins on the dorsum of the foot should be easily seen. The tributaries to the greater saphenous system can be located on the medial side of the first metatarsal. Outline the veins before exsanguinating the limb for tourniquet inflation.
- Exsanguinate the limb by wrapping or elevation and inflate the pneumatic tourniquet.
- Use straight, curved, or zigzag dorsal incisions to identify and preserve the dorsal veins and the dorsalis pedis artery and its distal continuation, the first dorsal metatarsal artery.
- If preoperative evaluation reveals the first metatarsal artery to be dorsal, proceed from proximal to distal, carefully protecting the artery. Ligate or clip the side branches.
- If the dominant artery has been shown to be plantar, dissect from the first web space proximally, extending a longitudinal plantar incision just lateral to the weight-bearing area of the plantar surface over the first metatarsal head.
- Dissect proximally to obtain a sufficient length of artery. At times, dividing the transverse metatarsal ligament is necessary to mobilize a plantar metatarsal artery.
- If the location of the dominant vessel is in doubt, begin the dissection in the first web space and dissect proximally. In the first web space, ligate the artery to the second toe and mobilize the first metatarsal artery proximally until it is determined whether it can be dissected from the dorsal or plantar aspect. Do not transect the proximal vessel attachments until vascularization through the arteriovenous pedicle to the great toe is ensured and until the hand dissection has been completed.
- Follow the dorsal artery to the extensor hallucis brevis, divide the extensor hallucis brevis, elevate it, and expose the deep peroneal nerve lateral to the dorsalis pedis artery. Preserve the deep peroneal nerve for suture to a recipient nerve in the thumb area.
- Follow the first metatarsal artery to the first web, leaving all branches attached to the great toe, and ligate or cauterize the branches to the second toe.
- Dissect and mobilize the superficial veins so that a long venous pedicle can be developed.
- In the first web, dissect the plantar digital nerve on the lateral side of the great toe and separate it from the digital nerve to the second toe by carefully dissecting proximally into the common digital nerve.
- Similarly, dissect the plantar digital nerve on the medial side of the great toe and mobilize it as far proximally as possible. Attempt to preserve both digital nerves.
- Obtain as much length as possible, depending on the requirements of the recipient thumb area. Occasionally, nerve grafts may be required.
- Determine the approximate tendon length requirements in the hand.

- Section the extensor hallucis longus tendon near the extensor retinaculum or more proximally through the same incision used for the vessel dissection.
- Make a transverse incision in the middle or proximal portion of the plantar surface of the foot to obtain adequate length of the flexor hallucis longus tendon.
- Dissect bluntly to locate the tendon and separate it from its connections to the flexor digitorum longus tendons in the foot. These attachments to other tendons make it extremely difficult to release the flexor hallucis longus tendon through an incision at the ankle.
- Separate the toe at the metatarsophalangeal joint. If an attempt is to be made to reconstruct the new metacarpophalangeal joint, the joint capsule may be taken with the toe.
- The plantar aspect of the metatarsal head should be preserved; however, the dorsal portion of the first metatarsal may be taken with the toe if an oblique osteotomy is made from the dorsal surface proximally to the plantar surface distally.
- Leave the vascular pedicle attached until the hand dissection has been completed and sufficient circulation to the toe is ensured.
- Release the tourniquet and achieve hemostasis in the foot.
- After separating the toe from the foot, close the foot incisions over small thin drains if needed.
- The skin flaps should be fashioned to allow side-to-side closure of the foot incision, leaving only small areas, if any, for skin grafting.
- After closure of the foot, apply a bulky, nonconstricting compression bandage.

HAND DISSECTION

- Two incisions usually are required for the hand dissection. Outline a curved incision in the dorsoradial aspect of the base of the thumb and a palmar incision along the thenar crease over the carpal tunnel and proximally into the distal forearm.
- Exsanguinate the limb by elevation or with an elastic wrap. Inflate the pneumatic tourniquet before beginning the dissection.
- Make a curved dorsal incision near the anatomic snuffbox, extending to the tip of the bony remnant of the thumb.
- Identify and mobilize the tendons of the extensor pollicis longus, extensor pollicis brevis, and abductor pollicis longus; the cephalic vein and its tributaries; the radial artery and its distal first metacarpal (princeps pollicis) extension; and the superficial radial nerve and its branches.
- Elevate skin flaps to expose the thumb remnant.
- Make a palmar incision parallel to the thenar crease, extending proximally and obliquely across the wrist flexion crease.
- Identify and expose branches of the digital nerves to the thumb, the flexor hallucis longus tendon, the adductor pollicis and abductor pollicis brevis tendons if available, and the palmar digital arteries if they are suitable for suture.
- Deflate the tourniquet and achieve satisfactory hemostasis. The remainder of the procedure can be done without inflating the tourniquet, or the tourniquet can

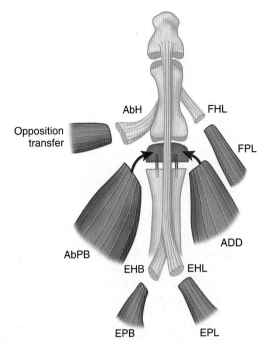

FIGURE 5.55 Transfer of great toe to thumb. Scheme suggested by May for reconstruction of available tendon attachments. *AbH,* Abductor hallucis; *AbPB,* abductor pollicis brevis; *ADD,* adductor hallucis; *EHB,* extensor hallucis brevis; *EHL,* extensor hallucis longus; *EPB,* extensor pollicis brevis; *EPL,* extensor pollicis longus; *FHL,* flexor hallucis longus; *FPL,* flexor pollicis longus. **SEE TECHNIQUE 5.28.**

be used intermittently to minimize blood loss and to aid in the completion of the anastomoses and neurorrhaphies.
- Achieve bony apposition of the transferred toe by making a hollow recess in the base of the proximal phalanx of the toe so that the thumb metacarpal or phalangeal remnant may be remodeled and inserted into the recess in the phalanx. Supplement this with additional internal fixation in the form of Kirschner wires as needed.
- Repair flexor and extensor tendons to balance forces on the transferred toe as much as possible. May et al. suggested a scheme for reconstruction of the available tendon attachments (Fig. 5.55).
- Ensure satisfactory flow through the recipient radial arterial branches and perform anastomoses between the dorsalis pedis artery and the first metacarpal or radial artery.
- Begin intravenous infusion of low-molecular-weight dextran (or heparin, depending on preference) after the arterial anastomosis has been completed.
- Anastomose the saphenous venous system to the cephalic system. Usually one arterial and one venous anastomosis are sufficient.
- Suture the lateral plantar digital nerve from the toe to the ulnar digital nerve of the thumb and the medial plantar digital nerve to the radial digital nerve. If it is available, the superficial radial nerve branches may be sutured to the deep peroneal nerve branches.
- Loosely close the wounds and drain them as needed with small, thin rubber drains.
- Apply skin grafts as needed.

- Apply a bulky, nonconstricting, noncompressing bandage, supporting the thumb, hand, and wrist with a plaster splint.

POSTOPERATIVE CARE The preferred postoperative anticoagulant therapy is continued. Low-molecular-weight dextran or heparin for 3 to 5 days has been recommended by various authors. The patient is kept quiet with the hand and foot elevated. Clinical observations and any available mechanical devices are used to monitor the circulation. Urinary output and serum hemoglobin and hematocrit determinations are monitored for the first 3 to 5 days until they have stabilized satisfactorily. Donor-site morbidity can be minimized by preventing walking on the involved foot for 2 to 4 weeks. Initially the foot is kept wrapped with an elastic bandage. After removal of the sutures, an elastic support stocking helps to reduce edema. If one foot remains unaffected, the patient may attempt to walk using a walker or crutches; however, care must be taken to avoid injuring the reconstructed thumb. If possible, bandage changes are delayed for 5 to 7 days. The thumb is protected for 3 to 4 weeks, and then gentle protected active motion is begun, graduating to more aggressive activities at 10 to 12 weeks. Most strenuous activities are delayed until there is evidence of sensory return.

TRIMMED-TOE TRANSFER

This modification was developed to solve the problem of an overly large digit after great-toe-to-hand transfer.

TECHNIQUE 5.29

(WEI ET AL.)

- Before surgery, obtain correct measurements, including the circumference of the normal thumb at the nail eponychium, the widest point at the interphalangeal joint, and the middle of the proximal phalanx. Carry the width measurement of the thumbnail over to the great toenail, placing the excess medially. From this point on the toenail, draw a longitudinal line proximally from the eponychium to the base of the proximal phalanx for reference. At this reference line, transpose the thumb measurements to their corresponding points on the great toe, with an additional 2 to 3 mm added to each measurement to ensure a tension-free closure.
- Taper the residual medial skin strip (the difference between the toe and thumb circumferences) to a point around the tip of the toe 2 mm below the nail to facilitate skin closure. The proximal incision line is determined by the level of thumb amputation.

DONOR-SITE DISSECTION

- Perform donor-site dissection under standard tourniquet control.
- Vascular identification and tendon and nerve dissection are as described in Technique 5.28.
- Incise and elevate the medial skin strip from distal to proximal and deepen the incision to the periosteum at the tip of the distal phalanx with minimal violation of the fibrous pulp septae. Continue the dissection plane proximally over the periosteum, medial collateral ligament, and joint capsule.
- Protect the medial neurovascular bundle retaining it in the harvested great toe.
- Dorsally, make a longitudinal incision in the periosteum, medial collateral ligament, and joint capsule. Elevate these tissues subperiosteally (hemicircumferential joint flap) to the midplantar surfaces of both the proximal and distal phalanges.
- Using an oscillating saw, perform a longitudinal osteotomy, removing 4 to 6 mm of width from the medial joint prominence and 2 to 4 mm of the phalangeal shafts. Rasp the osteotomy edges for a smooth contour.
- Drape the hemicircumferential flap, including the periosteum, medial collateral ligament, and joint capsule, over the raw bony surfaces and secure it with interrupted sutures after trimming.
- After approximating the medial skin incision, select the amputation level, leaving the donor great toe attached only by its vascular pedicle (Fig. 5.56).

RECIPIENT SITE PREPARATION

- A second team usually prepares the recipient site simultaneous to the donor-site dissection.
- For proper seating of the transferred great toe, skin incisions must be carefully planned and executed as well as possible joint arthrodesis or reconstruction, depending on the amputation level.
- Perform transfer of the trimmed toe as described in Technique 5.28.
- Close the donor site primarily, using the proximal portion of the remaining medial skin strip to assist in tension-free closure if needed.

POSTOPERATIVE CARE Postoperative care is the same as after Technique 5.29.

SECOND AND THIRD TOE TRANSPLANTATION

Although great toe transplantation, the wraparound procedure, and other more traditional procedures are useful for thumb reconstruction, a hand with the loss of the thumb and multiple digits or a hand with only the thumb intact is significantly impaired and requires more than thumb reconstruction alone. Transplant of multiple toes has been useful for hand reconstruction when more than one digit is lost. The second toe from one foot, second toes from both feet, or the second and third toes from one foot can be used as digits to restore opposition to the thumb. The latter can be used as a single neurovascular transplant. Leung classified patients with thumb loss into four categories suitable for second toe transplantation, preferring the second toe over the great toe (Fig. 5.57).

Gordon et al. evaluated a series of 16 patients who had 38 digits reconstructed with double toe transplantation from opposite feet. When one or two digits remained on the hand, toe transplantation improved function and appearance, while providing a broader and stronger surface for pinch and grip.

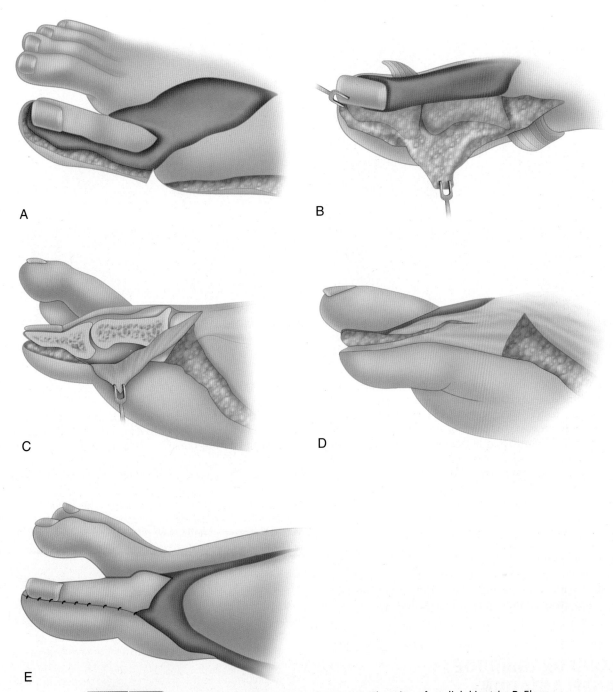

FIGURE 5.56 Wei et al. trimmed great toe harvest. **A,** Elevation of medial skin strip. **B,** Elevation of inferiorly based hemicircumferential joint flap. **C,** Longitudinal osteotomy of phalanges and joint. **D,** Repair of hemicircumferential joint flap. **E,** Closure of wound before transfer. **SEE TECHNIQUE 5.29.**

They found the range of motion to be functional, and hand function was significantly improved. Postoperative foot morbidity was minimal when a strict non–weight-bearing routine was followed. When sequential double toe transplantation procedures were compared with simultaneous double toe transplantation, these authors found an overall shortening of the operating time and the hospital stay after simultaneous double toe transplantation. Overall cost decreased if two toes, usually from separate feet, were transplanted to the hand simultaneously. The risk of impaired walking is lower if single

toes are removed from each foot compared with the removal of two toes with portions of the metatarsals.

■ **PREOPERATIVE PREPARATION**

As with all foot transplant procedures, the location of the arteries to the toes to be transplanted needs to be determined. Also, the adequacy of the remaining circulation to the foot needs to be determined using arteriography in two planes, in addition to the clinical assessment and the Doppler probe observations. The needs of the recipient hand should

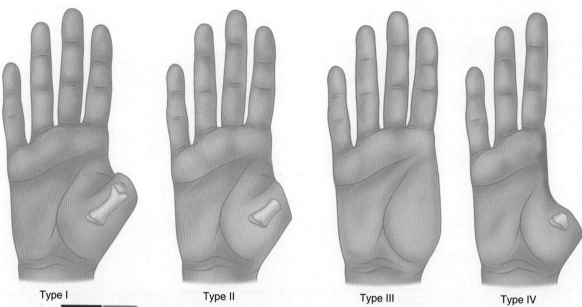

Type I   Type II   Type III   Type IV

FIGURE 5.57   Leung's classification of thumb loss, useful when considering different types of thumb reconstructive microsurgical procedures.

be evaluated to help decide which toes to use in specific locations. Buncke recommended clay models of the digits applied to the hand. Alternatively, plaster models created from alginate impressions of patients' toes can be used. The toe selected may be restricted by acquired posttraumatic or postural deformities, such as scarring and hammertoes, or by congenital anomalies and poor vascularization.

If a single toe is to be transplanted, two surgical teams are required, whereas if two toes are to be transplanted from separate feet, three teams are required—two to remove the toes and one to work on the hand.

Position the patient on a well-padded operating table with a heating and cooling blanket placed beneath so that both feet and the affected hand are easily accessible. Monitor the body temperature with an esophageal or rectal thermometer and urinary output with an indwelling urinary catheter.

SECOND OR THIRD TOE TRANSPLANTATION

TECHNIQUE 5.30

FOOT DISSECTION

- Outline the skin flaps on the foot, depending on the requirements for skin coverage in the hand (Fig. 5.58).
- If the reconstruction is to be done at or distal to the thumb metacarpophalangeal joint, usually no additional skin is required. If the level of reconstruction is at the carpometacarpal level, or if the thumb ray is totally lost, a skin flap from the dorsum of the foot may be incorporated with the toe to be transplanted. If the toe or toes are to be used for finger reconstruction, usually additional skin flaps are not required because the toe is placed on

top of the recipient finger or between existing fingers so that adjacent skin might suffice.
- Allow the dorsal veins to fill by hanging the foot over the edge of the table and outline with a skin pencil the tributaries of the greater and lesser saphenous venous systems.
- With an elastic wrap or elevation, exsanguinate the leg and inflate the pneumatic tourniquet.
- Elevate the skin flaps on the dorsum of the foot initially to identify and mobilize the saphenous tributaries.
- Carefully dissect and develop the venous pedicle.
- Locate the superficial peroneal nerve and include its branches with the toe.
- Transect the extensor digitorum longus and extensor digitorum brevis tendons proximally near the ankle through the same incision used to dissect the vessels.
- Identify the dorsalis pedis artery and mobilize it, leaving intact its branches passing laterally toward the second metatarsal. Divide the branches to the great toe at the first web space.
- The circulation to the second or to the second and third toes is supplied through the dorsalis pedis and first dorsal metatarsal arteries or through the communicating artery to the plantar metatarsal arteries and then to the plantar digital arteries. Use a plantar incision to identify and dissect the plantar digital nerves, the flexor digitorum longus and brevis tendons, the plantar digital arteries, and the distal portions of the plantar metatarsal arteries.
- Although dissection of the plantar structures is possible through the dorsal incision, a metatarsal osteotomy is required to allow exposure of the plantar structures, making the dorsal approach to the plantar structures more difficult.
- If the thumb or digital reconstruction is to be done at the metacarpophalangeal joint or more distally, remove the toe at the metatarsophalangeal joint.

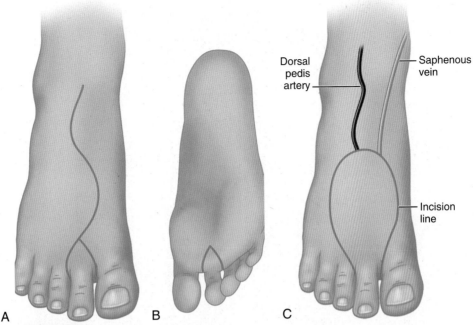

Dorsal pedis artery

Saphenous vein

Incision line

A   B   C

FIGURE 5.58   Second toe transplantation. **A,** Incisions outlined for removal of second toe. Dorsal foot incision allows access to neurovascular structures. **B,** Plantar incision for toe removal. **C,** Dorsal foot flap outlined if hand requires additional skin. **SEE TECHNIQUE 5.30.**

- If the level is more proximal, the distal metatarsal may be osteotomized at an appropriate length to meet the needs in the hand.
- Complete the dissection.
- Leave the vascular pedicles intact until the hand is ready to receive the transplanted digit.
- Deflate the tourniquet to ensure perfusion of the toes by the arterial pedicle.
- Use small vascular clamps to occlude the dorsalis pedis arterial system and the plantar metatarsal arteries to determine which arteries provide the best flow to the toes.
- When the hand is ready for the toes, ligate the arteries and veins and section the vessels.
- Close the foot wounds over small, thin drains as needed.
- Apply a bulky, nonconstricting compression bandage to the foot.

HAND DISSECTION

- If the thumb is to be reconstructed, at least two incisions are required, as described for the great toe and wrap-around procedures. Outline the skin incisions to be made.
- Exsanguinate the upper limb and inflate the pneumatic tourniquet.
- Make a curved dorsal incision extending from the anatomic snuffbox to the remnant of the thumb to expose the dorsal veins, the extensor tendons, the radial artery and its first metacarpal branch, and the branches of the superficial radial nerve.
- After making a palmar incision parallel with the thenar crease, dissect the digital nerves, the flexor pollicis longus tendon, and any available arterial branches.
- If the toe is to be transplanted to a finger distal to the metacarpophalangeal joint, develop dorsal and palmar skin flaps, exposing the dorsal digital veins, the extensor digitorum communis tendon, the volar digital arteries and nerves, and the flexor tendons.
- If the toe is to be transplanted with a portion of the metatarsal to replace a portion of lost metacarpal at or proximal to the metacarpophalangeal joint, make a dorsal curved incision to expose the dorsal venous tributaries on the hand, the extensor tendons, and the bony remnant of the metacarpal.
- On the palmar surface, make an incision crossing the palmar creases obliquely to expose the common digital arteries, the common and proper digital nerves, and the flexor tendons.
- Deflate the tourniquet and achieve adequate hemostasis.
- When the hand dissection has been completed and the hand prepared, ligate and transect the vessels to the toe or toes to be transplanted, close the foot wound as described previously, and begin the attachment of the toes to the thumb or digital position.
- Bone fixation with longitudinal Kirschner wires is easiest; however, combinations of Kirschner wires with wire sutures or small plates and screws also are satisfactory.
- Join the flexor and extensor tendons in the palm or near the wrist.
- The arterial anastomoses usually connect the dorsalis pedis of the first dorsal metatarsal artery to the radial or first metacarpal artery, although the plantar metatarsal arteries or plantar digital arteries to the toes may be anastomosed to the digital arteries of the fingers. It is important to show forceful pulsatile flow from the cut end of the recipient artery before arterial anastomoses are begun.
- When the arterial anastomoses have been completed, return bleeding through the dorsal veins should be unequivocal.

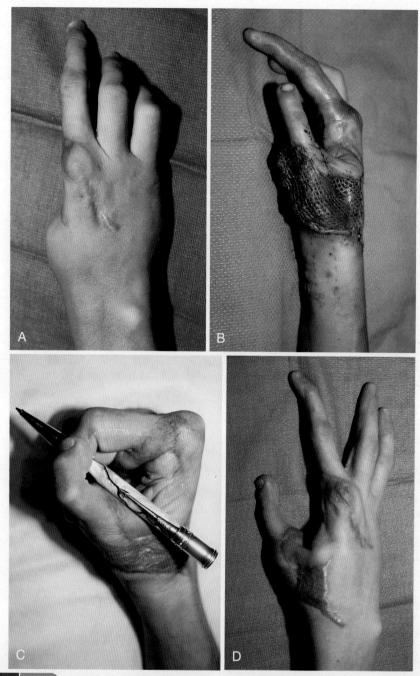

FIGURE 5.59 **A,** Amputated thumb and index finger after explosion injury. **B,** Delayed reconstruction with second toe to thumb free transfer and skin grafting. **C,** Useful pinch and acceptable appearance 6 months after surgery. **D,** Active interphalangeal joint extension. **SEE TECHNIQUE 5.30.**

- Suture the plantar digital nerves of the toes to the digital nerves of the fingers or thumb and, where available, suture dorsal cutaneous branches of the radial or ulnar nerves to the branches of the superficial or deep peroneal nerves that may accompany the transplanted toe or toes.
- Close the skin loosely, using small, thin rubber drains if needed.
- Supplemental skin grafting may be necessary as well (Fig. 5.59).
- Apply a bulky, nonconstricting bandage incorporating a plaster splint on the palmar side.

POSTOPERATIVE CARE The hand and foot are kept elevated. No smoking is allowed by patients or visitors. The room should be kept warm, and the patient should be sufficiently sedated so as to avoid emotional outbursts. A compression dressing is worn on the foot for 2 or more weeks, followed by an elastic stocking for 2 to 4 months to control edema. The circulation to the transplanted digit or digits is monitored closely for the first 1 to 3 days, and the patient is returned to the surgical suite for exploration of the anastomoses if evidence of circulatory compromise develops. The hand is immobilized for 3 to 4 weeks, followed by a graduated program of active mobilization of the transplanted digit. To minimize the morbidity associated with second toe removal, with second and third toe removal, or with the removal of second toes from each foot, the foot should be elevated for at least 2 weeks. If both feet have been donors, Gordon et al. have stressed the importance of using a wheelchair for an additional 2 weeks, at which time protected walking is begun with crutches or a walker until the patient can walk easily with minimal or no pain. Full use of the transplanted digit or digits is delayed until satisfactory motion and useful sensation return.

VASCULARIZED FREE FLAPS CONTAINING JOINTS AND EPIPHYSES

The clinical experiences of many surgeons suggest that whole joints, transplanted on a vascular pedicle, survive and function without deterioration. This procedure holds promise, especially in the area of allograft transplantation.

Clinical reports by Weiland et al. and Wray et al. suggest that growth continues after the vascularized transfer of physes. The careful experimental work of Brown et al. shows that long-term survival and useful growth can occur after free vascularized physeal transplantation. In their report of a small series, Singer et al. concluded that a vascularized transfer of the toe metatarsophalangeal joint to the finger metacarpophalangeal joint can provide painless, functional, stable motion with nearly normal growth potential. Transfers of the toe proximal interphalangeal joint to the finger proximal interphalangeal joint have not been as rewarding because of the difficulty in regaining motion and maintaining growth potential. Foo, Malata, and Kay reported that in three free joint transfers and one double joint transfer the joints were stable and maintained their growth potential, but range of motion of the proximal interphalangeal joint was limited to 30 degrees. Although this type of transplantation shows promise as a way of solving several difficult pediatric surgical problems, these authors cautioned that many questions remain unanswered and require research before the procedure can be widely applied to children.

REFERENCES

GENERAL MICROSURGERY

American College of Surgeons: resources for optimal care of the injured patient, Chicago, 2013, American College of Surgeons, Available at https ://www.facs.org/~/.../ vrc%20resources/resources%20for%20optimal%20 care.ashx, Accessed April 22, 2019.

Mours CM, Heule F, Lovius SE: A review of topical negative pressure therapy in wound healing sufficient evidence? Am J Surg 201:544, 2011.

Orgill DP, Gayer LR: Negative pressure wound therapy: past, present and future, Int Wound 10(Suppl 1):15, 2013.

Ridha H, Morritt AN, Wood SH: Spatulated end-to-end microvascular anastomosis: a useful technique for overcoming vessel size discrepancy, J Plast Reconstr Aesthet Surg 67:3254, 2014.

Wood BC, Molnar JA: Subatmospheric pressure therapy: basic science review, J Surg Orthop Adv 20:168, 2011.

NERVES

Chen C, Tang P, Zhao G: Bilaterally innervated dorsal digital flap for sensory reconstruction of digits, Injury 45:2018, 2014.

Fan A, Song L, Zhang H, et al.: Reconstruction of finger pulp defects with an innervated distally-based neurovascular flap, J Hand Surg Am, 2019, [Epub ahead of print].

Li M, Huang M, Yang Y, et al.: Preliminary study on functional and aesthetic reconstruction by using small artery-only free medial flap of the second toe for fingertip injuries, Clinics (Sao Paulo) 74:e1226, 2019.

REPLANTATION

Barzin A, Hernandez-Boussard T, Lee GK, et al.: Adverse events following digital replantation in the elderly, J Hand Surg Am 36:870, 2011.

Breahna A, Siddiqui A, Fitzgerald O'Connor E, et al.: Replantation of digits: a review of predictive factors for survival, J Hand Surg Eur 41:753, 2016.

Cavadas PC, Rubí C, Thione A, et al.: Immediate versus overnight-delayed digital replantation: comparative retrospective cohort study of survival outcomes, J Hand Surg Am 43:625e, 2018.

Chen KK, Hsieh TY, Chang KP: Tamai zone I fingertip replantation: is external bleeding obligatory for survival of artery anastomosis-only replanted digits? Microsurgery 34:535, 2014.

Cho HE, Zhong L, Kotsis S, et al.: Finger replantation optimization study (FRONT): update on national trends, J Hand Surg Am 43:903, 2018.

Fufa D, Calfee R, Wall L, et al.: Digit replantation: experience of two U.S. academic level-I trauma centers, J Bone Joint Surg 95A:2127, 2013.

Fufa DT, Lin CH, Lin YT, et al.: Survival and secondary surgery following lower extremity replantation, J Reconstr Microsurg 30:419, 2014.

Hahn HO, Jung SG: Results of replantation of amputated fingertips in 450 patients, J Reconstr Microsurg 22:407, 2006.

Hattori Y, Doi K, Sakamoto S, et al.: Fingertip replantation, J Hand Surg Am 32A:548, 2007.

Hustedt JW, Chung A, Bohl DD, et al.: Evaluating the effect of comorbidities on the success, risk, and cost of digital replantation, J Hand Surg Am 41:1145e, 2016.

Jeon BJ, Yang JW, Roh SY, et al.: Lateral nail fold incision technique for venous anastomosis in fingertip replantation, Ann Plast Surg 76:67, 2016.

Koshima I, Yamashita S, Sugiyama N, et al.: Successful delayed venous drainage in 16 consecutive distal phalangeal replantations, Plast Reconstr Surg 115:149, 2005.

Mahmoudi E, Huetteman HE, Chung KC: A population-based study of replantation after traumatic thumb amputation, 2007-2012, J Hand Surg Am 42:25, 2017.

Muneuchi G, Kurokawa M, Igawa K, et al.: Nonmicrosurgical replantation using a subcutaneous pocket for salvage of the amputated fingertip, J Hand Surg Am 30A:562, 2005.

Nishizuka T, Shauver MJ, Zhong L, et al.: A comparative study of attitudes regarding digit replantation in the United states and Japan, J Hand Surg Am 40:1646, 2015.

Panattoni JB, Ona IR, Ahmed MM: Reconstruction of fingertip injuries: surgical tips and avoiding complications, J Hand Surg Am 40:1016, 2015.

Patel AA, Blount AA, Owens PW, et al.: Functional outcomes of replantation following radiocarpal amputation, J Hand Surg Am 40:266, 2015.

Peterson SL, Peterson EL, Wheatley MJ: Management of fingertip amputations, J Hand Surg Am 39:2093, 2014.

Reavey PL, Stranix JT, Muresan H, et al.: Disappearing digits: analysis of national trends in amputation and replantation in the United States, Plast Reconstr Surg 141:857e, 2018.

Retrouvey H, Makerewich JR, Solaja O, et al.: Effect of vasopressor use on digit survival after replantation of revascularization—a large retrospective cohort study, Microsurgery 40:5, 2020.

Retrouvey H, Solaja O, Baltzer HL: The effect of increasing age on outcomes of digital revascularization or replantation, Plast Reconstr Surg 143:495, 2019.

Sabapathy SR, Venkatramani H, Bharathi RR, et al.: J Hand Surg Am 36:1104, 2011.

Sears ED, Chung KC: Replantation of finger avulsion injuries: a systematic review of survival and functional outcomes, J Hand Surg Am 36:686, 2011.

Shaterian A, Sayadi LR, Tiourin E, et al.: Predictors of hand function following digit replantation: quantitative review and meta-analysis, *Hand (N Y)*, 2019, [Epub ahead of print].

Tessler O, Bartow MJ, Tremblay-Champagne MP, et al.: Long-term health-related quality of life outcomes in digital replantation versus revision amputation, *J Reconstr Microsurg* 33:446, 2017.

Woo SH: Practical tips to improve efficiency and success in upper limb reimplantation, *Plast Reconstr Surg* 144:878e, 2019.

Zhpi M, Qi B, Yu A, et al.: Vacuum assisted closure therapy for treatment of complex wounds in replanted extremities, *Microsurgery* 33:620, 2013.

FREE SOFT-TISSUE TRANSFER

Al-Qattan MM, Al-Qattan AM: Defining the indications of pedicled groin and abdominal flaps in hand reconstruction in the current microsurgery era, *J Hand Surg Am* 41:917e, 2016.

Chang EI, Ibrahim A, Papazian N, et al.: Perforator mapping and optimizing design of the lateral arm flap: anatomy revisited and clinical experience, *Plast Reconstr Surg* 138:300e, 2016.

Del Pinal F, Klausmeyer M, Moraleda E, et al.: Foot web free flaps for single-stage reconstruction of hand webs, *J Hand Surg Am* 40:1152, 2015.

Giladi AM, Rinkinen JR, Higgins JP, et al.: Donor-site morbidity of vascularized bone flaps from the distal femur: a systematic review, *Plast Reconstr Surg* 142:363e, 2018.

Goh TL, Park SW, Cho Y, et al.: The search for the ideal thin skin flap: superficial circumflex iliac artery perforator flap—a review of 210 cases, *Plast Reconstr Surg* 135:592, 2015.

Heidekrueger PI, Denis E, Heing-Geldern A, et al.: One versus two venous anastomoses in microvascular lower extremity reconstruction using gracilis muscle or anterolateral thigh flaps, *Injury* 47:2828, 2016.

Higgins JP, Burger HK: Proximal scaphoid arthroplasty using the medial femoral trochlea flap, *J Wrist Surg* 2:228, 2013.

Kazmers NH, Thibaudeau S, Steinberger Z, et al.: Upper and lower extremity reconstructive applications utilizing free flaps from the medial funicular arterial system: a systematic review, *Microsurgery* 38:328, 2018.

Kim JT, Kim SW, Youn S, et al.: What is the ideal free flap for soft tissue reconstruction? A 10-year experience of microsurgical reconstruction using 334 latissimus dorsi flaps from a universal donor site, *Ann Plast Surg* 75:49, 2015.

Kokkalis ZT, Papanikos E, Mazis GA, et al.: Lateral arm flap: indications and techniques, *Eur J Orthop Surg Traumatol* 29:279, 2019.

Lee JC, St-Hilaire H, Christy MR, et al.: Anterolateral thigh flap for trauma reconstruction, *Ann Plast Surg* 64:164, 2010.

Lee KT, Mun GH: A systematic review of functional donor-site morbidity after latissimus dorsi muscle transfer, *Plast Reconstr Surg* 134:303, 2014.

Meyer A, Goller K, Horch RE, et al.: Results of combined vascular reconstruction and free flap transfer for limb salvage in patients with critical limb ischemia, *J Vasc Surg* 61:1239, 2015.

Philanddrianos C, Moullot P, Gay AM, et al.: Soft tissue coverage in distal lower extremity open fractures: comparison of free anterolateral thigh and free latissimus dorsi flaps, *Reconstr Microsurg* 34:121, 2018.

Schaverien MV, Hart AM: Free muscle flaps for reconstruction of upper limb defects, *Hand Clin* 30:165, 2014.

Song B, Chen J, Han Y, et al.: The use of fabricated chimeric flap for reconstruction of extensive foot defects, *Microsurgery* 36:303, 2016.

Wang HD, Alonso-Escalante JC, Cho BH, et al.: Versatility of free cutaneous flaps for upper extremity soft tissue reconstruction, *J Hand Microsurg* 9:58, 2017.

Zheng DW, Li ZC, Sun F, et al.: Use of a distal ulnar artery perforator-based bilobed free flap for repairing complex digital defects, *J Hand Surg Am* 39:2235, 2014.

FREE OSSEOUS TISSUE TRANSFER

Cavadas PC, Landin L: Treatment of recalcitrant distal tibial nonunion using the descending genicular corticoperiosteal free flap, *J Trauma* 64:144, 2008.

Gu JX, Pan JB, Liu HJ, et al.: Aesthetic and sensory reconstruction of finger pulp defects using free toe flaps, *Aesthetic Plast Surg* 38:156, 2014.

Higgins JP, Bürger HK: Osteochondral flaps from the distal femur: expanding applications, harvest sites, and indications, *J Reconstr Microsurg* 30:483, 2014.

Houdek MT, Wagner ER, Wyles CC, et al.: New options for vascularized bone reconstruction in the upper extremity, *Semin Plast Surg* 29:20, 2015.

Iorio ML, Masden DL, Higgins JP: Cutaneous angiosome territory of the medial femoral condyle osteocutaneous flap. *J Hand Surg Am* 37:1033, 2012.

Jones Jr DB, Burger H, Bishop AT, et al.: Treatment of scaphoid waist non-unions with an avascular proximal pole and carpal collapse: a comparison of two vascularized bone grafts, *J Bone Joint Surg* 90A:1616, 2008.

Larson AN, Bishop AT, Shin AY: Free medial femoral condyle bone grafting for scaphoid nonunions with humpback deformity and proximal pole avascular necrosis, *Tech Hand Up Extrem Surg* 11:246, 2007.

Yajima H, Maegawa N, Ota H, et al.: Treatment of persistent non-union of the humerus using a vascularized bone graft from the supracondylar region of the femur, *J Reconstr Microsurg* 23:107, 2007.

Zheng H, Liu J, Dai X, et al.: Free conjoined or chimeric medial sural artery perforator flap for the reconstuction of multiple defects in hand, *J Plast Reconstr Aesthet Surg* 68:565, 2015.

Zhou X, Wang L, Mi J, et al.: Thumb fingertip reconstruction with palmar V-Y flaps combined with bone and nail bed grafts following amputation, *Arch Orthop Trauma Surg* 135:589, 2015.

The complete list of references is available online at ExpertConsult.com.